THE AI FRONTIER IN MOLECULAR MODELLING AND DRUG DESIGNING

THE AI FRONTIER IN MOLECULAR MODELLING AND DRUG DESIGNING

Edited by

MANISH KUMAR GUPTA

SANJAY KUMAR

KRISHNA MISRA

ELSEVIER

ACADEMIC PRESS

An imprint of Elsevier

Academic Press is an imprint of Elsevier
125 London Wall, London EC2Y 5AS, United Kingdom
50 Hampshire Street, 5th Floor, Cambridge, MA 02139, United States

ISBN: 978-0-443-40338-5

For information on all Academic Press publications visit our website at https://www.elsevier.com/books-and-journals

Publisher: Megan Ball
Acquisitions Editor: Linda Buschman
Editorial Project Manager: Stuti Das
Production Project Manager: Fahmida Sultana
Cover Designer: Mark Rogers

Typeset by Integra Software Services

Dedication

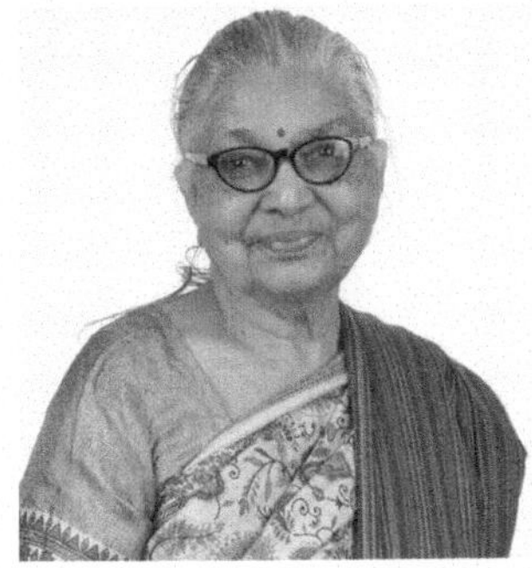

We dedicate this book to our beloved teacher, Late Prof. Krishna Misra, one of the editors of this book, a great teacher and research who not only supplied the most facts, but one in whose presence we became different people.

—Late Prof. Krishna Misra

Contents

Chapter 4 Drug target identification and validation using AI

Rubhashri Gurunathan, Rajaram Abhirami, Muthuraja Arun Pravin, and Sanjeev Kumar Singh

Chapter 5 AI based target-ligand binding methods

Muthuraja Arun Pravin, Saravanan Priyadharshini, Mohammad Aqueel Khan, Rajaram Abhirami, and Sanjeev Kumar Singh

Chapter 8 Natural language processing for drug discovery

Pankaj Tyagi, Ankish Arya, Prabhat Tripathi, Nidhi Dubey, Uma Shanker Tiwary, and Pritish Kumar Varadwaj

Chaper 9 Role of AI in predicting drug efficacy and toxicity

Neeraj Kumar, Manish Kumar Gupta, and Dev Brat Mishra

Contributors

Rajaram Abhirami Computer Aided Drug Design and Molecular Modelling Lab, Department of Bioinformatics, Alagappa University, Karaikudi, Tamil Nadu, India

Ankish Arya Systems Biology Lab, Department of Applied Sciences, Indian Institute of Information Technology Allahabad, Prayagraj, Uttar Pradesh, India

Himanshu Avashthi Department of Bioinformatics, Marwadi University, Rajkot, Gujarat, India

Kirtan Dave Bioinformatics Laboratory, Research and Development Cell, Parul University, Vadodara, Gujarat, India

Nidhi Dubey Systems Biology Lab, Department of Applied sciences, Indian Institute of Information Technology Allahabad, Prayagraj, Uttar Pradesh, India

Manish Kumar Gupta Department of Biotechnology , Faculty of Science, Veer Bahadur Singh Purvanchal University, Jaunpur, Uttar Pradesh, India

Rubhashri Gurunathan Computer Aided Drug Design and Molecular Modeling Lab, Department of Bioinformatics, Alagappa University, Karaikudi, Tamil Nadu, India

Atifa Hafeez Department of Biotechnology, Faculty of Science, Veer Bahadur Singh Purvanchal University, Jaunpur, Uttar Pradesh, India

Shriya Joshi Parul Institute of Applied Sciences, Parul University, Vadodara, Gujarat, India

Swarna Kanchan Joan C. Edwards School of Medicine, Marshall University, Huntington, WV, United States

Shruti Kapoor University of California Santa Cruz, Santa Cruz, CA, United States

Kushagra Kashyap Department of Life Sciences, School of Science and Mathematics, DES Pune University, Pune, Maharashtra, India

Aman Chandra Kaushik Technology Dissemination and Computational Biology Division, CSIR-Central Institute of Medicinal and Aromatic Plants, Lucknow, Uttar Pradesh, India

Minu Kesheri Marshall University, Huntington, WV, United States

Mohammad Aqueel Khan Computer Aided Drug Design and Molecular Modelling Lab, Department of Bioinformatics, Alagappa University, Karaikudi, Tamil Nadu, India

Neeraj Kumar Fish Biology Research Lab, Department of Zoology, T.D. P.G. College, Jaunpur, Uttar Pradesh, India

Sanjay Kumar Department of Structural & Molecular Biology, City College of New York, New York, NY, United States

Tapobrata Lahiri Department of Applied Sciences, Indian Institute of Information Technology Allahabad, Prayagraj, Uttar Pradesh, India

P.M. Mahitha University of California , San Diego, CA, United States

Dev Brat Mishra Fish Biology Research Lab, Department of Zoology, T.D.College, Jaunpur, India

Krishna Misra Systems Biology Lab, Department of Applied sciences, Indian Institute of Information Technology Allahabad, Prayagraj, Uttar Pradesh, India

Rajkrishna Mondal Biotechnolgy, Nagaland University, Kohima, Nagaland, India

Bharti Pandey Bioinformatics Lab, BTIS-Sub-Centre, Animal Biotechnology Division, ICAR—National Dairy Research Institute (Deemed University), Karnal, Haryana, India

Sapna Pandey INSACOG Genomics & Molecular Epidemiology Unit, NCDC, Delhi, India

Muthuraja Arun Pravin Computer Aided Drug Design and Molecular Modelling Lab, Department of Bioinformatics, Alagappa University, Karaikudi, Tamil Nadu, India

Saravanan Priyadharshini Computer Aided Drug Design and Molecular Modelling Lab, Department of Bioinformatics, Alagappa University, Karaikudi, Tamil Nadu, India

Shakti Sahi School of Biotechnology, Gautam Buddha University, Greater Noida, Uttar Pradesh, India

Ruchita Shelat Department of Physiology, The University of Tennessee Health Science Center, Memphis, TN, United States

Dev Bukhsh Singh Department of Biotechnology, Siddharth University, Siddharth Nagar, India

Manjusa Singh Department of Biotechnology, Faculty of Science, Veer Bahadur Singh Purvanchal University, Jaunpur, Uttar Pradesh, India

Naman Pratap Singh Department of Computer Science and Engineering, Jaypee University of Information Technology (JUIT), Solan, Himachal Pradesh, India

Pankaj Singh Department of Biotechnology, Dr. Rammanohar Lohia Avadh University, Ayodhya, Uttar Pradesh, India

Samvedna Singh School of Biotechnology, Gautam Buddha University, Greater Noida, Uttar Pradesh, India

Sanjeev Kumar Singh Computer Aided Drug Design and Molecular Modelling Lab, Department of Bioinformatics, Alagappa University, Karaikudi, Tamil Nadu, India

Satendra Singh Department of Computational Biology and Bioinformatics, Sam Higginbottom, University of Agriculture, Technology and Sciences, Prayagraj, India

Tiratha Raj Singh Department of Biotechnology and Bioinformatics, Centre of Healthcare Technologies and Informatics (CEHTI), Jaypee University of Information Technology (JUIT), Solan, Himachal Pradesh, India

Unnati Soni Systems Biology Lab, Department of Applied sciences, Indian Institute of Information Technology Allahabad, Prayagraj, Uttar Pradesh, India

Lakshmi Sonkusale Bioinformatics Lab, BTIS-Sub-Centre, Animal Biotechnology Division, ICAR—National Dairy Research Institute (Deemed University), Karnal, Haryana, India

Upasna Srivastava Department of Neurology , Yale University, New Haven, CT, United States

Destiny Sumani Department of Neurology, University of Texas Health Science Center, Houston, TX, United States

Uma Shanker Tiwary Department of Information Technology, Indian Institute of Information Technology Allahabad, Prayagraj, Uttar Pradesh, India

Prabhat Tripathi Systems Biology Lab, Department of Applied sciences, Indian Institute of Information Technology Allahabad, Prayagraj, Uttar Pradesh, India

Pankaj Tyagi Department of Information Technology, Indian Institute of Information Technology Allahabad, Prayagraj, Uttar Pradesh, India

Pritish Kumar Varadwaj Systems Biology Lab, Department of Applied sciences, Indian Institute of Information Technology Allahabad, Prayagraj, Uttar Pradesh, India

Deepak Verma Department of Oncology, Johns Hopkins Medicine, Baltimore, MD, United States

Shiv Kumar Yadav Department of Mathematics, Faculty of Engineering and Technology, Veer Bahadur Singh Purvanchal University, Jaunpur, Uttar Pradesh, India

Darshana Zujam Department of Life Sciences, School of Science and Mathematics, DES Pune University, Pune, Maharashtra, India

Foreword

The use of artificial intelligence (AI) in drug discovery and development has changed how scientists deal with one of the most important problems facing humanity: finding effective medicines. Drug development in the past took a lot of time, money, and resources, and it often failed a lot. But AI now gives us a remarkable opportunity to speed up discovery, cut costs, and make predictions about molecular behavior, drug–target interactions, and patient-specific responses more accurate than ever before.

This book puts together the main ideas, methods, and uses of AI in drug discovery in a clear and organized way. Not only does it cover the basics, but it also goes into more detail about advanced technologies like deep learning, natural language processing, and generative models. Each chapter shows how AI tools are being used in different fields, from early-stage molecule generation to clinical trials and personalized medicine. This is because experts have contributed their most up-to-date knowledge.

We are confident that this book will be useful and inspiring for students, researchers, and professionals in the fields of computational biology, structural biology, medicinal chemistry, and pharmaceutical sciences. This book imagines a future where AI speeds up the process of getting safe and effective drugs from idea to clinic, changing healthcare around the world. It does this by connecting science and technology.

The book titled *The AI Frontier in Molecular Modeling and Drug Designing* covers all the recent aspects of "AI" usage, which it covers in 16 chapters.

1. **Use of AI for Computer-Aided Drug Designing**: AI boosts up computer-aided drug design by figuring out the properties of molecules and improving libraries of compounds. It improves docking accuracy and cuts down on the need for trial and error in experiments. This chapter talks about how AI can be used in the drug design process.
2. **Use of AI for Analysis of Biological and Chemical Databases for Drug Discovery**: AI makes it possible to mine huge biological and chemical datasets quickly and easily. Machine learning finds hidden patterns that connect compounds to therapeutic results. This chapter talks about how AI will help to mine databases useful for drug discovery.
3. **Deep Learning for Protein Folding**: Deep learning breakthroughs have made it possible to accurately predict protein structures. This

information helps scientists make drugs that target proteins that are important for diseases. The chapter talks about protein models predicted from AI tools such as AlphaFold and how they have changed things.

4. **Drug Target Identification and Validation using AI**: AI algorithms look at omics and biological data to find new receptors. Predictive models confirm possible targets with great precision. The chapter examines methodologies that improve the reliability of drug targets.
5. **AI Based Target-Ligand Binding Methods**: AI enhances the accuracy of the prediction of binding affinities between ligands and receptors. Deep docking and other methods make it easier to study how ligands and receptors work together. The chapter talks about algorithms that are changing the way molecular interaction studies are done.
6. **Generative Models for Molecule Generation**: Generative AI makes new drug-like molecules that have the right properties. By creating chemical scaffolds, these models cut down on the time it takes to make new discoveries. The chapter deals with how Generative Adversarial Networks (GANs), Variational Autoencoders (VAEs), and reinforcement learning shall be useful to make molecules.
7. **AI Enabled Virtual Screening**: AI makes high-throughput virtual screening better for finding new drugs. Machine learning sifts through large compound libraries and finds more hits. The chapter describes how AI helps to find candidates quickly by describing protocols.
8. **Natural Language Processing (NLP) for Drug Discovery**: NLP gets information from scientific papers, patents, and clinical notes. AI-powered text mining finds possible targets and compounds. The chapter shows how language models help people learn new things faster.
9. **Role of AI in Predicting Drug Efficacy and Toxicity**: AI will enhance the prediction accuracy of how well drugs will work and what side effects they will have. Models look at both preclinical and clinical datasets to make safety evaluations more accurate. The chapter talks about how AI cuts down on expensive failures in the later stages.
10. **AI Enabled Tools Used in Drug Designing**: There are many AI-powered platforms that help with drug design and optimization. These tools use cheminformatics, bioinformatics, and machine learning all at once. The chapter looks at some of the most popular software and frameworks.

11. **AI Driven Clinical Trials**: AI makes clinical trial design and patient recruitment better. Predictive models make trials more successful and less expensive. The chapter explains how AI will assist in efficient clinical trials.
12. **AI, Network Biology and Multiomics Data in Drug Discovery**: AI combines genomics, transcriptomics, and proteomics with network biology. Multiomics data show how drugs affect the whole system. The chapter looks into network-based models using AI for drug discovery as a whole.
13. **AI-Driven Personalized Medicine and Biomarker Discovery**: AI helps to find biomarkers that may help doctors to choose the best treatments for each patient. Personalized models make treatments more accurate and effective. The chapter talks about how AI-based precision medicine has come a long way.
14. **AI Powered Precision Oncology**: AI makes it possible to correctly classify different types of cancer and predict how they will respond to treatment. Predictive algorithms help to choose the right therapy for a specific patient. The chapter shows how AI is changing oncology in a big way.
15. **AI Emergence in Nanomedicine, Pharmacogenomics and Biotechnology**: AI helps to design small particles, studying how genes and drugs interact, and coming up with new biotechnological ideas. It speeds up the process of bringing new fields together with drug development. The chapter talks about how AI can be useful in many different biological fields.
16. **AI in Medical Image Processing and Translational Science:** AI makes it easier to find diseases and check how well drugs work on patients by analyzing images. It connects what scientists learn in the lab with what they can do in the real world. The chapter talks about new imaging technologies that are helping drug science move forward.

Preface

Artificial intelligence (AI) is changing the way drug discovery works. In the past, developing drugs required several years of testing, high financial expenditure, and had a high chance of failure. Computational technologies, especially AI and machine learning, have given scientists powerful new tools to model, predict, and speed up almost every step of drug development, from finding targets to optimizing clinical trials.

The AI Frontier in Molecular Modeling and Drug Designing is a book that provides a comprehensive picture of how AI technologies are changing the development of new drugs. The chapters look at how AI can be used in different areas of modern science, including computer-aided drug design, predicting how proteins will fold, virtual screening, finding biomarkers, and improving clinical trials. It also shows how deep learning, natural language processing, and generative models can help solve some of the hardest problems in drug development.

The book has two main goals. First, it aims to give readers, students, researchers, and professionals a basic understanding of how AI is useful in drug discovery. Second, it wants to encourage new ideas by showing how the integration of biology, chemistry, data science, and computer science will lead to major improvements in healthcare.

We believe this book will be useful for those studying in research organizations, universities, and pharmaceutical companies all over the world. The authors have tried to make the information both useful and easy to understand so that professionals from diverse backgrounds can learn from the ideas shared here.

Lastly, we would like to thank everyone who helped us accomplish this book and made it possible, including contributors, reviewers, and coworkers. Their knowledge, hard work, and vision have made it possible for us to present this timely work at the crossroads of AI and drug discovery.

1

Use of artificial intelligence for computer aided drug designing

Upasna Srivastava[a], Manish Kumar Gupta[b], Swarna Kanchan[c], Minu Kesheri[d], Destiny Sumani[e], P.M. Mahitha[f], and Satendra Singh[g]

[a]*Department of Neurology , Yale University, New Haven, CT, United States*
[b]*Department of Biotechnology , Faculty of Science, Veer Bahadur Singh Purvanchal University, Jaunpur, Uttar Pradesh, India*
[c]*Joan C. Edwards School of Medicine, Marshall University, Huntington, WV, United States*
[d]*Marshall University, Huntington, WV, United States*
[e]*Department of Neurology, University of Texas Health Science Center, Houston, TX, United States*
[f]*University of California , San Diego, CA, United States*
[g]*Department of Computational Biology and Bioinformatics, Sam Higginbottom, University of Agriculture, Technology and Sciences, Prayagraj, India*

1 Introduction

The drug discovery process is changing very rapidly. Technological advancements save both cost and time in the development of new drugs. After the emergence of artificial intelligence (AI), the computer-assisted drug discovery and development process has been significantly enhanced. Various machine learning (ML) and AI-enabled algorithms are producing faster outputs. The following points must be taken into consideration to refine lead compounds, model molecular interactions, and predict therapeutic efficacy with unprecedented precision:

1.1 Computational tools in drug modeling

A multidisciplinary strategy called computer-aided drug design (CADD) uses computational tools and methods to speed up and improve the drug research and discovery process. CADD makes it easier to identify, model, and improve drug candidates more accurately and efficiently by combining concepts from computer science, chemistry, and biology. The two main approaches in CADD are ligand-based drug design (LBDD), which builds new therapeutic agents based on the activity profiles of existing compounds, and

The AI Frontier in Molecular Modelling and Drug Designing. https://doi.org/10.1016/B978-0-443-40338-5.00011-1

structure-based drug design (SBDD), which designs molecules that fit particular binding sites using the three-dimensional structure of a biological target. CADD can be used to estimate pharmacokinetics and possible toxicities, optimize lead compounds, repurpose current medications, and predict molecular interactions. CADD's capabilities are further enhanced by developments in AI and ML.

CADD can be used to estimate pharmacokinetics and possible toxicities, optimize lead compounds, repurpose current medications, and predict molecular interactions. CADD's capabilities are further enhanced by developments in AI and ML, which make it possible to analyze massive datasets and increase predictive accuracy (Leach and Gillet, 2007; Jumper et al., 2021). Combining these tools has revolutionized drug discovery, cutting down on the time and expense needed to launch novel treatments (Trott and Olson, 2010). However, there are still issues to be resolved, such as guaranteeing data quality, improving prediction models, and addressing privacy and AI ethics. Notwithstanding these challenges, CADD remains a vital component of contemporary pharmaceutical research, propelling the creation of novel and life-saving medications (Patel and Chalmers, 2003; Lipinski et al., 2001). The drug discovery process is shown in Fig. 1.1.

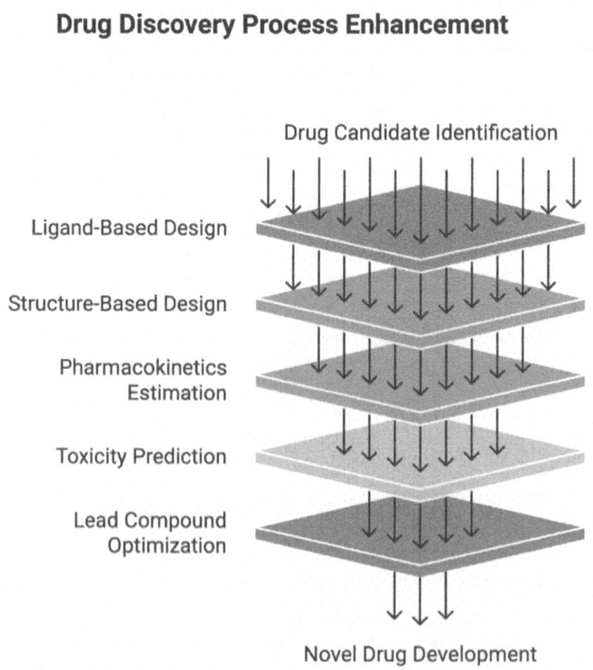

Fig. 1.1 Drug discovery enhancement. This layered diagram outlines key stages in the drug discovery pipeline, from candidate identification through design strategies, pharmacokinetic and toxicity assessment, to lead optimization, all culminating in the development of novel drugs.

It illustrates a layered approach to enhancing the drug discovery process, moving systematically from early-stage design to development. The process begins with Drug Candidate Identification, employing methods such as Ligand-Based Design and Structure-Based Design to pinpoint promising molecular scaffolds.

It then progresses through Pharmacokinetics Estimation to predict how compounds behave in the body, followed by Toxicity Prediction to assess safety profiles. The final stage is Lead Compound Optimization, which refines the chemical properties of candidates to improve efficacy and safety. Collectively, these stages support the advancement of Novel Drug Development, streamlining the journey from concept to clinically viable therapies.

1.2 Computer-aided drug design

1. **Simulation of molecular interactions:** Researchers can use CADD to model and forecast the interactions between pharmacological compounds and biological targets like DNA or proteins. According to (Jorgensen, 2004), these simulations shed light on possible medication efficacy, structural compatibility, and binding affinities.
2. **Drug design based on structure (SBDD)**. This method creates molecules that perfectly fit and attach to a target biomolecule's active sites by using its three-dimensional structure, which can be ascertained using methods such as cryo-electron microscopy or X-ray crystallography (Anderson, 2003; Jumper et al., 2021a).
3. **Drug design based on ligands (LBDD):** Without needing to know the target's three-dimensional structure, LBDD focuses on creating novel compounds using the structural and activity information of known ligands. To forecast biological activity, it uses quantitative structure-activity relationships (QSAR) (Leach and Gillet, 2007).
4. **Reasonable drug design**: CADD takes a focused approach by employing computational models and algorithms to rationalize drug design, maximizing properties prior to synthesis, in contrast to conventional trial-and-error methods (Lipinski et al., 1997).
5. **Virtual screening**: CADD greatly shortens the lead discovery time by enabling high-throughput virtual screening of sizable compound libraries to find possible therapeutic candidates (Trott and Olson, 2010).
6. **Lead compound optimization:** To improve efficacy and minimize side effects, CADD techniques refine possible leads by enhancing their pharmacological characteristics, stability, and binding affinities (Patel and Chalmers, 2003).

7. **Optimization of lead compounds:** Once potential leads are identified, CADD tools refine these compounds by optimizing their binding affinities, stability, and pharmacological properties to enhance efficacy and reduce side effects (Patel and Chalmers, 2003).
8. **Prediction of pharmacokinetics and toxicity:** In order to help with the early-stage removal of unsuitable candidates, computational methods in CADD can forecast a compound's absorption, distribution, metabolism, and excretion (ADME) characteristics, as well as any toxicological hazards (Daina et al., 2017).
9. **Integration with AI and ML:** Advanced AI-driven algorithms enhance CADD by analyzing complex biological data, identifying patterns, and improving predictive accuracy for drug discovery and optimization (Jumper et al., 2021).
10. **Cost and time efficiency:** By replacing certain experimental processes with computational simulations, CADD reduces the financial and temporal burdens of drug development, streamlining the path from discovery to clinical trials (Schneider et al., 2018).
11. **Collaborative capabilities:** CADD tools often integrate cloud computing and shared platforms, facilitating collaboration among researchers worldwide and democratizing access to drug discovery technologies. These features position CADD as a transformative tool in modern drug development, enabling faster, more precise, and cost-effective solutions for complex therapeutic challenges (Cavasotto and Orry, 2007).

Fig. 1.2 shows the stages of CADD, and Table 1.1 provides the description of the tools for AI-driven CADD.

1.3 History and evolution of computational drug discovery

1.3.1 Initial years (1960s–1980s)

I. **Structure-activity relationships (SAR):** QSAR, an approach used to forecast a compound's biological activity based on its chemical structure, were first analyzed using computational techniques in the 1960s.
II. **Molecular docking:** This approach was developed in the 1970s to simulate the interactions of tiny molecules with biological targets, such as proteins.
III. **Algorithm development:** To approximate chemical interactions, simple computational tools and techniques have been established, such as energy minimization for molecular structures.

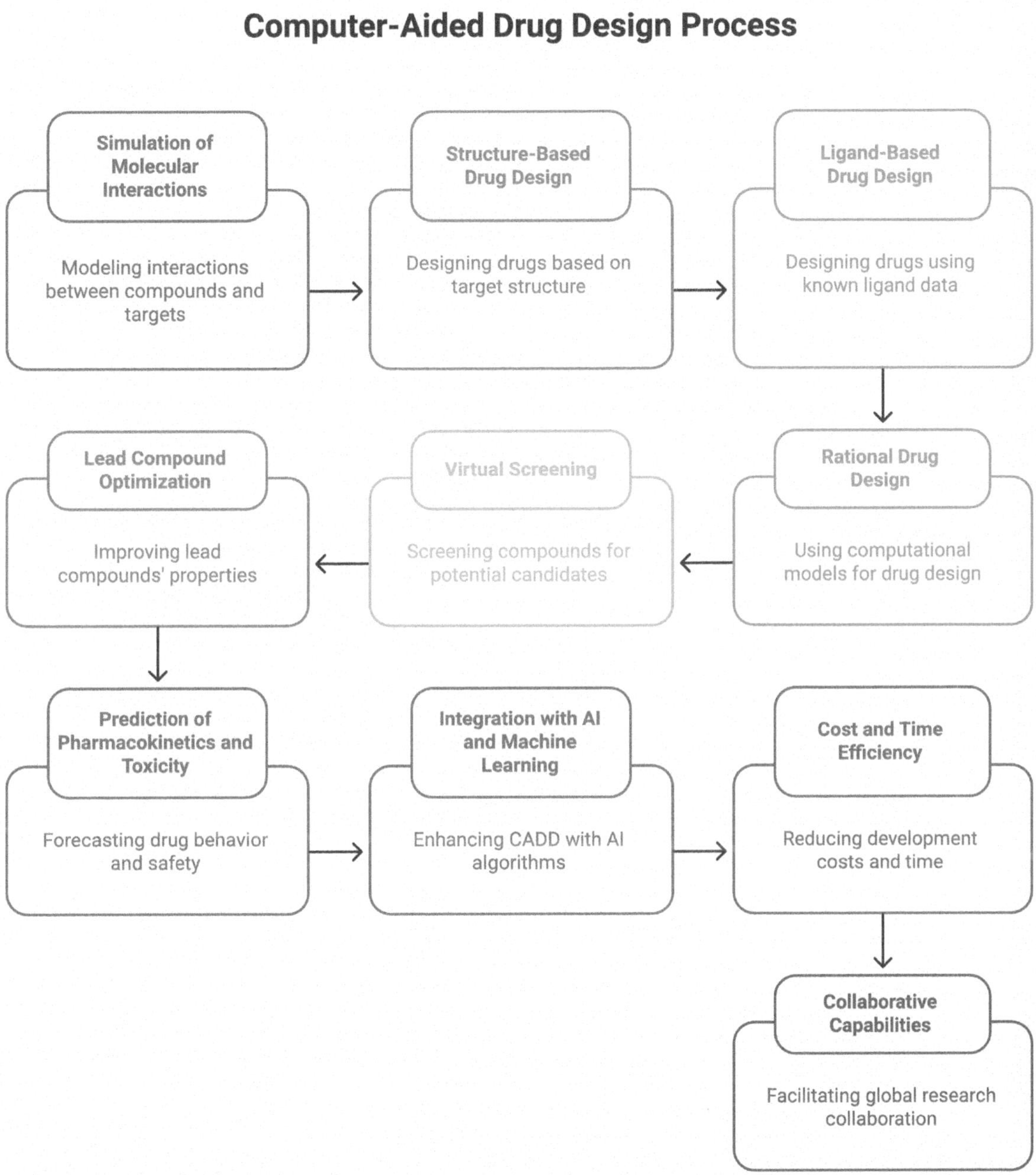

Fig. 1.2 This diagram illustrates the stages of computer-aided drug design, from simulating molecular interactions and structure or ligand-based design to virtual screening, lead optimization, and safety prediction. Integration with machine learning improves predictions, supporting cost-effective, collaborative drug development.

Table 1.1 Tools and frameworks for AI-driven CADD.

Tool	Description	Key features	References
DeepChem	Open-source platform for applying deep learning to chemical and biological datasets.	Molecular property prediction, protein-ligand binding, QSAR modeling.	Wu et al. (2018), DeepChem Documentation
RDKit	A chemical informatics toolkit for cheminformatics and molecular descriptor calculations.	Feature generation, molecular fingerprinting, substructure search, and visualization.	RDKit documentation
Schrödinger AI Suite	Comprehensive software suite integrating AI with molecular modeling for drug discovery.	Molecular docking, binding affinity prediction, pharmacophore modeling, ADME/Tox screening.	Schrödinger website
AlphaFold	DeepMind's AI system predicts 3D protein structures with atomic accuracy.	Predicts protein folding and aids in target identification for drug design.	Jumper et al. (2021), DeepMind AlphaFold.
Chemprop	A ML tool for predicting molecular properties using message-passing neural networks (MPNNs).	Property prediction, including solubility, toxicity, and bioavailability.	Yang et al., 2019), Chemprop GitHub
OpenEye Toolkit	Suite of cheminformatics and molecular modeling tools for drug discovery and lead optimization.	Molecular docking, shape-based screening, and ligand-based virtual screening.	OpenEye website
MolBERT	Pretrained deep learning model for chemical structure representations, based on natural language models.	Predicts molecular properties and performs molecule classification tasks.	MolBERT
PyTorch and TensorFlow	ML frameworks for building and training AI models.	Supports deep learning tasks such as QSAR modeling, generative drug design, and feature extraction.	Paszke et al. (2019) (PyTorch), Abadi et al. (2016) (TensorFlow), TensorFlow.
ChEMBL	Database of bioactive molecules with drug-like properties.	Provides bioactivity data for ML models and supports QSAR and virtual screening tasks.	Gaulton et al. (2017), ChEMBL database
PubChem	Public database for chemical compounds and their biological activities.	Large-scale chemical dataset for training AI models includes bioactivity assays and pharmacological data.	Kim and Rush (2016), PubChem
Basilisk	AI-driven de novo drug design platform for generating novel chemical structures.	Generative models, such as GANs and VAEs, are used for automated molecule creation.	Kadurin et al. (2017), Basilisk Reference.
Exscientia Platform	AI-powered drug discovery platform, combining knowledge graphs with generative AI models.	Multitarget optimization, prioritization of compounds for lead selection, and rapid drug discovery cycles.	Hopkins et al. (2004), Exscientia
AtomNet	Deep learning-based framework for structure-based drug discovery.	Predicts binding affinities, performs ligand-based screening, and optimizes lead compounds.	Wallach et al. (2015), AtomNet

1.3.2 The development of advanced techniques in the 1990s and 2000s

I. **High-performance computing:** Large-scale molecular interaction simulations have been made possible by advancements in hardware and software.
II. **Structural databases:** Many 3D structures for potential pharmacological targets are available in databases such as the Protein Data Bank (PDB).
III. **Virtual screening:** Using virtual screening techniques, scientists were able to computationally screen millions of molecules and rank those that were most likely to bind to the target.

1.3.3 Modern era (2000s-present)

- **AI and ML in CADD**: ML algorithms now analyze complex datasets to predict drug efficacy, toxicity, and pharmacokinetics.
- **Molecular dynamics simulations**: These simulations explore the time-dependent behavior of drug-target interactions in realistic biological environments.
- **Cloud computing and big data**: The integration of cloud platforms and big data analytics has enabled the handling of massive datasets for drug discovery.

1.3.4 Cost efficiency

- Traditional drug discovery is resource-intensive and expensive, with an average cost of $1–2 billion per drug.
- CADD drastically cuts these costs by focusing on virtual simulations and reducing the number of failed experiments.

1.3.5 Precision and targeted therapies

1. CADD uses molecular docking and dynamics to design drugs that precisely bind to specific biological targets, improving their effectiveness and reducing side effects.
2. This approach is particularly useful for developing drugs against diseases with complex mechanisms, like cancer or neurological disorders.

1.3.6 Enhancing drug safety

Predictive models in CADD assess ADME and Toxicity (ADME/Tox) properties, identifying potentially harmful compounds before clinical trials.

1.3.7 Facilitating personalized medicine

CADD supports the development of personalized drugs by analyzing patient-specific genetic and molecular data. For example, drugs can be tailored to target mutations unique to an individual's cancer cells.

1.3.8 Key success stories in CADD

HIV protease inhibitors: Computational tools have helped design inhibitors that effectively bind to the HIV protease enzyme, leading to successful antiretroviral therapies.

Imatinib (Gleevec): A pioneering cancer drug developed for chronic myeloid leukemia using SBDD.

Oseltamivir (Tamiflu): An antiviral drug designed using CADD to target the neuraminidase protein in influenza viruses.

2 AI for drug target identification and validation

AI is significantly transforming the process of identifying and validating drug targets, providing enhanced speed, precision, and new perspectives on disease mechanisms. By integrating AI with technologies such as Alpha Fold, DeepChem, and Benevolent AI, researchers are able to identify and confirm therapeutic targets more quickly and effectively than previously possible. These developments are leading to the creation of innovative treatments that address unmet medical needs in the fields of precision medicine and complex diseases. Table 1.2 outlines the dataset for drug target identification and validation as an example.

Table 1.2 Example dataset for drug target identification and validation.

Drug	Protein sequence	Interaction	Description
CCO	MGHHHHHHGS	1	Interaction detected
CCN	MEKKLRRQR	0	No interaction
CCC	MGHHHHHHGS	1	Interaction detected
CCCC	MGHQTRPQR	0	No interaction
CCCN	MGHMMRQGS	1	Interaction detected
CCCO	MGHPRLQRS	1	Interaction detected
CCOCC	MAKKRQHLS	0	No interaction
CCOCCN	MGHHKLRRG	1	Interaction detected
CCCCCC	MGHPTLRRQ	0	No interaction
CCOCCCN	MGHHPLRQS	1	Interaction detected

2.1 Protocol for AI in drug target identification and validation using Python tools

Python programming is used to identify and verify drug targets. It has been examined how drugs bind to proteins, predict likely targets, and test those predictions using computational approaches.

Workflow steps

A simplified dataset containing drug molecular features and protein sequences for demonstration purposes was used in the study.

Dataset:

1. **Drugs**: Represented using the Simplified Molecular Input Line Entry System (SMILES) notation.
2. **Proteins**: Represented by their amino acid sequences.

Box 1.1 defines the steps to load and explore drug and protein data.

Box 1.1 Load and explore drug and protein data

#Install rdkit package

To get started, install RDKit if you haven't yet

```
!pip install rdkit
```

#Confirm it is installed

```
import rdkit
```

#Bring in basic data libraries

```
import pandas as pd import numpy as np
```

#RDKit tools for working with chemical structures and calculating descriptors

```
from rdkit import Chem from rdkit.Chem import Descriptors
```

#Tools for building and evaluating machine learning models

```
from sklearn.preprocessing import OneHotEncoder from sklearn.ensemble import RandomForestClassifier from sklearn.model_selection import train_test_split from sklearn.metrics import accuracy_score, classification_report, ConfusionMatrixDisplay
```

#Libraries for creating plots

```
import matplotlib.pyplot as plt import seaborn as sns
```

#A small demo dataset for checking drug–protein interactions

Bring in needed Python libraries

```
import pandas as pd import numpy as np from rdkit import Chem from rdkit.Chem import Descriptors from sklearn.preprocessing import OneHotEncoder from sklearn.ensemble import RandomForestClassifier from sklearn.model_selection import train_test_split from sklearn.metrics import accuracy_score, classification_report, ConfusionMatrixDisplay import matplotlib.pyplot as plt import seaborn as sns
```

#Make a simple table with example drugs, proteins, and whether they interact

```
interaction_data = pd.DataFrame({ 'Drug': ['CCO', 'CCN', 'CCC', 'CCCC', 'CCCN', 'CCOCC', 'CCOCCN', 'CCCCCC', 'CCCO', 'CCCCN'], 'Protein': [ 'MGHHHHHHGS', 'MEKKLRRQR', 'MGHHHHHHGS', 'MGHQTRPQR', 'MGHMMRQGS', 'MAKKRQHLS', 'MGHHKLRRG', 'MGHPTLRRQ', 'MGHPRLQRS', 'MGHHPLRQS' ], 'Interaction': [1, 0, 1, 0, 1, 0, 1, 0, 1, 1] })
```

print("Here's our example interaction table:") print(interaction_data)

#Step 1: Calculate basic properties for drug molecules

def get_molecular_features(smiles_string): mol = Chem.MolFromSmiles(smiles_string) if mol: return [Descriptors. MolWt(mol), # Molecular weight Descriptors.NumHAcceptors(mol), # Number of H-bond acceptors Descriptors. NumHDonors(mol) # Number of H-bond donors] else: return [np.nan, np.nan, np.nan]

#Apply the function to each drug entry

drug_features = data['Drug'].apply(get_molecular_features) features_df = pd.DataFrame(drug_features.tolist(), columns=['Molecular Weight', 'Hbond Acceptor', 'Hbond Donors'])

#Add the features back to the main dataset

data = pd.concat([data, features_df], axis=1) print("

Data with Computed Drug Features:

", data)

#Step 2: Turn protein sequences into one-hot encoded vectors with fixed length

def encode_protein_sequence(seq, max_len=10): amino_acid_list = 'ACDEFGHIKLMNPQRSTVWY' encoder = OneHot Encoder(categories=[list(amino_acid_list)], sparse=False, handle_unknown='ignore')

#Adjust sequence length (truncate or pad)

chars = list(seq[:max_len]) + [''] * (max_len - len(seq)) chars_array = np.array(chars).reshape(-1, 1)

#Perform one-hot encoding

encoded = encoder.fit_transform(chars_array) return encoded.flatten()

#Apply encoding to all proteins

data['EncodedProtein'] = data['Protein'].apply(encode_protein_sequence) print("

Data with Encoded Protein Sequences:

", data[['Protein', 'EncodedProtein']].head())

#Step 3: Combine drug features and protein encoding into a single matrix

X = np.hstack([features_df.values, np.vstack(data['EncodedProtein'].values)]) y = data['Interaction'].values print("

Shape of Feature Matrix:", X.shape)

#Step 4: Split into training and testing sets

X_train, X_test, y_train, y_test = train_test_split(X, y, test_size=0.3, random_state=42)

#Step 5: Build and train a random forest model

rf = RandomForestClassifier(n_estimators=100, random_state=42) rf.fit(X_train, y_train)

#Step 6: Test the model and show results

predictions = rf.predict(X_test) print("

Model Accuracy:", accuracy_score(y_test, predictions)) print("Detailed Report:

", classification_report(y_test, predictions))

#Visualization: Plot confusion matrix

ConfusionMatrixDisplay.from_estimator(rf, X_test, y_test, cmap='Blues') plt.title("Confusion Matrix") plt.show()

#Visualization 3: Data Distribution by Molecular Weight#

Plot: Checking how molecular weights are distributed

plt.figure(figsize=(10, 6))sns.histplot(data['MolecularWeight'], bins=10, kde=True, color='green')

plt.title("Molecular Weight Distribution")

plt.xlabel("Molecular Weight")

```
plt.ylabel("Count")
plt.show()
#Visualization 4: Protein Sequence Lengths
#Plotting the lengths of protein sequences in our data
protein_seq_lengths = data['Protein'].apply(len) plt.figure(figsize=(10, 6)) sns.histplot(protein_seq_lengths,
bins=10, kde=True, color='purple') plt.title("Protein Sequence Length Distribution") plt.xlabel("Sequence Length") plt.
ylabel("Count") plt.show()
#Step 7: Predict New Drug-Target Pair
#Step 7: Make a prediction for a new drug–protein combination
#Define a new example
test_drug = "CCCN" test_protein = "MGHHLQLRRS"
#Generate features for this new pair
test_drug_features = get_molecular_features(test_drug) test_protein_encoded =
encode_protein_sequence(test_protein)
#Combine all features into one array
test_input = np.hstack([test_drug_features, test_protein_encoded])
#Use the trained model to predict interaction
predicted_result = rf.predict([test_input]) print(" \n
Prediction for New Drug–Protein Pair (1 = Interaction, 0 = No Interaction):", predicted_result[0])
```

```
#To get started, install RDkit package
pip install rdkit
import rdkit
#check installation of
import pandas as pd
import numpy as np
from rdkit import Chem
from rdkit.Chem import Descriptors
from sklearn.preprocessing import OneHotEncoder
from sklearn.ensemble import RandomForestClassifier
from sklearn.model_selection import train_test_split
from sklearn.metrics import accuracy_score, classification_report,
ConfusionMatrixDisplay
import matplotlib.pyplot as plt
import seaborn as sns
```

Fig. 1.3 depicts the visualization of the output in the form of graphs.

2.2 Understanding disease mechanisms with AI

Fig. 1.4 represents workflows for simulating protein interactions, predicting docking using ML, and visualizing compound predictions.

Computational pipeline: Understanding disease mechanisms using protein-protein docking and molecular simulations

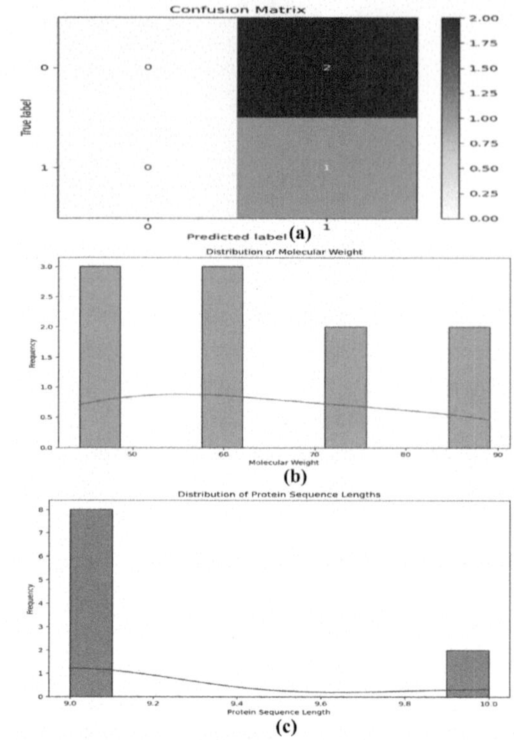

Fig. 1.3 Visualization of the output. (A) Graph illustrates the confusion matrix, (B) distribution of molecular weight, and (C) distribution of protein sequence lengths visualization.

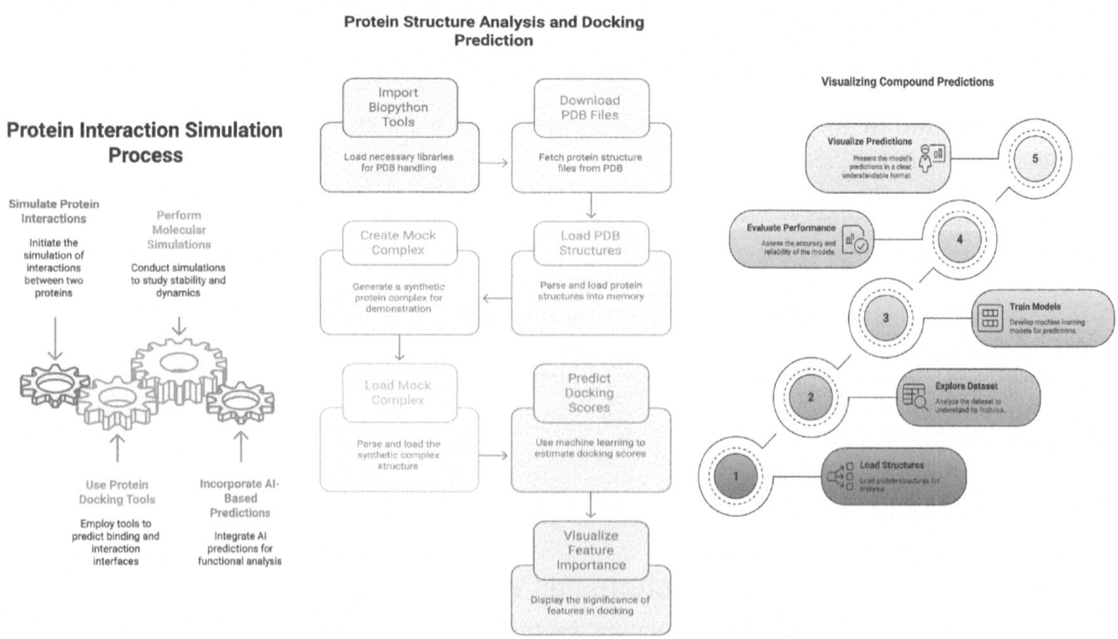

Fig. 1.4 Multistep framework for protein interaction modeling and compound prediction. Steps include molecular simulations, docking analysis, AI integration, dataset exploration, model training, and performance evaluation for informed drug discovery.

1. **Simulate interactions between two proteins** related to a disease.
2. **Use protein docking tools** to predict binding and interaction interfaces.
3. Perform **molecular simulations** to study stability and dynamics.

Incorporate **AI-based docking score predictions** for functional analysis.

2.3 Multistep framework for protein interaction modeling and compound prediction

Box 1.2 defines the steps to perform protein interaction modeling and compound interaction analysis.

Box 1.2 Install the following Python Libraries

#Install Required Libraries: Install the following **Python Libraries.** pip install biopython pip install matplotlib pip install seaborn pip install scikit-learns

from Bio.PDB import PDBList, PDBParser

#Set up the downloader

pdb_downloader = PDBList()# Download Beta-Amyloid (PDB ID: 1IYT) and Tau (PDB ID: 6NTR) pdb_downloader.retrieve_pdb_file('1IYT', pdir='/Users/us74/Desktop', file_format='pdb') pdb_downloader.retrieve_pdb_file('6NTR', pdir='/Users/us74/Desktop', file_format='pdb') **Step 3: Load Structures from Files#Once downloaded, load the structures using Biopython parser.**

#Initialize the parser

structure_parser = PDBParser()

#Load the Beta-Amyloid structure

beta_amyloid = structure_parser.get_structure("BetaAmyloid", "/Users/us74/Desktop/pdb1iyt.ent")

#Load the Tau structure

tau_protein = structure_parser.get_structure("Tau", "/Users/us74/Desktop/pdb6ntr.ent")

#Confirm loading

print("Beta-Amyloid Loaded:", beta_amyloid) print("Tau Protein Loaded:", tau_protein) #Example output: Downloading PDB structure '1iyt'. Downloading PDB structure '6ntr'. Beta-Amyloid Loaded: <Structure id=BetaAmyloid> Tau Protein Loaded: <Structure id=Tau> **#Step 4: Visualize the Protein Structures.** You can use py3Dmol for easy interactive visualization in notebooks. import py3Dmol def visualize_pdb(pdb_path): with open(pdb_path, 'r') as file: pdb_content = file.read() view = py3Dmol.view(width=800, height=600) view.addModel(pdb_content, 'pdb') view.setStyle({'cartoon': {'color': 'spectrum'}}) view.zoomTo() return view

#Show the Beta-Amyloid structure

visualize_pdb('/Users/us74/Desktop/pdb1iyt.ent')

#import Biopython tools for working with PDB structures

from Bio.PDB import PDBList, PDBParser

#Step 1: Download PDB files to a chosen location

```
downloader = PDBList()
```

#Fetch Beta-Amyloid (PDB ID: 1IYT) and Tau (PDB ID: 6NTR)

```
downloader.retrieve_pdb_file('1IYT', pdir='/Users/us74/Desktop', file_format='pdb') downloader.retrieve_pdb_file('6NTR', pdir='/Users/us74/Desktop', file_format='pdb')
```

#Step 2: Load the downloaded PDB structures

```
parser = PDBParser() beta_amyloid_structure = parser.get_structure("BetaAmyloid", "/Users/us74/Desktop/pdb1iyt.ent") tau_structure = parser.get_structure("Tau", "/Users/us74/Desktop/pdb6ntr.ent")
#Show confirmation in output
print("Loaded Beta-Amyloid Structure:", beta_amyloid_structure) print("Loaded Tau Structure:", tau_structure)
```

#Step 3: Create a simple, fake "docked" complex for demonstration

```
mock_complex_content = """ HEADER FAKE COMPLEX ATOM 1 N ALA A 1 11.104 9.104 8.174 1.00 20.00 N ATOM 2 CA ALA A 1 12.104 9.504 9.174 1.00 20.00 C ATOM 3 C ALA A 1 13.304 8.704 9.574 1.00 20.00 C ATOM 4 O ALA A 1 13.804 7.804 9.074 1.00 20.00 O ATOM 5 CB ALA A 1 11.604 10.904 9.574 1.00 20.00 C TER END """ mock_complex_path = "/Users/us74/Desktop/Amyloid_Tau_Complex.pdb" with open(mock_complex_path, "w") as file: file.write(mock_complex_content) print(f"Mock complex file saved at: {mock_complex_path}")
```

#Step 4: Load and examine the fake docked complex

```
complex_structure = parser.get_structure("AmyloidTauComplex", mock_complex_path) print("
Residue details in the loaded complex:")
for model in complex_structure: for chain in model: for residue in chain: print("Residue:", residue.get_resname(), "Chain ID:", chain.id)
```

#Step 5: Use machine learning to predict docking scores

```
import pandas as pd from sklearn.ensemble import RandomForestRegressor from sklearn.model_selection import train_test_split
```

#Example dataset of features and docking scores

```
features_data = pd.DataFrame({ 'Hydrophobicity': [0.6, 0.8, 0.5, 0.7], 'HydrogenBonds': [5, 8, 3, 6], 'InterfaceArea': [1200, 1400, 1100, 1300], 'DockingScore': [-150, -160, -120, -140] })
print("
Sample Docking Features Data:") print(features_data)
```

#Separate predictors and target

```
X = features_data[['Hydrophobicity', 'HydrogenBonds', 'InterfaceArea']] y = features_data['DockingScore']
```

#Split data for training/testing

```
X_train, X_test, y_train, y_test = train_test_split(X, y, test_size=0.3, random_state=42)
```

#Train a RandomForest model

```
rf_model = RandomForestRegressor(n_estimators=100, random_state=42) rf_model.fit(X_train, y_train)
#Predict score for a new example
new_sample = [[0.7, 6, 1250]] predicted_docking_score = rf_model.predict(new_sample) print("
Predicted Docking Score for new complex:", predicted_docking_score[0])
```

```
#Step 6: Visualize which features matter most
import matplotlib.pyplot as plt import seaborn as sns feature_importance = rf_model.feature_importances_ feature_names = ['Hydrophobicity', 'HydrogenBonds', 'InterfaceArea'] plt.figure(figsize=(10, 6)) sns.barplot(x=feature_importance, y=feature_names, palette='viridis') plt.title("Importance of Features in Docking Score Prediction") plt.xlabel("Importance Value") plt.ylabel("Feature") plt.show()
#Step 7: Visualize Example Molecular Dynamics RMSD Data
#Example time (ns) and RMSD (nm) values
simulation_time = [0, 10, 20, 30, 40, 50] rmsd_values = [0.1, 0.15, 0.12, 0.13, 0.14, 0.11]
#Create a plot of RMSD over time
plt.figure(figsize=(8, 6)) plt.plot(simulation_time, rmsd_values, marker='o', label='RMSD') plt.title("RMSD Across Molecular Dynamics Simulation") plt.xlabel("Time (nanoseconds)") plt.ylabel("RMSD (nanometers)") plt.legend() plt.show()
```

Step 1: Load and Visualize Protein Structures

Fig. 1.5 portrays the loading and visualization of the protein structures. Biopython is used to automatically download the PDB files for Beta-Amyloid (1IYT) and Tau (6NTR).

Step 2: Download and Load Protein Structure

#This will download the PDB files directly into the current directory. **Biopython is used** to automatically fetch PDB files for the Beta-Amyloid and Tau proteins.

Structure exists: '/Users/us74/Desktop/pdb1iyt.ent'

Structure exists: '/Users/us74/Desktop/pdb6ntr.ent'

Beta-Amyloid Structure Loaded: <Structure id=Amyloid>

Tau Structure Loaded: <Structure id=Tau>

Mock docked complex created at /Users/us74/Desktop/Amyloid_Tau_Complex.pdb

Residues in Docked Complex:

Residue: ALA Chain: A

Docking Features Dataset has been shown in Table 1.3.

Predicted Docking Score for New Interaction: -143.4

2.3.1 Docking via cluspro or HADDOCK

Protein-protein docking is performed using online tools like ClusPro or HADDOCK. The basic workflow is as follows:

1. **Upload the protein structures**
   a. Upload the beta-amyloid structure (pdb1iyt.ent).
   b. Upload the Tau structure (pdb6ntr.ent).
2. **Submit the Docking Job**
   a. For HADDOCK, specify interacting residues (optional).
   b. Download the resulting docked complex (e.g., Amyloid_Tau_Complex.pdb).
3. **Visualize the Docked Complex**: Use **PyMOL** or **Py3Dmol** to visualize the interaction.

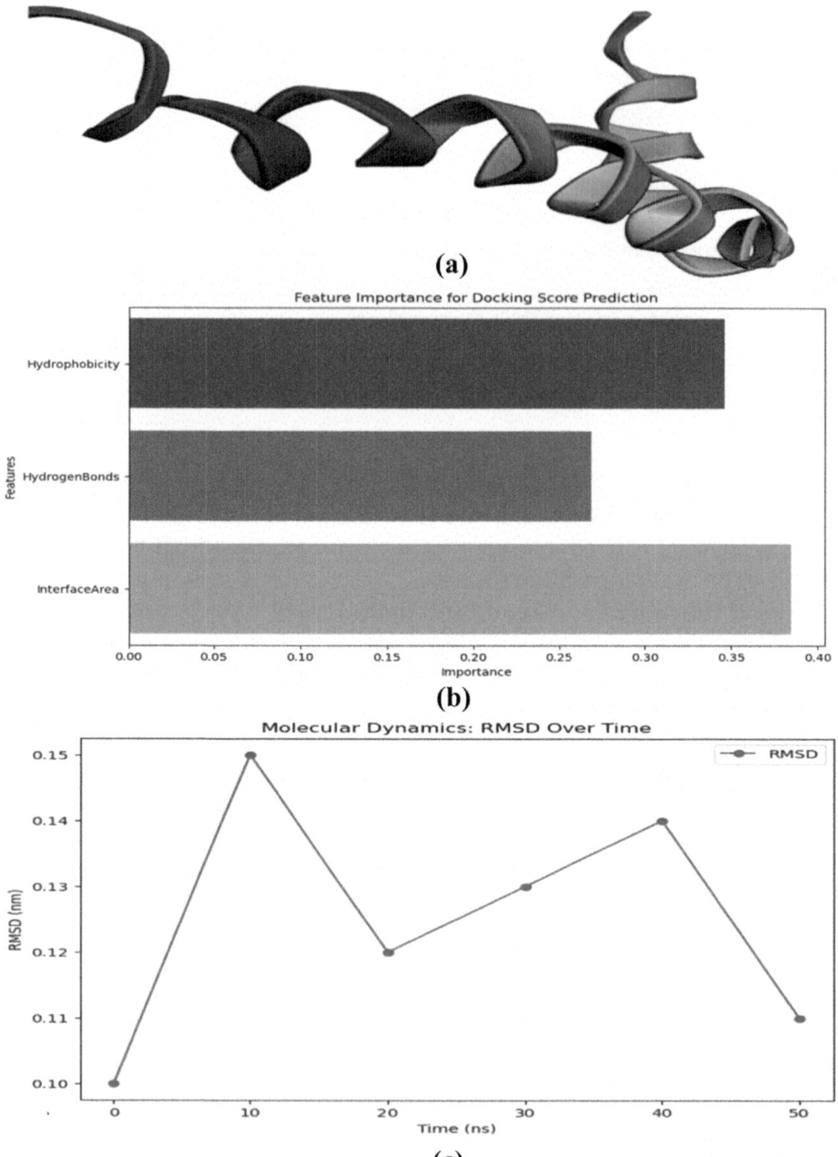

Fig. 1.5 Graphical representation of loading and visualization of protein structure. (A) Structure of the Alzheimer's disease amyloid beta-peptide (PDB ID: 1IYT), (B) Feature importance for docking score prediction, and (C) Molecular dynamics root mean square deviation over 50 ns.

Table 1.3 Feature importance for docking score prediction.

Features importance	Hydrophobicity	HydrogenBonds	InterfaceArea	DockingScore
0	0.6	5	1200	− 150
1	0.8	8	1400	− 160
2	0.5	3	1100	− 120
3	0.7	6	1300	− 140

2.3.2 ADME or Tox predictions with AI

Predicting **ADME/Tox** profiles using AI provides a powerful tool for early-stage drug discovery. By leveraging ML models and molecular descriptors, AI accelerates the screening of drug candidates, helping to reduce time and cost in pharmaceutical development.

Computational Pipeline: Predicting ADME/Tox Profiles Using AI.

To build a predictive model for bioavailability and toxicity prediction using a ML approach, the code is shown in Box 1.3, and its output is displayed in Fig. 1.6.

Box 1.3 Computational pipeline for predicting ADME/Tox profiles using AI

Step 1: Install Required Libraries pip install pandas scikit-learn matplotlib seaborn

Step 2: Import Libraries and Load the Dataset import pandas as pd import seaborn as sns import matplotlib.pyplot as plt from sklearn.model_selection import train_test_split from sklearn.ensemble import RandomForestClassifier from sklearn.metrics import classification_report, confusion_matrix, accuracy_score

#Create the dataset

data = pd.DataFrame({ 'MolecularWeight': [250.3, 320.5, 180.2, 295.4, 215.3, 350.7, 150.1, 270.3, 310.0, 290.5], 'LogP': [3.2, 2.8, 1.5, 3.9, 1.8, 4.5, 0.9, 3.1, 3.6, 3.0], 'HBA': [4, 5, 3, 6, 3, 8, 2, 4, 6, 5], 'HBD': [1, 2, 0, 2, 1, 3, 0, 1, 2, 1], 'RotatableBonds': [6, 4, 2, 7, 3, 10, 1, 5, 8, 6], 'Bioavailability': [1, 1, 1, 0, 1, 0, 1, 1, 0, 1], # Target for absorption 'Toxicity': [0, 1, 0, 1, 0, 1, 0, 0, 1, 1] # Target for toxicity })

#Split features and targets

X = data[['MolecularWeight', 'LogP', 'HBA', 'HBD', 'RotatableBonds']] y_bioavailability = data['Bioavailability'] y_toxicity = data['Toxicity']

Step 3: Explore the Dataset#Plot feature distributions and correlations:

#Visualize distributions of features

sns.pairplot(data, vars=['MolecularWeight', 'LogP', 'HBA', 'HBD', 'RotatableBonds'], hue='Toxicity') plt.suptitle('Feature Distributions (Hue=Toxicity)', y=1.02) plt.show()

#Correlation heatmap

correlation_matrix = data.corr() sns.heatmap(correlation_matrix, annot=True, fmt='.2f', cmap='coolwarm') plt.title('Feature Correlation Heatmap') plt.show()

Step 4: Split the Dataset

Train-test split for bioavailability and toxicity models

X_train, X_test, y_train_bio, y_test_bio = train_test_split(X, y_bioavailability, test_size=0.3, random_state=42) X_train, X_test, y_train_tox, y_test_tox = train_test_split(X, y_toxicity, test_size=0.3, random_state=42)

Step 5: Train machine learning models

#Bioavailability Model

#Train Random Forest for Bioavailability

bio_model = RandomForestClassifier(n_estimators=100, random_state=42) bio_model.fit(X_train, y_train_bio)

#Predict

y_pred_bio = bio_model.predict(X_test)

#Train Random Forest for Toxicity

tox_model = RandomForestClassifier(n_estimators=100, random_state=42) tox_model.fit(X_train, y_train_tox)

#Predict

y_pred_tox = tox_model.predict(X_test)

Step 6: Evaluate Model Performance

#Evaluate Bioavailability Model

#Accuracy and Classification Report

bio_acc = accuracy_score(y_test_bio, y_pred_bio) print(f"Bioavailability Prediction Accuracy: {bio_acc * 100:.2f}%") print("Bioavailability Classification Report:

", classification_report(y_test_bio, y_pred_bio))

#Confusion Matrix

cm_bio = confusion_matrix(y_test_bio, y_pred_bio) sns.heatmap(cm_bio, annot=True, fmt='d', cmap='Blues', xticklabels=['Poor', 'Good'], yticklabels=['Poor', 'Good']) plt.title('Confusion Matrix - Bioavailability') plt.xlabel('Predicted') plt.ylabel('Actual') plt.show()

#Evaluate Toxicity Model

#Accuracy and Classification Report

tox_acc = accuracy_score(y_test_tox, y_pred_tox) print(f"Toxicity Prediction Accuracy: {tox_acc * 100:.2f}%") print("Toxicity Classification Report:

", classification_report(y_test_tox, y_pred_tox))

#Confusion Matrix

cm_tox = confusion_matrix(y_test_tox, y_pred_tox) sns.heatmap(cm_tox, annot=True, fmt='d', cmap='Reds', xticklabels=['Non-Toxic', 'Toxic'], yticklabels=['Non-Toxic', 'Toxic']) plt.title('Confusion Matrix - Toxicity') plt. xlabel('Predicted') plt.ylabel('Actual') plt.show()

Step 7: Feature Importance Visualization

#Feature importance for bioavailability model

bio_importances = pd.Series(bio_model.feature_importances_, index=X.columns) bio_importances.sort_ values(ascending=True).plot(kind='barh', color='teal') plt.title('Feature Importance - Bioavailability') plt.xlabel('Importance Score') plt.ylabel('Features') plt.show()

#Feature importance for toxicity model

tox_importances = pd.Series(tox_model.feature_importances_, index=X.columns) tox_importances.sort_ values(ascending=True).plot(kind='barh', color='darkred') plt.title('Feature Importance - Toxicity') plt.xlabel('Importance Score') plt.ylabel('Features') plt.show()

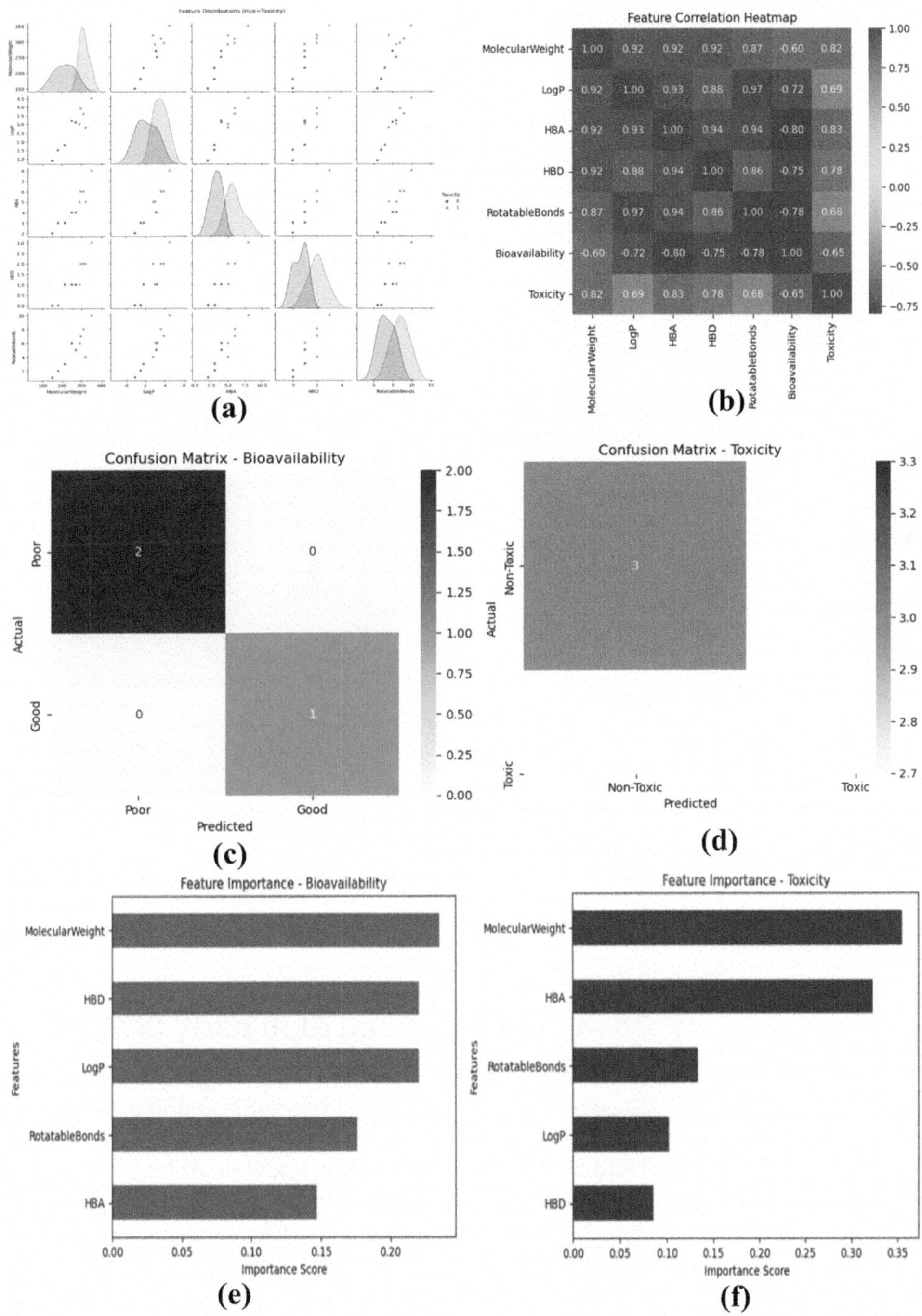

Fig. 1.6 The graphical visualization of the output. (A) Feature distribution and correlation for toxicity, (B) Feature correlation heatmap, (C) Confusion matrix for bioavailability, (D) Confusion matrix for toxicity, (E) Feature importance: Bioavailability, (F) Feature importance: Toxicity.

Table 1.4 Bioavailability classification report.

	Precision	recall	f1-score	support
0	1.00	1.00	1.00	2
1	1.00	1.00	1.00	1
Accuracy			1.00	3
macro avg	1.00	1.00	1.00	3
weighted avg	1.00	1.00	1.00	3

Table 1.5 Toxicity classification report.

	Precision	recall	f1-score	support
1	1.00	1.00	1.00	3
Accuracy			1.00	3
macro avg	1.00	1.00	1.00	3
weighted avg	1.00	1.00	1.00	3

#Output

Predicted Bioavailability (1=Good, 0=Poor): 1Predicted Toxicity (1=Toxic, 0=Non-Toxic): 0

Bioavailability Prediction Accuracy: 100.00%, as shown in Table 1.4.

Toxicity prediction accuracy: 100.00%, as shown in Table 1.5.

3 Advantages of using AI in early drug design

Combining AI with CADD brings clear benefits, especially at the start of drug development. Early discovery aims to find potential drug candidates and study their properties, a process that is often slow, expensive, and complicated. By working together, AI and CADD help make these steps quicker and more efficient, saving both time and money while improving results. Table 1.6 outlines the benefits for early-stage drug development.

Table 1.6 Benefits for early-stage drug development.

Benefit	Description	Applications	Tools	References
1. Faster candidate identification	AI can screen millions of compounds virtually, predicting their potential as drug candidates and significantly reducing the time spent on manual screening.	Insilico Medicine identified a fibrosis drug candidate in just 46 days.	DeepChem Chemprop RDKit	Wu et al. (2018) (DeepChem) Yang et al., 2019) (Chemprop)
2. Cost reduction	AI reduces the need for costly experiments by predicting compound properties (e.g., binding affinity, toxicity) and eliminating weak candidates early.	AI-powered platforms reduce R&D costs by 15%–20%, according to Deloitte.	Exscientia Schrödinger	Gaulton et al. (2017) (ChEMBL)
3. Improved prediction accuracy	AI predicts key properties like ADME/Tox, bioavailability, and binding affinity with high precision.	AtomNet predicts protein-ligand interactions with high accuracy for structure-based drug discovery.	AtomNet PyTorch TensorFlow	Wallach et al. (2015) (AtomNet)
4. Multiproperty optimization	AI optimizes multiple drug properties simultaneously (e.g., efficacy, selectivity, safety), ensuring drug candidates meet all desired criteria.	Exscientia used multiobjective optimization to develop a drug for obsessive-compulsive disorder, which entered clinical trials within 12 months.	Exscientia Basilisk Schrödinger	Kadurin et al. (2017)
5. Rapid de novo drug design	AI generates novel molecules using generative models like GANs and VAEs, optimizing them for specific properties.	Insilico Medicine used AI to design a new kinase inhibitor in 18 months, compared to the typical 4–6 years.	Basilisk DeepChem RDKit	Kadurin et al. (2017)
6. Enhanced safety profiles	AI predicts potential toxic effects of compounds early, reducing failure rates in preclinical and clinical trials.	Toxicity prediction models help eliminate harmful candidates early, reducing costs associated with failed trials.	Chemprop DeepChem ChEMBL	Yang et al. (2019)
7. Facilitating drug repurposing	AI identifies new uses for existing drugs by analyzing biological data, reducing the time to market.	BenevolentAI repurposed Baricitinib (for arthritis) to treat COVID-19 during the pandemic.	BenevolentAI Exscientia	Hopkins et al. (2004)
8. Enabling precision medicine	AI integrates patient-specific data (e.g., genomics, proteomics) to design personalized treatments.	AI developed tailored cancer therapies by targeting unique mutations in patient subgroups.	AlphaFold DeepChem	Jumper et al. (2021) (AlphaFold Database)

4 The role of AI in health and diseases

4.1 AI in machine learning

AI helps advance drug discovery by using ML to recognize patterns and predict outcomes in complicated datasets (Vamathevan et al., 2019). ML can process vast amounts of biological, chemical, and clinical data to reveal patterns that might go unnoticed by humans (Chen et al., 2018). For instance, ML can forecast how a drug will bind to its target by studying data from similar compounds and targets (Gawehn et al., 2016). This capability significantly accelerates the identification of potential drug candidates, reducing the time and cost traditionally required for this process This ability speeds up finding promising drug candidates while cutting down the usual time and costs involved (Zhavoronkov et al., 2019). In addition, ML models can also estimate how effective a drug will be, its safety, and possible side effects by analyzing preclinical and clinical data (Schneider, 2018). ML techniques like supervised and unsupervised learning also help classify diseases based on genetic and phenotypic data, enabling the development of targeted therapies (Chen et al., 2018).

Recent advancements, such as reinforcement learning, are being applied to optimize molecular design, leading to the creation of compounds with improved pharmacological properties (Segler et al., 2018). In current research, ML has been instrumental in identifying new antiviral compounds, streamlining vaccine development, and advancing the discovery of drugs for rare diseases (Vamathevan et al., 2019). As the field evolves, ML continues to be a cornerstone of AI's transformative impact on drug discovery. The example dataset of treated cancer patient has been taken in study and shown in Table 1.7.

The datasets shows following features as:

1. **PatientID**: Unique identifier for each patient
2. **Age**: Age of the patient in years
3. **Gender**: Gender of the patient (Male/Female)
4. **TumorSize (cm)**: Size of the tumor in centimeters
5. **TreatmentType**: Type of treatment received by the patient
   - **Surgery**: Surgical removal of the tumor
   - **Radiation**: Radiation therapy
   - **Chemotherapy**: Chemical-based therapy
6. **LymphNodesAffected**: Number of lymph nodes affected by the cancer
7. **Stage**: Cancer stage (1, 2, 3, or 4)
8. **Recurrence**: Target variable indicating if the cancer recurred (1 = Yes, 0 = No)

Computational Pipeline: Predicting Cancer Recurrence Using ML

Table 1.7 The dataset of cancer treated patients.

PatientID	Age	Gender	TumorSize (cm)	Treatment type	LymphNodes affected	Stage	Recurrence (1 = Yes, 0 = No)
1	45	Male	3.2	Chemotherapy	1	2	1
2	52	Female	5.1	Radiation	2	3	0
3	38	Female	2.3	Surgery	0	1	0
4	60	Male	4.8	Chemotherapy	3	3	1
5	47	Female	3	Surgery	0	2	0
6	55	Male	6	Radiation	4	4	1
7	42	Female	2.9	Surgery	0	1	0
8	65	Male	4.5	Chemotherapy	2	2	1
9	50	Female	3.5	Radiation	1	2	0
10	58	Male	5.5	Chemotherapy	3	3	1

The dataset is used to predict the likelihood of cancer recurrence using a Random Forest Classifier as given in Box 1.4 and visualization has been represented in Fig. 1.7.

Box 1.4 Computational pipeline for predicting cancer recurrence using machine learning

Step 8: Predict for New Compounds

#New compound data: MolecularWeight=300, LogP=3.0, HBA=4, HBD=1, RotatableBonds=5

new_compound = [[300, 3.0, 4, 1, 5]]

#Predict bioavailability and toxicity

bio_pred = bio_model.predict(new_compound) tox_pred = tox_model.predict(new_compound) print(f"Predicted Bioavailability (1=Good, 0=Poor): {bio_pred[0]}") print(f"Predicted Toxicity (1=Toxic, 0=Non-Toxic): {tox_pred[0]}")

Step-9: Visualization of New Compound Predictions import matplotlib.pyplot as plt

Predicted outcomes for the new compound

labels = ['Bioavailability', 'Toxicity'] predictions = [bio_pred[0], tox_pred[0]] # Bioavailability: 1=Good, Toxicity: 1=Toxic

Map predictions to descriptive labels

descriptions = ['Good' if predictions[0] == 1 else 'Poor', 'Toxic' if predictions[1] == 1 else 'Non-Toxic']

Visualization

plt.figure(figsize=(6, 4)) colors = ['teal' if p == 1 else 'gray' for p in predictions] plt.bar(labels, predictions, color=colors, alpha=0.8, width=0.5)

Add descriptive labels to the x-axis

plt.xticks(range(len(labels)), [f"{labels[i]} ({descriptions[i]})" for i in range(len(labels))])

Add labels and title

plt.ylabel('Prediction Outcome') plt.title('Predictions for New Compound') plt.ylim(0, 1.5) # Limit y-axis for better visualization plt.show()

Step-9: Visualization of New Predictions import matplotlib.pyplot as plt

#Predicted outcomes for the new sample

labels = ['Feature A', 'Feature B'] predictions = [pred_a[0], pred_b[0]] # Example: 1=Positive, 0=Negative

Map predictions to descriptive labels

descriptions = ['Positive' if predictions[0] == 1 else 'Negative', 'Positive' if predictions[1] == 1 else 'Negative']

Visualization

plt.figure(figsize=(6, 4)) colors = ['teal' if p == 1 else 'gray' for p in predictions] plt.bar(labels, predictions, color=colors, alpha=0.8, width=0.5)

Add descriptive labels to the x-axis

plt.xticks(range(len(labels)), [f"{labels[i]} ({descriptions[i]})" for i in range(len(labels))])

Add labels and title

plt.ylabel('Prediction Score') plt.title('Predictions for New Sample') plt.ylim(0, 1.5) # Limit y-axis for better visualization plt.show()

#Step 1: Import libraries

import pandas as pd from sklearn.model_selection import train_test_split from sklearn.ensemble import RandomForestClassifier from sklearn.metrics import accuracy_score, confusion_matrix, classification_report import seaborn as sns import matplotlib.pyplot as plt

#Step 2: Load and prepare the data

import pandas as pd from sklearn.model_selection import train_test_split

#Step 1: Load and prepare the data

data = pd.DataFrame({ 'PatientID': [1, 2, 3, 4, 5, 6, 7, 8, 9, 10], 'Age': [45, 52, 38, 60, 47, 55, 42, 65, 50, 58], 'Gender': ['Male', 'Female', 'Female', 'Male', 'Female', 'Male', 'Female', 'Male', 'Female', 'Male'], 'TumorSize': [3.2, 5.1, 2.3, 4.8, 3.0, 6.0, 2.9, 4.5, 3.5, 5.5], 'TreatmentType': ['Chemotherapy', 'Radiation', 'Surgery', 'Chemotherapy', 'Surgery', 'Radiation', 'Surgery', 'Chemotherapy', 'Radiation', 'Chemotherapy'], 'LymphNodesAffected': [1, 2, 0, 3, 0, 4, 0, 2, 1, 3], 'Stage': [2, 3, 1, 3, 2, 4, 1, 2, 2, 3], 'Recurrence': [1, 0, 0, 1, 0, 1, 0, 1, 0, 1]

})

#Step 2: Encode categorical variables

data['Gender'] = data['Gender'].replace({'Male': 0, 'Female': 1}) data['TreatmentType'] = data['TreatmentType'].replace({'Surgery': 0, 'Radiation': 1, 'Chemotherapy': 2})

#Step 3: Define features and target

features = ['Age', 'Gender', 'TumorSize', 'TreatmentType', 'LymphNodesAffected', 'Stage'] X = data[features] y = data['Recurrence']

#Step 4: Split into training and testing sets

X_train, X_test, y_train, y_test = train_test_split(X, y, test_size=0.3, random_state=42)

#Convert categorical data into numerical format

data['Gender'] = data['Gender'].map({'Male': 0, 'Female': 1}) data['TreatmentType'] = data['TreatmentType'].map({'Surgery': 0, 'Radiation': 1, 'Chemotherapy': 2})

#Features and target variable

X = data[['Age', 'Gender', 'TumorSize', 'TreatmentType', 'LymphNodesAffected', 'Stage']] y = data['Recurrence']

#Split into training and testing sets

X_train, X_test, y_train, y_test = train_test_split(X, y, test_size=0.3, random_state=42)

#Step 3: Build and Train the Random Forest Model

#Initialize the Random Forest Classifier

rf_model = RandomForestClassifier(n_estimators=100, random_state=42) rf_model.fit(X_train, y_train)

#Make predictions

y_pred = rf_model.predict(X_test)

#Step 4: Evaluate the model

#Accuracy

accuracy = accuracy_score(y_test, y_pred) print(f"Accuracy: {accuracy * 100:.2f}%")

#Confusion Matrix

cm = confusion_matrix(y_test, y_pred) print("Confusion Matrix:

", cm)

#Classification Report

print("Classification Report:

", classification_report(y_test, y_pred))

#Visualize the Confusion Matrix

sns.heatmap(cm, annot=True, fmt='d', cmap='Blues', xticklabels=['No Recurrence', 'Recurrence'], yticklabels=['No Recurrence', 'Recurrence']) plt.title('Confusion Matrix') plt.xlabel('Predicted') plt.ylabel('Actual') plt.show()

#Step 5: Feature Importance

#Plot feature importance

importances = rf_model.feature_importances_ feature_names = X.columns

plt.barh(feature_names, importances, color='teal') plt.title('Feature Importance') plt.xlabel('Importance Score') plt.show()

#Step 6: Predict for new patients

Predict recurrence for a new patient

new_patient = [[50, 1, 4.0, 2, 1, 2]] # Age=50, Female, TumorSize=4.0, Chemotherapy, 1 Lymph Node, Stage 2

prediction = rf_model.predict(new_patient)

print("Recurrence Prediction (1=Yes, 0=No):", prediction[0])

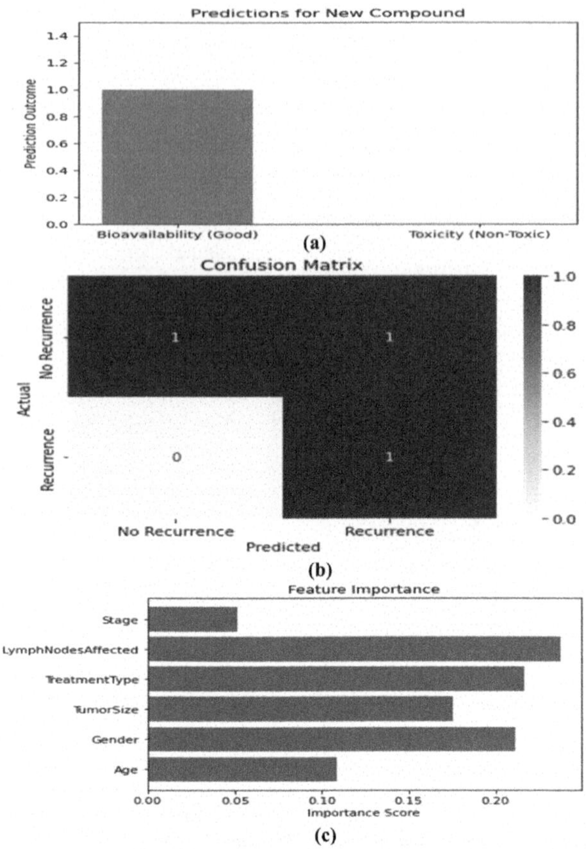

Fig. 1.7 Graphical visualization of the output. (A) Prediction outcome for new compounds Bioavailability and Toxicity, (B) Confusion matrix actual vs predicted, and (C) Feature importance vs importance Score.

#Output

Recurrence Prediction (1=Yes, 0=No): 1

This example demonstrates how to analyze cancer treatment data and predict recurrence using a Random Forest Classifier. The same principles can be extended to larger datasets with more features, advanced ML models, and domain-specific optimizations.

4.2 AI in deep learning

it is a subset of ML, and ML is a subset of AI. Deep learning is a powerful tool for analyzing health data, especially for tasks like disease detection, medical image classification, and patient risk prediction. In this tutorial, a deep learning model built with TensorFlow/Keras to classify health data is used (e.g., predicting diabetes risk).

Table 1.8 Example dataset for Alzheimer's prediction.

Age	MMSE (cognitive score)	Hippocampus volume (mm^3)	APOE4 gene (1 = Present)	Years of education	Outcome (0 = No Alzheimer's, 1 = Alzheimer's)
72	24	4500	1	12	1
65	27	4800	0	16	0
80	18	4200	1	10	1
74	22	4400	1	12	1
60	29	5000	0	18	0
67	26	4700	0	14	0
85	16	4100	1	8	1
70	23	4550	1	12	1
63	28	4900	0	15	0
78	20	4300	1	10	1

Here's an example dataset (Table 1.8) designed for Alzheimer's disease (AD) prediction. This dataset is synthetic and includes features commonly associated with Alzheimer's risk factors, such as age, cognitive test scores, and brain volume metrics.

Table above mentioned table shows following features as

1. **Age**: The patient's age in years.
2. **Mini-mental state examination (MMSE) (cognitive score)**: The MMSE score, ranging from 0 to 30 (lower scores indicate greater cognitive impairment).
3. **Hippocampus volume (mm^3)**: A brain region crucial for memory, measured in cubic millimeters (lower volume is associated with Alzheimer's).
4. **APOE4 gene**: Presence of the APOE4 allele, a known genetic risk factor for Alzheimer's (1 = Present, 0 = Not Present).
5. **Years of education**: Total years of formal education (higher education levels may offer protective cognitive reserves).
6. **Outcome**: Target variable, indicating whether the patient has Alzheimer's (1 = Alzheimer's, 0 = No Alzheimer's).

Deep learning computational pipeline with this dataset:

This dataset and pipeline (Box 1.5) provide a foundation for building deep learning models to predict Alzheimer's risk. Modify the dataset and model as needed for real-world applications, such as including more clinical or genetic data. The output of this analysis has been shown in Fig. 1.8.

Box 1.5 Computational pipeline for deep learning models to predict Alzheimer's risk

Step 1: Load the Data

#Save the dataset as a CSV file (e.g., alzheimers_data.csv) or create it directly in Python: import pandas as pd

#Create the Alzheimer's dataset

data = pd.DataFrame({ 'Age': [72, 65, 80, 74, 60, 67, 85, 70, 63, 78], 'MMSE': [24, 27, 18, 22, 29, 26, 16, 23, 28, 20], 'HippocampusVolume': [4500, 4800, 4200, 4400, 5000, 4700, 4100, 4550, 4900, 4300], 'APOE4': [1, 0, 1, 1, 0, 0, 1, 1, 0, 1], 'YearsOfEducation': [12, 16, 10, 12, 18, 14, 8, 12, 15, 10], 'Outcome': [1, 0, 1, 1, 0, 0, 1, 1, 0, 1] })

#Split features and target

X = data[['Age', 'MMSE', 'HippocampusVolume', 'APOE4', 'YearsOfEducation']].values y = data['Outcome'].values

Step 2: Preprocess the data

#Normalize the features for better model performance: from sklearn.preprocessing import StandardScaler from sklearn.model_selection import train_test_split

#Standardize the features

scaler = StandardScaler() X = scaler.fit_transform(X)

#Split into training and test sets

X_train, X_test, y_train, y_test = train_test_split(X, y, test_size=0.3, random_state=42)

Step 3: Build the deep learning model

#Create a simple feedforward neural network for binary classification: import tensorflow as tf from tensorflow.keras.models import Sequential from tensorflow.keras.layers import Dense

Define the model

model = Sequential([Dense(16, activation='relu', input_shape=(X_train.shape[1],)), Dense(8, activation='relu'), Dense(1, activation='sigmoid') # Output layer for binary classification])

#Compile the model

model.compile(optimizer='adam', loss='binary_crossentropy', metrics=['accuracy'])

#Train the model

history = model.fit(X_train, y_train, validation_data=(X_test, y_test), epochs=50, batch_size=4, verbose=1)

Step 4: Evaluate the model

#Evaluate on the test set

test_loss, test_accuracy = model.evaluate(X_test, y_test) print(f"Test Accuracy: {test_accuracy * 100:.2f}%")

Step 5: VisualizeTrainingimport matplotlib.pyplot as plt

#Plot training and validation accuracy

plt.plot(history.history['accuracy'], label='Training Accuracy') plt.plot(history.history['val_accuracy'], label='Validation Accuracy') plt.xlabel('Epochs') plt.ylabel('Accuracy') plt.legend() plt.title('Model Training Performance') plt.show()

Step 6: Make predictions

#Predict for a new patient

new_patient = scaler.transform([[75, 21, 4350, 1, 11]]) # Replace with real patient data

prediction = (model.predict(new_patient) > 0.5).astype(int)

print("Prediction (1 = Alzheimer's, 0 = No Alzheimer's):", prediction[0][0])

import numpy as np import pandas as pd from sklearn.model_selection import train_test_split from sklearn.preprocessing import MinMaxScaler

#Generate example data for BMI and blood pressure

data = pd.DataFrame({ 'BMI': [18.5, 24.9, 30.0, 35.0, 22.0, 27.5, 33.0, 19.0, 25.5, 31.5], 'BloodPressure': [80, 75, 90, 100, 85, 88, 92, 78, 82, 96], 'Risk': [0, 0, 1, 1, 0, 1, 1, 0, 0, 1] # 0 = Low Risk, 1 = High Risk })

#Separate input variables and target

features = data[['BMI', 'BloodPressure']].values labels = data['Risk'].values

#Scale features to [0, 1] range

scaler = MinMaxScaler() features_scaled = scaler.fit_transform(features)

#Split data into training and testing sets

X_train, X_test, y_train, y_test = train_test_split(features_scaled, labels, test_size=0.3, random_state=42)

#Display training data

print("Training Feature Set:

", X_train) print("Training Labels:

", y_train)

Step 3: Define the quantum feature mapping. This mapping transforms classical input into a quantum representation. Here, a ZZFeatureMap is utilized. from qiskit.circuit.library import ZZFeatureMap

#Initialize a feature map for two variables (BMI and blood pressure).

feature_map = ZZFeatureMap(feature_dimension=2, reps=2, entanglement='full')

Step 4: Configure the quantum simulation environment. We will use the qasm_simulator backend in Qiskit to emulate quantum computation on a classical machine.

pip install qiskit pip install qiskit-machine-learning

from qiskit import Aer from qiskit.utils import QuantumInstance

#Initialize the simulator backend

backend = Aer.get_backend('qasm_simulator') quantum_instance = QuantumInstance(backend, shots=1024)

Step 5: Train the quantum support vector machine. Next, we will build and fit a Quantum Support Vector Classifier (QSVC) using the training data.

from qiskit_machine_learning.algorithms import QSVC

#Create and train the QSVC model.

qsvc = QSVC(quantum_instance=quantum_instance, feature_map=feature_map) qsvc.fit(X_train, y_train)

Step 6: Evaluate the model performance. We will use the test data to make predictions and calculate the classification accuracy.

from sklearn.metrics import accuracy_score

3 Generate predictions on the test set

y_pred = qsvc.predict(X_test)

#Compute and display accuracy

accuracy = accuracy_score(y_test, y_pred) print(f"QSVM Model Accuracy: {accuracy * 100:.2f}%")

import pandas as pd from rdkit import Chem from rdkit.Chem import Descriptors

#Step 2.1: Create a sample dataset with SMILES representations and activity outcomes

data = pd.DataFrame({ 'SMILES': ['CCO', 'CCN', 'CCCC', 'CCOC', 'CCCN'], # SMILES strings for simple molecules 'Activity': [1, 0, 1, 0, 1] # Activity labels: 1 = Active, 0 = Inactive })

#Step 2.2: Function to calculate molecular descriptors

def calculate_descriptors(smiles): mol = Chem.MolFromSmiles(smiles) if mol: return [Descriptors.MolWt(mol), **# Molecular Weight** Descriptors.NumHAcceptors(mol), **# Number of Hydrogen Bond Acceptors** Descriptors.NumHDonors(mol) **# Number of Hydrogen Bond Donors**] return [None, None, None]

#Apply descriptor calculation to the dataset

descriptor_values = data['SMILES'].apply(calculate_descriptors) descriptor_df = pd.DataFrame(descriptor_values.tolist(), columns=['MolWt', 'HBA', 'HBD'])

#Merge the descriptor data with the original dataframe

data = pd.concat([data, descriptor_df], axis=1)

print("Dataset with Calculated Molecular Descriptors:" \n, data)

Step 3: Train a machine learning model

Train-Test Split and Model Training We will train a **Random Forest classifier** to predict whether a molecule is active (1) or inactive (0) based on its molecular descriptors. from sklearn.ensemble import RandomForestClassifier from sklearn.model_selection import train_test_split from sklearn.metrics import accuracy_score, classification_report

#Step 3.1: Define Features (X) and Target (y)

X = data[['MolWt', 'HBA', 'HBD']] # Molecular descriptors as features y = data['Activity'] # Activity labels as the target

#Step 3.2: Split the data into training and testing sets

X_train, X_test, y_train, y_test = train_test_split(X, y, test_size=0.3, random_state=42)

#Step 3.3: Train a Random Forest model

rf_model = RandomForestClassifier(n_estimators=100, random_state=42) rf_model.fit(X_train, y_train)

#Step 3.4: Evaluate the model

y_pred = rf_model.predict(X_test) print("Accuracy:", accuracy_score(y_test, y_pred)) print("Classification Report:" \n, classification_report(y_test, y_pred))

#Step 4.1: Define new molecules (in SMILES format)

new_molecules = ['CCC', 'CCOCC', 'CCCN']

#Step 4.2: Compute descriptors for new molecules

new_descriptors = [compute_descriptors(smiles) for smiles in new_molecules]

#Step 4.3: Predict activity for the new molecules

predictions = rf_model.predict(new_descriptors) for smiles, pred in zip(new_molecules, predictions): print(f"Molecule: {smiles}, Predicted Activity: {'Active' if pred == 1 else 'Inactive'}")

Molecule: CCC, Predicted Activity: ActiveMolecule: CCOCC, Predicted Activity: InactiveMolecule: CCCN, Predicted Activity: Inactive

Step 5: Visualize results

#Visualize molecular weight distribution

Plot the distribution of molecular weights in the dataset.

import seaborn as sns import matplotlib.pyplot as plt

#Distribution of molecular weights plt.figure(figsize=(10, 6)) sns.histplot(data['MolWt'], kde=True, bins=10, color='blue') plt.title("Distribution of Molecular Weight") plt.xlabel("Molecular Weight") plt.ylabel("Frequency") plt.show()

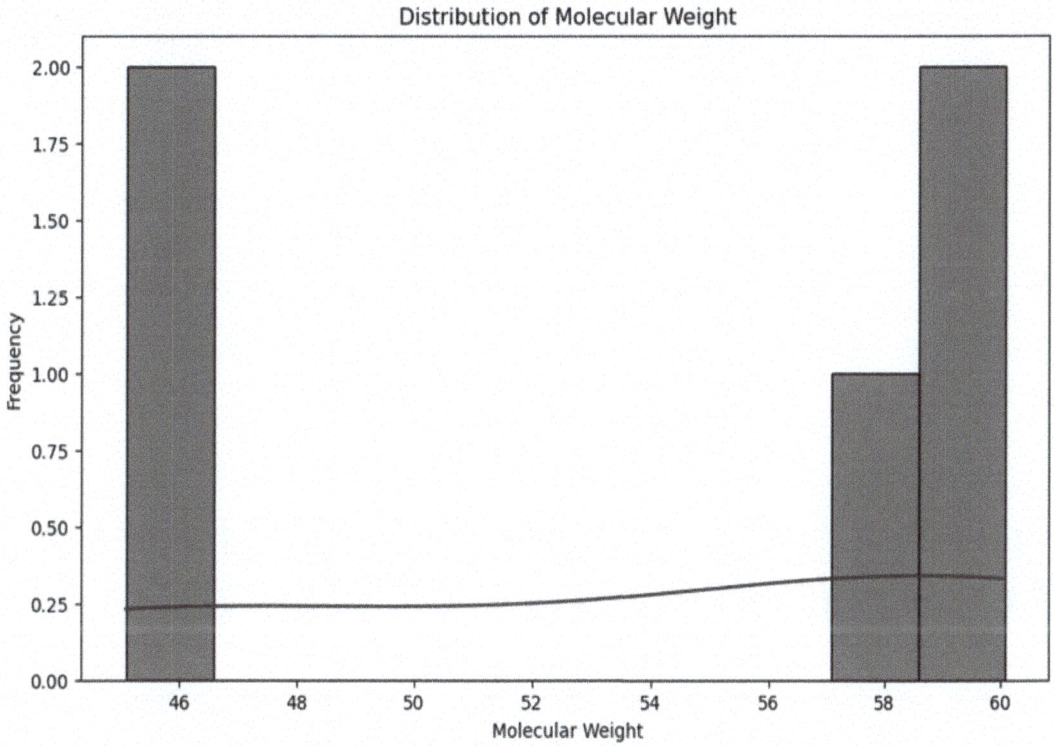

Fig. 1.8 Graphical visualization of the output. Distribution of molecular weight.

5 Emerging trends in AI and drug discovery

5.1 Quantum computing with AI

Quantum computing leverages the principles of quantum mechanics, such as superposition and entanglement, to process information in fundamentally new ways, offering potential speedups over traditional computational approaches (Biamonte et al., 2017). This technology holds promise for transforming data-driven disciplines by enabling faster and more efficient analysis of large and complex datasets. For example, uncovering subtle patterns in data could support progress in healthcare, finance, and climate modeling (Cerezo et al., 2021). A key application involves classification tasks, where quantum algorithms help distinguish among different categories of information. One notable example is the Quantum Support Vector Machine (QSVM), which can perform binary classification using quantum resources. These methods can be implemented with quantum programming frameworks such as Qiskit (Abbas et al., 2021).

5.2 QML in healthcare

In healthcare, adapting QSVMs to analyze health data is feasible with proper preprocessing, feature selection, and quantum encoding. By leveraging QML techniques, health researchers and practitioners can uncover deeper insights from datasets, leading to improvements in diagnostics and treatment outcomes (Verdon et al., 2019).

5.3 Computational workflow: Quantum support vector machine in health data classification

This section outlines the use of a quantum support vector machine (QSVM), implemented with Qiskit, for categorizing health-related data. A simulated dataset is employed to estimate diabetes risk using features such as body mass index (BMI) and blood pressure. Box 1.6 outlines the required steps of the workflow, and the visualization of the output is depicted in Fig. 1.9.

Box 1.6 Computational workflow for QSVM in health data classification

import os import pandas as pd import numpy as np

Step 1: Create a folder on the desktop desktop_path = os.path.join(os.path.expanduser("~"), "Desktop") folder_name = "ProteomicsData" folder_path = os.path.join(desktop_path, folder_name) os.makedirs(folder_path, exist_ok=True) Folder created at: {folder_path}

Step 2: Create a small dataset proteins = ["Alpha_synuclein", "DJ_1", "PINK1", "Parkin", "UCHL1", "LRRK2", "Tau", "Beta_spectrin", "Hsp70", "ATPA13A2"] np.random.seed(42) num_patients = 50 #Small dataset for efficient execution

data = DataFrame(np.random.rand(num_patients, len(proteins)) * 100, columns = proteins)

data['Parkinsons'] = np.random.choice([0, 1], size = num_patients, p = [0.5, 0.5]) data.insert(0, "Patient_ID", ["Patient_{i+1}" for i in range(num_patients)])

Save the dataset to the folder csv_file_path = os.path.join(folder_path, "parkinsons_proteomics_data.csv") data.to_csv(csv_file_path, index = False) Dataset saved at: {csv_file_path}

#Output Folder created at: /Users/usr/Desktop/ProteomicsData Dataset saved at: /Users/usr/Desktop/ProteomicsData/parkinsons_proteomics_data.csv

#Step 2: Load and Preprocess the Dataset from sklearn.preprocessing import StandardScaler from sklearn.model_selection import train_test_split data = pd.read_csv(csv_file_path)

#Separate features and labels X = data.iloc[:, 2:-1] #Exclude Patient_ID and Parkinsons columns y = data['Parkinsons']

#Normalize the features scaler = StandardScaler() X_scaled = scaler.fit_transform(X)

#Split into training and testing sets X_train, X_test, y_train, y_test = train_test_split(X_scaled, y, test_size=0.2, random_state=42)

#Step 3: Train a Neural Network for Classification using Logistic Regression from sklearn.linear_model import LogisticRegression from sklearn.metrics import accuracy_score, confusion_matrix, classification_report

#Initialize and train Logistic Regression log_reg = LogisticRegression(random_state=42, max_iter=200) log_reg.fit(X_train, y_train)

#Evaluate on the test set y_pred = log_reg.predict(X_test) accuracy = accuracy_score(y_test, y_pred)

#Print metrics print(f"Logistic Regression Test Accuracy: {accuracy:.2f}") print("Confusion Matrix:") print(confusion_matrix(y_test, y_pred)) print("Classification Report:") print(classification_report(y_test, y_pred))

#Step-4 Clustering and PCA Visualization from sklearn.decomposition import PCAfrom sklearn.cluster import KMeansimport matplotlib.pyplot as plt import seaborn as sns **#Reduce dimensionality with PCA** pca = PCA(n_components=2) X_pca = pca.fit_transform(X_scaled) **#Perform K-means** clusteringkmeans = KMeans(n_clusters=2, random_state=42) clusters = kmeans.fit_predict(X_scaled) **#Add clusters to the original dataset** data['Cluster'] = clusters **#Plot the clusterspIt.figure(figsize=(8, 6))** sns.scatterplot(x=X_pca[:, 0], y=X_pca[:, 1], hue=clusters, palette='viridis', s=100) plt.title('K-means Clustering of Parkinson's Proteomics Data') plt.xlabel('PCA Component 1') plt.ylabel('PCA Component 2') plt.legend(title='Cluster') plt.show()

#Step6-Protein-Protein Interaction Network Visualization import networkx as nx

#Define protein-protein interactions (example connections)

edges = [("Alpha_synuclein", "LRRK2"), ("DJ_1", "PINK1"), ("Parkin", "ATP13A2"), ("Alpha_synuclein", "UCHL1"), ("Tau", "Beta_spectrin"), ("Hsp70", "LRRK2")]

#Build the graph

G = nx.Graph() G.add_nodes_from(proteins) G.add_edges_from(edges)

#Draw the graph

plt.figure(figsize=(10, 8))

nx.draw_networkx(G, with_labels=True, node_color='lightblue', edge_color='black', node_size=1200, font_size=16)

plt.title('Protein-Protein Interaction Network')

plt.show()

#Step7-boxplots for multiple proteins import seaborn as sns import matplotlib.pyplot as plt

```
#Melt the dataset for plotting
melted_data = data.melt(id_vars=['Parkinsons'], value_vars=proteins, var_name='Protein', value_name='Expression')
#Boxplot for multiple proteins
plt.figure(figsize=(12, 8)) sns.boxplot(x='Protein', y='Expression', hue='Parkinsons', data=melted_data, palette='coolwarm') plt.title('Boxplot of Protein Expressions by Parkinsons Status') plt.xlabel('Proteins')plt.ylabel('Expression Levels') plt.xticks(rotation=45, ha='right') plt.legend(title='Parkinsons (0=Control, 1=Disease)') plt.grid(axis='y') plt.tight_layout() plt.show()
```

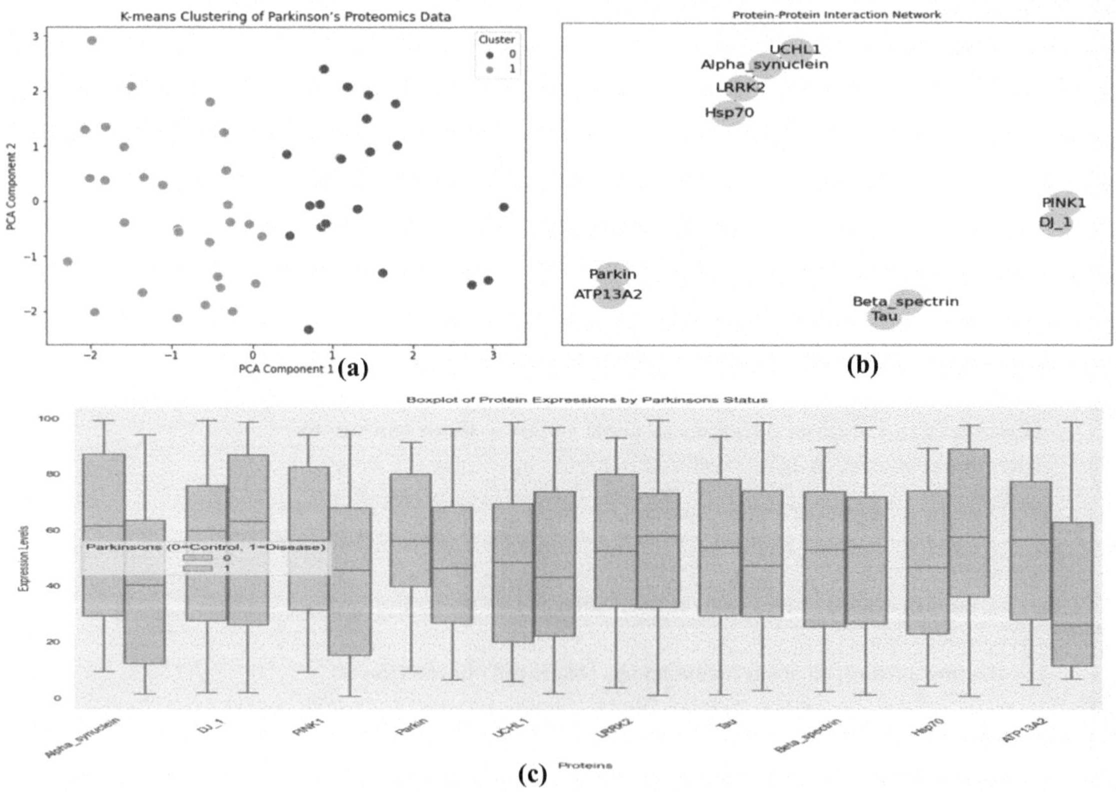

Fig. 1.9 Graphical representation of the output. (A) K-means clustering of Parkinson's proteomics data, (B) Protein-protein interaction outcome, and (C) Various protein expressions by Parkinson's status.

Step 1: Set up the environment

Verify that the following packages are installed on the system: pip install qiskit qiskit-machine-learning scikit-learn matplotlib

Step 2: Generate and prepare the data

In this step, a health dataset for a two-class problem (e.g., diabetes risk, where 0 indicates low risk and 1 indicates high risk) has been created. A synthetic health dataset for binary classification (e.g., risk of diabetes: 0 = No Risk, 1 = High Risk) has been created.

AI-driven molecule screening combines all necessary steps in a clear and cohesive format. This section describes an end-to-end process for screening molecules: data preparation, model training, and visualization. It uses a simple example dataset, but you can replace it with real-world data sources.

5.4 Datasets for molecule screening

For real-world applications, you can replace the synthetic dataset with large-scale datasets:

Public Databases:

1. **ZINC database**:
   a. https://zinc.docking.org/
   b. Curated catalog of purchasable compounds for virtual screening
   c. Contains millions of molecules in SMILES format
2. **ChEMBL**:
   a. https://www.ebi.ac.uk/chembl/
   b. Contains bioactivity data (e.g., IC50, EC50, Ki values) for drug-like compounds
3. **III. PubChem**:
   a. https://pubchem.ncbi.nlm.nih.gov/
   b. Offers chemical property data, including 3D structures

A synthetic dataset of molecules is used with **SMILES strings**, their **activity labels**, and computed molecular descriptors such as **molecular weight (MolWt), hydrogen bond acceptors (HBA),** and **hydrogen bond donors (HBD), as shown in** Table 1.9 (console output) and Table 1.10 (accuracy output).

Table 1.9 Dataset with calculated molecular DESCRIPTORS.

	SMILES	ACTIVITY	MOLWT	HBA	HBD
0	CCO	1	46.069	1	1
1	CCN	0	45.085	1	1
2	CCCC	1	58.124	0	0
3	CCOC	0	60.096	1	0
4	CCCN	1	59.112	1	1

Table 1.10 Accuracy classification report.

	Precision	recall	f1-score	support
0	0.00	0.00	0.00	1.0
1	0.00	0.00	0.00	1.0
Accuracy			0.00	2.0
macro avg	0.00	0.00	0.00	2.0
weighted avg	0.00	0.00	0.00	2.0

6 Computational models for proteomics data analysis

Proteomics, the large-scale exploration of proteins and their functions, has been significantly advanced through the use of computational modeling approaches. These methods are crucial for interpreting complex, high-dimensional proteomics datasets. ML and deep learning models, in particular, are widely applied to identify patterns, predict protein functions, and study protein-protein interactions. Notably, tools such as AlphaFold (Jumper et al., 2021a) have transformed the field of protein structure prediction by delivering highly accurate three-dimensional models, supporting research in drug design and disease mechanisms. Beyond structure prediction, computational models are also leveraged to identify biomarkers for early disease diagnosis, with oncology being a prominent area of application (Zhang et al., 2022) Several databases and software resources support these computational approaches. **UniProt** provides extensive protein sequence and functional annotations, while Proteomics Identification Database (**PRIDE**) enables the sharing and analysis of mass spectrometry-based proteomics data. Analysis platforms like **MaxQuant** and **Perseus** are widely used for quantitative proteomics and are increasingly integrated with ML methods for deeper insights. In addition, tools such as **DeepLC** apply deep learning for precise retention time prediction in liquid chromatography–mass spectrometry workflows.

Integrative computational strategies have enabled multiomics analyses that merge proteomics data with genomics, transcriptomics, and metabolomics, offering a more comprehensive understanding of biological systems. Tools such as **OmicsNet** and **Pathway Commons** allow researchers to combine information across these various omics levels, using ML techniques to identify molecular networks and disease-associated pathways. In addition, data-driven software solutions like **Spectronaut** and **Scaffold data-independent acquisition (DIA)** are incorporating advanced modeling approaches to support the analysis of DIA mass spectrometry experiments—an area that is rapidly expanding within proteomics research. Recent research emphasizes how computational modeling is advancing proteomics. For instance, deep learning techniques have been applied to data from the **PRIDE** repository to predict protein posttranslational modifications, contributing to new findings in areas such as cancer and neurodegenerative disorders. In addition, natural language processing (NLP) methods are being used to analyze scientific literature databases like **PubMed**, helping to extract information relevant to proteomics and supporting faster hypothesis development and testing.

These developments in computational methods, data resources, and analytical tools are greatly expanding the reach and depth of proteomics research. They support the identification of potential therapeutic targets, the discovery of disease-related biomarkers, and progress in precision medicine, ushering in a new era for understanding human health and disease.

6.1 AI for Parkinson's proteomics data analysis

AI to proteomics data related to Parkinson's disease. This will include data preparation, classification using neural networks, clustering, and visualization through plots and a protein-protein interaction (PPI) network.

Logistic regression test accuracy: 0.40 Table 1.11

Confusion Matrix:

[[0 5]

[1 4]]

Table 1.11 Classification report of accuracy.

	Precision	recall	f1-score	support
0	0.00	0.00	0.00	5
1	0.44	0.80	0.57	5
Accuracy			0.40	10
macro avg	0.22	0.40	0.29	10
weighted avg	0.22	0.40	0.29	10

6.2 Integration of computational methods for understanding Alzheimer's disease mechanisms

Advanced computational techniques, including ML and deep learning, are enhancing traditional CADD workflows by enabling the development of therapeutic molecules that specifically target proteins involved in AD pathology (Jumper et al., 2021). These approaches help streamline drug discovery by reducing both time and costs, offering effective strategies to address complex neurological conditions.

6.2.1 Computational approaches in Alzheimer's disease mechanism analysis

AD is marked by the presence of amyloid-beta (Aβ) plaques, tau protein tangles, and neuroinflammatory responses. Computational modeling has been instrumental in dissecting these pathological mechanisms by integrating multiomics datasets. For example, advanced analytical approaches have identified important genetic and epigenetic factors, such as the APOE ε4 allele, that contribute to amyloid and tau abnormalities (Zhou et al., 2022).

6.2.2 Biomarker identification and target validation in AD

Computational methods, such as random forests and convolutional neural networks, have been used to detect early biomarkers for AD, including plasma neurofilament light chain and glial fibrillary acidic protein (GFAP) (Nakamura et al., 2020). These biomarkers aid in early diagnosis and guide the development of targeted treatment strategies. In addition, analyses of PPI networks using computational models have confirmed kinases like CDK5 and GSK3β as relevant targets for addressing tau hyperphosphorylation, supporting the rational design of new therapeutic agents.

6.2.3 Novel compound design and optimization for AD

Advanced computational strategies have facilitated the development of new compounds targeting critical mechanisms in AD. Techniques such as reinforcement learning and generative adversarial networks are used in tools like **REINVENT** to optimize molecules aimed at enzymes, including beta-secretase (BACE1) and tau kinases. These methods help design compounds with desirable pharmacokinetic and pharmacodynamic profiles (Olivecrona et al., 2017).

6.2.4 Case study: BACE1 inhibitor development

AI-driven de novo drug design has identified inhibitors for BACE1, a critical enzyme involved in Aβ production. ChemTS, a reinforcement learning platform, was used to generate compounds that selectively bind to BACE1, improving their specificity and reducing off-target effects. This process shortened the discovery timeline and reduced experimental costs (Olivecrona et al., 2017).

6.2.5 Case study: Alphafold for tau aggregation targets

AI tools like AlphaFold have elucidated the structures of tau proteins, which aggregate in AD. Using these structures, AI models have facilitated the design of inhibitors that stabilize tau's native conformation, potentially preventing its pathological aggregation (Jumper et al., 2021).

6.3 AI for virtual screening and drug repurposing in Alzheimer's

AI-enhanced virtual screening enables the rapid identification of high-affinity molecules from large chemical libraries. In addition, AI facilitates drug repurposing, where approved drugs are screened for new therapeutic applications.

6.3.1 Case study: Riluzole for Alzheimer's

An AI-based study identified riluzole, an FDA-approved ALS drug, as a potential therapy for Alzheimer's. By targeting amyloid aggregation pathways, riluzole demonstrated neuroprotective effects in preclinical models, showcasing how AI can uncover new uses for existing drugs (Aliper et al., 2016).

6.3.2 Case study: Multitarget screening for Alzheimer's and Parkinson's

AI models integrating Alzheimer's and Parkinson's disease datasets have identified multitarget compounds that modulate neuroinflammation and oxidative stress. These compounds, discovered through virtual screening, offer therapeutic potential for neurodegenerative conditions with overlapping pathologies.

6.3.3 Integration of multiomics data to study AD mechanisms

Advanced computational approaches support the integration of proteomics, genomics, and metabolomics data to achieve a comprehensive understanding of AD mechanisms. For example, analyses of single-cell RNA sequencing (scRNA-seq) data using computational models have identified distinct microglial subpopulations involved in regulating amyloid plaque formation and neuroinflammatory responses.

6.3.4 Case study: Microglial subtypes in neuroinflammation

AI-driven analysis of scRNA-seq data from Alzheimer's patients identified pro-inflammatory and antiinflammatory microglial states. This discovery led to the development of immunomodulatory compounds targeting microglial activation, offering a novel approach to mitigate neurodegeneration.

6.3.5 Case study: Multiomics integration for Alzheimer's pathways

An AI-based integrative analysis of AMP-AD datasets revealed interactions between amyloid, tau, and metabolic pathways. This study highlighted the role of mitochondrial dysfunction in Alzheimer's progression and suggested potential metabolic drug targets.

7 Discussion

The integration of advanced computational techniques with CADD represents a transformative shift in pharmaceutical research, improving both the efficiency and accuracy of drug discovery workflows. This chapter examines how tools based on ML, deep learning, and NLP streamline essential stages of drug development—from target identification through lead optimization to ADME/Tox prediction. Despite these significant advantages, challenges remain, including maintaining data quality, addressing biases in training data, and managing ethical and regulatory considerations.

8 Challenges and opportunities

Data challenges: AI models depend on the accuracy and completeness of data. Poorly curated datasets can lead to inaccurate predictions, emphasizing the importance of robust databases like ChEMBL and PubChem.

Ethical and regulatory hurdles: Applying advanced computational methods in drug design introduces concerns related to data privacy, intellectual property rights, and the interpretability of model predictions. Addressing these challenges will require coordinated efforts across the industry and the development of clear regulatory guidelines to promote responsible and compliant use.

Next-generation technologies: Advances like quantum computing have the potential to significantly improve molecular modeling and lead optimization by overcoming the limitations of classical computational techniques.

9 Impact on healthcare

CADD, enhanced by advanced computational methods, is reshaping healthcare by streamlining the discovery of treatments for cancer, neurodegenerative conditions, and rare genetic disorders. It enables faster identification of promising drug candidates, improves the precision of predictive models, and supports the development of personalized therapies tailored to individual patients. These innovations help lower costs and shorten development timelines, effectively addressing important unmet medical needs.

9.1 Relevance to brain diseases and human health

The application of AI-driven CADD is particularly impactful in addressing complex brain diseases, where traditional approaches often fall short. Neurodegenerative diseases such as Alzheimer's, Parkinson's, and Huntington's are characterized by complex molecular processes that can be explored using advanced computational tools like Alpha-fold and molecular dynamics simulations. These approaches enable researchers to uncover new therapeutic targets, design compounds with improved blood–brain barrier permeability, and minimize neurotoxic effects.

AI-enhanced CADD also facilitates precision medicine by analyzing patient-specific genetic and molecular data to develop therapies tailored to unique disease profiles. In addition, AI-driven platforms such as Exscientia and Benevolent AI accelerate drug repurposing, offering new treatment avenues for conditions with limited therapeutic options, including ALS and rare genetic brain disorders.

9.2 Empowering researchers and scientists

By automating labor-intensive processes such as virtual screening and lead discovery, AI allows researchers to focus on hypothesis generation and experimental validation. Open-source tools and collaborative platforms like DeepChem and RDKit foster innovation and global cooperation among scientists, democratizing access to advanced technologies. Tutorials and practical examples provided in this chapter also serve as a valuable resource for early-career researchers, bridging the gap between traditional methodologies and modern AI-driven approaches.

10 Conclusion

This chapter explores how advanced computational approaches are revolutionizing CADD, with the potential to redefine drug discovery and healthcare delivery. By addressing key challenges such as data quality, ethical concerns, and regulatory barriers, these methods pave the way for more efficient, cost-effective, and personalized therapies. In the realm of neurological disorders and broader medical applications, these technologies present powerful opportunities to decode complex brain conditions, facilitate early diagnosis, and foster novel treatment strategies. As these tools continue to evolve and gain traction, they hold immense potential to meet global health challenges and improve overall well-being.

References

Abadi, M., Agarwal, A., Barham, P., Brevdo, E., Chen, Z., Citro, C., et al., 2016. TensorFlow: Large-Scale Machine Learning on Heterogeneous Distributed Systems. Proceedings of the 12th USENIX Symposium on Operating Systems Design and Implementation (OSDI). arXiv:1603.04467.

Abbas, A., Sutter, D., Zoufal, C., Lucchi, A., Figalli, A., Woerner, S., 2021. The power of quantum neural networks. Nat. Comput. Sci. 2662-8457. 1 (6), 403–409. doi:10.1038/s43588-021-00084-1.

Aliper, A., Plis, S., Artemov, A., Ulloa, A., Mamoshina, P., Zhavoronkov, A., 2016. Deep learning applications for predicting pharmacological properties of drugs and drug repurposing using transcriptomic data. Mol. Pharm. 13 (7), 2524–2530. doi:10.1021/acs.molpharmaceut.6b00248.

Anderson, A.C., 2003. The process of structure-based drug design. Chem. Biol. 1074-5521. 10 (9), 787–797. doi:10.1016/j.chembiol.2003.09.002.

Biamonte, J., Wittek, P., Pancotti, N., Rebentrost, P., Wiebe, N., Lloyd, S., 2017. Quantum machine learning. Nature. 0028-0836. 549 (7671), 195–202. doi:10.1038/nature23474.

Cavasotto, C.N., Orry, A.J.W., 2007. Ligand docking and structure-based virtual screening in drug discovery. Curr. Top. Med. Chem. 1568-0266. 7 (10), 1006–1014. Available from: http://www.ingentaconnect.com/content/ben/ctmc/2007/00000007/00000010/art00013. doi:10.2174/156802607780906753.

Cerezo, M., Arrasmith, A., Babbush, R., Benjamin, S.C., Endo, S., Fujii, K., McClean, J.R., Mitarai, K., Yuan, X., Cincio, L., Coles, P.J., 2021. Variational quantum algorithms. Nat. Rev. Phys. 2522-5820. 3 (9), 625–644. doi:10.1038/s42254-021-00348-9.

Chen, H., Engkvist, O., Wang, Y., Olivecrona, M., Blaschke, T., 2018. The rise of deep learning in drug discovery. Drug Discov. Today. 1359-6446. 23 (6), 1241–1250. doi:10.1016/j.drudis.2018.01.039.

Daina, A., Michielin, O., Zoete, V., 2017. SwissADME: a free web tool to evaluate pharmacokinetics, drug-likeness and medicinal chemistry friendliness of small molecules. Sci. Rep. 2045-2322. 7 (1). doi:10.1038/srep42717.

Gaulton, A., Hersey, A., Nowotka, M., et al., 2017. The ChEMBL database in 2017. Nucleic Acids Res. 45, D945-D954.

Gawehn, E., Hiss, J.A., Schneider, G., 2016. Deep learning in drug discovery. Mol. Inform. 1868-1751. 35 (1), 3–14. Available from: http://onlinelibrary.wiley.com/journal/10.1002/(ISSN)1868-1751. doi:10.1002/minf.201501008.

Hopkins, A.L., Groom, C.R., Alex, A., 2004. Ligand efficiency: a useful metric for lead selection. Drug Discov. Today 9 (10), 430–431. doi:10.1016/S1359-6446(04)03069-7.

Jorgensen, W.L., 2004. The many roles of computation in drug discovery. Science 303 (5665), 1813–1818. doi:10.1126/science.1096361.

Jumper, J., Evans, R., Pritzel, A., Green, T., Figurnov, M., Ronneberger, O., Tunyasuvunakool, K., Bates, R., Žídek, A., Potapenko, A., Bridgland, A., Meyer, C., Kohl, S.A.A., Ballard, A.J., Cowie, A., Romera-Paredes, B., Nikolov, S., Jain, R., Adler, J., Back, T., et al., 2021. Highly accurate protein structure prediction with AlphaFold. Nature 596 (7873), 583–589. doi:10.1038/s41586-021-03819-2.

Kadurin, A., Nikolenko, S., Khrabrov, K., Aliper, A., Zhavoronkov, A., 2017. druGAN: an advanced generative adversarial autoencoder model for de novo generation of new molecules with desired molecular properties in silico. Mol. Pharm. 14 (9), 3098–3104. doi:10.1021/acs.molpharmaceut.7b00346.

Kim, Y., Rush, A.M., 2016. Sequence-level knowledge distillation. In Proceedings of the 2016 Conference on Empirical Methods in Natural Language Processing. Austin, Texas: Association for Computational Linguistics, pp. 1317–1327.

Leach, A.R., Gillet, V.J., 2007. An Introduction to Chemoinformatics. Springer Netherlands, United Kingdom, pp. 1–255. Available from: http://www.springerlink.com/openurl.asp?genre=book&isbn=978-1-4020-6290-2. doi:10.1007/978-1-4020-6291-9.

Lipinski, C.A., Lombardo, F., Dominy, B.W., Feeney, P.J., 2001. Experimental and computational approaches to estimate solubility and permeability in drug discov ery and development settings. Adv. Drug Deliv. Rev. 46 (1–3), 3–26. doi:10.1016/s0169-409x(00)00129-0.

Nakamura, Y., Tamaoki, J., Nagase, H., Yamaguchi, M., Horiguchi, T., Hozawa, S., Ichinose, M., Iwanaga, T., Kondo, R., Nagata, M., Yokoyama, A., Tohda, Y., 2020. Japanese guidelines for adult asthma 2020. Allergology International, 69 (4), 519–548. doi:10.1016/j.alit.2020.08.001.

Olivecrona, M., Blaschke, T., Engkvist, O., Chen, H., 2017. Molecular de-novo design through deep reinforcement learning. J. Cheminform. 1758-2946. 9 (1). doi:10.1186/s13321-017-0235-x.

Paszke, A., Gross, S., Massa, F., Lerer, A., Bradbury, J., Chanan, G., 2019. PyTorch: An imperative style, high-performance deep learning library. Advances in Neural Information Processing Systems (NeurIPS) 32, 8024–8035.

Patel, D.R., Chalmers, R.K., 2003. Computational approaches to drug discovery. Pharm. Res. 20 (4), 515–526. doi:10.1023/A:1023268409786.

Schneider, G., 2018. Automating drug discovery. Nat. Rev. Drug Discov. 1474-1776. 17 (2), 97–113. doi:10.1038/nrd.2017.232.

Schneider, G., Walters, W.P., Plowright, A.T., 2018. Prospects for artificial intelligence in drug discovery. Drug Discov. Today 23 (5), 892–900. doi:10.1016/j.drudis.2018.01.005.

Segler, M.H.S., Preuss, M., Waller, M.P., 2018. Planning chemical syntheses with deep neural networks and symbolic AI. Nature. 1476-4687. 555 (7698), 604–610. Available from: http://www.nature.com/nature/index.html. doi:10.1038/nature25978.

Trott, O., Olson, A.J., 2010. AutoDock Vina: improving the speed and accuracy of docking with a new scoring function, efficient optimization, and multithreading. J. Comput. Chem. 31 (2), 455–461. doi:10.1002/jcc.21334.

Vamathevan, J., Clark, D., Czodrowski, P., Dunham, I., Ferran, E., Lee, G., Li, B., Madabhushi, A., Shah, P., Spitzer, M., Zhao, S., 2019. Applications of machine learning in drug discovery and development. Nat. Rev. Drug Discov. 1474-1776. 18 (6), 463–477. doi:10.1038/s41573-019-0024-5.

Verdon, G., Broughton, M., Biamonte, J., 2019. A universal training algorithm for quantum deep learning. arXiv preprint arXiv:1901.03592.

Wallach, I., Dzamba, M., Heifets, A., 2015. AtomNet: A deep convolutional neural network for bioactivity prediction in structure-based drug discovery. arXiv preprint arXiv:1510.02855. Available from: https://arxiv.org/abs/1510.02855 (Accessed 6 August 2026).
Wu, Z., Ramsundar, B., Feinberg, E.N., et al. 2018. MoleculeNet: a benchmark for molecular machine learning. Chem. Sci. 9, 513–530.
Yang, G.R., Joglekar, M.R., Song, H.F., Newsome, W.T., Wang, X.J., 2019. Task representations in neural networks trained to perform many cognitive tasks. Nat. Neurosci. 22 (2), 297-306. doi:10.1038/s41593-018-0310-2.
Zhang, Q., Li, X., Liu, X., Liu, S., Zhang, M., Liu, Y., Zhu, C., Wang, K., 2022. The effect of non-invasive brain stimulation on the downregulation of negative emotions: A meta-analysis. Brain Sciences, 12 (8), 1107. doi:10.3390/brainsci12081107.
Zhavoronkov, A., Ivanenkov, Y.A., Aliper, A., Veselov, M.S., Aladinskiy, V.A., Aladinskaya, A.V., Terentiev, V.A., Polykovskiy, D.A., Kuznetsov, M.D., Asadulaev, A., Volkov, Y., Zholus, A., Shayakhmetov, R.R., Zhebrak, A., Minaeva, L.I., Zagribelnyy, B.A., Lee, L.H., Soll, R., Madge, D., Xing, L., Guo, T., Aspuru-Guzik, A., 2019. Deep learning enables rapid identification of potent DDR1 kinase inhibitors. Nat. Biotechnol. 1546-1696. 37 (9), 1038–1040. Available from: http://www.nature.com/nbt/index.html. doi:10.1038/s41587-019-0224-x.

2

Use of AI for analysis of biological and chemical databases for drug discovery

Nidhi Dubey, Prabhat Tripathi, Unnati Soni, Ankish Arya, Krishna Misra, and Pritish Kumar Varadwaj
Systems Biology Lab, Department of Applied Sciences, Indian Institute of Information Technology Allahabad, Prayagraj, Uttar Pradesh, India

1 Introduction

The incorporation of artificial intelligence (AI) into pharmaceutical and biomedical sciences represents a major advancement, improving multiple phases of the drug discovery and development process. Through the adoption of AI, researchers are able to streamline processes, reduce expenditures, and boost the safety and efficacy of therapeutic compounds (Mitchell, 2018). Over the years, AI has evolved from a promising concept to an essential component of pharmaceutical data analysis, powered by progress in natural language processing (NLP) and machine learning (ML) (Kolluri et al., 2022). Its growing application across the drug discovery pipeline, including target identification, predictive modeling, virtual screening, and trial design, has transformed how effective candidates for complex diseases are identified. Importantly, AI's capability to accurately process large-scale biological and chemical information positions it as a critical enabler of precision medicine (Koromina et al., 2019).

1.1 Importance of biological and chemical databases

Extensive biological and chemical databases, for example, GeneCards and PubChem, consist of large datasets that help in informed decision-making in drug discovery and the selection of data. These databases comprise massive repositories that assist researchers in discovering promising drug compounds and analyzing their interactions within biological and chemical systems. By combining data from these datasets, a superior approach can

The AI Frontier in Molecular Modelling and Drug Designing. https://doi.org/10.1016/B978-0-443-40338-5.00013-5

be acknowledged for an improved drug discovery process, consisting of information on intricate biological phenomena, leading to potential drug candidates and druggable targets (Noorain et al., 2023). Combining chemical and biological databases allows researchers to investigate how molecular structures relate to biological functions, providing insights into their interaction mechanisms within physiological systems. By adopting this approach, decision-making regarding drug efficacy and safety can be ensured through predictive analytics using AI. In addition, risks associated with drug development can be significantly minimized this way (Bender and Cortes-Ciriano, 2021). By leveraging data from multiple sources, scientists can prioritize research directions, minimizing the risks associated with drug development. Personalized medicine approaches can be facilitated by integrating biological and chemical data. These combined data can be tailored to specific patient populations, considering genetic, environmental, and lifestyle factors affecting drug responses. Well-versed decision-making obtained from datasets empowers the design of operative therapies, reducing side effects and improving overall treatment results (Mak et al., 2024).

1.2 Objectives of the chapter

This chapter explores and delves into the role of AI in advancing drug discovery, emphasizing enhanced analysis of biomedical and chemical databases. It outlines various data sources, their classifications, and approaches for organizing and managing data within structured repositories. In addition, it covers key statistical methods used in molecular data interpretation, including clustering algorithms and regression models. The discussion extends to ML strategies, detailing concepts such as model deployment, integration, supervised and unsupervised learning, as well as reinforcement learning (RL) frameworks.

2 Data types for machine learning applications in drug discovery

Successful implementation of ML in drug discovery relies strongly on the diversity, accuracy, and integration of accessible datasets. These data-centric methodologies have transformed traditional drug development workflows by enabling faster and more precise identification of potential drug candidates, predicting therapeutic targets, and uncovering relevant biomarkers.

2.1 Biological data types

Different biological types are needed to understand the molecular basis of diseases and potential therapeutic targets. These data types include genomic, proteomic, metabolomic, and clinical data types, which provide different insights into the system (Shah et al., 2024). Next-generation sequencing produces genomic data that can generate enormous data sets of DNA sequences, genetic variations, and gene expression profiles. This data helps identify potential drug targets that are disease-associated genes and pathways by analyzing the mutation and gene expression profiles. ML algorithms predict how gene variations might modify the drug response to better assist in personalized medicine. However, the proteomic data generated using more modern technologies, such as mass spectrometry, offers high resolution for protein structures and interactions. ML thus provides a way to accurately predict proteins' structures and their probable interactions in the prediction step of drug discovery with candidate lead compounds. Metabolic data provide insights into the small molecules and metabolites of biological systems, which are critical for understanding disease states, metabolic pathways, and drug metabolism. Thus, with the analysis of metabolic data, we can assess the pharmacokinetics and pharmacodynamics of drug candidates, thereby optimizing drug targets and development. The clinical data include patients' medical histories, treatment results, and demographics. Phenotypic data, on the other hand, includes observable traits. All these data are essential for grouping patients and predicting drug responses with ML models. Fig. 2.1 shows the types of data used in ML for the process of drug discovery.

2.2 Chemical data types

Chemical data would include the functional and structural properties of the compound, forming the basis of drug design and discovery. This relationship helps model the structures against their biological properties, furthering the drug discovery processes. Large datasets of compounds generated by high throughput screening against biological targets can be implemented in ML models for virtual screening, which will identify lead compounds from a vast library of compounds. Molecular descriptors include structural features like bond types and atomic charges, which are crucial inputs for virtual screening. The molecular structure is encoded as 3D molecular structures or simplified molecular input line entry system (SMILES) strings, where ML models predict the relationships between molecular features and biological properties. These ML models predict properties like toxicity, lipophilicity, solubility, and

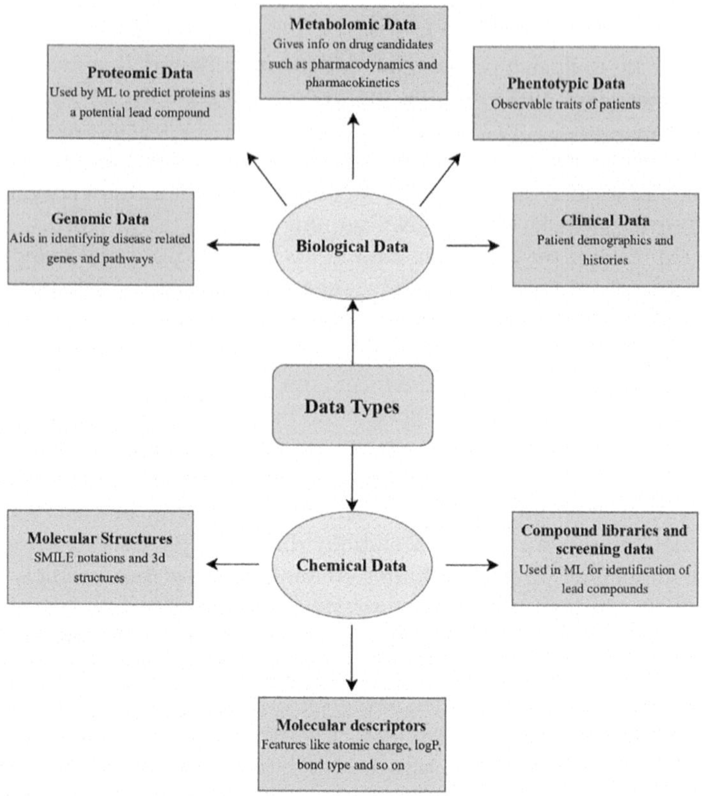

Fig. 2.1 Overview of biological and chemical data types used in machine learning for drug discovery. Key biological and chemical data types are used in machine learning for drug discovery, supporting target identification and compound optimization.

bioactivity, as well as their values, such IC50 EC50 in compound libraries, which reduces experimental time and expenses. Such large compound libraries are generated from datasets. High throughput screening is used against biological targets and can be implemented for virtual screening in an ML model, which identifies leads in a vast library.

2.3 Data formats and standards

Database data comes in different forms that reflect the complexity and variations of information kept within databases. Thus, standardization is a prerequisite for establishing compatibility and consistency in other datasets. Structure Data File is a widely used cheminformatics chemical file format. It presents chemical structure records of bond types and other data, such as compound attributes. It has emerged as a popular standard for importing chemical data and exporting chemical information. Single-letter codes express base pairs or amino acids in the text-based representation known as FASTA, which is used for representing protein or nucleotide sequences. Thus, this format makes integration into workflows for similarity searches, annotation, and sequence alignment easier. Other formats include MOL2, which is used for molecular modeling, and Protein Data Bank (PDB), which is used for 3D structure representations of biomolecular data. CSV/TSV is used to store information in tabular formats. **Standardization protocols and ontologies:** Data standardization is very important for drug development as it ensures uniformity of data across platforms. IUPAC (International Union of Pure and Applied Chemistry) nomenclature names chemical compounds worldwide and offers consistency and clarity in different data sets used in drug discovery. Databases such as ChEMBL and PubChem offer data on biology and chemistry at a standard level. In addition, formats such as JSON (JavaScript Object Notation) and XML (Extensible Markup Language), when used with schemas, facilitate data sharing across AI tools and systems. In particular, ontologies such as Gene Ontology (GO) and Chemical Entities of Biological Interest (ChEBI) describe and classify biological and chemical entities in a structured manner. Several specialized file formats are commonly employed in molecular modeling and structural analysis, including:

- InChI—International chemical identifier for representing chemical substances in a standardized text format
- mmCIF—Macromolecular crystallographic information file used in structural biology
- PQR—A variation of the PDB format adapted for electrostatics computations
- SMILES—For encoding molecular structures as strings
- CIF—Crystallographic information file for storing crystallographic data
- XYZ—A straightforward format for representing atomic coordinates and molecular geometries
- MMTF—Macromolecular transmission format designed for efficient data exchange of 3D structures
- GRO—GROMACS file format for molecular simulation input
- MDL Molfile—A structure file format for representing molecules and their properties
- MOL2—A widely used format in computational chemistry and molecular docking studies

Here, the CIF, mmCIF, and PDB formats are important in crystallographic and structural analysis. SMILES and InChI offer simplified versions of molecular structures in text form to facilitate data sharing and computational processing. Advanced formats such as GRO and MMTF use detailed modeling and simulation to help predict molecular dynamics and interactions accurately.

2.4 Challenges in data diversity and heterogeneity

Data inconsistency and integration problems in data domains such as genomics, proteomics, cheminformatics, and clinical studies involved in drug discovery exhibit high data diversity and heterogeneity, which present a significant challenge. Differing nomenclature and units of measurement in multiple datasets make them unusable in drug discovery. Molecules have different data formats, which require the necessary preprocessing steps for standardization. Chemical datasets often contain duplicate or redundant information, while biological datasets usually have missing entries. Datasets derived from highthroughput screening may exhibit variations in quality and structure, making their integration difficult. There are some strategies to harmonize diverse data types, which address heterogeneity and solve problems through systematic approaches. Removing duplicates, converting data to standardized formats, and imputing missing values should be done. For preprocessing tasks, tools such as OpenBabel for chemical data and Biopython for biological data can be used (O'Boyle et al., 2011; Cock et al., 2009). Furthermore, ML models can also identify patterns and align incomplete and inconsistent data, especially in instances of ambiguous annotations.

3 Sources and acquisition of biological and chemical data

Scientific and medicinal advances primarily depend on the sources and collection of biological and chemical data. Chemical data originates from sources such as laboratory analyses, chemical libraries, and computer simulations, while biological data is typically gathered through experiments, clinical research, and genomic sequencing. Public databases like GenBank, PubChem, and the PDB greatly aid the centralization and dissemination of this data. Drug discovery, disease research, and the creation of innovative therapeutics are made easier by the efficient collection and analysis of large datasets, made possible by advanced technologies like mass spectrometry, bioinformatics tools, and high-throughput screening.

3.1 Publicly available databases

A wide array of open-access databases offers rich and diverse datasets that significantly support the application of ML in drug discovery and biomedical research. For instance, the National Center for Biotechnology Information (NCBI) [https://www.ncbi.nlm.nih.gov/] provides critical tools such as PubMed for accessing biomedical literature and GenBank for nucleotide sequence data. The UniProt database [https://www.uniprot.org/] functions as a central hub for protein-related data, delivering open-access insights into protein sequences and functions. At the European Bioinformatics Institute (EMBL-EBI) [https://www.ebi.ac.uk/], platforms like Ensembl offer genome annotation, while ChEMBL supplies curated information on chemical structures, nomenclature, and pharmacological relevance. PubChem [https://pubchem.ncbi.nlm.nih.gov/] serves as one of the most extensive chemical databases, providing detailed profiles on the physical, chemical, and biological attributes of small molecules, along with 3D structural data. These resources frequently include additional metadata such as toxicity assessments, patent filings, and literature links. ChEMBL [https://www.ebi.ac.uk/chembl/] also acts as a chemogenomic repository tailored to druglike compounds. Likewise, DrugBank [https://www.drugbank.ca/] compiles extensive pharmaceutical information, integrating data on drug mechanisms, molecular targets, and pharmacogenomics. A comprehensive summary of these databases is presented in Table 2.1.

3.2 Open-source platforms and repositories

Open-source platforms collaborate worldwide and help in community-driven data curation and analysis. These platforms enable researchers to collaborate voluntarily and showcase their expertise to tackle a common problem among researchers, leading to increased

Table 2.1 Summary of publicly available databases.

Databases	Nature of the database	Links
NCBI	GenBank, PubMed	https://www.ncbi.nlm.nih.gov/
UniProt	Protein sequences and their functional data	https://www.uniprot.org/
EMBL-EBI	Ensembl (genomic annotations), ChEMBL (chemical structures)	https://www.ebi.ac.uk/
PubChem	Chemical and biological properties of small molecules	https://pubchem.ncbi.nlm.nih.gov/
DrugBank	Pharmaceutical data on drugs	https://go.drugbank.com/
ZINC	Chemical database for virtual screening	https://zinc.docking.org/
PDB	Structural data of biological macromolecules	https://www.rcsb.org/
KEGG	Pathways, genomes, diseases	https://www.genome.jp/kegg/

productivity. GitHub [https://github.com/] is a developer platform that allows hosting scripts and storing, sharing, and managing datasets and computational workflows. It also provides a structured platform for experiment organization for researchers, allowing them to use issues and project boards to track and manage their progress. Community-driven initiatives include projects like Open Targets [https://www.opentargets.org/], which put forward a platform for multidisciplinary experts to curate and validate. It is a freely available, comprehensive tool that groups multiple public data sources and helps researchers identify and categorize data for potential therapeutic drug targets for further research.

3.3 Commercial databases

The proprietary and commercial databases are mainly designed to provide a well-curated dataset for developing new drugs, advanced drug discovery, and enhanced drug delivery processes. Databases such as Clarivate Analytics Integrity [https://clarivate.com/], which provides drug information, including detailed development data, mechanisms of action, and clinical trial results, and GOSTAR [https://www.excelra.com/gostar/], a database from Excelra containing in silico and experimental data on small molecules, including pharmacodynamic and pharmacokinetic properties, are key resources. Moreover, these commercial databases have various advantages compared to public databases. They offer higher quality due to strict curation and validation, which enhances the precision and reliability of the data. These databases also feature extensive and comprehensive datasets, which may include exclusive information not available on other platforms. Their regular maintenance and professional technical support are critical factors ensuring relevance and reliability. Lastly, they also provide proprietary insights, allowing users to access novel or patented compounds, including their experimental results, thereby accelerating users' research processes.

3.4 Data mining and extraction techniques

To automate, automated data extraction from online sources is commonly achieved using web scraping tools such as Beautiful Soup [https://www.crummy.com/software/BeautifulSoup/] and Scrapy [https://scrapy.org/], which facilitate the collection of information from digital repositories. For unstructured textual data found in scientific publications and patent records, NLP libraries like NLTK (Natural Language Toolkit) and TextBlob are utilized to identify and interpret relevant content. In addition, domain-specific platforms such as Patent Lens [https://www.lens.org/] provide specialized tools for extracting pharmaceutical data directly from global patent sources.

4 Data organization and management

Drug development initiatives that are successful in the big data and AI era depend significantly on efficient data management and organization. To guarantee data integrity, accessibility, and security, current pharmaceutical research generates and analyzes enormous amounts of biological and chemical data, making robust systems and procedures necessary. This section focuses on the key principles of organizing and managing data within AI-based drug discovery frameworks.

4.1 Dataset preparation and quality refinement

The process of curating data serves as an essential foundation for ensuring the quality and usability of datasets in AI-driven analysis. It involves identifying and addressing various data anomalies that can impact the quality and reliability of AI models. Anomalies are instances within a dataset that deviate from the general patterns and do not fit into the usual trends. Most of the time, the concept of anomalies is poorly defined, ambiguous, and considered domain-specific. Several crucial actions are involved in data cleaning, each with the specific goal of resolving a particular issue in a dataset.

Locating and rectifying outliers is another critical approach to data cleaning to enhance the reliability of information. Missing values, outliers, unaccounted duplicates, and inconsistencies are some types of anomalies, and they interfere with the analysis and model's performance. Enhanced handling of anomalies leads to better data quality and, therefore, results that are highly reliable. The most basic techniques employed in the detection of these anomalies are statistical techniques. These include the exploitation of descriptive statistics and visual tools to check for abnormal values and patterns. Domain expertise also plays a role, where trained individuals in the specific field point out data that doesn't make sense biologically or chemically. In addition, automated tools are used to apply well-trained algorithms to find these anomalies mathematically. At this stage, the data identified as an anomaly is treated using a wide range of techniques. These techniques include data cleaning, which encompasses simple processes such as filling in missing values for data that was not captured in full; deletion, which removes duplicate values or extreme differences that fall outside acceptable limits; and formatting, which helps standardize different formats within the dataset. Lastly, there is alteration, a process that involves removing or correcting typographical errors or inconsistent data, either manually or through automated systems.

It is important to maintain data quality and integrity in order to build trustworthy AI models. In drug discovery, researchers can implement several traceability measures that improve AI model analysis by enhancing data quality, thereby improving outcomes and the repeatability of the analysis. Some of these measures include—data verification and data cross-checking, where the accuracy of data is confirmed while the model is checked against several measures by referencing different works or experiments. Such SOPs should encompass quality control mechanisms for uniformity. For instance, adherence to a data entry SOP ensures this consistency. There are routine inspections that also add to the assurance of quality consistency over time, together with time-based reviews, while provenance-based tracking describes the input source, changes made, and the transformations done, promoting openness and traceability in the process.

4.2 Data storage solutions

The complexity of modern software applications is increasing and becoming more intricate, which makes them harder to maintain and extend. Database systems need to adapt to this new trend as well. Moreover, the choice of a data storage solution is crucial for efficient data management and retrieval in AI-driven drug discovery. The three main categories of data storage solutions are listed below:

4.2.1 Relational databases

Relational databases organize data into structured tables with predefined relationships. The attributes of the various entities that each table represents are contained in its fields. These tables require the identification of the data that will serve as both their foreign keys and their primary keys. It is also necessary to establish the relationships between them. This enables the RDBMS to accurately reflect the actual configuration of the elements that are being studied (Trillo-Montero et al., 2023). Drug repurposing is a developing area in the science of drug discovery that offers new uses for already-approved drugs. Relational databases provide several advantages, including: (1) an accessible and intuitive way to search for and retrieve drug-related information without technical hurdles, (2) support for drug repurposing approaches such as single-agent, combination, and context-dependent repurposing strategies, and (3) the option to filter by target categories, enabling users to identify drug candidates relevant to particular diseases or molecular targets. However, they may face challenges with scalability for very large datasets and flexibility for handling diverse and rapidly changing data types.

4.2.2 Nonrelational databases

Nonrelational (NoSQL) databases provide greater adaptability in data structuring, making them particularly suitable for managing large-scale unstructured or semistructured datasets. In the context of drug discovery, commonly used NoSQL systems include document-oriented databases such as MongoDB [https://www.mongodb.com] and CouchDB [https://couchdb.apache.org/]; key-value stores like Redis [https://redis.io] and Amazon DynamoDB [https://aws.amazon.com/dynamodb]; and wide-column databases such as Apache Cassandra [https://cassandra.apache.org/] and Google Bigtable [https://cloud.google.com/bigtable]. These platforms offer notable benefits over traditional relational databases, including enhanced scalability, high performance with massive datasets, flexible data models, and compatibility with distributed computing frameworks. Nonetheless, they may fall short in terms of strict consistency enforcement and lack a universal querying language, which are typical strengths of relational database systems.

4.2.3 Cloud-based storage and management systems

Cloud computing has emerged as a key enabler of modern drug discovery workflows, offering scalable infrastructure, cost-effective solutions, and streamlined deployment for handling large-scale biomedical data. Major providers offer a variety of storage and database services tailored for biomedical applications. For instance, Amazon Web Services (AWS) supports solutions like S3[https://aws.amazon.com/s3], RDS [https://aws.amazon.com/rds], and DynamoDB [https://aws.amazon.com/dynamodb], enabling efficient handling of structured and unstructured datasets. Google Cloud Platform contributes with Cloud Storage [https://cloud.google.com/storage], Cloud SQL-[https://cloud.google.com/sql], and Bigtable-[https://cloud.google.com/bigtable], which facilitate high-throughput data processing and management. Microsoft Azure also provides robust options such as Blob Storage [https://azure.microsoft.com/en-us/products/storage/blobs], Azure SQL Database-[https://azure.microsoft.com/en-us/products/azure-sql/database], and Cosmos DB-[https://azure.microsoft.com/en-us/products/cosmos-db], offering global distribution and real-time access capabilities. These services collectively support the storage, analysis, and sharing of large-scale datasets in modern drug development workflows. The use of these cloud-based systems for AI-driven drug discovery has several advantages, such as scaling to meet demands where more storage space and computing power resources are required, seamlessly connecting to cloud-based AI and ML, being cost-efficient through pay-as-you-use strategies, utilizing fewer infrastructure management resources, and integrating with advanced analysis and ML models available in the cloud.

4.3 Data annotation and the of metadata management

Metadata, defined as 'information about data within any data environment,' plays a crucial role in making biological and chemical datasets useful for AI analysis. End users can use it to check the data's quality and determine its value for use in drug discovery. The ability of metadata to filter out nonessential information during searches enhances the precision of algorithmic results. It is also essential for ensuring consistency and harmonization throughout different datasets.

4.3.1 Tools and standards for effective annotation

Effective data annotation depends on reliable tools and well-defined standards that support accuracy, consistency, and scalability. Modern annotation platforms often include functionalities such as automated tagging, collaborative workflows, and built-in validation mechanisms, making them suitable for annotating diverse data types, including textual, visual, and auditory content. Standardized frameworks, such as taxonomies and ontologies, serve as shared references that facilitate uniform data labeling and promote compatibility across systems. Within the drug discovery domain, several specialized tools and annotation standards have been introduced to maintain the integrity and uniformity of metadata annotations.

Ontologies and controlled vocabularies

a. GO [https://www.geneontology.org] is extensively used for annotating gene functions.
b. ChEBI [https://www.ebi.ac.uk/chebi] provides detailed classifications and relationships among chemical compounds relevant to biological systems (Hastings et al., 2016)
c. EFO (Experimental Factor Ontology) [https://www.ebi.ac.uk/efo] is designed to standardize the representation of experimental variables and conditions, thereby improving consistency in the annotation of experimental designs (Malone et al., 2010)

Metadata standards

a. ISA-Tab (Investigation, Study, Assay) [https://isa-tools.org/isa-tab] is used for describing biological experiments (Sansone et al., 2012)
b. CHELM (Hierarchical Editing Language for Macromolecules) for representing complex biomolecules [https://www.ebi.ac.uk/chelm](Zhang et al., 2012)

Annotation tools

a. OpenRefine: A powerful tool for cleaning and transforming data, including metadata annotation [https://openrefine.org].
b. Annotator: A web-based tool for collaborative annotation of scientific datasets [https://annotator.org].
c. CEDAR Workbench: A platform for creating and managing metadata templates compliant with community standards [https://cedar.stanford.edu/].

4.4 Version control and reproducibility

Version control plays a critical role in managing modifications to datasets, analysis code, and AI models throughout the lifecycle of a project. It supports collaborative workflows, maintains a history of changes, and enhances the reproducibility of scientific research. Although initially developed for software engineering, version control systems are now commonly used in data science and drug discovery efforts. Tools such as Git, a distributed version control system known for its flexibility and widespread adoption, and Mercurial, which offers comparable distributed versioning capabilities, are frequently employed to organize and track project evolution.

5 Understanding molecular features and engineering for molecular data

Molecular features are fundamental to drug discovery, providing the core input for predictive models and investigations into structure activity relationships. These features encompass a wide range of properties that characterize molecules, from their structural attributes to their physicochemical properties and biological activities.

5.1 Structural features and molecular fingerprints

Structural features encapsulate the fundamental aspects of a molecule's architecture, which can be categorized into three main types: topological, geometrical, and electronic features. Topological features describe the connectivity of atoms within a molecule, geometrical features represent the three-dimensional (3D) arrangement of atoms, and electronic features characterize the distribution of electrons within the molecule. Apart from these structural features, molecular fingerprints—frequently bit strings—act as condensed and encoded representations of molecular structures. Molecular fingerprints were first created for substructure searching in chemical databases, but they are now valuable tools for classification, clustering, and similarity searches. Common types of molecular fingerprints include Extended-Connectivity Fingerprints (ECFP), MACCS keys, and Topological Torsion (TT) fingerprints. ECFPs focus on capturing circular substructures around each atom and were explicitly developed for modeling structure-activity relationships. MACCS (Molecular ACCess System) keys, based on predefined atom symbols, bond types, and other molecular properties, employ bit keysets such as 166 bit and 960 bit configurations for substructure identification and molecular similarity. Although they appear to be used less frequently than other fingerprint types, TT fingerprints, which are classified as 2D structural fingerprints, provide excellent computational efficiency and superior performance. When combined, these molecular fingerprints and structural characteristics offer strong instruments for describing and evaluating molecular structures.

5.1.1 Physicochemical traits and bioactivity profiles

Physicochemical properties play a vital role in determining how a molecule behaves within biological environments. Fundamental characteristics such as molecular weight, lipophilicity (commonly expressed as LogP), topological polar surface area, and counts of hydrogen bond donors, acceptors, and rotatable bonds are routinely assessed. These attributes underpin several widely accepted druglikeness filters, including Lipinski's Rule of Five. On the other hand, biological activity data—typically derived from experimental assays—offer valuable insights into a compound's potential therapeutic relevance. Such data may include binding affinities to biological targets, modulation of enzymatic activity, and results from various cell-based functional assays.

5.2 Strategies for feature extraction

It is a critical step in data preprocessing, transforming raw data into meaningful formats that improve the effectiveness of ML models. These methods are designed to reduce data dimensionality, improve clarity, and identify critical patterns that contribute to accurate predictions.

5.2.1 Descriptor calculation methods

Numerical values that quantify different aspects of a molecule's structure and characteristics are called molecular descriptors. Statistical metrics, structural patterns, and molecular characteristics are among the quantitative features that are extracted from molecular data to create these descriptors. Descriptor calculation methods, such as physicochemical computations, fingerprints, and

ML-based feature extraction, are crucial in summarizing complex molecular information into formats suitable for modeling and analysis. Molecular descriptors can be broadly categorized into several types. Constitutional descriptors represent basic structural features of a molecule, including counts of atoms, bonds, or specific molecular fragments. Topological descriptors provide insights into atomic connectivity patterns, utilizing indices such as Wiener and Zagreb to quantify molecular structure. In contrast, geometrical descriptors emphasize the 3D aspects of molecules, capturing metrics like surface area and molecular volume. Finally, quantum chemical descriptors are derived from electronic structure calculations and include properties such as HOMO-LUMO (Highest Occupied Molecular Orbital-Lowest Unoccupied Molecular Orbital) energies. Together, these descriptors provide comprehensive insight into molecular properties and are essential for computational chemistry and molecular modeling. Lastly, features like HOMO-LUMO energies are among the quantum chemical descriptors that are obtained from electronic structure calculations. When combined, these descriptors offer a thorough understanding of molecular properties and are essential for molecular modeling and computational chemistry.

5.2.2 Use of software tools

Various software packages, both open-source and commercial, calculate molecular descriptors and fingerprints to predict drug responses. Liu et al. (2018) used a recommender system based on cell line or drug similarity, while Wei et al. (2019) employed a complex network with gene expression and drug similarity data. A network-based framework for predicting drug synergy was proposed by Cheng et al. (2019). These methods highlight the potential of integrating genomic data and chemical fingerprints in drug development. Table 2.2 lists these software programs or systems that can produce chemical fingerprints and descriptors.

5.3 Techniques for feature selection

Selecting features involves identifying the most relevant variables within a dataset to enhance model accuracy and minimize computational complexity. Techniques used for this purpose may involve assessing the correlation between features and the target variable, evaluating different feature combinations to determine the optimal subset, or leveraging embedded methods within ML models that inherently perform feature selection. This step not only simplifies model interpretation and accelerates training time but also helps prevent overfitting. Broadly, feature selection techniques are divided into three broad categories based on their methodology:

Table 2.2 Chemoinformatics software tools for fingerprint and molecular descriptor analysis.

Software tools	Description	References
RDKit OpenBabel Mordred PaDEL PubChem	A comprehensive cheminformatics toolkit that offers a wide range of descriptor calculations A chemical toolbox designed to speak many languages of chemical data A molecular descriptor calculator that can generate over 1800 descriptors 875 descriptors (including 431 3D and 1444 1D and 2D descriptors), and 12 different fingerprint kinds (a total of 16, 092 bits) 881 bits long fingerprints for 2D structures	https://www.rdkit.org/ https://openbabel.org/ https://github.com/mordred-descriptor/mordred http://padel.nus.edu.sg/software/padeldescriptor (Yap, 2011) https://pubchem.ncbi.nlm.nih.gov/

5.3.1 Filter methods

Filter methods for feature selection evaluate each feature independently to assess its relevance to the target variable. These techniques choose the most essential features to be included in the model by ranking them according to their individual importance. Filter approaches are especially well-suited for initial feature selection because of their simplicity, speed, and model-agnostic nature. They rely on the statistical properties of features rather than the specifics of any ML algorithm. Filter-based techniques commonly utilize methods such as correlation analysis to remove features with high interdependence, thereby reducing redundancy in the dataset. Mutual information is another commonly applied metric that quantifies how much information a feature contributes to predicting the target variable. In parallel, the chi-square test evaluates whether categorical features and the target variable are statistically independent. These approaches help streamline preprocessing by refining the feature set, ultimately enhancing both model accuracy and interpretability.

5.3.2 Model-guided wrapper techniques

Wrapper methods assess different combinations of features by iteratively training and validating a ML model to identify the subset that yields the best performance. These methods iteratively identify the subset that delivers the highest predictive performance. Unlike filter methods, which are model-agnostic, wrapper approaches incorporate the learning algorithm itself to assess feature relevance, often resulting in better accuracy but with greater computational demands. Notable examples include Recursive Feature Elimination (RFE), which systematically eliminates the least significant features using model-driven evaluation, while stepwise approaches, such as forward and backward selection, incrementally include or exclude features based on their influence on the model's accuracy. While resource-intensive, wrapper methods are particularly valuable when tuning feature sets for specific ML algorithms.

5.3.3 Embedded feature selection methods

By incorporating feature selection directly into the model training process, embedded methods offer an effective compromise between accuracy and computational cost. These approaches refine feature selection as part of learning, making them generally more efficient than wrapper methods and less susceptible to overfitting. Lasso regression is one example that uses L1 regularization to reduce some feature coefficients to zero, eliminating less significant features from the model. Another example is the importance of random forest features, which evaluates the significance of features based on the mean decrease in impurity across decision trees. By combining feature selection with model training, embedded methods streamline the process and produce robust feature sets tailored to the chosen algorithm.

5.4 Dimensionality reduction techniques

Dimensionality reduction aims to simplify datasets by minimizing the number of input features while retaining the most significant patterns and structures. Techniques like Principal Component Analysis (PCA) and t-SNE (t-distributed Stochastic Neighbor Embedding) transform high-dimensional data into a more compact form, improving the efficiency of analysis, interpretation, and visualization of complex data. Table 2.3 compares dimensionality reduction techniques for visualizing a molecular dataset. These methods lower computational complexity and enhance model performance by eliminating redundant or unnecessary features. While effective for handling large datasets, they

Table 2.3 Comparison of PCA, t-SNE, and autoencoder-based dimensionality reduction for visualizing a molecular dataset.

Characteristics	PCA	t-SNE	Autoencoder-based
Type of algorithm: Unique solution, computation time, projection type, type of approach, interpretation, purpose.	Deterministic? Yes. 0.29 s. Linear global PCA is just a rotation of axes. Dimensionality reduction	Stochastic No. 109.50 s nonlinear local/global subjective interpretation Data visualization in low dimensions (typically 2D)	Deterministic: No 30–120 s linear or nonlinear global subjective interpretation Simplify complex data, enhance interpretability, and facilitate exploration of relationships.

can sometimes lead to a loss of interpretability, as the new features may not have precise meanings in the context of the source data. These techniques are essential for handling high-dimensional molecular data, improving computational efficiency, and aiding in data visualization.

5.4.1 *Principal component analysis)*

PCA is a popular dimensionality reduction method that transforms high-dimensional data into a smaller number of uncorrelated variables called principal components while preserving the majority of the dataset's variance. It works by identifying the axes along which the data shows the greatest variation and projecting the data onto these directions. Through orthogonal transformation, PCA transforms correlated features into linearly independent components. This technique is commonly used in ML workflows as a preprocessing step to reduce complexity, enhance computational speed, and minimize overfitting. Furthermore, PCA facilitates the visualization of complex, high-dimensional datasets in two or three dimensions, aiding in the discovery of underlying structures and patterns.

5.4.2 *t-distributed stochastic neighbor embedding*

t-SNE is a nonlinear technique for dimensionality reduction that excels at maintaining local relationships in data, making it particularly useful for visualizing complex datasets. In contrast to linear approaches like PCA, t-SNE preserves intricate data relationships by focusing on maintaining the relative distances between neighboring data points, which helps reveal patterns and clusters in high-dimensional spaces. This characteristic makes it particularly effective for exploring intricate datasets, such as those in molecular research, where uncovering clusters is essential. However, its computational demands can pose challenges when applied to large datasets, potentially limiting its scalability. Nonetheless, due to its strength in highlighting local similarities, t-SNE remains a preferred method for exploratory analysis and visual interpretation. In addition to t-SNE, dimensionality reduction can also be achieved using autoencoders and deep learning (DL) techniques, which offer scalable and model-driven alternatives for capturing complex data structures.

5.4.3 *Autoencoders and deep learning approaches*

Autoencoders are a type of neural network that compress input data into a lower-dimensional format and then reconstruct it, allowing the model to learn efficient, compact representations of the original information. In contrast to linear approaches, autoencoders are very effective at handling complicated datasets because they can learn complex, nonlinear correlations. They are frequently employed to reduce dimensionality and extract features, which makes it possible to represent data more effectively for downstream tasks. Denoising autoencoders, designed to eliminate noise from input data while maintaining its essential structure, exemplify how autoencoders can be modified to serve specific uses. This versatility makes autoencoders a valuable tool in data preprocessing and analysis.

5.5 Handling feature collinearity and redundancy

High correlation between two or more features in a dataset causes feature collinearity and redundancy, which impairs interpretability and makes the model unstable. This leads to multicollinearity, which hinders model performance and makes it difficult to determine the distinct contribution of each feature. To mitigate redundancy, strategies such as eliminating one of the correlated variables, implementing dimensionality reduction methods like PCA, or applying regularization techniques such as Lasso can be employed. These methods contribute to better model performance by minimizing overfitting, enhancing interpretability, and ensuring that each selected feature contributes distinct and meaningful information to the analysis.

Resolving these problems is essential to creating reliable prediction models. Multiple strategies can be used to address multicollinearity in order to enhance model performance and provide more trustworthy interpretations. Reducing duplication in the dataset by eliminating one of the highly associated features is a popular strategy. Another choice is to use domain-specific information to combine correlated features into a single composite feature, which simplifies the data and reduces multicollinearity. Removing one feature from a pair of highly correlated variables using correlation analysis and measuring the degree of multicollinearity for each feature using the Variance Inflation Factor are important methods to reduce multicollinearity. L1 (Lasso) and L2 (Ridge) regularization methods are used to manage model complexity by applying penalties to overly complex models, which helps prevent overfitting and improves generalization. By discouraging reliance on less informative features, these methods improve both the robustness and interpretability of the model while minimizing issues related to multicollinearity.

5.5.1 Feature set optimization to maximize model performance

Achieving an optimal feature set for model performance involves selecting variables that minimize noise and redundancy while maximizing predictive value. This process retains only the most influential features that significantly enhance the model's accuracy. A refined feature set not only reduces the risk of overfitting but also results in more efficient models that are smaller, faster, and better at generalizing to new data. Techniques such as feature importance ranking—commonly implemented using model-specific measures like those from random forests—help prioritize the most relevant inputs. Methods RFE with Cross-Validation further support this by evaluating performance across different feature subsets to determine the ideal number of variables. Moreover, incorporating expert domain knowledge can guide the selection process by preserving features that are biologically or contextually meaningful.

Case studies in practical feature engineering highlight the transformative role of carefully crafted input features in improving ML model performance. For example, engineered features such as patient age groups, disease progression rates, or symptom patterns have enhanced predictive accuracy in disease diagnosis models. Combining transaction frequency with geo-location trends in financial fraud detection has led to more robust anomaly detection systems. Similarly, techniques like word embeddings and sentiment scores have significantly improved sentiment analysis tasks in NLP. In order to maximize model accuracy and interpretability, these case studies highlight the value of domain expertise and repeated testing in deriving features that capture significant insights.

5.5.2 Quantitative structure-activity relationship modeling for drug-target binding affinity

Utilizing a comprehensive feature engineering strategy to maximize model performance, ML models were developed in a study by Ballester and Mitchell (2010) to predict protein-ligand binding affinities. Using RDKit and MOE software, the authors computed over 1500 chemical descriptors, giving the model a rich set of features. They used correlation-based feature selection to exclude strongly correlated descriptors in order to resolve redundancy and guarantee a more effective feature set. The most important descriptors were identified by using Random Forest for feature importance ranking. In addition, to identify an optimal subset of features, they also used cross-validated recursive feature removal. The effectiveness of their feature selection and model optimization strategy was demonstrated by the considerable improvement in the final model's prediction performance after selecting 60 critical characteristics compared to traditional scoring methods.

5.5.3 DL for molecular property prediction

The introduction of graph convolutional networks (GCNs) for the prediction of chemical characteristics by Duvenaud et al. (2015) marked a significant breakthrough in ML for chemistry. They depicted atoms as nodes, molecules as graphs, and bonds as edges, using a feature engineering technique. This made it possible for the model to utilize the structural information already present in the molecules. They developed a specialized neural network architecture that directly learns to extract relevant information from these molecular graphs in order to produce more accurate predictions. They significantly improved the model's capacity to capture important molecular features by adding domain information and initializing atom features with relevant chemical properties. By demonstrating the capacity of GCNs to forecast molecular properties, this innovative technique set a new standard for computational chemistry.

5.6 Lessons learned and best practices

The performance and dependability of models in data analysis and ML can be significantly improved by applying essential lessons and best practices. Extensive data preparation and cleaning are required to ensure high-quality inputs, addressing issues such as outliers, redundancy, and missing values. The process of feature engineering for molecular data in drug discovery is illustrated as a flowchart in Fig. 2.2. By focusing on the most relevant characteristics, techniques like feature selection and dimensionality reduction, such as PCA, enhance the model's accuracy and efficiency.

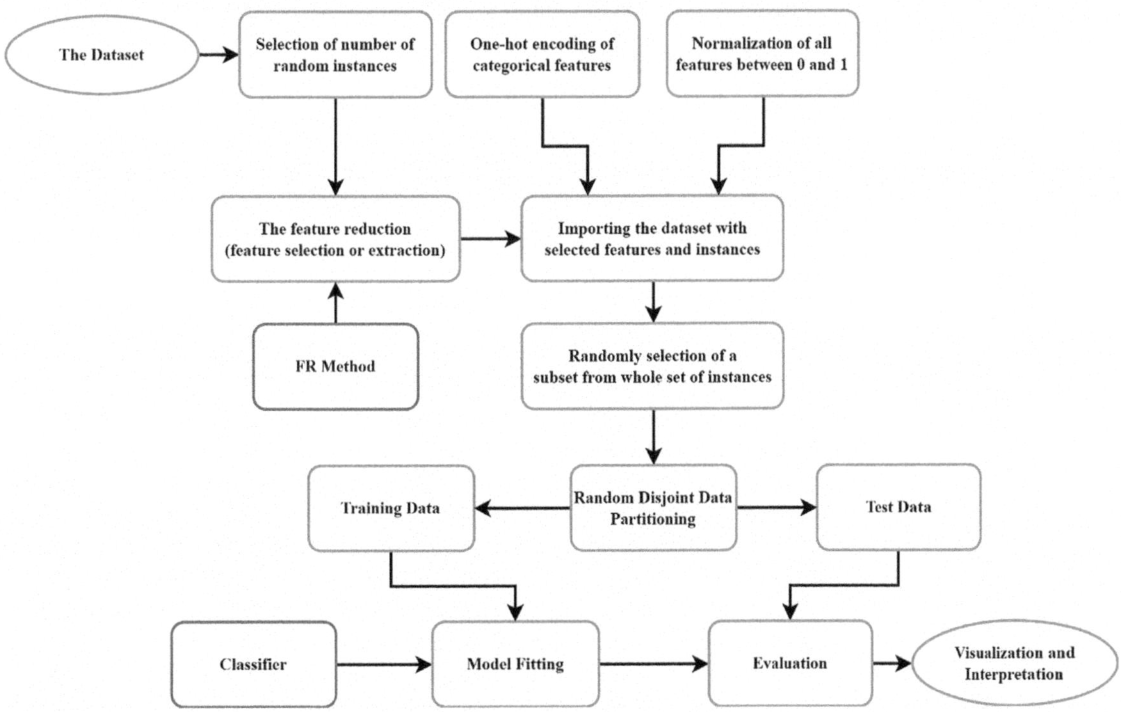

Fig. 2.2 Standardized workflow for feature reduction and model evaluation in ML-based drug discovery. A typical machine learning pipeline highlighting data preprocessing, feature reduction, model training, and performance evaluation for robust and interpretable outcomes.

To ensure generalizability and avoid over fitting, regular validation and cross-validation are crucial. In addition, models are continuously evaluated and improved as new data becomes available to ensure adaptability and long-term performance. Interpretability and robustness are enhanced by combining data-driven methods with domain expertise, as automated feature selection techniques can be improved with chemical intuition. It's critical to consider how feature engineering and model selection interact; deep neural networks (DNNs) are an example. Validating feature importance using techniques such as permutation importance ensures real-world relevance while avoiding data leakage by performing feature selection only on the training set to prevent overly optimistic performance estimates. Continuous improvement based on new insights and model performance is necessary for iterative feature engineering. Lastly, performance and interpretability must be balanced, particularly in drug discovery, where more straightforward characteristics can reveal crucial information about underlying mechanisms. Together, these practices enable the development of reliable, interpretable, and effective machine-learning models.

6 Statistical tools and methods for molecular data analysis

Many statistical tools and methods have been used to analyze molecular data in drug discovery. These methods help identify patterns, relationships, and significant findings, facilitating drug development. By combining powerful statistical methods with computational power, these tools help researchers make better decisions and advance discoveries in the field of molecular biology and precision medicine as well. They are all given below as:

6.1 Exploratory data analysis

It is a very important part of biological data analysis because it helps the researcher understand the structure and relationships in complex datasets without preconceived hypotheses. It allows exploratory data analysis (EDA) to look at the data in a holistic manner, where a better understanding of relationships, trends, and anomalies would eventually inform deeper statistical analyses. One of the main advantages of EDA is the use of visual representation techniques to make complex biological data simpler. Such tools assist in the detection of patterns, correlations, and anomalies hidden in data at a preliminary stage. Often-used visualization techniques include heatmaps and scatter plots. Heatmaps provide a color coded representation of data values, which helps identify correlations and patterns across different variables. In biological data, this can be particularly useful for examining gene expression patterns, protein interactions, or metabolic activities (Blbas, 2024). Scatter plots serve as an effective tool for examining relationships between two continuous variables. They can reveal trends, groupings, and outliers, offering insights into potential correlations or anomalies within the data. For instance, in experimental studies, scatter plots may be used to explore associations between gene expression levels and observable phenotypic characteristics (Kaur et al., 2018).

EDA focuses on visualizing data and leverages graphical methods to detect underlying structures that may be overlooked through traditional analyses. It helps reveal clusters and trends, which provide insight into how biological entities interact or differ under certain conditions. EDA often utilizes dimensionality reduction and clustering techniques, for instance, PCA, hierarchical clustering, and k-means, to uncover patterns and structure within complex datasets. These techniques are beneficial in reducing the dimensionality of large-scale biological data, such as single-cell RNA sequencing or genomic datasets, making it easier to uncover significant biological patterns, such as cell populations or genetic variants. PCA efficiently reduces the complexity of the data and retains as much of the variance as possible. It simplifies high-dimensional biological data into a more compact form, making it easier to detect patterns associated with disease progression and treatment response. Clustering techniques such as k-means and hierarchical clustering are used to group data instances based on shared characteristics, making them valuable for detecting biologically relevant clusters such as distinct cell types or genetic variants with shared traits. While EDA is a powerful approach for revealing patterns and generating hypotheses, it is essential to interpret visual outputs with caution. Visualizations can be deceptive if not supported by contextual understanding; for example, observed correlations do not necessarily imply causation, and some patterns may arise from biases in data collection rather than genuine biological phenomena. Therefore, pairing EDA with rigorous statistical validation is critical to ensure the reliability of insights and to prevent drawing unwarranted conclusions.

6.2 Descriptive and inferential statistics

Statistics plays a fundamental role in data analysis, enabling researchers to quantify patterns, draw interpretations, and communicate results across diverse scientific domains. Descriptive statistics help condense large datasets by summarizing key attributes through measures of central tendency and variability. Central tendency is commonly represented by the mean, median, and mode. The mean represents the average and is obtained by dividing the sum of all values by the total number of entries. The mode refers to the value that appears most often, making it helpful for analyzing datasets with frequent repetitions. The median, which represents the central value in a sorted dataset, is especially useful when outliers might skew the average. Variability measures, on the other hand, provide insight into how widely the data values are dispersed. Common measures of variability include the range, which reflects the gap between the highest and lowest values; variance, which calculates the average of the squared differences from the mean; and standard deviation, the square root of the variance, which indicates how much the data points typically deviate from the mean using the same unit as the original values. Together, these statistics provide a comprehensive summary of the dataset's distribution and structure (Blbas, 2024). For example, descriptive statistics summarize gene expression levels across different populations or analyze survival rates in clinical trials (Selvamuthu and Das, 2024).

To illustrate these concepts, consider a study measuring the expression levels of a specific gene in cancer patients. The mean provides an overall average of gene expression across all individuals, giving a general sense of expression within the group. The mode highlights the most frequently observed expression level, similar to determining the value that appears most frequently in the data. The median, representing the middle value when all expression levels are sorted, is particularly valuable when the dataset includes extremely high or low values, as it is less affected by outliers. The standard deviation indicates how much variability exists among patients—whether most individuals show similar gene expression levels or if there's significant variation across the group. If we look at how long patients survive during a drug trial, the mean gives us a general sense of the average survival time. The mode shows the survival time that appears most frequently. The median tells us the point where half the patients lived longer and half lived less. And again, the standard deviation helps us understand whether most patients had similar survival times or if the outcomes were quite different from one another.

Inferential statistics is concerned with drawing conclusions about an entire population based on a sample that accurately reflects the larger group. By leveraging probability theory and various statistical models, this approach allows researchers to make informed generalizations, estimate population parameters, and test hypotheses even when direct observation of the full population is not feasible. It relies on data samples to estimate population parameters; observed patterns in the sample are statistically significant and likely present in the entire population. A central aspect is hypothesis testing, where researchers propose a null hypothesis and use statistical tests to determine whether to reject or accept it. This procedure is also used to test scientific hypotheses. For example, researchers might want to find out how effective a new drug is for treating a specific disease or whether certain genetic markers are associated with certain diseases (Marshall and Jonker, 2011). They test the drug on a group of patients and use statistical methods to determine if the results are strong enough to suggest that the drug truly works, rather than the observed effects being due to chance. Similarly, they may study whether certain genetic markers, such as specific changes in a person's DNA, are linked to a higher risk of developing a disease. These kinds of questions are answered using inferential statistics, which help scientists make informed conclusions based on sample data.

6.3 Regression analysis

This statistical method is used to analyze how one or more independent variables influence a dependent variable. It serves two main purposes: to interpret how variables are associated and to predict outcomes based on known inputs. This method is widely applied across disciplines such as biological data analysis, environmental sciences, and medical research for modeling trends and making data-driven predictions.

6.3.1 Types of regression

There are three types of regression analyses available. Simple linear regression utilizes one independent variable, which helps to predict the dependent variable. The use of simple linear regression is applied in modeling the regulatory interactions between genes. It helps to understand genetic networks based on expression data. Multiple linear regression (MLR) employs the use of multiple independent variables for prediction, making the model more accurate. In stable-isotope-labeled mass spectrometry studies, MLR models can quantify peptide abundances while considering specific isotope incorporation rates, improving the accuracy of protein expression measurements. Nonlinear regression models relationships that do not strictly follow a straight line; hence, it is especially useful in biological and chemical applications where complicated interactions are common. In pharmacokinetics, longitudinal data is analyzed using nonlinear mixed-effects models to evaluate the concentration of drugs at given time intervals. In chemistry, nonlinear mapping techniques establish structure-activity relationships in acaricide studies with physicochemical descriptors (Domine et al., 1993).

6.4 Classification analysis

Classification analysis in biological and chemical contexts involves assigning data points to predefined categories based on their distinguishing features. This is the most important approach to understanding complex data, such as genomics or chemical compositions. There are various techniques used for the classification and prediction of data in biological and chemical fields. Statistical methods like decision trees simplify complex decision-making by splitting data based on key characteristics. Bayesian Networks classify data using probabilistic relationships, while support vector machines (SVMs) create optimal hyperplanes for separating classes, excelling in high-dimensional datasets (Phyu, 2009). Within chemical databases utilized for drug discovery, compounds are grouped according to their bioactivity against specific targets—for example, a protein implicated in cancer pathways. For instance, the prediction of whether a compound is "active" or "inactive" is based on its chemical features, such as molecular weight, logP, hydrogen bond donors, and acceptors. While classification analysis provides powerful tools, it has the potential to oversimplify complex biological and chemical phenomena, which may lead to the loss of basic associations within the data because some methods may fail to recognize important interactions between variables. Despite offering robust tools, classification analysis has the potential to oversimplify intricate chemical and biological processes. Since some approaches may fail to detect small but significant interactions among variables, this could result in the loss of critical relationships within the data.

6.5 Clustering in biological and chemical data

Clustering methods are essential in drug development, as they help organize large chemical datasets into meaningful groups, thereby streamlining compound selection and enhancing virtual screening efforts. These techniques help identify structurally similar compounds, which could exhibit very similar biological activities. The primary clustering methods used in drug development include hierarchical, nonhierarchical, and neural network-based approaches (Frades and Matthiesen, 2009). Clustering in biological and chemical data identifies patterns by grouping similar types of cells or similar types of compounds on the basis of a few extracted features called data points. In biology, it helps in gene expression analysis, protein classification, and the discovery of different disease subtypes. Drug discovery is streamlined for chemical datasets by grouping various substances according to distinct molecular characteristics.

6.6 Use of statistical software and tools

Programming languages such as Python and R, along with specialized tools like Stata, Statistical Package for the Social Sciences (SPSS), and Statistical Analysis System (SAS), provide diverse capabilities for statistical analysis. Python is especially suited for general-purpose programming and excels in handling large datasets, ML, and advanced analytics through its rich ecosystem of libraries, including SciPy, pandas, and scikit-learn. R is a favorite in academic and research environments because of its proficiency in statistical modeling and data visualization, as well as its extensive packages like ggplot2. Specialized applications like SAS, SPSS, and Stata are designed for industries that require regulatory compliance and user-friendly interfaces, and they have strong capabilities for specific statistical approaches and large datasets (Abatan and Olayemi, 2014).

7 Applications of ML in drug development

ML is transforming the field of drug discovery by allowing rapid and effective analysis of intricate biological and chemical datasets. By processing large volumes of information such as molecular structures, biological networks, and multiomics data, ML models can predict drug-target interactions, identify promising lead compounds, and optimize therapeutic properties, including safety and efficacy. Frequently used methods include supervised learning for tasks such as classification as well as regression, unsupervised learning for clustering compounds in chemical libraries, and DL approaches for advanced molecular modeling and representation learning. Fig. 2.3 represents the classification of ML along with specific applications in drug discovery. The following are the primary ML approaches applied in drug discovery, along with broad explanations and examples for each.

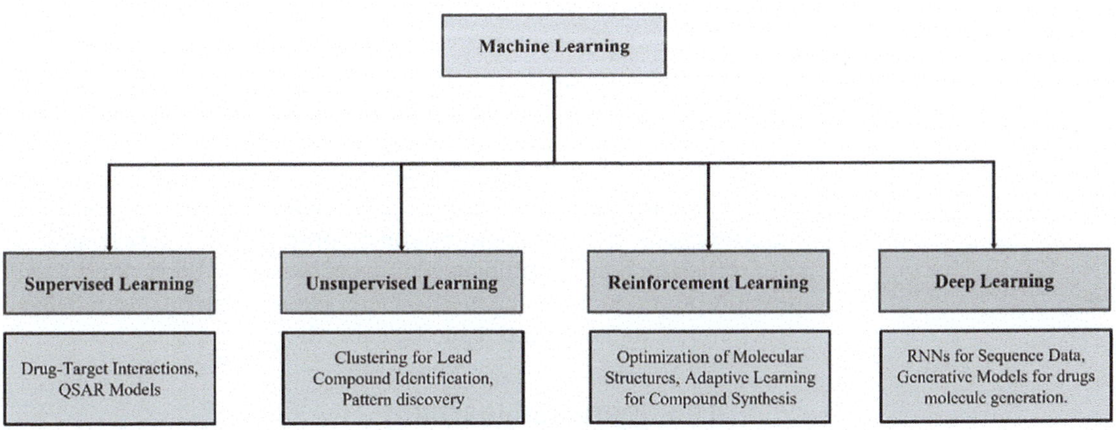

Fig. 2.3 Overview of machine learning paradigms in drug development. Different machine learning approaches—supervised, unsupervised, reinforcement, and deep learning—support diverse tasks in drug discovery, from target prediction to molecular generation.

7.1 Supervised learning

It is an ML approach in which algorithms are trained on datasets that include both input features and known output labels. Through the process, the model learns to associate specific input patterns with corresponding outcomes, enabling it to make accurate predictions on new, unseen data. It typically involves two main tasks: regression, which predicts continuous outcomes, and classification, which assigns inputs to specific predefined classes. Model performance is typically evaluated by comparing predicted outputs to actual values in a separate test set and further improved using techniques such as cross-validation and hyperparameter optimization. In the context of drug discovery, this is widely applied in applications like predicting drug-target binding affinities and developing Quantitative structure-activity relationship (QSAR) models.

7.1.1 Predictive modeling for drug-target interactions

Identifying interactions between drug compounds and biological targets, such as proteins or genes, is a fundamental aspect of the drug discovery process. Supervised ML models, such as random forests, DNNs, and SVMs, are commonly trained on validated drug target interaction datasets to predict new, previously untested relationships (You et al., 2019). For example, a random forest model built using data from sources like ChEMBL can be used to infer potential interactions for novel compounds. This approach may help identify small molecules with a high likelihood of binding to disease-associated targets, such as cancer-related proteins, thereby guiding future experimental validation efforts.

7.1.2 QSAR models

QSAR uses supervised ML techniques to establish correlations between the structural features of chemical compounds and their biological activities. These models enable the prediction of a compound's bioactivity based on its molecular descriptors (Fisher et al., 2024). For instance, a QSAR model utilizing SVMs could be trained to forecast the inhibitory potential of molecules against a specific enzyme, such as acetylcholinesterase. Input features may consist of properties such as lipophilicity, counts of hydrogen bond donors and acceptors, and molecular weight—factors that capture essential physicochemical traits impacting biological activity.

7.2 Unsupervised learning

It is a branch of ML that analyzes data without relying on predefined labels or output values. Its primary objective is to uncover hidden patterns, structures, or groupings within datasets, making it especially useful for lead discovery and interpreting complex biological data. Common methods include clustering, where similar data points are grouped together using algorithms like hierarchical clustering or k-means, and dimensionality reduction, which transforms high-dimensional datasets into simpler, lower-dimensional representations. Unlike supervised learning, unsupervised techniques work without known outcomes, allowing for the exploration of data to reveal novel insights. Clustering methods are generally categorized into three main types:

- **K-means clustering:** This method partitions data into a specified number of clusters (k) by grouping points based on similarity. The algorithm begins by selecting k initial centroids and assigning each data point to the nearest one. The centroids are then recalculated as the average of all points in each cluster, and the process repeats until the assignments no longer change. K-means is computationally efficient and performs well with datasets that have clearly separated clusters.
- **Hierarchical clustering:** It creates a nested sequence of clusters by progressively combining or dividing data points. It usually begins by treating each data point as its own cluster, gradually merging the nearest pairs until all points are combined into one overarching cluster. This process is visualized through a dendrogram, which illustrates the hierarchical structure and allows for interpretation at different levels of granularity.
- **DBSCAN (Density-based spatial clustering of applications with noise):** It groups points that are closely located based on a defined density threshold, while marking isolated points in sparse regions as outliers. In contrast to K-means, this method does not require defining the number of clusters in advance and can detect clusters of varying shapes and sizes. This method is particularly effective in identifying irregular patterns and handling noisy datasets.

7.2.1 Clustering for lead compound identification

Clustering techniques are applied to group chemical compounds based on shared physicochemical characteristics or similar biological responses. This helps identify leads with potential druglike properties. For example, by using k-means clustering to group a large library of compounds based on molecular fingerprints, researchers can focus on clusters containing compounds with known therapeutic potential for diseases like diabetes.

7.2.2 Pattern discovery in biological data

Patterns in biological datasets, like gene expression or protein interactions, can be found via unsupervised learning. These trends can point to potential treatment targets or disease-related mechanisms.

For example, when applied to transcriptome data, PCA can help design targeted treatments by detecting patterns of gene expression associated with specific cancer subtypes.

7.3 Reinforcement learning in drug design

RL is also a type of ML that enhances decision-making by learning from trial-and-error experiences within a given environment. In the context of drug discovery, RL is applied to tasks such as optimizing molecular structures and guiding synthesis pathways. The model, referred to as the agent, explores the chemical space and obtains evaluative signals as rewards or penalties depending on how well the generated molecules meet specified criteria like binding strength or toxicity levels. Over successive iterations, the agent refines its strategy to enhance outcomes related to drug effectiveness and safety.

7.3.1 Optimization of molecular structures

RL-based models explore chemical space to optimize molecular structures for desired properties, such as increased binding affinity or reduced toxicity. These models balance exploration (trying new structures) and exploitation (refining known promising candidates). Example: The REINVENT algorithm uses RL to design molecules with high activity against a specific protein target, such as kinase inhibitors. The model generates structures, tests their properties in silico, and iteratively refines them.

7.3.2 Adaptive learning strategies for compound synthesis

RL directs compound synthesis by adjusting strategies to maximize yield, efficiency, or other factors in response to experimental feedback. This is very beneficial for complex synthetic routes. For example, RL can be used to optimize the synthesis route for a potential antibiotic, reducing reaction steps while increasing yield. Each synthesis attempt teaches the system something, and its strategy improves over time.

7.4 DL techniques in drug discovery

DL techniques have revolutionized drug discovery by enabling sophisticated, complex data analysis. These techniques leverage multilayered neural networks to process various data types, such as chemical structures, biological sequences, and high-dimensional datasets. Below are key applications of DL in drug discovery.

7.4.1 Convolutional neural networks in biomedical imaging

Convolutional neural networks (CNNs) are extensively utilized for image analysis because of their capacity to identify and learn spatial hierarchies and visual patterns within the data. In drug discovery, they are applied to process and analyze microscopy images, protein-ligand binding interactions, and chemical structures represented as images (De Cao and Kipf, 2018). CNNs predict drug efficacy by analyzing phenotypic screening images, enhancing decision-making. They also aid in studying protein structures and drug binding through advanced techniques like cryo-EM and X-ray crystallography images, accelerating drug development. For example, a CNN can be used to analyze microscopy images of cells treated with different compounds. The model identifies morphological changes induced by effective drug candidates, which may indicate cytotoxicity or other desired biological effects.

7.4.2 Leveraging RNNs for sequential data analysis

RNNs are well-suited for handling sequential data due to their ability to retain information across time steps. In drug discovery, RNNs are commonly employed to predict the bioactivity of peptide or protein sequences and to model chemical reactions. They can also be used to forecast reaction outcomes by learning patterns within sequential molecular data. For example, an LSTM (Long Short-Term Memory) network trained on SMILES representations of compounds predicts molecular properties such as solubility or toxicity. Similarly, an RNN can analyze amino acid sequences to predict the antimicrobial activity of peptides.

7.4.3 Generative models (e.g., generative adversarial networks, variational autoencoders) for molecule generation

Models such as variational autoencoders (VAEs) and generative adversarial networks are gaining traction for generating new chemical compounds tailored to desired therapeutic effects. By learning underlying patterns from existing chemical structures or sequences, these models can generate new molecules that are tailored to exhibit optimized pharmacological characteristics (e.g., potency, Absorption, Distribution, Metabolism, and Excretion properties) and expand chemical libraries by generating diverse, novel compounds. MolGAN is one tool that generates valid and diverse molecular graphs by learning from existing drug datasets. For instance, it can create kinase inhibitors with optimized binding affinity (Salih et al., 2025). A VAE model trained on SMILES strings generates novel drug-like molecules that are chemically feasible and align with therapeutic goals, such as reducing off-target effects.

8 Designing patient-friendly medicinal tools using AI

The use of AI in designing patient-friendly medical devices transforms how people engage with healthcare systems. AI-powered solutions, like devices with sensors, virtual health assistants, and user-friendly mobile health apps, are designed to track health indicators, provide patients with immediate feedback, and help them manage long-term illnesses. These tools make complex medical information accessible to people with varying degrees of health literacy by using adaptive interfaces and NLP. AI can also tailor reminders and recommendations according to patient preferences and behavior, increasing patient involvement and adherence to treatment plans. Through the integration of innovation and user-focused design, AI is transforming healthcare into a more inclusive system, enabling individuals to actively participate in managing their own health.

8.1 Personalized medicine and AI

AI's introduction into healthcare has opened the door to more personalized and effective medical treatments. Personalized medicine, or precision medicine, seeks to customize medical decisions, practices, and supplies products to particular patients based on their environmental, lifestyle, and genetic factors. AI expedites this process by examining enormous datasets, finding patterns, and making remarkably accurate predictions. ML algorithms enhance the drug discovery process by identifying disease-related genetic markers and facilitating the creation of individualized therapies that enhance treatment effectiveness and reduce the likelihood of side effects.

8.1.1 Personalized therapeutics using patient-specific data

AI algorithms are capable of processing large volumes of patient data, ranging from genetic profiles and clinical records to lifestyle habits and environmental influences, to uncover patterns and predict the most suitable treatment strategies for each individual. This strategy allows for several benefits: Identification of genetic markers that predict treatment response, drug dosage optimization based on individual metabolism, and selection of medications with the highest likelihood or best chance of success for each patient. For instance, IBM Watson for Oncology analyzes clinical research, guidelines, and patient medical records using NLP and ML to provide evidence-based therapy recommendations that are specific to each cancer patient. This increases the process's speed and dependability. Figure 2.4 shows the process of using AI in customized medicine.

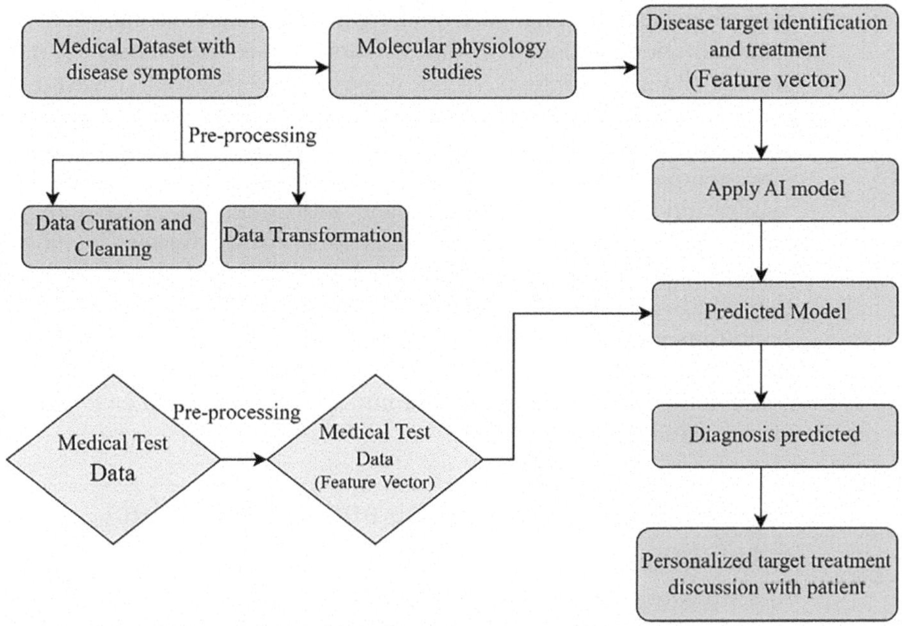

Fig. 2.4 AI-driven workflow for personalized medicine. An end-to-end pipeline illustrating how AI leverages curated medical and physiological data to generate personalized treatment recommendations.

8.1.2 Predictive analytics for treatment outcomes

AI-powered predictive analytics can predict treatment results, giving patients reasonable expectations and clinicians additional information to make more informed decisions. These analytics can forecast long-term prognosis based on treatment choices, estimate the chance of treatment effectiveness, and predict potential complications or adverse effects. According to Rajkomar et al. (2018), DL models trained on electronic health record (EHR) data have shown strong capability in forecasting clinical outcomes such as in-hospital mortality, unplanned readmissions within 30 days, extended hospital stays, and discharge diagnoses.

8.2 Development of decision support systems

Clinical Decision Support Systems (CDSS) are designed to aid healthcare professionals in making well-informed, data-driven choices about patient treatment and management. With the integration of AI, these systems have become more advanced, offering improved accuracy, usability, and contextual understanding. AI-enabled CDSS can assist in selecting appropriate medications and optimizing dosages by evaluating individual patient characteristics, such as age, weight, renal function, and genetic information, while also incorporating current clinical guidelines, recent research, and potential drug interactions. For instance, the pharmacogenomics Clinical Annotation Tool (PharmCAT) recommends dosages for drugs with known pharmacogenomic associations based on genetic data. Patient-facing applications leverage AI to empower individuals to manage their health and medications. These tools can provide various benefits, such as medication reminders and adherence tracking, customized to the individual's health status and therapy, enabling them to track symptoms and side effects for improved monitoring. An example is the AiCure mobile app, which uses AI and smartphone cameras to confirm medication ingestion and improve adherence in clinical trials and patient care.

8.3 AI in drug repurposing and adverse effect prediction

AI is transforming adverse effect prediction and drug repurposing by using sophisticated algorithms and large biomedical datasets to find new therapeutic uses for already-approved medications and predict possible negative effects. In drug repurposing, AI models analyze complex data, such as molecular structures, genetic profiles, and clinical outcomes, to identify promising drug-disease associations more efficiently than traditional methods. AI techniques, including NLP and ML, integrate data from different external sources, such as clinical trial results, EHRs, and molecular interaction datasets, to predict potential risks and adverse drug reactions. By accelerating the identification of repurposing opportunities and enhancing safety assessments, AI is transforming the drug development pipeline, reducing costs, and improving patient outcomes.

8.3.1 Identifying new uses for existing drugs

Drug repurposing, or repositioning, is the process of discovering new medical uses for already approved drugs, aiming to shorten the timeline and reduce costs in drug development. However, confirming the effectiveness and safety of a drug in a different disease setting remains a major challenge. In this context, AI offers powerful solutions by leveraging large-scale datasets to predict and optimize various drug attributes, ultimately aiding in the development of repurposed treatments that are both safer and more effective. AI can support this process by analyzing extensive databases that include protein structures, drug-target interaction networks, and disease-specific pathways to identify potential new targets for existing compounds. This data-driven approach can significantly increase the chances of success in new therapeutic areas. A notable example is the use of AI by BenevolentAI to identify baricitinib, a drug initially approved for rheumatoid arthritis, as a candidate therapy for COVID-19, highlighting the real-world effectiveness of AI-driven drug repurposing approaches.

8.3.2 Forecasting and mitigating potential side effects

While faster and cheaper than traditional drug discovery, drug repurposing faces challenges like poor target specificity, limited candidate pools, and the need for further optimization and clinical studies. Intellectual property issues can also hinder progress. AI algorithms help overcome these challenges by processing large-scale chemical and biological datasets to reveal previously unknown relationships between drugs and diseases. For example, Dey et al. (2018) used DL to predict drug-induced liver injury with high accuracy, surpassing traditional methods. Figure 2.5 depicts the process of AI-driven drug repurposing.

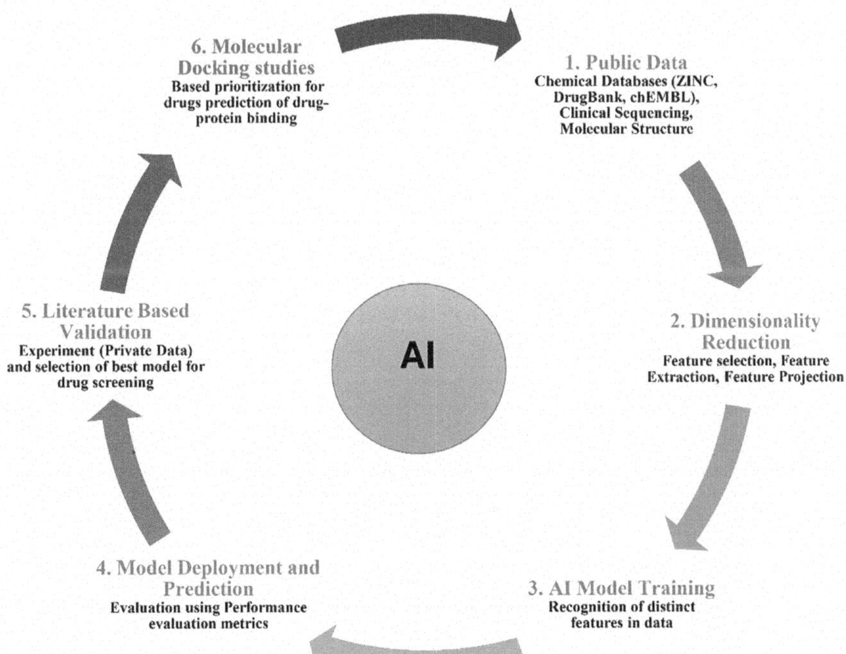

Fig. 2.5 AI-driven workflow for drug repurposing and screening: A circular framework illustrating the stages of AI-based drug repurposing, from public data acquisition and dimensionality reduction to model training, prediction, validation, and molecular docking studies.

8.4 User-centric design principles

Creating medicinal tools that prioritize patient needs involves emphasizing user experience and accessibility. AI-driven digital symptom checkers can assist individuals in receiving timely and appropriate care by assessing symptoms and suggesting suitable levels of medical attention. Applying user-centered design principles ensures that these AI tools are not only accurate and reliable but also intuitive and comfortable for patients to interact with. Key considerations for designing accessible and user-friendly AI medicinal tools include intuitive interfaces that require minimal training; clear and concise language, avoiding medical jargon when possible; customizable features to accommodate different user preferences and abilities; and compatibility with assistive technologies for users with disabilities. For example, the Ada Health app uses a conversational AI interface to guide users through a symptom assessment, making the process more engaging and less intimidating. Continuous improvement of AI medicinal tools depends on patient feedback, quality metrics, and benchmarking. Internal benchmarking monitors practices within an organization over time, while external benchmarking compares performance across organizations to identify best practices. Tools like control charts are useful for tracking data trends and ensuring continuous improvement in user-centric design. Involving end-users, as shown by Aziz et al. (2024), enhances the adoption and satisfaction of CDSS.

8.5 Case studies of successful medicinal AI tools

Successful medical AI tool case studies demonstrate how they are revolutionizing healthcare. For instance, IBM Watson Health has been used to analyze vast datasets of clinical trials and research papers, providing oncologists with tailored treatment options for cancer patients. In a similar advancement, Google's DeepMind created an AI system capable of forecasting acute kidney failure up to 48 hours before it occurs, allowing clinicians to intervene earlier and potentially prevent critical outcomes. Likewise, platforms such as PathAI enhance the accuracy of pathology diagnoses by detecting intricate patterns in medical imaging data, often surpassing the diagnostic precision of human experts. These examples demonstrate how AI-powered tools enhance diagnostic accuracy, personalize treatment plans, and optimize patient care, paving the way for smarter as well as more efficient healthcare systems.

8.5.1 Analysis of real-world applications and their impact

The cutting-edge and dominant field of information technology is AI, which can imitate the human state of mind and cognitive functions.

CDSS with intelligent diagnostic functions has emerged as one of the key scientific concerns for medical information with the advancement of AI and medical diagnosis technologies.

1. **IBM Watson for oncology:** It is an AI-based decision support system developed to help clinicians formulate individualized cancer treatment plans using patient data and current medical research. Used in over 80 Chinese hospitals since 2016, it provides counseling for most cancer patients. A study in India showed 93% concordance with tumor board recommendations for breast cancer. Key points regarding IBM are:
   a. Application: AI-powered clinical decision support for cancer treatment
   b. Impact: A study in India showed a 93% concordance with tumor board treatment recommendations for breast cancer cases.
   c. Challenges: One major challenge is the "black box" nature of its decisions. Regular updates are also essential to keep models aligned with current medical research and guidelines.
2. **Babylon Health:** The Babylon Triage and Diagnostic System is designed to provide users with guidance on appropriate levels of medical care while offering transparent explanations for its recommendations. This includes presenting a list of potential causes for the reported symptoms and identifying any warning signs that may require urgent attention (Baker et al., 2020). The following section outlines the system's impact, practical applications, and the key challenges associated with its implementation.
   a. Application: AI-powered virtual medical assistant and symptom checker.
   b. Impact: Proved to be as accurate as human physicians in the case of diagnosing common conditions.
   c. Challenges: Manages the constraints of remote diagnostics and further guarantees patient safety.
3. **DeepMind's AI for eye disease diagnosis:** The most recent example of real-world applications of AI tools is from London, where scientists at Moorfields Eye Hospital, University College London (UCL), and DeepMind developed an AI system using 3D optical coherence tomography (OCT) scans to detect over 50 eye diseases and recommend treatments. The software is built on well-established DL principles, which find common patterns in data by using algorithms. Here, the data consists of 3D scans of the patients' eyes created with OCT technology. It takes around ten minutes to create these scans, which involve reflecting near-infrared light off the inside surfaces of the eyes. In doing so, a 3D image of the tissue is created, which is a standard

method of evaluating eye health. The application, impact, and challenges are:

a. Application: AI system for analyzing eye scans and detecting over 50 eye diseases.
b. Impact: Achieved expert-level performance in diagnosing and recommending referrals for over 50 sight-threatening eye diseases (De Fauw et al., 2018).
c. Challenges: Integration into existing healthcare workflows and ensuring consistent performance across diverse patient populations.

8.6 Lessons learned and future improvement areas

Several challenges must be addressed when implementing AI in healthcare, such as problems with data quality, infrastructure constraints, ethical dilemmas, and legal restrictions. While digitizing health records has been a major priority over the last ten years, the upcoming years will be devoted to analyzing this abundance of data to produce new insights, enhance clinical results, and create cutting-edge solutions. Expanding translational AI research and providing medical practitioners with the tools to use AI technology efficiently are necessary to overcome these challenges. Leaders and practitioners can adopt AI-augmented systems thanks to digital upskilling, which will promote innovation and improve patient care. To successfully integrate AI into healthcare, several crucial factors must be considered. To minimize bias and enhance their ability to generalize across populations, AI models should be trained on datasets that are both representative and diverse. Figure 2.6 shows an infographic highlighting key success factors and challenges in implementing patient-friendly medicinal AI tools, based on case study insights.

AI decision-making procedures must be transparent and explicable to gain patients' and clinicians' trust. Adoption will be promoted, and operations will be streamlined with seamless integration into current procedures, such as clinical practices and EHR systems. Maintaining performance, integrating new medical information, and tackling new difficulties all depend on the ongoing assessment and updating of AI technologies. Robust frameworks that protect data and address ethical issues must prioritize ethical concerns and patient privacy. Lastly, encouraging cooperation among AI researchers, medical professionals, and patients ensures that AI technologies align with the requirements and preferences of the real world. Healthcare may use AI to provide ethical, efficient, and patient-friendly solutions by addressing these issues.

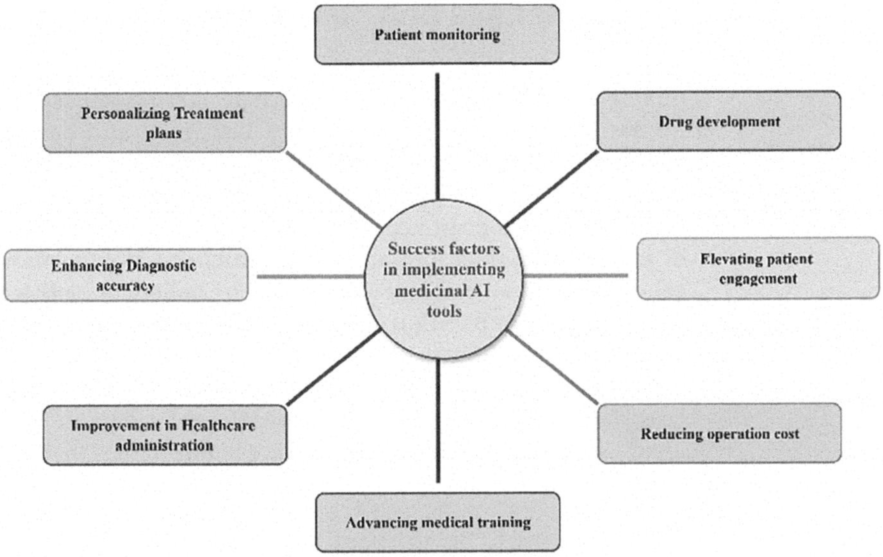

A

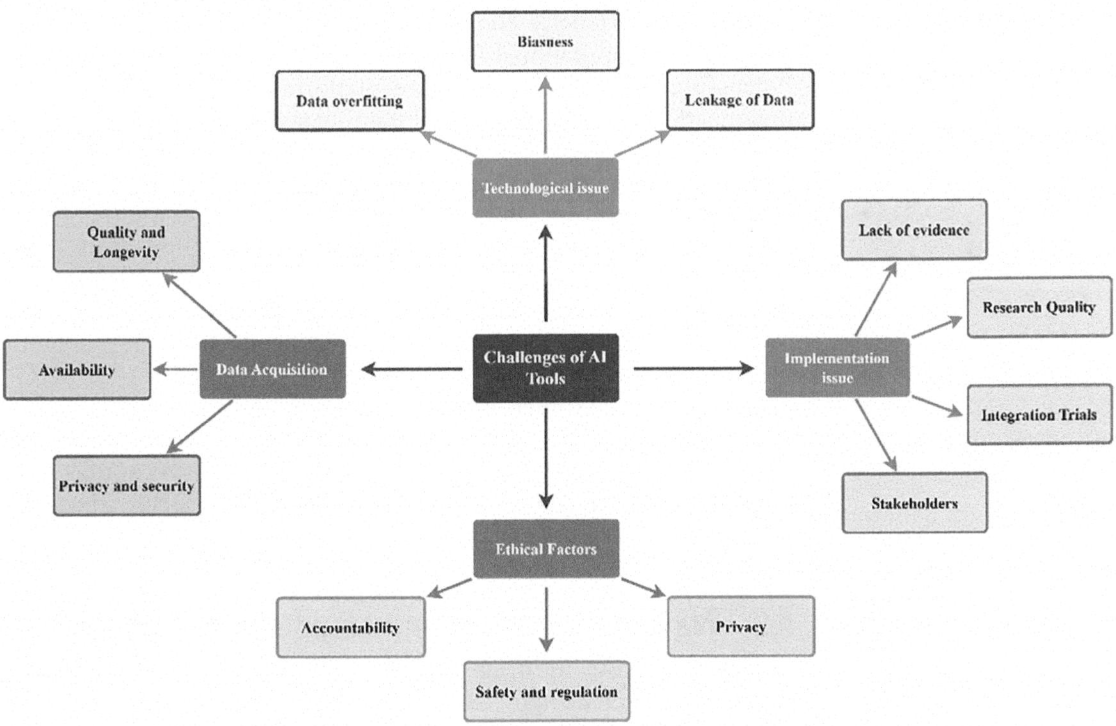

Fig. 2.6 Key factors and barriers in deploying patient-centric AI tools in healthcare: A dual-framework illustrating critical success factors and major challenges—technological, ethical, and operational—in implementing AI-driven solutions in clinical settings.

9 Challenges and limitations

AI-based drug discovery faces significant obstacles related to data quality and completeness. Issues such as missing values, inconsistent formatting, and inaccuracies within biological and chemical databases can greatly hinder the reliability and effectiveness of AI models, ultimately impacting predictive accuracy and research outcomes. For example, incorrect predictions resulting from missing annotations or inconsistent data formats can obstruct the identification of critical drug candidates. To overcome these challenges, substantial data cleaning and imputation approaches are necessary. Furthermore, ensuring data validity and reliability is crucial, as datasets from multiple sources can vary in quality. Standardizing data collection processes and validating datasets are essential for guaranteeing that AI algorithms operate with accurate and reliable data.

9.1 Computational and resource constraints

The computational demands of AI in drug discovery are substantial, particularly when processing large-scale datasets such as genomic sequences or extensive chemical libraries. These tasks often require advanced computational resources, including GPUs (Graphics Processing Unit) and cloud-based platforms. However, for smaller organizations, accessing and maintaining such infrastructure can be both challenging and cost-prohibitive. Another concern is the limited transparency of certain AI models, especially DL architectures, which are often perceived as "black boxes" due to the difficulty in interpreting their decision-making processes. The absence of interpretability in drug discovery models may reduce confidence and hinder proper verification. To tackle this issue, interpretation tools such as SHapley Additive Explanations (SHAP) and Local Interpretable Model-Agnostic Explanations (LIME) have been developed. SHAP assigns numerical values to each feature to quantify its impact on the model's output, while LIME constructs an interpretable model in the vicinity of a particular prediction to mimic the behavior of the complex model, making it easier to understand how that specific decision was reached (Zhu et al., 2024).

9.2 Navigating ethical and compliance challenges

Implementing AI in drug discovery introduces significant ethical and legal challenges, especially around patient privacy, algorithmic fairness, and regulatory adherence. It is essential to comply with stringent standards set by authorities such as the United States Food and Drug Administration (US FDA) to ensure drug safety and effectiveness. In addition, safeguarding sensitive health data requires alignment with privacy regulations like the General Data Protection Regulation and the Health Insurance Portability and Accountability Act, emphasizing responsible data handling and patient confidentiality. Building trust in AI systems involves proactively addressing algorithmic bias, securing sensitive data, and promoting transparency. It is the duty of researchers and developers to build AI systems that uphold fairness, undergo thorough validation, and adhere strictly to relevant ethical and legal standards, promoting accountable and trustworthy innovation in the healthcare sector.

10 Future directions and emerging trends

AI and ML are expected to revolutionize drug discovery and development. These technologies enable the rapid analysis of large-scale biological and chemical datasets, expediting the design of new compounds, forecasting drug-target and drug-drug interactions, and advancing disease insights through multiomics integration. Moving forward, the continued progress of AI-driven drug discovery will rely on robust partnerships between academic institutions and the pharmaceutical industry, promoting more precise disease modeling and the creation of highly targeted therapeutic interventions.

10.1 Advancements in AI technologies

AI has made significant advancements in various aspects of drug discovery. It comprises various path-breaking changes, such as virtual screening of large datasets and drug repurposing of small molecules and proven drugs. Also, many advancements can be observed in the areas of DL, RL, and other technologies.

10.1.1 Influence of quantum computing on drug discovery

Molecular simulation of complexes is a vital step for the study of their dynamic behavior; therefore, it's an important parameter for drug discovery. In this process, quantum computing can be an imperative factor that transforms it to the next level. Quantum computers utilize qubits to execute the superposition and entanglement of the simulation precisely and rapidly, which helps researchers study and model intricate biomolecular interactions. With the help of quantum computing, rapid treatment with a personalized approach can be facilitated.

10.1.2 Effect of edge computing and federated learning

Combining quantum computing with edge computing and federated learning offers a transformative pathway for drug discovery, particularly by strengthening data privacy and security while enabling decentralized, high-performance analysis across diverse research environments. These technologies are expected to aid in a more personalized approach to disease treatment by curating and securing patient data and suggesting predictive analyses using AI.

10.2 Combination with other omics technologies

A combination of several omics methodologies can be a revolutionary step in drug discovery. This will help in understanding the complex and intricate biological data and will facilitate a more personalized and advanced approach to disease treatment.

10.2.1 Integrating genomics, proteomics, and metabolomics data

The analysis of combined data from different omics layers can be a holistic way to identify a drug target or a pathway that may have been overlooked due to focusing on a single layer, and it will help in understanding intricate biological processes within cellular systems more precisely. This integrative and comprehensive approach will aid in accurate drug target and pathway prediction, which will help in reducing off-target drug delivery and the toxicity produced thereafter.

10.2.2 Multimodal data analysis

The vast datasets of the drug discovery process can be effectively analyzed and evaluated using multimodal data analysis approaches of AI/ML technologies. This approach can streamline data preparation by automating tasks such as preprocessing, normalization, and dataset integration, thereby significantly reducing the time and effort required in early-stage data handling. In addition, AI algorithms are able to examine numerous data streams simultaneously, uncovering intricate biological correlations that may help design new therapeutics or repurpose old ones while reducing adverse effects.

11 Conclusion

This chapter concludes by highlighting the revolutionary impact of AI in drug discovery and healthcare, which is driving a fundamental shift in the way pharmaceutical research and patient care are approached. AI is accelerating the typically prolonged and complex drug development processes through data-driven solutions, enabling precise predictions and spurring innovation at an unprecedented level. Molecular research and the development of new therapeutics have been made possible by integrating various chemical and biological data sets using standardized formats and sophisticated data mining techniques. AI-driven drug development will only be successful if obstacles like data heterogeneity, quality problems, and ethical issues are resolved. Effective data management and organization, which include robust curation, security, annotation, and version control processes, are necessary for maximizing the value of data assets. By prioritizing data security and privacy, pharmaceutical companies can protect intellectual property, ensure regulatory compliance, and even build stakeholder trust. AI promises to revolutionize the way people manage their health, and its influence extends beyond drug discovery into the realm of patient-centric healthcare. The development of personalized and user-centric medical technologies, informed by continuous real-world data, holds the promise to redefine healthcare delivery, enhance patient outcomes, and foster greater patient empowerment. Realizing these benefits, however, requires addressing key challenges such as effective data integration, ethical governance, and maintaining high standards of quality. Unlocking the full capabilities of AI will depend on fostering interdisciplinary collaboration and aligning technological innovation with real clinical demands. By focusing on both advanced computational tools and the human dimensions of healthcare, AI can transform global health systems into more inclusive, efficient, and equitable models. Embracing AI as a catalyst for innovation while upholding trust, transparency, and ethical responsibility will be vital for shaping the future of drug discovery and healthcare. This chapter has underscored these critical principles and offers a strategic vision for leveraging AI to create a more connected and health-empowered world.

References

Abatan, S.M., Olayemi, M., 2014. The role of statistical software in data analysis. Int. J. Appl. Res. Stud. 3, 2278–9480.

Aziz, M.H.A., Rowe, C., Southwood, R., Nogid, A., Berman, S., Gustafson, K., 2024. A scoping review of artificial intelligence within pharmacy education. Am. J. Pharm. Educ. 1553-6467. 88 (1). Available from: https://pdf.sciencedirectassets.com/783535/1-s2.0-S0002945924X00029/1-s2.0-S0002945923045539/main.pdf?. doi:10.1016/j.ajpe.2023.100615.

Baker, A., Perov, Y., Middleton, K., Baxter, J., Mullarkey, D., Sangar, D., Butt, M., DoRosario, A., Saurabh Johri, A., 2020. Comparison of artificial intelligence and human doctors for the purpose of triage and diagnosis. Front. Artif. Intell. 2624-8212. 3. doi:10.3389/frai.2020.543405.

Ballester, P.J., Mitchell, J.B.O., 2010. A machine learning approach to predicting protein-ligand binding affinity with applications to molecular docking. Bioinformatics. 1460-2059. 26 (9), 1169–1175. doi:10.1093/bioinformatics/btq112.

Bender, A., Cortes-Ciriano, I., 2021. Artificial intelligence in drug discovery: what is realistic, what are illusions? Part 2: a discussion of chemical and biological data. Drug Discov. Today. 1359-6446. 26 (4), 1040–1052. doi:10.1016/j.drudis.2020.11.037.

Blbas, H.T.A., 2024. Descriptive statistics. Recent Advances in Biostatistics. doi:10.5772/intechopen.1002179.

Cheng, F., Kovács, I.A., Barabási, A.L., 2019. Network-based prediction of drug combinations. Nat. Commun. 2041-1723. 10 (1). Available from: http://www.nature.com/ncomms/index.html. doi:10.1038/s41467-019-09186-x.

Cock, P.J.A., Antao, T., Chang, J.T., Chapman, B.A., Cox, C.J., Dalke, A., Friedberg, I., Hamelryck, T., Kauff, F., Wilczynski, B., De Hoon, M.J.L., 2009. Biopython: freely available Python tools for computational molecular biology and bioinformatics. Bioinformatics. 1460-2059. 25 (11), 1422–1423. doi:10.1093/bioinformatics/btp163.

De Cao, N., Kipf, T., 2018. MolGAN: an implicit generative model for small molecular graphs. arXiv. 2331-8422. Available from: https://arxiv.org. doi:10.48550/arxiv.1805.11973.

De Fauw, J., Ledsam, J.R., Romera-Paredes, B., Nikolov, S., Tomasev, N., Blackwell, S., Askham, H., Glorot, X., O'Donoghue, B., Visentin, D., van den Driessche, G., Lakshminarayanan, B., Meyer, C., Mackinder, F., Bouton, S., Ayoub, K., Chopra, R., King, D., Karthikesalingam, A., Hughes, C.O., Raine, R., Hughes, J., Sim, D.A., Egan, C., Tufail, A., Montgomery, H., Hassabis, D., Rees, G., Back, T., Khaw, P.T., Suleyman, M., Cornebise, J., Keane, P.A., Ronneberger, O., 2018. Clinically applicable deep learning for diagnosis and referral in retinal disease. Nat. Med. 1546-170X. 24 (9), 1342–1350. Available from: http://www.nature.com/nm/index.html. doi:10.1038/s41591-018-0107-6.

Dey, S., Luo, H., Fokoue, A., Jianying, H., Zhang, P., 2018. Predicting adverse drug reactions through interpretable deep learning framework. BMC Bioinformatics. 1471-2105. 19 (S21). doi:10.1186/s12859-018-2544-0.

Domine, D., Devillers, J., Chastrette, M., Karcher, W., 1993. Non-linear mapping for structure-activity and structure-property modelling. J. Chemom. 0886-9383. 7 (4), 227–242. doi:10.1002/cem.1180070402.

Duvenaud, D., Maclaurin, D., Aguilera-Iparraguirre, J., Gómez-Bombarelli, R., Hirzel, T., Aspuru-Guzik, A., Adams, R.P., 2015. Convolutional networks on graphs for learning molecular fingerprints. In: Advances in Neural Information Processing Systems. 10495258. Neural information processing systems foundation, United States, pp. 2224–2232.

Fisher, J.L., Williams, K.T., Schneider, L.J., Keebaugh, A.J., German, C.L., Hott, A.M., Singh, N., Clewell, R.A., 2024. Evaluation of QSAR models for tissue-specific predictive toxicology and risk assessment of military-relevant chemical exposures: a systematic review. Comput. Toxicol. 2468-1113. 32. Available from: https://www.sciencedirect.com/science/journal/24681113. doi:10.1016/j.comtox.2024.100329.

Frades, I., Matthiesen, R., 2009. Overview on techniques in cluster analysis. In: Methods in Molecular Biology, Vol. 593. Springer Science and Business Media LLC, pp. 81–107. doi:10.1007/978-1-60327-194-3_5.

Hastings, J., Owen, G., Dekker, A., Ennis, M., Kale, N., Muthukrishnan, V., Turner, S., Swainston, N., Mendes, P., Steinbeck, C., 2016. ChEBI in 2016: improved services and an expanding collection of metabolites. Nucleic Acids Res. 0305-1048. 44 (D1), D1214. doi:10.1093/nar/gkv1031.

Kaur, P., Stoltzfus, J., Yellapu, V., 2018. Descriptive statistics. Int. J. Acad. Med. 2455-5568. 4 (1), 60. doi:10.4103/ijam.ijam_7_18.

Kolluri, S., Lin, J., Liu, R., Zhang, Y., Zhang, W., 2022. Machine learning and artificial intelligence in pharmaceutical research and development: a review. AAPS J. 1550-7416. 24 (1). doi:10.1208/s12248-021-00644-3.

Koromina, M., Pandi, M.T., Patrinos, G.P., 2019. Rethinking drug repositioning and development with artificial intelligence, machine learning, and omics. OMICS. 1557-8100. 23 (11), 539–548. Available from: www.liebertonline.com/omi. doi:10.1089/omi.2019.0151.

Liu, H., Zhao, Y., Zhang, L., Chen, X., 2018. Anti-cancer drug response prediction using neighbor-based collaborative filtering with global effect removal. Mol. Ther. Nucleic Acids. 2162-2531. 13, 303–311. doi:10.1016/j.omtn.2018.09.011.

Mak, K.-K., Wong, Y.-H., Pichika, M.R., 2024. Artificial intelligence in drug discovery and development. In: Drug Discovery and Evaluation: Safety and Pharmacokinetic Assays. Springer Science and Business Media LLC, pp. 1461–1498. doi:10.1007/978-3-031-35529-5_92.

Malone, J., Holloway, E., Adamusiak, T., Kapushesky, M., Zheng, J., Kolesnikov, N., Zhukova, A., Brazma, A., Parkinson, H., 2010. Modeling sample variables with an experimental factor ontology. Bioinformatics. 1367-4811. 26 (8), 1112–1118. doi:10.1093/bioinformatics/btq099.

Marshall, G., Jonker, L., 2011. An introduction to inferential statistics: a review and practical guide. Radiography. 1078-8174. 17 (1), e1. doi:10.1016/j.radi.2009.12.006.

Mitchell, J.B., 2018. Artificial intelligence in pharmaceutical research and development. Future Med. Chem. 1756-8927. 10 (13), 1529–1531. Available from: http://www.future-science.com/loi/fmc. doi:10.4155/fmc-2018-0158.

Noorain, V.S., Parveen, B., Parveen, R., 2023. Artificial intelligence in drug formulation and development: applications and future prospects. Curr. Drug Metab. 1389-2002. 24 (9), 622–634. doi:10.2174/0113892002265786230921062205.

O'Boyle, N.M., Banck, M., James, C.A., Morley, C., Vandermeersch, T., Hutchison, G.R., 2011. Open Babel: an open chemical toolbox. J. Cheminform. 1758-2946. 3 (10). Available from: http://www.jcheminf.com/content/pdf/1758-2946-3-33.pdf. doi:10.1186/1758-2946-3-33Ireland.

Phyu, T.N., 2009. Citeseer Survey of classification techniques in data mining. In: Proceedings of the international multiconference of engineers and computer scientists, Vol. 1. pp. 727–731.

Rajkomar, A., Oren, E., Chen, K., Dai, A.M., Hajaj, N., Hardt, M., Liu, P.J., Liu, X., Marcus, J., Sun, M., Sundberg, P., Yee, H., Zhang, K., Zhang, Y., Flores, G., Duggan, G.E., Irvine, J., Le, Q., Litsch, K., Mossin, A., Tansuwan, J., Wang, D., Wexler, J., Wilson, J., Ludwig, D., Volchenboum, S.L., Chou, K., Pearson, M., Madabushi, S., Shah, N.H., Butte, A.J., Howell, M.D., Cui, C., Corrado, G.S., Dean, J., 2018. Scalable and accurate deep learning with electronic health records. Npj Digit. Med. 2398-6352. 1 (1). Available from: https://www.nature.com/npjdigitalmed/. doi:10.1038/s41746-018-0029-1.

Salih, A., Raisi-Estabragh, Z., Galazzo, I.B., Radeva P. Petersen S.E., Lekadir, K. Menegaz G., 2025. A Perspective on Explainable Artificial Intelligence Methods: SHAP and LIME. Adv. Intell. Syst. 7, 2400304. doi:10.1002/aisy.202400304 .

Sansone, S.A., Rocca-Serra, P., Field, D., Maguire, E., Taylor, C., Hofmann, O., Fang, H., Neumann, S., Tong, W., Amaral-Zettler, L., Begley, K., Booth, T., Bougueleret, L., Burns, G., Chapman, B., Clark, T., Coleman, L.A., Copeland, J., Das, S., De Daruvar, A., De Matos, P., Dix, I., Edmunds, S., Evelo, C.T., Forster, M.J., Gaudet, P., Gilbert, J., Goble, C., Griffin, J.L., Jacob, D., Kleinjans, J., Harland, L., Haug, K., Hermjakob, H., Sui, S.J.H., Laederach, A., Liang, S., Marshall, S., McGrath, A., Merrill, E., Reilly, D., Roux, M., Shamu, C.E., Shang, C.A., Steinbeck, C., Trefethen, A., Williams-Jones, B., Wolstencroft, K., Xenarios, I., Hide, W., 2012. Toward interoperable bioscience data. Nat. Genet. 1546-1718. 44 (2), 121–126. doi:10.1038/ng.1054.

Selvamuthu, D., Das, D., 2024. Introduction to probability, statistical methods, design of experiments and statistical quality control. In: University Texts in the Mathematical Sciences. Springer Nature Singapore. doi:10.1007/978-981-99-9363-5.

Shah, P., Thakkar, D., Panchal, N., Jha, R., 2024. Artificial intelligence and machine learning in drug discovery. In: Converging Pharmacy Science and Engineering in Computational Drug Discovery. IGI Global, India, pp. 54–75. Available from: https://www.igi-global.com/book/converging-pharmacy-science-engineering-computational/334222. doi:10.4018/979-8-3693-2897-2.ch003.

Trillo-Montero, D., Cosano-Lucena, S., Gonzalez-Redondo, M., Luna-Rodriguez, J.J., Santiago, I., 2023. Design and development of a relational database management system (RDBMS) with open source tools for the processing of data monitored in a set of photovoltaic (PV) plants. Appl. Sci. 2076-3417. 13 (3), 1357. doi:10.3390/app13031357.

Wei, D., Liu, C., Zheng, X., Li, Y., 2019. Comprehensive anticancer drug response prediction based on a simple cell line-drug complex network model. BMC Bioinformatics. 1471-2105. 20 (1). doi:10.1186/s12859-019-2608-9.

Yap, C.W., 2011. PaDEL-descriptor: an open source software to calculate molecular descriptors and fingerprints. J. Comput. Chem. 1096-987X. 32 (7), 1466–1474. doi:10.1002/jcc.21707.

You, J., McLeod, R.D., Hu, P., 2019. Predicting drug-target interaction network using deep learning model. Comput. Biol. Chem. 1476-9271. 80, 90–101. doi:10.1016/j.compbiolchem.2019.03.016.

Zhang, T., Li, H., Xi, H., Stanton, R.V., Rotstein, S.H., 2012. HELM: a hierarchical notation language for complex biomolecule structure representation. J. Chem. Inf. Model. 1549-960X. 52 (10), 2796–2806. Available from: http://pubs.acs.org/journal/jcisd8. doi:10.1021/ci3001925.

Zhu, Q., Cai, Y., Fang, Y., Yang, Y., Chen, C., Fan, L., Nguyen, A., 2024. Samba: semantic segmentation of remotely sensed images with state space model. Heliyon. 2405-8440. 10 (19), e38495. doi:10.1016/j.heliyon.2024.e38495.

3

Deep learning for protein folding

Tapobrata Lahiri[a] **and Rajkrishna Mondal**[b]
[a]*Department of Applied Sciences, Indian Institute of Information Technology Allahabad, Prayagraj, Uttar Pradesh, India*
[b]*Biotechnolgy, Nagaland University, Kohima, Nagaland, India*

1 Backdrop

If proteins function as the fundamental molecular machinery within living cells, then the complex process of protein folding stands as the most important determinant in achieving their biologically active, three-dimensional conformation. For a long time, it has been very hard for computers to figure out a protein's native, functional structure just by utilizing its linear amino acid sequence.

In the past, progress in this field has oscillated between stagnation and advancement. However, there has been a significant breakthrough in the last few years. The extraction of intramolecular communication constraints from evolutionary trajectories, the distillation of sequence-structure correlations derived from preexisting structural datasets, the integration of homology templates from protein data banks (PDBs), and the iterative refinement of coarsely predicted molecular structures to high-resolution conformations—each of these aspects, once governed by traditional energy-based models and stochastic sampling heuristics, has now been revolutionized by the paradigm-shifting adoption of deep neural networks (DNNs).

Here in, we will undertake a rigorous reassessment of deep learning (DL)-driven structural prediction methods, study their underlying classifications in depth, elucidate the mysterious computational foundations within the so-called black box, and explore the transition from monomeric to ensemble-level structural interpretation. Furthermore, we will critically interrogate the inherent limitations and computational hurdles that constrain the effectiveness and applicability of these pioneering methods.

The AI Frontier in Molecular Modelling and Drug Designing. https://doi.org/10.1016/B978-0-443-40338-5.00015-9

2 Protein folding: The problem

During the complex translation process, the genetic blueprint is converted into a polypeptide chain. Subsequently, this nascent chain undergoes a hierarchical cascade of structural transformations, which are determined by a wide range of intermolecular interactions, including both short-range and long-range contacts. These interactions create next-level structural motifs such as α-helices and β-sheets, which then come together to form tertiary architectures that define the protein's three-dimensional shape, as depicted in Fig. 3.1.

For multisubunit protein complexes, the coordinated assembly of the discrete polypeptide chains culminates in the formation of a quaternary structure, which is essential for functional integrity. This complex sequence of folding events can either proceed autonomously, governed by intrinsic physicochemical principles, or require the intervention of molecular chaperones and auxiliary cofactors, which ensure precise orchestration of structural maturation.

Structural biologists have elucidated the three-dimensional architecture of over 200,000 proteins across all domains of life using empirical techniques like protein X-ray crystallography, nuclear magnetic resonance spectroscopy, and cryo-electron microscopy. These experimentally obtained structures, archived in the PDB, encode the Cartesian coordinates of atomic positions in three-dimensional space, providing an invaluable framework for structural and functional insights. Despite these advances, predicting protein 3D structure from sequence information alone remains the most complex and daunting challenge in molecular biology. Computational biologists have used progressively refined algorithmic approaches to fill this gap, starting with homology modeling, which assumes that proteins that share significant sequence similarity will adopt similar structural folds. Subsequent advances have incorporated coevolutionary principles,

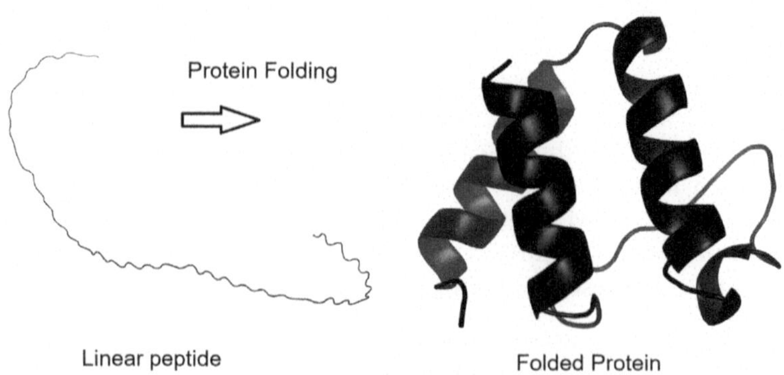

Fig. 3.1 Protein folding definition. The process of transforming a straight chain of amino acids into a unique and functional three-dimensional shape defines protein folding.

according to the empirical reflection that spatially proximal residues within a protein often undergo correlated evolutionary changes. By examining coevolutionary patterns across multiple sequence alignments (MSA), researchers have inferred residue-residue contact maps, exploiting these constraints to improve structural predictions. Over the years, predictive methods have evolved through incremental refinement, integrating advanced homology-based modeling techniques and residue distance constraints derived from MSAs. These iterative improvements have gradually strengthened the precision and consistency of computational structure predictions, ultimately leading to the emergence of sophisticated DL frameworks that now define the forefront of the field. A comparison flowchart between DL-based and conventional approaches for predicting the protein 3D structure is shown in Fig. 3.2.

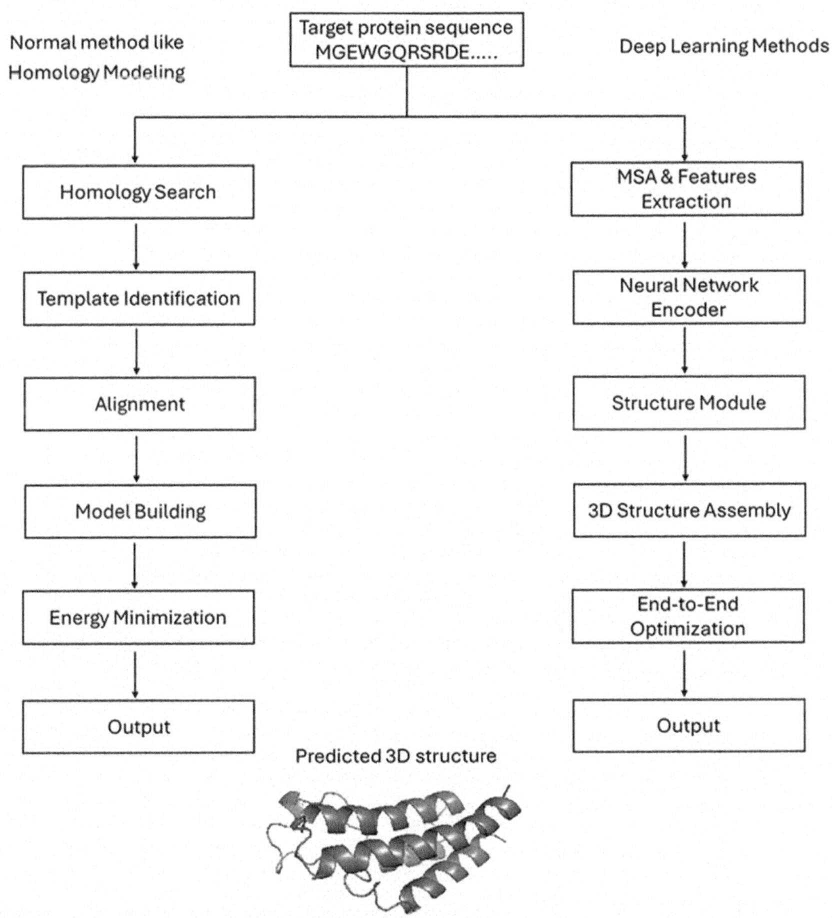

Fig. 3.2 Homology modeling vs. deep learning-based method. Flowchart: Traditional vs. deep learning protein structure prediction.

3 Complexity linked with protein-folding

Levinthal's paradox (Levinthal, 1968), a thought experiment that demonstrates the gigantic number of possible conformations a protein could theoretically adopt, is the best example of the complexity of the protein folding problem. The paradox emphasizes that it would take more time than the age of the universe for a protein to discover its proper shape if it were to randomly search through every potential structure.

Following straightforward mathematical illustrations based on a condensed protein model can demonstrate the complexity:

3.1 Exponential conformational space—levinthal-style

Assume that, on average, each amino acid residue can take on s different pertinent conformations (rotamer/backbone states). The number of potential global conformations for a protein with x residues.

$$N_{conf} = s^{x}$$

Hypothetically, assume the protein has 100 residues, and each residue has 1000 possible local states.

$$N_{conf} = 1000^{100}$$

$$N_{conf} = 10^{300}$$

Suppose a computer tests 10^{13} conformations/second. Therefore, the required time for the computer to complete the task will be.

$$T = \frac{10^{300}}{10^{13}} \text{ seconds} = \sim 1.4 \times 10^{10} \text{ years}$$

The worst-case search space is astronomically large, as demonstrated by the above math. Actually:

The physical energy landscape is not random; rather, it has a funnel-like structure that directs folding.

To avoid a thorough search, folding makes use of kinetics, local interactions, and hierarchical assembly.

For many proteins, algorithms use physics, heuristics, machine learning, and coarse-graining to efficiently find native states; however, worst-case hardness is still a crucial theoretical limit.

4 Deep learning

DL, a definitive category of machine learning, usually works with big data sets that have labels. DL algorithms can make predictions about what follows based on new data they haven't seen before.

These algorithms help solve many problems, such as recognizing images, processing natural language, and recognizing speech. DL uses multilayered artificial neural networks to find and comprehend complex patterns in data. The fact that DL models can learn hierarchical representations of data is one of the main reasons they are superior to traditional machine learning algorithms. The application of DNN architectures to protein structure prediction is typically tailored to the nature and format of the input data. In this field, the most popular types of DNNs are convolutional neural networks (CNNs), recurrent neural networks (RNNs), graph neural networks (GNNs), long short-term memory (LSTM) networks, transformers, and generative adversarial networks (GANs) (Qin et al., 2024).

4.1 DL architecture

4.1.1 Convolutional neural networks

CNNs were first designed to recognize images, but they have also been very effective at learning complicated spatial patterns in biological data across one, two, and three dimensions. Pertaining to protein structure prediction, CNNs are particularly useful for analyzing protein sequences, contact maps, and spatial morphology.

A emblematic CNN architecture harbors several key components:

- The convolutional layer uses filters to extract local features from the input data.
- Pooling layers, which reduce spatial dimensions, improve computational efficiency, and enable the learning of hierarchical features.

Activation functions, which introduce nonlinearities to capture complex relationships in the data, are essential components in neural networks.

Fully connected layers, which combine the learned features and make the final forecasts.

CNNs can be adapted to various representations of protein data:

- 1D CNNs are useful for linear amino acid sequence analysis and extracting local sequence motifs.
- 2D CNNs are commonly applied for predicting t contact or distance maps, which represent residue-residue relationships as 2D matrices.
- 3D CNNs can model the spatial transformation of proteins by operating directly on a 3D voxelized representation of the atomic structure.

Overall, CNNs provide a powerful framework for hierarchical feature extraction and have become a fundamental component in modern protein structure prediction pipelines.

4.1.2 Recurrent neural networks

RNNs are good at working with data that comes in a sequence. RNNs are a good choice for modeling protein folding because it occurs in a sequence. Recurrent connections, hidden states, and shared weights are some of the most important components of RNNs. The hidden states serve as a type of memory, enabling the network to identify dependencies and patterns within sequences. LSTM networks and gated recurrent units are the two main types of RNNs. Both use a gating mechanism to regulate the flow of information, which allows them to retain or discard data over long sequences.

4.1.3 Generative adversarial networks

GANs are DL models that are exceptionally robust, consisting of two neural networks: a generator and a discriminator. They can create very realistic data when they work together. GANs aren't direct competitors to models like AlphaFold2 or RoseTTAFold, but they do open up new possibilities in areas such as creating new protein designs, filling in gaps in structural data, and improving experimental data.

4.1.4 Transformers

The self-attention mechanism remains the most important part of the Transformer architecture. It has changed the way we predict protein structures, especially with models like DeepMind's AlphaFold2 and Baker Lab's RoseTTAFold. The self-attention mechanism effectively captures complex interactions between amino acids, regardless of their position in the sequence. This is different from traditional RNNs, which have trouble with long-range dependencies. In addition, Transformers can be trained quickly on large datasets because they can run multiple processes at once. This makes them great for computational biology tasks.

5 DL for sequence-based structure prediction

The outstanding performance of AlphaFold2 (Jumper et al., 2021) at the 14th Critical Assessment of Techniques for Protein Structure Prediction (CASP14) in December 2020 initiated a global research surge aimed at enhancing sequence-based protein three-dimensional structure prediction via DL methodologies (Pereira et al., 2021). New methods have tried to overcome the conventional constraints of in silico techniques. There are two main types of DL models workable for predicting protein structure: alignment-based and protein language model-based (Jänes and Beltrao, 2024), a few of which are listed in Table 3.1. Alignment-based predictors, including AlphaFold2 and RoseTTAFold (Baek et al., 2021), produce input

Table 3.1 List of deep learning-based protein structure prediction tools.

Name of the tool	Feature	References, Year
MetaPSICOV	Coevolution-based prediction of residue contacts in proteins	Jones et al. (2015)
DeepCov	Improved contact prediction in nonhomologous protein complexes	Jones and Kandathil (2018)
DeepFragLib	Building protein-specific fragment libraries from amino acid residues	Wang et al. (2019)
AlphaFold2	Reliable prediction and quality scoring of protein monomer and complex structures	Jumper et al. (2021)
TrRosetta	Fast and precise de novo modeling of protein monomers	Yang et al. (2020)
CopulaNet	Protein complex modeling using coevolution signals from sequence alignments	Ju et al. (2021)
RGN2	Fast protein structure prediction from single sequences with language models	Chowdhury et al. (2022)
SPOT-Contact-LM	The protein contact map narrows the accuracy gap in predicting homologous and nonhomologous complexes	Singh et al. (2022)
ColabFold	Efficient and scalable modeling of large protein complexes	Mirdita et al. (2022)
Umol	Evoformer processes protein sequences and ligand SMILES to model protein-ligand complexes	Bryant et al. (2024)
ESMFold	Faster atomic-level protein structure predictions with protein language modeling, replacing MSA input	Lin et al. (2023)
IgFold	Deep learning for predicting 3D structures of antibody variable regions	Ruffolo et al. (2022)

features that encompass MSA depth data and pairwise distance maps, frequently supplemented by homologous proteins with established structures. Table 3.2 lists common datasets used for training and validation. The next step in the structural module shows the three main-chain atoms (nitrogen, alpha-carbon, and carbon) of each residue as a triangle. The neural network learns to adjust the positions of these triangles to correctly form the protein structure. The goal is to get the most out of coevolutionary information from MSAs while using as little known structural template data as possible. After making a rough first model, AlphaFold2 uses a repeated refinement process to improve the accuracy of the protein's 3D structure by optimizing all model parameters at once from start to finish. Even though all alignment-based DL predictors use MSA and coevolutionary data, they still show differences in how well they work. Therefore, there is a lot of room to explore important decision-making factors that could help improve performance.

Table 3.2 Datasets used for training and validation for deep learning-based structure predictors.

Ruffolo et al. (2022) PDB (protein data bank)	**Experimentally determined 3D protein structures**	**>220,000 entries (2025)**	**Supervised learning, training/test sets**
UniProt	Protein sequence database with annotations	>250 M sequences	Pretraining large protein LMs
UniRef50/90	Clustered UniProt at 50% or 90% sequence identity	Millions of sequences	Efficient model training, reduces redundancy
CASP (Critical Assessment of Structure Prediction)	Biennial blind challenge for structure prediction	~100 targets per round	Benchmarking DL models
CATH/SCOPe	Structural classification databases	~150 K domains	Evaluating fold-level generalization
PDB (Protein Data Bank)	Experimentally determined 3D protein structures	>220,000 entries (2025)	Supervised learning, training/test sets

Alignment-based predictors depend on the depth of MSA, which is a key part of how they work. However, many proteins, particularly newly evolved or engineered ones, have shallow MSAs, which makes these methods less useful. Protein language model-based predictors solve this problem by using large datasets to train on masked amino acid predictions from many input sequences. Some of these models are RGN2 (Chowdhury et al., 2022), ESMFold (Lin et al., 2023), OmegaFold (Wu et al., 2022), and EMBER2 (Weissenow et al., 2022). These language-based methods are usually faster than AlphaFold2, but they cannot achieve the same level of accuracy when deep MSA is available. For proteins with shallow MSA depth, language-based predictors often perform better than alignment-based methods, though.

6 Network architecture of alphafold2

AlphaFold2's network architecture is an avant-garde DL system that can predict the protein 3D structure with higher accuracy (Jumper et al., 2021), as shown in Fig. 3.3. It is often said to have two main parts that are connected to each other, with the first part being data processing:

6.1 Input processing and feature engineering

MSA generation: This is a crucial first step. AlphaFold2 takes the protein sequence information of the query and searches massive protein sequence databases (e.g., UniRef, Big Fantastic Database (BFD),

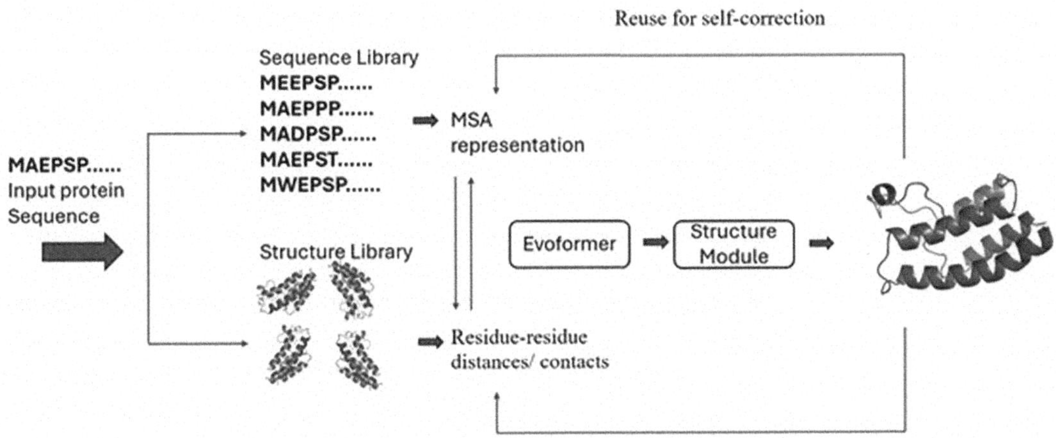

Fig. 3.3 AlphaFold2 workflow. Schematic representation of AlphaFold2 network architecture.

MGnify) to find evolutionarily related sequences. These similar sequences are then aligned, creating an MSA. The idea is that amino acids important for protein function and structure tend to coevolve across species, providing important clues about which residues are nearby in the 3D structure.

Template search (optional but helpful): AlphaFold2 also searches the PDB for existing protein structures that are similar to the query sequence. While it may predict new structures, templates can provide valuable initial structural information.

Feature representation: The MSA and, if available, template information are converted into numerical "features" that the neural network can understand. These include information about amino acid identity, sequence relationships, and predicted residue-residue distances or contacts.

Evoformer blocks ("trunks"): This is the core of AlphaFold2's prediction engine—a series of stacked neural network blocks (often 48 in the original model).

Transformer-like architecture: Evoformer is based on the Transformer architecture, which is highly effective at processing natural language. The "attention process" helps it learn how protein sequences and sequences in the MSA are connected over long distances.

Joint reasoning on MSA and pairwise representations: One important new feature of Evoformer is that it can improve two main models simultaneously and repeatedly.

MSA representation: Information about individual amino acid sequences in the MSA.

Pairwise representation: A 2D matrix representing the relationship (e.g., distance or contact) between every pair of residues in the target protein.

Information exchange: Evoformer blocks are designed to allow a continuous flow of information between the MSA and the pairwise representations. Updates to one representation inform and refine the other, enabling the model to "reason" in a coherent manner about evolutionary relationships and spatial constraints. This iterative refinement is crucial for accuracy.

Triangle multiplier and self-attention update: Within each Evoformer block, various attention and multiplier operations are performed to update these representations, ensuring that geometric constraints (such as triangle inequalities for distances) are implicitly learned and enforced.

Structure module: After refining the Evoformer MSA and pairwise representations, this module takes the processed information and translates it directly into a 3D protein structure.

Irreversible point attention: The Structure module uses a special form of attention that is "equivalent" to 3D rotations and translations. This means that it implicitly understands that the internal geometry of the protein should not change if the entire protein is rotated or displaced. This makes the learning task significantly easier.

Iterative 3D coordinate generation: The module iteratively refines every amino acid's 3D coordinates, builds the protein backbone, and then adds side chains.

Reuse: A powerful technique used in AlphaFold2 is "reuse". The predicted 3D structure and refined representation from one pass through Evoformer and the Structure Module can be fed back as input for the next pass. This allows the model to gradually refine its predictions, essentially self-correcting and improving accuracy over a number of iterations (typically 3 in the original model).

In short, AlphaFold2's architecture combines evolutionary information from MSA with advanced DL techniques (particularly attention processes) to create a sophisticated internal representation of protein interactions, which it translates directly into highly accurate 3D structures.

7 RoseTTAFold network architecture

The Baker Lab at the University of Washington created RoseTTAFold, a highly significant DL model for predicting the structure of proteins (Baek et al., 2021). It employs a different core architectural philosophy compared to AlphaFold2, particularly its "three-track" approach, yet it achieves similarly high accuracy.

A brief description of its network architecture is given below:

7.1 Three-track neural network

The defining feature of RoseTTAFold is its three parallel "tracks," or streams of information, that continuously exchange data:

1D sequence track: This track examines information about each residue in the protein sequence. It deals with features derived from MSA, such as patterns of amino acids, conservation, and predicted secondary structure. This track primarily works with one-dimensional sequences.

2D pairwise interaction track (distance map track): This track focuses on the relationships between pairs of amino acids. It learns to predict distances and orientations between residues, which are often derived from coevolutionary signals in an MSA. This information is represented as a 2D grid (a "distance map").

3D coordinate track: This is a new feature that makes RoseTTAFold stand out. This track works directly with the 3D atomic coordinates of the protein backbone. It improves the accuracy and timeliness of the real spatial positions of amino acids.

7.2 Information flow and communication

The key to RoseTTAFold's success is the two-way and iterative exchange of information between these three tracks. Unlike some previous models that may process 1D, then 2D, then 3D in a sequential manner, RoseTTAFold allows information to flow between all three tracks simultaneously.

For example, insights gained from the 1D sequence context can refine predicted 2D distances, which, in turn, can guide the refinement of 3D coordinates. Conversely, the geometric constraints and emerging patterns of 3D structures can help improve the understanding of 1D sequence features and 2D interactions.

This "collective reasoning" across different levels of abstraction (sequence, pairwise interactions, and 3D coordinates) allows the network to build a more coherent and accurate overall model of the folded state of the protein.

7.3 Transformer-like attention mechanisms

RoseTTAFold employs attention mechanisms akin to AlphaFold2, specifically utilizing "axial attention" and "triangular attention." However, the initial publication on RoseTTAFold delineates distinct attention mechanisms in contrast to AlphaFold2's exclusive "invariant point attention" and "triangular multiplicative update" within its Evoformer. These attention layers allow the model to determine the importance of different parts of the input data when making predictions. This enables it to identify long-range relationships between proteins.

7.4 Integration of templates (optional)

While RoseTTAFold can predict new structures, it effectively integrates information from known homologous protein structures (templates) when available. This can further improve accuracy, especially for proteins with close evolutionary relatives.

7.5 Iterative refinement (recycling)

Like AlphaFold2, RoseTTAFold uses iterative refinement, sometimes known as "recycling". The output from one pass through the network can be fed back as input for the next pass, allowing the model to progressively improve its predictions.

In short, RoseTTAFold's architecture is characterized by its innovative "three-track" design, which enables a rich, bidirectional flow of information between sequence, pairwise interactions, and 3D coordinate representation. This integrated approach, combined with modern attention mechanisms, allows it to collectively reason about protein structures at multiple levels simultaneously, resulting in highly accurate predictions.

8 Unpacking the black box of DL

People often call DL models "black boxes" because they are hard to understand, and it's difficult to figure out how they make predictions based on input data. The OpenFold team's analysis shows that the learning process progresses in steps: it starts with 1D representations, then moves on to 2D and 3D structural representations, and finally captures secondary structural elements, even though these can often be predicted from sequence information alone (Ahdritz et al., 2022). In another test, OpenFold demonstrated that their system could evaluate structural templates without using MSAs, just like classical structure prediction methods that use energy functions to rank models. This suggests that the model may have implicitly learned an energy-like function during training (Roney and Ovchinnikov, 2022).

9 CASP: A platform for showcasing the transformative power of DL

When it comes to protein structure prediction, structural biologists view the Critical Assessment of Structure Prediction (CASP) as the Olympics. Since 1994, a community-wide experiment has been carried out every two years with the main goal of assessing what we know about protein structure prediction right now. DL techniques demonstrated a notable improvement at CASP13 (2018), especially when it came to predicting the distances between amino acids. At CASP14 (2020), DeepMind's AlphaFold2 model made history by achieving previously unheard-of levels of accuracy. Many experts in the field said that the long-standing "protein folding problem" was virtually resolved for single-chain proteins because its predictions were so similar to the structures found through experimentation. This was a significant turning point in the history of science.

From the most challenging to the simplest, CASP has expanded over time to incorporate a number of prediction categories:

Template-based modeling: For proteins that can be used as templates and have a known, comparable structure.

"New Fold" or template-free modeling: Proteins without a comparable known structure necessitate a new prediction. DL has had the largest impact in this category, which is the most difficult.

Refinement: Enhancing an existing model that has flaws.

Protein complexes: Forecasting the interactions and assembly of several protein chains.

10 Performance metrics for protein-folding models

Assessing the accuracy and dependability of protein folding models requires evaluating their performance. A lot of different computational measures have been developed to objectively compare a predicted structure to the experimentally determined "ground truth" structure, although experimental validation is still the gold standard. Table 3.3 lists a few important performance indicators for protein folding models.

Table 3.3 Popular performance metrics for protein folding models.

Metric	Description	Typical use	References
GDT_TS (Global distance test—total score)	Percentage of residues within the distance cutoff of the native structure	Benchmarking accuracy in CASP	Zemla et al. (1999)
RMSD (Root mean square deviation)	Mean distance between anticipated and experimental coordinates.	Structural similarity	Kabsch (1978)
TM-score (Template modeling score)	Scale-independent similarity metric (0–1)	Fold-level comparison	Zhang and Skolnick (2004)
lDDT (Local distance difference test)/ pLDDT(predicted protein structure confidence score without needing a reference structure)	Local accuracy of predicted interatomic distances	Evaluating fine-grained accuracy	Mariani et al. (2013), Jumper et al. (2021).
Confidence/PAE (Predicted aligned error)	Model's internal reliability estimate	Filtering low-confidence predictions	Jumper et al. (2021)

11 Predicting protein structure with multiple conformations

Some proteins can have more than one biologically active shape in cells. One major problem with AlphaFold2 and other current structure predictors is that they usually only provide one best conformation for a protein. The Cfold tool (Bryant and Noé, 2024) addresses this issue by grouping structural templates together and creating separate MSAs for each group. Then, structures are predicted based on these MSAs, which are specific to each cluster. This approach makes it possible to identify different conformations. Molecular dynamics (MD) simulations are another method to explore different protein conformations. MD can generate many distinct conformational states, but these changes are often driven by physiological factors, such as ligand binding or posttranslational modifications, which are difficult to accurately replicate in silico. Consequently, capturing these dynamic transitions in a digital environment remains a significant challenge.

12 Predicting protein complex structures through subunit assembly

Protein complex structure prediction is a key area within DL-based structural biology. With the subsequent introduction of the direct coupling analysis method (Weigt et al., 2009), coevolutionary information has played a central role in predicting protein-protein interactions. Building on the achievements of AlphaFold2 in forecasting individual protein structures, AlphaFold2-Multimer (Evans et al., 2022) extended these capabilities to model interactions within multimeric complexes. The recent release of AlphaFold3 (Abramson et al., 2024) marks a significant advancement, with enhanced capabilities to predict interactions among multiple molecular entities—including proteins, nucleic acids, and small molecules—surpassing its predecessors in scope and accuracy. Despite these advancements, the prediction accuracy for protein-protein interactions remains limited, typically achieving reliable results in only 50%–70% of cases where interaction data is available. Consequently, its performance is expected to drop further in large-scale proteome studies aimed at identifying previously uncharacterized interactions. Moreover, modeling protein complexes with a large number of subunits continues to pose significant challenges, primarily due to the substantial computational resources required. As such, efficient and scalable methods remain an area of ongoing research.

13 Protein design using DL

Protein design, commonly known as inverse folding, entails the conception of a sequence of amino acids that will assume a designated three-dimensional backbone conformation. As a fundamental discipline within synthetic biology, protein design concentrates on engineering proteins with customized functions, enhanced stability, or other specific attributes (Defresne et al., 2021).

There are two primary methodologies in protein design: de novo design and protein redesign. De novo design aims to fabricate entirely new proteins from the ground up, incorporating folds and functions absent in nature. Conversely, protein redesign focuses on modifying existing protein structures to improve or alter their functional and structural properties.

The primary objective of protein design is to predict a suitable sequence for a target backbone while simultaneously ensuring that the resulting protein meets specific biochemical and biophysical characteristics, including catalytic activity, binding affinity, or thermal stability.

Traditionally, computational protein design (CPD) has relied on optimization-based methods that attempt to find sequences minimizing an energy function, ensuring correct folding and desired traits. To make the problem tractable—since it is NP-hard—these methods often employ simplifications such as fixed backbone conformations and rotamer libraries for side-chain modeling.

But the rise of DL has given us a strong, data-driven option. DL models are great at finding complicated patterns in big datasets. They have already transformed areas such as computer vision and natural language processing (NLP). In protein design, they learn the basic rules of how proteins fold and function by analyzing huge amounts of sequence and structure data. They don't need to be explicitly programmed to do this.

AlphaFold2's significant achievement in predicting protein structures with near-atomic precision has accelerated the application of DL throughout the CPD process. DL is now ready to change the way we design proteins, from inverse folding to function-driven generation, bringing new levels of efficiency, accuracy, and creativity.

In CPD, generating protein sequences relies on effective representations of either the sequence itself or the associated structure. When focusing on sequence-based representations, the training datasets can be extremely large, encompassing millions of sequences—only a small fraction of which may be functionally characterized.

To process and learn from these sequences, DL models require appropriate encoding techniques. Among the most commonly used are the following:

13.1 One-hot encoding

This method uses a binary vector, usually of size 20, to represent each amino acid. Sometimes, the vector is made longer to fill in gaps or unknown residues. These vectors are put together into an n × 20 matrix for a protein that is n long. DL models trained on these kinds of matrices often use data from MSAs to learn the statistical distribution of residues so they can create new sequences with similar biochemical properties.

13.2 Learned embeddings

These methods extract task-relevant information from protein sequences that have been converted into fixed-size numerical representations. They draw inspiration from NLP concepts, perceiving protein sequences as "sentences" and amino acids as "words." These models predict the next residue in a sequence, much like next-word prediction in NLP. UniRep (Alley et al., 2019), SeqVec (Heinzinger et al., 2019), and ProtTrans (Elnaggar et al., 2020) are examples of methods that generate dense vector embeddings, capturing the structural and semantic properties of amino acids and entire protein sequences.

13.3 Position-specific scoring matrices(PSSMs)

PSSMs are a very useful tool for designing proteins. They indicate the probability of each amino acid occurring at a specific place, derived from numerous sequence alignments. PSSMs use evolutionary information to make a position-wise profile that shows how residues are conserved and how they change over time. This makes it easier to predict and design sequences.

14 Protein function prediction using DL

High-throughput genome sequencing and annotation are causing protein sequence databases to grow very quickly. However, using experimental methods like biochemical assays and structural analysis to infer what newly discovered proteins do is still time-intensive and extravagant. As a result, computational methods, such as DL methods, are showing promising results for predicting protein function.

In recent years, DL-based approaches have conceptualized protein function prediction as a multilabel classification challenge, frequently employing Gene Ontology (GO) terms as standardized functional labels. As shown in Fig. 3.4, modern DL tools use a wide range of input features, including protein sequence, structure, interaction data, domain information, and textual descriptions. These features are processed by architectures like CNNs, RNNs, transformers, and GNNs.

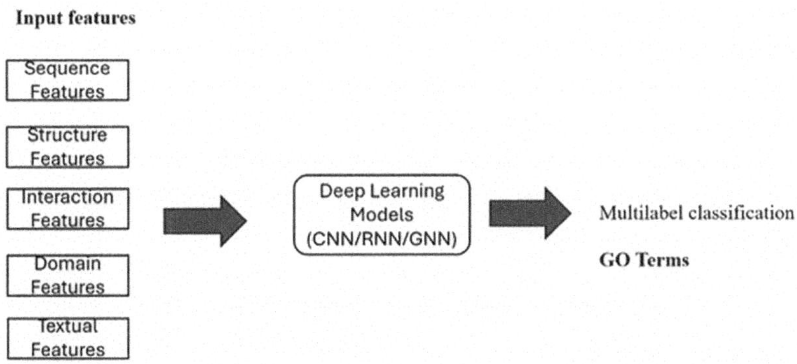

Fig. 3.4 Protein function classification. Workflow for protein function prediction as a multilabel classification.

14.1 Sequence-based methods

For function prediction based solely on amino acid sequences, techniques such as CNNs, RNNs, DNNs, and transformer models are widely used. For example, ProLanGO (Cao et al., 2017) converts protein sequences into GO terms using an RNN-based language translation approach. Another tool, DeepGOPlus (Kulmanov et al., 2020), performs functional annotation by combining CNN-based motif detection with sequence similarity. TALE (Cao et al., 2021) enhances prediction performance by integrating attention mechanisms and hierarchical regularization to jointly embed sequences and functional labels.

Recent tools like TEMPROT (Oliveira et al., 2023) and ATGO (Zhu et al., 2022) incorporate pretrained protein language models (e.g., ESM-1b (Rives et al., 2021), ProtBERT-BFD (Elnaggar et al., 2020) to generate high-quality sequence embeddings, which significantly improve prediction accuracy.

14.2 Structure-based methods

Protein structure prediction is also important for figuring out what proteins do. Structural information, frequently acquired through contemporary DL tools like AlphaFold2 and RoseTTAFold, augments functional annotation by supplying essential spatial context. These techniques often utilize GNNs to depict proteins as graphs derived from their contact maps. DeepFRI (Gligorijević et al., 2021), TransFun (Boadu et al., 2023), and Struct2GO (Jiao et al., 2023) are significant methodologies that employ structural information to predict protein function.

14.3 Protein-protein interaction-based methods

Numerous proteins perform their functions by assembling into multimeric complexes. Consequently, protein-protein interaction (PPI) data can be utilized to enhance protein function prediction. Methods such as NetQuilt, DeepGO, and STRING2GO use DL architectures to enhance prediction performance by combining sequence data with PPI networks (Boadu et al., 2025).

15 DL-inspired protein structure prediction in drug discovery

The three-dimensional conformation of a protein provides a definitive understanding of its interactions with other molecules, including prospective pharmaceutical compounds. The bottleneck of structure-based drug discovery has traditionally been the high cost and time required to obtain the target protein's structure through experimental methods. The ability to accurately and rapidly predict protein structures through DL-based methods has had the following transformative impact on drug discovery:

- **Faster target identification:** DL-based protein prediction methods have made it easier to find and confirm potential drug targets, especially for proteins that were difficult to study in the lab previously.
- **Rational drug design:** Understanding the target protein's 3D structure is very helpful for "structure-based drug design," and here are some of the reasons why:
  - Virtual screening: This makes it easy to quickly find powerful drug molecules from compound libraries that are most likely to bind to the target protein's active site.
  - De novo drug design: The target protein's three-dimensional shape can also be used to create new drug-like molecules that fit the shape and chemical features of the target's binding pocket.
  - Lead optimization: The target protein's 3D structure can be used to improve existing drug candidates by enhancing their binding affinity, increasing their specificity, and optimizing their pharmacokinetic properties.
- **Learning about protein–ligand interactions:** AlphaFold 3, the next version of AlphaFold2, not only gives you accurate protein structures from sequence input, but it also predicts protein interaction patterns with other molecules, such as small molecules, ions, DNA, and RNA.

16 Future aspects

AlphaFold2 and its sequel have undoubtedly advanced the prediction of single-domain protein structures and significantly enhanced our comprehension of protein interactions. Nonetheless, significant challenges remain in precisely predicting the structures of large, multidomain proteins, proteins capable of adopting several conformations, and protein complexes including numerous subunits.

Also, protein engineering, especially figuring out how mutations affect things and predicting the structures of synthetic proteins, are other areas where DL-based methods could be useful. New techniques like protein language models try to make it so that we don't have to rely on MSAs and structural templates as much, but they still aren't very accurate.

Combining different data sources is one promising way to make things better. We can improve the accuracy of predictions for both individual proteins and protein complexes by combining results from biochemical and low-resolution structural experiments with current DL-based in silico methods.

AI disclosure

During the preparation of this work, the author(s) used Google Gemini in order to improve the readability and language of the chapter. After using this tool/service, the author(s) reviewed and edited the content as needed and take(s) full responsibility for the content of the publication.

References

Abramson, J., Adler, J., Dunger, J., Evans, R., Green, T., Pritzel, A., Ronneberger, O., Willmore, L., Ballard, A.J., Bambrick, J., Bodenstein, S.W., Evans, D.A., Hung, C.-C., O'Neill, M., Reiman, D., Tunyasuvunakool, K., Wu, Z., Žemgulytė, A., Arvaniti, E., Beattie, C., Bertolli, O., Bridgland, A., Cherepanov, A., Congreve, M., Cowen-Rivers, A.I., Cowie, A., Figurnov, M., Fuchs, F.B., Gladman, H., Jain, R., Khan, Y.A., Low, C.M.R., Perlin, K., Potapenko, A., Savy, P., Singh, S., Stecula, A., Thillaisundaram, A., Tong, C., Yakneen, S., Zhong, E.D., Zielinski, M., Žídek, A., Bapst, V., Kohli, P., Jaderberg, M., Hassabis, D., Jumper, J.M., 2024. Accurate structure prediction of biomolecular interactions with AlphaFold 3. Nature. 0028-0836. 630 (8016), 493–500. doi:10.1038/s41586-024-07487-w.

Ahdritz, G., Bouatta, N., Floristean, C., Kadyan, S., Xia, Q., Gerecke, W., O'Donnell, T.J., Berenberg, D., Fisk, I., Zanichelli, N., Zhang, B., Nowaczynski, A., Wang, B., Stepniewska-Dziubinska, M.M., Zhang, S., Ojewole, A., Guney, M.E., Biderman, S., Watkins, A.M., Ra, S., Lorenzo, P.R., Nivon, L., Weitzner, B., Ban, Y.E.A., Sorger, P.K., Mostaque, E., Zhang, Z., Bonneau, R., AlQuraishi, M., 2022. OpenFold: retraining AlphaFold2 yields new insights into its learning mechanisms and capacity for generalization. bioRxiv. 2692-8205. Available from: https://www.biorxiv.org. doi:10.1101/2022.11.20.517210.

Alley, E.C., Khimulya, G., Biswas, S., AlQuraishi, M., Church, G.M., 2019. Unified rational protein engineering with sequence-based deep representation learning. Nat. Methods. 1548-7105. 16 (12), 1315–1322. Available from: http://www.nature.com/nmeth/. doi:10.1038/s41592-019-0598-1.

Baek, M., DiMaio, F., Anishchenko, I., Dauparas, J., Ovchinnikov, S., Lee, G.R., Wang, J., Cong, Q., Kinch, L.N., Schaeffer, R.D., Millán, C., Park, H., Adams, C., Glassman, C.R., DeGiovanni, A., Pereira, J.H., Rodrigues, A.V., Van Dijk, A.A., Ebrecht, A.C., Opperman, D.J., Sagmeister, T., Buhlheller, C., Pavkov-Keller, T., Rathinaswamy, M.K., Dalwadi, U., Yip, C.K., Burke, J.E., Garcia, K.C., Grishin, N.V., Adams, P.D., Read, R.J., Baker, D., 2021. Accurate prediction of protein structures and interactions using a three-track neural network. Science. 1095-9203. 373 (6557), 871–876. Available from: https://science.sciencemag.org/content/373/6557/871.full. doi:10.1126/science.abj8754.

Boadu, F., Cao, H., Cheng, J., 2023. Combining protein sequences and structures with transformers and equivariant graph neural networks to predict protein function. Bioinformatics. 1367-4803. 39 (Supplement_1), i318. doi:10.1093/bioinformatics/btad208.

Boadu, F., Lee, A., Cheng, J., 2025. Deep learning methods for protein function prediction. Proteomics. 1615-9861. 25 (1-2). Available from: http://onlinelibrary.wiley.com/journal/10.1002/(ISSN)1615-9861. doi:10.1002/pmic.202300471.

Bryant, P., Noé, F., 2024. Structure prediction of alternative protein conformations. Nat. Commun. 15 (1). doi:10.1038/s41467-024-51507-2.

Bryant, P., Kelkar, A., Guljas, A., Clementi, C., Noé, F., 2024. Structure prediction of protein-ligand complexes from sequence information with Umol. Nat. Commun. 2041-1723. 15 (1). doi:10.1038/s41467-024-48837-6.

Cao, R., Freitas, C., Chan, L., Sun, M., Jiang, H., Chen, Z., 2017. ProLanGO: protein function prediction using neural machine translation based on a recurrent neural network. Molecules. 1420-3049. 22 (10), 1732. doi:10.3390/molecules22101732.

Cao, Y., Shen, Y., Valencia, A., 2021. TALE: Transformer-based protein function Annotation with joint sequence–Label Embedding. Bioinformatics, 37 (18), 2825–2833. doi:10.1093/bioinformatics/btab198.

Chowdhury, R., Bouatta, N., Biswas, S., Floristean, C., Kharkar, A., Roy, K., Rochereau, C., Ahdritz, G., Zhang, J., Church, G.M., Sorger, P.K., AlQuraishi, M., 2022. Single-sequence protein structure prediction using a language model and deep learning. Nat. Biotechnol. 1087-0156. 40 (11), 1617–1623. doi:10.1038/s41587-022-01432-w.

Defresne, M., Barbe, S., Schiex, T., 2021. Protein design with deep learning. Int. J. Mol. Sci. 1422-0067. 22 (21), 11741. doi:10.3390/ijms222111741.

Elnaggar, A., Heinzinger, M., Dallago, C., Rehawi, G., Wang, Y., Jones, L., Gibbs, T., Feher, T., Angerer, C., Steinegger, M., Bhowmik, D., Rost, B., 2020. ProtTrans: towards cracking the language of life's code through self-supervised deep learning and high performance computing. bioRxiv. 2692-8205. Available from: https://www.biorxiv.org. doi:10.1101/2020.07.12.199554.

Evans, R., O'Neill, M., Pritzel, A., Green, T., Figurnov, M., Ronneberger, O., Jumper, J., 2022. Protein complex prediction with AlphaFold-multimer. Science 377 (6607), eadd5699. doi:10.1126/science.add5699.

Gligorijević, V., Renfrew, P.D., Kosciolek, T., Leman, J.K., Berenberg, D., Vatanen, T., Chandler, C., Taylor, B.C., Fisk, I.M., Vlamakis, H., Xavier, R.J., Knight, R., Cho, K., Bonneau, R., 2021. Structure-based protein function prediction using graph convolutional networks. Nat. Commun. 2041-1723. 12 (1). Available from: http://www.nature.com/ncomms/index.html. doi:10.1038/s41467-021-23303-9.

Heinzinger, M., Elnaggar, A., Wang, Y., Dallago, C., Nechaev, D., Matthes, F., Rost, B., 2019. Modeling aspects of the language of life through transfer-learning protein sequences. BMC Bioinformatics. 1471-2105. 20 (1). doi:10.1186/s12859-019-3220-8.

Jänes, J., Beltrao, P., 2024. Deep learning for protein structure prediction and design—progress and applications. Mol. Syst. Biol. 1744-4292. 20 (3), 162–169. doi:10.1038/s44320-024-00016-x.

Jiao, P., Wang, B., Wang, X., Liu, B., Wang, Y., Li, J., Wren, J., 2023. Struct2GO: protein function prediction based on graph pooling algorithm and AlphaFold2 structure information. Bioinformatics. 1367-4811. 39 (10). doi:10.1093/bioinformatics/btad637.

Jones, D.T., Kandathil, S.M., 2018. High precision in protein contact prediction using fully convolutional neural networks and minimal sequence features. Bioinformatics. 1460-2059. 34 (19), 3308–3315. Available from: http://bioinformatics.oxfordjournals.org/. doi:10.1093/bioinformatics/bty341.

Jones, D.T., Singh, T., Kosciolek, T., Tetchner, S., 2015. MetaPSICOV: combining coevolution methods for accurate prediction of contacts and long range hydrogen bonding in proteins. Bioinformatics. 1460-2059. 31 (7), 999–1006. Available from: http://bioinformatics.oxfordjournals.org/. doi:10.1093/bioinformatics/btu791.

Ju, F., Zhu, J., Shao, B., Kong, L., Liu, T.Y., Zheng, W.M., Bu, D., 2021. CopulaNet: learning residue co-evolution directly from multiple sequence alignment for protein structure prediction. Nat. Commun. 2041-1723. 12 (1). Available from: http://www.nature.com/ncomms/index.html. doi:10.1038/s41467-021-22869-8.

Jumper, J., Evans, R., Pritzel, A., Green, T., Figurnov, M., Ronneberger, O., Tunyasuvunakool, K., Bates, R., Žídek, A., Potapenko, A., Bridgland, A., Meyer, C., Kohl, S.A.A., Ballard, A.J., Cowie, A., Romera-Paredes, B., Nikolov, S., Jain, R., Adler, J., Back, T., Petersen, S., Reiman, D., Clancy, E., Zielinski, M., Steinegger, M., Pacholska, M., Berghammer, T., Bodenstein, S., Silver, D., Vinyals, O., Senior, A.W., Kavukcuoglu, K., Kohli, P., Hassabis, D., 2021. Highly accurate protein structure prediction with AlphaFold. Nature. 0028-0836. 596 (7873), 583–589. doi:10.1038/s41586-021-03819-2.

Kabsch, W., 1978. A discussion of the solution for the best rotation to relate two sets of vectors. Acta Crystallogr. Sect. A. 0567-7394. 34 (5), 827–828. doi:10.1107/s0567739478001680.

Kulmanov M, Hoehndorf R and Cowen L. (2020). DeepGOPlus: improved protein function prediction from sequence. Bioinformatics, 36(2), 422–429. 10.1093/bioinformatics/btz595

Levinthal, C., 1968. Are there pathways for protein folding?. J. Chim. Phys. 0021-7689. 65, 44–45. doi:10.1051/jcp/1968650044.

Lin, Z., Akin, H., Rao, R., Hie, B., Zhu, Z., Wenting, L., Smetanin, N., Verkuil, R., Kabeli, O., Shmueli, Y., Dos Santos Costa, A., Fazel-Zarandi, M., Sercu, T., Candido, S., Rives, A., 2023. Evolutionary-scale prediction of atomic-level protein structure with a language model. Science. 0036-8075. 379 (6637), 1123–1130. doi:10.1126/science.ade2574.

Mariani, V., Biasini, M., Barbato, A., Schwede, T., 2013. lDDT: a local superposition-free score for comparing protein structures and models using distance difference tests. Bioinformatics. 1367-4803. 29 (21), 2722–2728. doi:10.1093/bioinformatics/btt473.

Mirdita, M., Schütze, K., Moriwaki, Y., Heo, L., Ovchinnikov, S., Steinegger, M., 2022. ColabFold: making protein folding accessible to all. Nat. Methods. 1548-7091. 19 (6), 679–682. doi:10.1038/s41592-022-01488-1.

Oliveira, G.B., Pedrini, H., Dias, Z., 2023. TEMPROT: protein function annotation using transformers embeddings and homology search. BMC Bioinformatics. 1471-2105. 24 (1). Available from: https://bmcbioinformatics.biomedcentral.com/. doi:10.1186/s12859-023-05375-0.

Pereira, J., Simpkin, A.J., Hartmann, M.D., Rigden, D.J., Keegan, R.M., Lupas, A.N., 2021. High-accuracy protein structure prediction in CASP14. Proteins: Struct., Funct. Bioinf. 1097-0134. 89 (12), 1687–1699. Available from: http://onlinelibrary.wiley.com/journal/10.1002/(ISSN)1097-0134. doi:10.1002/prot.26171.

Qin, Y., Chen, Z., Peng, Y., Xiao, Y., Zhong, T., Yu, X., 2024. Deep learning methods for protein structure prediction. MedComm. 2769-6456. 3 (3). doi:10.1002/mef2.96.

Rives, A., Meier, J., Sercu, T., Goyal, S., Lin, Z., Liu, J., Guo, D., Ott, M., Zitnick, C.L., Ma, J., Fergus, R., 2021. Biological structure and function emerge from scaling unsupervised learning to 250 million protein sequences. Proc. Natl. Acad. Sci. U. S. A. 1091-6490. 118 (15). Available from: https://www.pnas.org/content/118/15/e2016239118. doi:10.1073/pnas.2016239118.

Roney, J.P., Ovchinnikov, S., 2022. State-of-the-art estimation of protein model accuracy using AlphaFold. Phys. Rev. Lett. 1079-7114. 129 (23). Available from: https://journals.aps.org/prl/abstract/10.1103/PhysRevLett.129.238101. doi:10.1103/PhysRevLett.129.238101.

Ruffolo, J.A., Chu, L.S., Mahajan, S.P., Gray, J.J., 2022. Fast, accurate antibody structure prediction from deep learning on massive set of natural antibodies. bioRxiv. 2692-8205. Available from: https://www.biorxiv.org. doi:10.1101/2022.04.20.488972.

Singh, J., Litfin, T., Singh, J., Paliwal, K., Zhou, Y., Martelli, P.L., 2022. SPOT-contact-LM: improving single-sequence-based prediction of protein contact map using a transformer language model. Bioinformatics. 1367-4803. 38 (7), 1888–1894. doi:10.1093/bioinformatics/btac053.

Wang, T., Qiao, Y., Ding, W., Mao, W., Zhou, Y., Gong, H., 2019. Improved fragment sampling for ab initio protein structure prediction using deep neural networks. Nat. Mach. Intell. 2522-5839. 1 (8), 347–355. doi:10.1038/s42256-019-0075-7.

Weigt, M., White, R.A., Szurmant, H., Hoch, J.A., Hwa, T., 2009. Identification of direct residue contacts in protein–protein interaction by message passing. Proc. Natl. Acad. Sci. 0027-8424. 106 (1), 67–72. doi:10.1073/pnas.0805923106.

Weissenow, K., Heinzinger, M., Rost, B., 2022. Protein language-model embeddings for fast, accurate, and alignment-free protein structure prediction. Structure. 0969-2126. 30 (8), 1169. doi:10.1016/j.str.2022.05.001.

Wu, R., Ding, F., Wang, R., Shen, R., Zhang, X., Luo, S., Su, C., Wu, Z., Xie, Q., Berger, B., Ma, J., Peng, J., 2022. High-resolution de novo structure prediction from primary sequence. bioRxiv. 2692-8205. Available from: https://www.biorxiv.org. doi:10.1101/2022.07.21.500999.

Yang, J., Anishchenko, I., Park, H., Peng, Z., Ovchinnikov, S., Baker, D., 2020. Improved protein structure prediction using predicted interresidue orientations. Proc. Natl. Acad. Sci. U. S. A. 1091-6490. 117 (3), 1496–1503. Available from: https://www.pnas.org/content/pnas/117/3/1496.full.pdf. doi:10.1073/pnas.1914677117.

Zemla, A., Venclovas, Č., Moult, J., 1999. Krzysztof fidelis, processing and analysis of CASP3 protein structure predictions. Proteins: Struct., Funct., Genet. 0887-3585. 37 (S3), 22–29. doi:10.1002/(SICI)1097-0134(1999)37:3+<22::AID-PROT5>3.3.CO;2-N.

Zhang, Y., Skolnick, J., 2004. Scoring function for automated assessment of protein structure template quality. Proteins: Struct., Funct., Bioinf. 0887-3585. 57 (4), 702–710. doi:10.1002/prot.20264.

Zhu, Y.H., Zhang, C., Yu, D.J., Zhang, Y., 2022. Integrating unsupervised language model with triplet neural networks for protein gene ontology prediction. PLoS Comput. Biol. 1553-7358. 18 (12). Available from: https://journals.plos.org/ploscompbiol/article?id=10.1371/journal.pcbi.1010793. doi:10.1371/journal.pcbi.1010793.

4

Drug target identification and validation using AI

Rubhashri Gurunathan, Rajaram Abhirami, Muthuraja Arun Pravin, and Sanjeev Kumar Singh
Computer Aided Drug Design and Molecular Modelling Lab, Department of Bioinformatics, Alagappa University, Karaikudi, Tamil Nadu, India

1 Introduction

The drug design and development process is a multifaceted, expensive, time-intensive, laborious, complex, and resource-intensive procedure that embarks upon identifying and validating a therapeutic target—steps that intensely affect the success of subsequent stages of the drug discovery pathway. The typical discovery process involves identifying target proteins that are causally linked to pathophysiology and developing a plausible framework for therapeutic intervention (Selvaraj et al., n.d.). Generally, a drug discovery process involves numerous stages, including target selection, screening, in vitro and in vivo evaluation, and medical trials, which typically require significant investments of time and resources—around $2 billion and 10 years to deliver a novel therapeutic to market (Pun et al., 2023). Zhou et al. (2022) reported that by the year 2022, more than 500 drugs had been successfully developed, which represents a smaller fraction of the estimated drug targets within the human body. Despite extensive clinical optimization, drug development faces significant challenges. The typical failure rate in clinical trials was staggering—84.6% from 2009 to 2018. The principal cause behind the failure of clinical trials, mainly in phase I and phase II, is the lack of clinical efficacy. This results in substantial financial losses and wasted resources (Sun et al., 2022). The traditional "one gene, one drug, one disease" hypothesis of the drug discovery process may have contributed to the low rate of success in drug discovery and development (Zeng et al., 2020). Initially, drug discovery requires validation and the building of hypotheses, which is perilous due to the inconclusive information about the target and drug (Yoo et al., 2023). Furthermore, the rate of success in advancing a drug undergoing phase I clinical evaluation to market is very low, with fewer than 10% receiving approval. Population aging, unhealthy

The AI Frontier in Molecular Modelling and Drug Designing. https://doi.org/10.1016/B978-0-443-40338-5.00012-3

routines, and unmet medical needs in chronic diseases, coupled with late-stage drug failure, have driven transformative breakthroughs in drug development. The accomplishment of any drug development program centers on precisely identifying targets involved in chronic diseases and validating their role in disease mechanisms. Drug target identification is a crucial yet highly complex step in the drug development process (Madhukar et al., 2019). A drug target is conventionally a biological molecule—commonly a protein, enzyme, gene, or signaling pathway—that is critically involved in the pathophysiology of a disease and whose alteration can elicit chronic disease progression and symptoms. By inhibiting or down regulating this target, it is possible to diminish disease pathology and enable the restoration of normal cellular, tissue, and organ functions. In early-stage research, animal models, such as transgenic and knockout organisms, are widely employed for target identification and validation processes. The discovery and development of promising and affordable treatments for human diseases represent a considerable challenge in the absence of comprehensive knowledge regarding drug targets (Zeng et al., 2020). Hence, the identification of the right drug target and its validation is important for improving the probability of developing clinically effective treatments.

However, traditional approaches for drug target identification and validation relied heavily on experimental techniques such as biochemical assays, genetic studies, and high-throughput screening. Though reliable, the process is time-intensive, resource-intensive, and frequently limited in its capability to manage the intricate nature of biological systems and the vast quantity of data generated by current high-throughput technologies. However, advancements in artificial intelligence (AI) technology have brought a revolution to the arena of drug discovery and development, contributing unprecedented solutions to hasten the procedure and reduce costs over the past few years (Wang, 2024; Huang et al., 2024). Fig. 4.1 summarizes the key differences and benefits of traditional and ML/artificial neural networks (ANN) approaches in drug target validation. AI, also known as computer-based intelligence, can potentially surpass human capabilities, encompassing the ability to acquire information, develop rules for its utilization, draw definitive conclusions, perform corrections, and execute complex tasks, such as recognizing patterns and images, understanding language, and learning from experience, sometimes with accuracy exceeding that of human beings (Bharadwaj et al., 2024). It has been utilized across numerous divisions, such as revolutionizing educational methods and streamlining and automating business processes.

With the advent of AI, researchers are widely applying AI in drug discovery for tasks such as virtual screening, retrosynthesis, de novo design, reaction prediction, and de novo protein design, which are divided into two groups: predictive and generative tasks (Deng et al., 2022; Shiammala et al., 2023). In drug discovery, the opportunity for

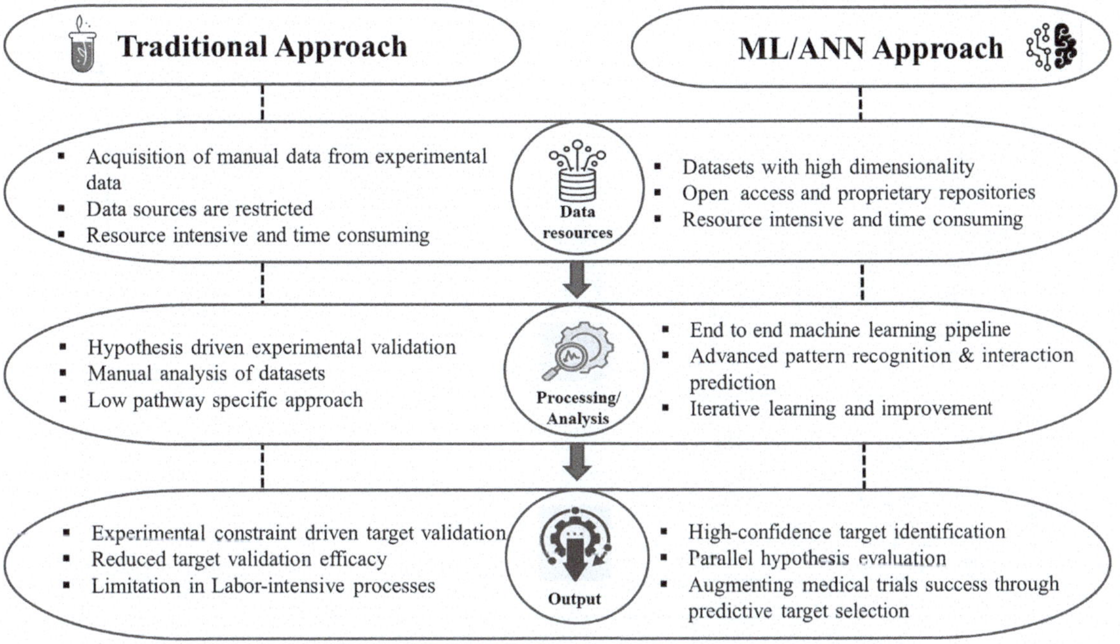

Fig. 4.1 Comparative analysis of traditional vs. AI-powered target identification and validation.

the application of AI has expanded to encompass the entire early drug discovery process (Yoo et al., 2023). AI leverages computational algorithms such as deep learning (DL), machine learning (ML), geometric learning, graph-based learning in biological and molecular systems, few-shot learning, and generative models for molecular design to analyze massive datasets, recognize patterns, extract valuable information, and make predictions with high precision and efficiency. It improves the effectiveness and accuracy of drug target identification and validation, as well as offers novel ideas and directions for the further drug development process (Blair et al., 2006). The processes of target identification and validation leveraging AI techniques are illustrated in Fig. 4.2. The combination of AI and drug discovery procedures has transfigured target identification and validation, bringing exceptional innovation and efficiency to the process. Target identification and validation are known to be the first key steps in the drug discovery process that are efficacious, safe, and druggable (Wang et al., 2004). Target identification involves detecting the precise cellular pathways or biological molecules that can be altered by drugs (from traditional small molecules and peptides to emerging short RNAs and antibodies) to achieve therapeutic benefits. This has become progressively vital in modern drug discovery and the dominant strategy in drug discovery (Pun et al., 2023; Yoo et al., 2023).

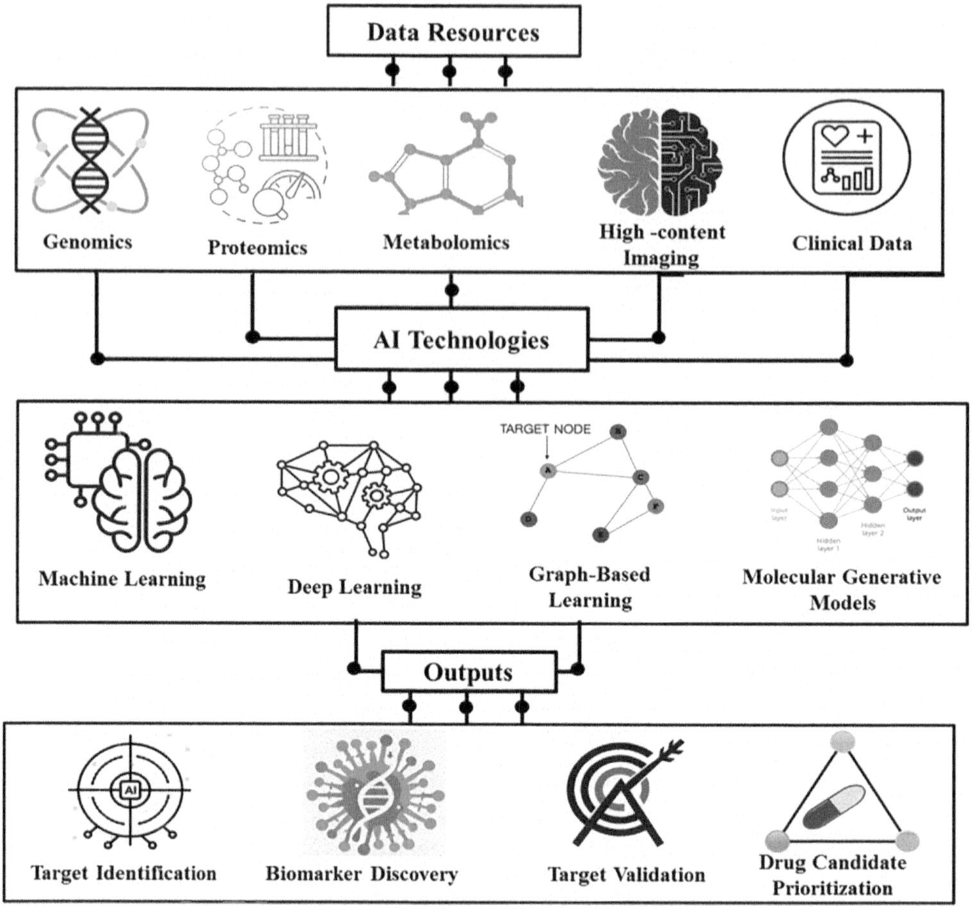

Fig. 4.2 AI-powered target identification and validation.

Validation includes assessing the structural, functional, and biological relevance of the identified targets. AI-driven target identification and validation have enabled the discovery of new druggable targets and the development of targeted therapies for a wide range of diseases such as cancer, cardiovascular disorders, viral infections, bacterial infections, and neurological conditions. It provides automated analysis of textual data through supervised learning models, unsupervised learning models, and natural language processing (NLP), a subset of AI, which accelerates potential drug target identification by reducing the dependency on manual curation and improving the drug discovery process. This is among the crucial advantages of using AI in drug discovery, as it helps navigate the extensive search space of potential targets. In recent years, the amount of data has expanded expressively, consisting of high-content imaging of clinical materials, human genetic information from large populations, and genomic, proteomic, transcriptomic, and metabolic analyses of healthy and infected individuals. This has created remarkable new possibilities for early target identification and validation through the rigorous analysis of biomedical data, encompassing elementary research on disease mechanisms to clinical investigations (Pun et al., 2023). The power to collect and harness colossal datasets via diverse types of databases has been transformative. However, the multidimensional nature and complexity of the datasets represent substantial challenges for analysis. Advanced analytical techniques are required to produce statistically robust models that can generate reliable predictions for target identification (Santos et al., 2022). This is where AI plays a central role. The capability of AI to process and interpret multifaceted biomedical networks enables the identification of patterns and relationships within the data that may remain subtle when analyzed using conventional procedures. AI algorithms empower researchers to gain profound insights into disease mechanisms, enabling a better understanding of disease processes, accelerating biomarker discovery, and facilitating the identification of promising therapeutic targets (Mamoshina et al., 2018; Zhavoronkov et al., 2019; Muslu et al., 2022). ML algorithms, particularly DL models, are widely used to investigate multiomics data such as proteomics, genomics, and transcriptomics to discover promising therapeutic targets. These advancements underscore the critical contributions of AI to contemporary drug discovery by permitting the efficient integration and understanding of large-scale datasets for the identification and validation of therapeutic targets (Huang et al., 2024). Recently, the integration of AI and ML approaches into biologic-based therapies (biopharmaceuticals) has gained substantial traction (Wang et al., 2024). Furthermore, a crucial aspect of this chapter emphasizes the application of AI in the drug discovery process, specifically target identification and validation, which have a substantial impact on the drug discovery process. It also explores the methodologies and concepts used in AI-driven drug target identification, focusing on specific algorithms and their application in uncovering disease-specific pathways. The ability of AI to forecast the interactions among genes, proteins, enzymes, peptides, and small molecules has unlocked new avenues for precise drugs or medicines. This advancement enables researchers to identify and design highly targeted therapeutic interventions. The structure of this chapter aims to provide an inclusive summary of how AI is reforming the realm of drug target identification and validation. It explores a wide range of key AI techniques, algorithms, tools, and software used, ranging from conventional ML models like random forest (RF) to advanced DL methods, highlighting their role in the identification of targets and their validation. Table 4.1 highlights the role of AI in drug

Table 4.1 AI-driven approaches in drug target identification and validation.

Phases	AI Techniques/ Models	Application	Benefits
Data analysis and integration	ML, natural language processing (NLP), DL	• Information extraction from biomedical recourse • Multiomics data integration	• Extract valuable information from massive datasets. • Determines critical disease biomarkers and related pathways
Target identification	support vector machine (SVM), Neural Networks, RF	• Diseased protein or pathway identification. • *Predicting drug target ligand interaction*	• Enhances the reliability of target identification and validation. • Minimize false positive
Biological pathway analysis	Molecular Graph Learning, Graph Neural Networks (GNNs)	• Signaling pathway analysis and identification linked to disease. • Molecular interaction mapping	• Explore the disease pathophysiology at the mechanistic level.
Target validation	Reinforcement Learning (RL), Generative Adversarial Networks (GANs)	• Predicting protein-ligand interaction • Evaluating predicted targets using validated datasets	• Improves the support for target selection.
Biomarker characterization	Feature selection method, Clustering algorithms	• Identification of biological markers for disease diagnosis and personalized medicine	• Enables personalized medicine
Drug effectiveness prediction	Deep neural networks (DNNs), Bayesian models	• Assessing the potential therapeutic drug target • Evaluating drug effectiveness and risk ratio	• Prioritizes the potential target
Clinical validation	AI-driven data mining tools, NLP	• Examining and analyzing medical records and clinical trials. • Assessing findings with real-world data	• Streamline research from lab to patient care

target identification and validation. Moreover, the validation of these targets, often a bottleneck in drug discovery, is being transformed through computational techniques that evaluate the relevance and efficacy of identified targets. By examining these, researchers will gain an understanding of the practical implementation of AI in drug discovery and its effectiveness in the development of novel therapeutics against chronic diseases. The sections will also underscore the progression of AI-driven methodologies over traditional approaches, emphasizing their ability to analyze high-dimensional data, leading to significant time and cost reductions while advancing predictive accuracy. By the end of this chapter, AI's pivotal role in addressing some of the most persistent challenges in contemporary biomedical research will be emphasized.

2 Unveiling disease pathways with AI using bioinformatics

The introduction of AI has significantly transformed an extensive array of scientific disciplines, including bioinformatics. The capability of AI to analyze complex biological data and detect intricate patterns has established it as a vital instrument for elucidating disease pathways (Singh et al., 2023). This chapter examines the use of AI in bioinformatics, aiming to uncover disease pathways and provide deeper insights into the fundamental mechanisms underlying various diseases. Overall, AI in unveiling disease pathways is denoted in Fig. 4.3.

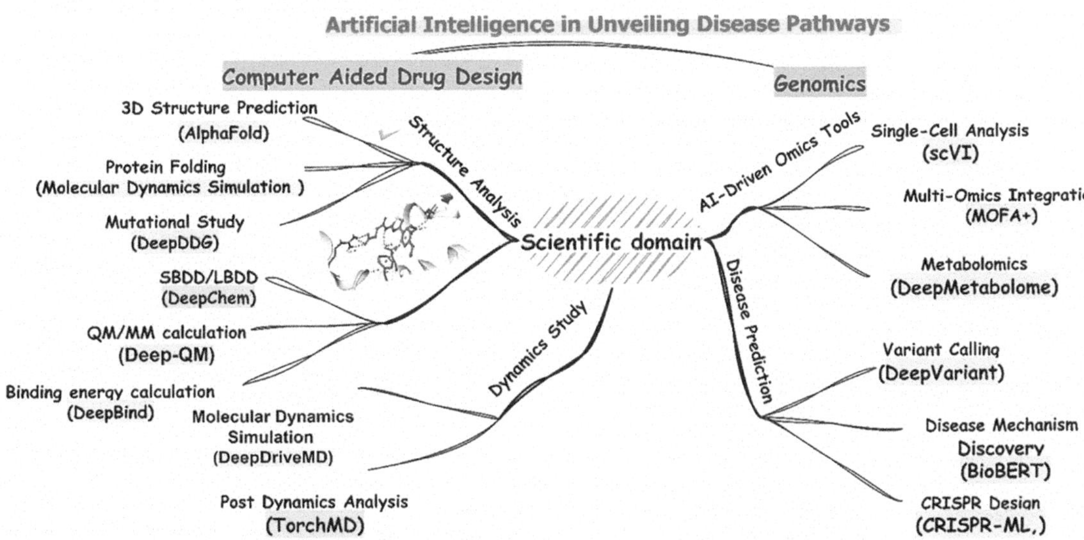

Fig. 4.3 AI in unveiling disease pathways.

2.1 Bioinformatics and AI: A synergistic partnership

Bioinformatics is a multidisciplinary domain that integrates computer science, statistics, and biology, playing a vigorous role in managing and analyzing biological data. The emergence of advanced high-throughput technologies has substantially increased biological data, encompassing genomic sequences, gene expression profiles, and protein structures (Singh et al., 2024). This surge in data necessitates the use of advanced computational tools for effective analysis and interpretation, a requirement adequately fulfilled by AI/ML. AI algorithms, particularly those in DL and ML, demonstrate exceptional proficiency in identifying multifaceted patterns and relationships within extensive datasets, rendering them indispensable for research in bioinformatics (Li et al., 2023). Tables 4.2 and 4.3 present an overview of the AI-driven tools and the algorithms for unveiling disease pathways.

AI is driving significant transformations within the healthcare sector, mostly in the domains of medical visual data analysis, personalized treatment, and disease pathway analysis (Bajwa et al., 2021). DL, which is a subset of AI, has demonstrated exceptional

Table 4.2 AI-driven tools for unveiling disease pathways.

Tools	Description	References
scVelo	Infers RNA velocity based on single-cell RNA-sequencing data to model cell trajectories and dynamics.	(Bergen et al., 2020)
DeepVariant	Uses deep learning for accurate genomic variant calling from sequencing data.	(Poplin et al., 2018)
DeepCell	Analyzing single-cell imaging data using deep learning for cellular phenotyping.	(Magness et al., 2024)
MOFA (Multiomics Factor Analysis)	Incorporates multiple omics datasets (e.g., genomics, transcriptomics, proteomics).	(Argelaguet et al., 2018)
MetaboAnalyst	A robust tool designed for metabolomics analysis and pathway enrichment interpretation.	(Pang et al., 2024)
AlphaFold	DL-based tool to predict protein three dimensional structures, vital for understanding protein-ligand interactions in disease pathways.	(Uzoeto et al., 2024)
DeepLigand	Employs convolutional neural networks (CNNs) to predict binding sites and potential ligands for protein targets.	(Zeng and Gifford, 2019)
DeepChem	Applies ML models to forecast binding affinities and molecular interactions in drug discovery.	(Singh, 2021)
DeltaDock	Uses reinforcement learning to model ligand flexibility and refine docking scores for dynamic systems.	(Yan et al., 2024)
GNN-DTI	Leverages GNN to model protein-ligand complexes and predict interaction pathways.	(Sun et al., 2024)

Table 4.3 AI-driven algorithm for unveiling disease pathways.

Tools	Algorithm
scVelo	ML—Probabilistic modeling
DeepVariant	Artificial neural network (ANN)—Convolutional neural network (CNN)
DeepCell	1) CNNs 2) Recurrent neural networks (RNNs)
MOFA	ML—Probabilistic, Bayesian and multiview learning
MetaboAnalyst	Deep learning and k-Nearest neighbors (KNN)
AlphaFold	Deep learning—Transformers based neural network
DeepLigand	ANN-CNN
DeepChem	Various ML algorithm 1) Graph Convolutional Networks (GCNs) 2) CNN 3) RNNs
DeltaDock	Geometric deep learning (GDL)
GNN-DTI	GNNs

efficacy in analyzing complex medical visual data, such as biomedical imaging and signal processing, thereby facilitating more accurate diagnosis and classification of medical conditions. AI enhances personalized treatment by synthesizing diverse medical data types, such as imaging, genomic data, and clinical history, while concurrently reducing costs and mitigating human error. Nonetheless, several challenges persist. The reliance of AI on extensive, high-quality datasets is constrained by privacy concerns and data heterogeneity. Furthermore, the lack of interpretability within AI models, particularly those rooted in DL, often classified as "black boxes," limits their applicability in clinical settings due to issues of trust and transparency. Ethical considerations regarding algorithmic bias and data privacy further complicate the integration of AI into healthcare. Nevertheless, the prospects of AI in disease pathway analysis are optimistic. Initiatives are underway to develop models that exhibit greater interpretability, thereby providing transparent and reliable predictions. AI's capacity to amalgamate multiomics data, including genomics, proteomics, and other omics platforms, affords a holistic understanding of disease mechanisms, which may lead to novel discoveries (Gao et al., 2022). Moreover, AI is anticipated to transform personalized medicine by customizing therapies based on an individual's genetic and medical history. AI and ML are also expected to enhance the functionality of diagnostic laboratories by improving early disease detection, increasing diagnostic accuracy, and optimizing laboratory operations (Quazi, 2022). As advancements in algorithms, data availability, and processing power continue to evolve, AI stands poised to address existing challenges and redefine the future landscape of healthcare.

3 AI-driven drug target identification

Drug target identification is a critical and indispensable component of the drug discovery pipeline, paving the way for the development of novel therapeutic solutions. This multifaceted process involves identifying specific biomolecules, such as proteins, nucleic acids, or other molecular entities, that are pivotal in disease pathways and can be modulated by therapeutic agents to achieve desired clinical outcomes (Schenone et al., 2013). The accurate identification of drug targets is crucial for ensuring the efficacy and safety of potential therapeutics, significantly influencing the success ratio of subsequent drug development stages (Ezike et al., 2023). Historically, the identification of drug targets relied on experimental methodologies, including high-throughput screening and genetic manipulation. High-throughput screening allows the rapid assessment of a multitude of compounds against a biological target to identify active candidates, while genetic manipulation techniques, including gene knockouts and gene editing, enable the exploration of the functional significance of specific genes or proteins within cellular systems (Ayon, 2023). These methods, complemented by molecular biology techniques, have been influential in advancing the understanding of biomolecular functions and their relevance to disease mechanisms.

Despite these advancements, traditional methods are time and resource-intensive, and often hindered by the complexity of biological systems. The recent emergence of AI has introduced transformative possibilities into the arena of drug target identification (Abbas et al., 2024). AI-driven approaches leverage vast biological datasets and sophisticated algorithms to analyze complex biological information with unparalleled speed and precision. By employing ML and NLP methods, AI can identify patterns, predict interactions, and uncover novel insights into disease mechanisms and drug-target relationships (Bajwa et al., 2021; Yadav et al., 2024). AI has become an integral tool in the process of target identification by leveraging large-scale omics datasets such as proteomics, genomics, metabolomics, and transcriptomics. Through advanced algorithms, AI processes these datasets to reveal key biomarkers and prioritize druggable targets with high therapeutic potential. For example, AI tools like DeepTarget and DeepBind, which utilize DL frameworks, are instrumental in predicting target interactions and binding affinities, significantly streamlining the identification of relevant disease-associated targets (Abbas et al., 2024). A key benefit of AI in target identification is rooted in its capability to forecast drug-target interactions with high precision. By analyzing molecular structures and binding dynamics, AI enables the assessment of the viability of specific biomolecules as therapeutic targets. This precision is particularly valuable for repurposing existing drugs, as it uncovers novel interactions with potential therapeutic applications. AI models have demonstrated success in predicting small molecule-protein binding using structure-based methods, including molecular docking and ML-driven scoring functions, enhancing the efficiency of target evaluation (Bajwa et al., 2021).

AI significantly contributes to identifying novel targets through disease network analysis. By mapping and examining molecular networks, AI identifies critical nodes or hubs that drive disease progression. This network-based approach uncovers the interconnected pathways underlying diseases, revealing targets that remain undetected by conventional approaches. In addition, AI-powered tools can simulate perturbations in these networks to forecast the effects of target modulation, providing valuable insights into the therapeutic potential of candidate targets (Yadav et al., 2024). The adoption of AI in drug target identification has also been supported by advancements in computational infrastructure and the accessibility of large-scale biological datasets (Le et al., 2025). Public repositories, including the Human Protein Atlas, UniProt, and The Cancer Genome Atlas, provide comprehensive data resources that AI models can utilize for training and validation (Askr et al., 2023; Croft et al., 2023; López-Cortés et al., 2024). Furthermore, AI-based platforms such as AlphaFold have revolutionized structural biology by predicting protein structures with remarkable accuracy, enabling researchers to study the structural basis of drug-target interactions in unprecedented detail (Nussinov et al., 2022). Table 4.4 represents an outline of AI tools and platforms for target identification.

In summary, AI-driven drug target identification is transforming drug discovery by offering unprecedented efficiency, accuracy, and insight. By harnessing AI technologies, the process of identifying potential therapeutic targets becomes quicker and more economical compared to conventional methods. This cutting-edge approach not only increases the chances of developing effective treatments for complex diseases but also provides a deeper understanding of biological systems. As AI continues to develop, its integration with experimental techniques will expand the possibilities in drug discovery, ultimately transforming the face of modern healthcare.

Table 4.4 Outline of AI tools and platforms for target identification.

Tool names	Pathways	Algorithms/ Methods used	Applications	Uses in disease prediction	References
GeneMANIA	Gene/protein interaction pathways	Machine learning (ML), coexpression data	Predict gene function, network relationships	Cancer, neurodegenerative diseases, cardiovascular diseases	(Mostafavi et al., 2008)
OmicsNet	Multiomics networks	Graph theory, network biology	Multiomics data integration for biomarker and target identification	Cancer, metabolic disorders, infectious diseases	(Zhou and Xia, 2018)
OpenTargets	Transcriptomic, proteomics pathways	Integrated data analysis, scoring systems	Aggregates data to prioritize disease-specific targets	Cancer, rare diseases, metabolic disorders	(Koscielny et al., 2017)
DeepChem	Protein-ligand interaction pathways	Deep learning (DL), convolutional networks	Predict molecular interactions, docking, and binding affinity	Cancer, viral infections, and rare genetic diseases	Singh (2021)
AlphaFold by DeepMind	Protein folding and structural pathways	AI-based protein 3D structure prediction	High-accuracy protein structure prediction for target identification	Infectious diseases, genetic disorders, and cancer	Jumper et al. (2021)
DeepVariant	Variant analysis pathways	Deep neural networks (DNNs)	Identifies genetic variants linked to diseases	Genetic disorders, cancer	(Poplin et al. (2018)
Base Space Correlation Engine	Genomic and transcriptomic pathways	Correlation analysis, bioinformatics tools	Identifies disease-related genes and their associations	Cancer, autoimmune diseases, neurodegeneration	(Khurana et al., 2021)
GEMINI	GWAS and SNP analysis pathways	AI-based GWAS tools, regression analysis	Links genetic mutations to diseases for target discovery	Cancer, cardiovascular diseases, rare disorders	(Paila et al., 2013)
Pharos	Protein interaction pathways	Big data, clustering algorithms	Identifies understudied proteins (dark genome) as potential drug targets	Rare diseases, cancer, neurological disorders	(Nguyen et al., 2017)
AI-GCN	Molecular network pathways	GCNs	Predicts potential targets using molecular graphs and networks	Cancer, infectious diseases	(Lu et al., 2020)

GANs for Drug Discovery	Protein-ligand interaction pathways	Generative adversarial networks (GANs)	Proposes novel targets and small molecules for therapeutic development	Cancer, infectious diseases, genetic disorders	(Kadurin et al., 2016)
BioXcel AI	Multiomics and drug-target pathways	AI-based multiomics analysis	Integrates omics data to identify actionable disease targets	Cancer, metabolic disorders, autoimmune diseases	(Chakraborty et al., 2023)
H_2O.ai	Multiomics and pathway analysis	ML and DL	Analyzes large datasets for target prediction	Cancer, rare diseases, infectious diseases	(Cook, 2016)
Metascape	Pathway enrichment and network analysis	Bioinformatics-based pathway analysis	Identifies disease pathways and links them to therapeutic targets	Cancer, autoimmune diseases, cardiovascular diseases	Zhou et al., 2019 (Zhou et al., 2019)
PANDA	Transcriptional regulation, immune response pathways, and metabolic networks	Message-passing algorithm to integrate multiple biological networks	Transcription factors, genes driving disease phenotypes	Cancer, diabetes, and autoimmune disorders	(Sonawane et al., 2019)

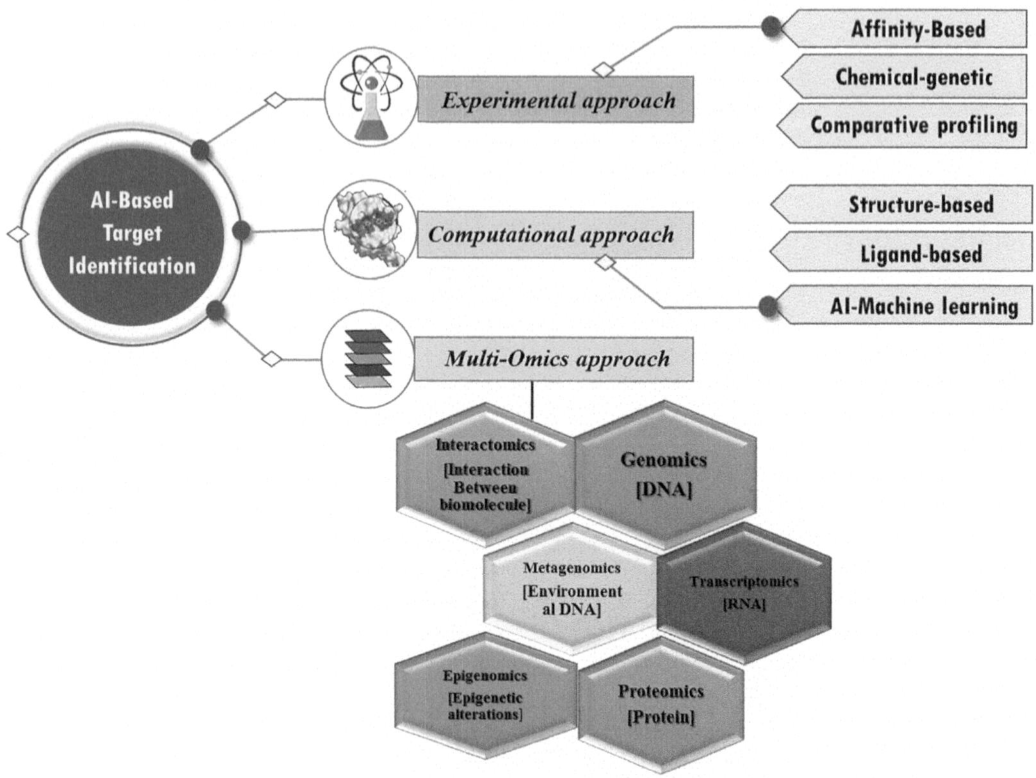

Fig. 4.4 Strategies of AI in target identification.

3.1 The AI role in drug target identification

AI encompasses computational algorithms and ML techniques that allow machines to imitate human intelligence, learning patterns from vast datasets and making predictions or automated decisions with minimal human interference. In the context of drug target identification, AI leverages omics data, literature mining, and structural biology to unravel complex biological networks and identify potential drug targets. This approach contrasts with conventional methods, which are often time and labor-intensive and also prone to experimental biases. Fig. 4.4 elaborates on various strategies of AI in target identification.

3.1.1 Accelerating the discovery process

AI facilitates the rapid analysis of extensive datasets, such as genome-wide association studies (GWAS), proteomics, metabolomics, and transcriptomics to identify biomarkers and potential therapeutic targets. For instance, DL algorithms can investigate gene expression profiles to predict disease-associated genes and pathways. A notable example is the usage of convolutional neural networks (CNNs) to analyze histopathological data for identifying cancer biomarkers (Esteva et al., 2017). Such advancements significantly reduce the timeline for identifying viable targets, which previously spanned years.

3.1.2 Enhancing predictive accuracy

Traditional drug discovery methods often struggle with false positives and false negatives due to the complexity of biological systems. AI addresses these challenges by integrating multiomics datasets and employing predictive modeling to enhance target validation accuracy. For example, AI-driven algorithms like DeepBind predict protein-DNA interactions with remarkable precision, aiding in target discovery (Alipanahi et al., 2015).

3.2 AI techniques and data types in drug target identification

Several AI methodologies have demonstrated remarkable efficacy in drug target identification. These include ML, DL, NLP, and reinforcement learning (RL).

ML: ML algorithms learn from historical data and make forecasts based on patterns. Techniques involving support vector machines (SVMs), RFs, and gradient boosting are widely used for analyzing gene-disease associations. For instance, SVMs have been applied to GWAS data to identify genetic loci linked with diseases like Alzheimer's and diabetes.

DL: DL, a subgroup of ML, utilizes ANNs with multiple layers to capture complex data relationships. RNNs and CNNs have been instrumental in analyzing genomic sequences and protein structures. AlphaFold, an AI model developed by DeepMind, exemplifies DL's potential by forecasting the structures of proteins with accuracy on par with experimental data (Jumper et al., 2021).

NLP: NLP assists AI systems in examining unstructured text sources, such as scientific literature and electronic health documentation. Tools like BioBERT and PubMed...

RL: RL algorithms optimize decision-making by learning from interactions with the environment. In target identification, RL has been employed to design molecules with specific binding affinities to target proteins (Popova et al., 2018).

3.3 Applications of AI in target identification

AI's versatility has facilitated its application across several phases of drug target discovery, from disease pathway elucidation to structural prediction.

Multiomics data integration: Diseases often result from the interaction between genetic, epigenetic, and environmental influences. AI integrates multiomics data to construct comprehensive disease models, identifying key drivers of pathogenesis. For example, AI-based tools like TensorFlow and PyTorch have been employed to integrate transcriptomic and proteomic datasets for cancer target discovery (Cheng, 2021).

Network biology: Network-based approaches, powered by AI, analyze protein–protein interaction (PPI) networks to categorize hub proteins crucial for disease progression. Algorithms like DeepGraphMine analyze PPI networks to predict novel drug targets, particularly in complex diseases like neurodegenerative disorders (Wang, 2020)

Structural biology: AI enhances structure-based drug design by envisioning the three-dimensional structures of target proteins and their interactions with ligands. The success of **AlphaFold** in accurately predicting protein folding has opened innovative avenues for understanding protein function and designing targeted therapies (Jumper et al., 2021).

Modeling and predicting molecular interactions for drug development: AI algorithms, including SVMs and CNNs, are employed to classify PPIs, predict drug-binding sites, and model protein structures (Dhakal et al., 2022).

Personalized medicine: AI models, including RFs and logistic regression, are applied to forecast disease risk through the analysis of personal genetic information and clinical data (Rezayi et al., 2022). DL algorithms also analyze biomarkers and clinical imaging data to assist in disease diagnostic determination and prognosis.

Medical image analysis: DL algorithms, particularly CNNs, are used for segmenting clinical imaging, identifying aberrations, and classifying diseases. Medical image features are extracted using computer vision techniques for deeper evaluation.

Medical image analysis: DL algorithms, particularly CNNs, are used for segmenting clinical imaging, identifying aberrations, and classifying diseases. Medical image features are extracted using computer vision techniques for deeper evaluation.

Biomedical text mining: NLP methods are employed to derive information from biomedical literature, encompassing scientific literature and experimental records. ML models, including topic modeling and sentiment analysis, facilitate the identification of relevant information and the classification of documents (Rojas-Carabali et al., 2024).

4 AI-assisted validation of identified drug targets

Drug target validation is a vital step in drug discovery and development, ensuring that the identified targets, such as biomolecules, proteins, genes, enzymes, or pathways, have a direct and significant role in the mechanism of disease. To alter the disease mechanism, modifying the activity of the molecular target is the fundamental approach in drug discovery. Developing a novel drug is initiated from target identification through the adoption of advanced methodologies. Target discovery requires a therapeutic rationale aimed at modulating target regulation and involves identifying evidence associating a target with a disease. Then, validation of the identified targets is carried out using in vivo and ex vivo models, with clinical data playing an important role (Dara et al., 2022). the drug target in cell and animal models is crucial for reducing project failure and minimizing the overall cost of drug discovery, which may not translate into effective therapies within the pharmaceutical industry (Pun et al., 2023). However, the drug development process begins with identifying and prioritizing targets based on the available information and literature studies. Once the target is identified, its role in the specific disease is confirmed using various experimental models, a process known as target validation. Initial validation of the identified target is critical to directing resources toward promising molecules with a higher likelihood of success (Failli et al., 2019). Today, in modern biology, massive datasets are generated through various sources, including clinical imaging, transcriptomics, proteomics, metabolomics analyses, and genetic information from large populations, which have paved the way for new possibilities in early target discovery and validation. AI is gradually being utilized to analyze these complex datasets and provide predictions for target selection and validation in data-driven experiments and animal models (Yoo et al., 2023). AI offers a robust framework for potential drug target validation by combining various data-driven approaches with computational models and experimental models. Traditional and conventional target validation methods rely on extensive experimental studies or assays, which are nonautomated, power-intensive, and limited when dealing with the intricacies of biological systems. AI is increasingly successful in identifying drug targets that are validated (Pun et al., 2023). For instance, in a Drosophila model that mimics amyotrophic lateral sclerosis (ALS), 28 AI—identified targets were found for ALS treatment. This study revealed eight novel targets that were previously reported and found to significantly reduce neurodegeneration in the Drosophila's eyes when their function was suppressed (Pun et al., 2022). Within the same therapeutic domain, an ML-based approach was utilized to recognize KANK1 as a new target gene linked with ALS. Subsequently, the neurotoxicity effect of KANK1 mutation was validated using CRISPR-Cas9 in human neurons (Zhang et al., 2022). In addition, using DL methods, CDK20 was acknowledged as a potential target for hepatocellular carcinoma (HCC) treatment. A highly potent novel molecular inhibitor, created by generative AI, exhibited selective antiproliferative activity in HCC cell growth (Ren et al., 2023). Following this, through the use of DL methodologies, histone deacetylase 6 (HDAC6) inhibition emerged as a potential cardioprotective strategy, which was then validated using BAG3 cardiomyocyte-knockout mouse model of heart disease (Yang et al., 2022). In addition, deepDTnet was developed—a system that integrates 15 data types, including chemical, phenotypic, cellular, and genomic information—to facilitate the computational identification of new molecular drug targets for existing medications (Zeng et al., 2020).

AI—assisted target validation methods employ ML to assimilate diverse data types, including pathway analysis, gene expression profiles, and information derived from scientific literature (Zhou et al., 2024). They are known to be prevailing tools, demonstrating significant utility in the validation of identified drug targets, improving research and development effectively, facilitating the analysis of wide-ranging biomedical data, and augmenting the decision-making processes involved in patient recruitment for clinical trials. AI uses ML, DL, and other advanced techniques for target validation by processing multidimensional data from proteomic, transcriptomic, genomic, and metabolomic sources.

4.1 ML in drug target validation

ML methods are increasingly implemented in target identification and validation due to the escalating prevalence of data-driven experimentation within the field. Identifying therapeutic drug targets starts with understanding how diseases are caused by manipulating complex biological systems, either through natural or experimental validation. ML approaches, such as decision-tree classifiers, are utilized to examine protein–protein interaction networks. This analysis enables the identification of critical factors, such as transcription pathways and metabolic processes, involved in cellular functions (Costa et al., 2010). Utilizing genomic data, Jeon and his colleagues developed an SVM-based classifier to differentiate druggable and nondruggable proteins in ovarian and breast cancers (Jeon et al., 2014). This classifier approach identified considerable potential drug targets across a wide range of multiple cancer types. Validation through peptide inhibitors exposed significant antiproliferative properties, with breast cancer cells exhibiting a twofold increase compared to other methods.

Target identification and validation have been substantially advanced through ML approaches and their associated methodologies. LASSO (L1 regularization) and regression models are utilized to construct a genome-scale model of 718 transcription factors within the mouse striatum, identifying early intervention in Huntington's disease (Ament et al., 2018). Following a similar strategy, Mamoshina et al. (2018) utilize supervised ML models, such as SVM, to recognize biomarkers and molecular targets decisive for the development of antiaging therapies. NLP techniques have been utilized to extract biological entities such as genes, diseases, drugs, and drug targets from biomedical databases such as Medline and European Union Adverse Drug Reaction (Bravo et al., 2015; Kim et al., 2017). In Alzheimer's disease research, DL splicing signal models have been utilized to predict alternative splicing events and integrate RNA sequence data to gain deeper therapeutic insights (Leung et al., 2014; Vaquero-Garcia et al., 2016). RF, logical models, analysis of variance (ANOVA), and many other ML techniques were employed to predict drug responses based on molecular features (Iorio et al., 2016). These tools validate the possible use of AI in the identification and validation of therapeutic targets and their complex biological systems.

4.2 Artificial neural networks on target validation

While using ANN, target validation in drug discovery faces significant challenges. High-dimensional datasets, characterized by tens to thousands of features, are vulnerable to the "curse of dimensionally", necessitating significant training data to explore the input space sufficiently (Heux et al., 2012). In addition, the selection of ANN architecture considerably influences both the training period and categorization accuracy. Different ANN algorithms can create different outcomes despite utilizing identical datasets. For instance, Bernick established that the polynomial learning machine (PLM) performs better than SVM in training and testing times while maintaining comparable accuracy, with PLMs being significantly faster for large datasets (Bernick, 2006). ANN offers an advancement over traditional statistical methods. Unlike linear models like linear discriminant analysis, most ANNs, such as multilayer perceptrons (MLPs) and SVMs, are intrinsically nonlinear, enabling them to model complex relationships. Furthermore, ANN can generalize from incomplete data lacking predefined models, and with adequate hidden neurons, an MLP can approximate any nonlinear function (Chauhan et al., 2016). ANN is implemented in various software packages, such as commercial tools like Mathematica and MATLAB, and specialized programs like JavaNNS and Neural Labs. A comparison of ANN software is available on the University of Colorado's website. Several users also develop custom ANN programs, often using fast, compiled languages like C, C++, or C#. In target validation, ANNs are employed across multiple stages, such as target discovery, compound screening, and hit evaluation. Notably, significant overlap exists between these stages.

AI algorithms possess the capability to analyze intricate biological networks and pathways, thereby identifying crucial molecules and interactions implicated in the progression of diseases. This insight can be leveraged to develop targeted therapies and personalized treatment strategies. For instance, AI can be utilized to assess stroke treatments and predict the risk of intracranial hemorrhage.

AI is significantly advancing the drug discovery pipeline by systematically examining biological data, genetic information, and disease pathways to identify potential drug targets. Furthermore, AI algorithms are capable of predicting drug interactions, thereby reducing the time required for new medications to reach the market.

5 Algorithmic approaches for target identification and validation

ML algorithms can examine genomic data to identify genes that are linked to discover four pivotal genes that hold prognostic significance for juvenile idiopathic arthritis, thereby offering valuable insights into the immune dysregulation present in autoimmune disorders (Dudek et al., 2024). Moreover, these algorithms can predict the progression of autoimmune diseases in individuals who exhibit preclinical symptoms by examining electronic health records alongside genetic information. ML algorithms can examine genomic data to identify genes that are linked with specific diseases. For example, researchers have successfully utilized ML techniques to discover four pivotal genes that hold prognostic significance for juvenile idiopathic arthritis, thereby offering valuable insights into the immune dysregulation present in autoimmune disorders (Dudek et al., 2024). Moreover, these algorithms can predict the progression of autoimmune diseases in individuals who exhibit preclinical symptoms by examining electronic health records alongside genetic information.

5.1 ML algorithms

ML algorithms serve a pivotal role in the field of bioinformatics, allowing researchers to analyze intricate biological data and uncover disease pathways (Auslander et al., 2021). Various ML techniques are employed for these purposes, each offering unique strengths in data analysis and pattern recognition.

SVMs: SVMs are robust algorithms employed for both classification and regression domains (Brereton and Lloyd, 2010). Their effectiveness is particularly pronounced in high-dimensional spaces, and they exhibit resilience to outliers. In the field of bioinformatics, SVMs are exploited for various applications, such as the classification of PPIs, the estimation of drug-binding sites, and the identification of differentially expressed genes.

K-nearest neighbors (KNN): The KNN algorithm is a straightforward yet efficient method that organizes data points based on the classes of their nearby neighbors. Within bioinformatics, KNN is applied to tasks such as gene expression analysis and disease prediction.

RF: The RF algorithm is a communal learning technique that amalgamates multiple decision trees to augment prediction accuracy. It is extensively applied in bioinformatics for tasks including the identification of genes-associated with diseases, anticipating the course of disease progression, and the classification of diseases.

Decision trees: Decision trees are graded models that formulate predictions by traversing a series of decisions derived from input features. They are characterized by their interpretability and can be utilized for both classification and regression problems (Blockeel et al., 2023). In bioinformatics, decision trees are employed for applications such as predicting disease risk and classifying patient outcomes.

5.2 Deep learning algorithms

DL algorithms, which represent a subset of ML, have exhibited significant success in a variety of bioinformatics applications. The following are some of the most frequently employed DL algorithms:

ANNs: ANNs are modeled after the structure and functionality of the human brain (Puri et al., 2016). They comprise interconnected nodes, often referred to as neurons, which are organized into multiple layers. In the field of bioinformatics, ANNs are applied to tasks such as predicting disease status, analyzing medical images, and identifying potential drug targets.

CNNs: CNNs are specialized neural networks designed for the processing of grid-like data, including images. Their architecture is particularly effective in feature extraction from images, making them valuable for bioinformatics applications, including medical image analysis, disease classification, and drug discovery.

Recurrent neural networks (RNNs): RNNs are specialized for the interpretation of sequential data, including natural language and time series. They possess a memory mechanism that enables them to retain past information for predictive purposes. In bioinformatics, RNNs find applications in analyzing gene sequences, predicting protein structures, and processing biomedical text (Tunkiel et al., 2022). This synthesis of DL algorithms underscores their pivotal role in advancing research and applications within the bioinformatics landscape.

5.3 NLP techniques

NLP methods are essential for the extraction and interpretation of information from various forms of text data, including scientific publications, healthcare records, and patents. These advanced techniques facilitate significant progress within bioinformatics and allied disciplines (Hao et al., 2021). A critical component of NLP is Named Entity Recognition, which focuses on classifying and categorizing precise entities like proteins, genes, diseases, and medications within textual content. This capability is instrumental in the development of knowledge graphs, which are invaluable for advancing drug development and scientific inquiry. Another vital NLP technique is word embeddings, which represent words as dense numerical vectors that encapsulate semantic relationships and contextual meanings. This representation enhances models' abilities to comprehend intricate associations among words, thereby improving various processes, such as text classification, information retrieval, and sentiment analysis. Furthermore, relation extraction advances this process by identifying and extracting significant associations between entities, such as drug-target interactions, gene-disease associations, and PPIs. Such analyses are critical for constructing comprehensive knowledge bases in the field. In addition, topic modeling is employed to uncover latent themes or patterns within extensive document collections (Jim et al., 2024). This technique enables the examination of trends in scientific literature and the identification of emerging health concerns in patient data. Collectively, these methodologies not only enhance data-driven decision-making but also promote innovation in bioinformatics, drug development, and personalized medicine.

6 Challenges and opportunities in AI-based target identification

6.1 Challenges in AI-based target identification

6.1.1 Data limitation and biases

AI-based drug target identification depends heavily on large, high-quality datasets. However, these datasets are often incomplete or biased, reflecting skewed population representations. Publicly available datasets are typically aggregated from predominantly well-represented groups, leading to the underrepresentation of diverse populations. Such biases may result in treatments that are effective in certain populations but not others, causing disparities in health outcomes. For example, therapies that work well in predominantly studied groups may have reduced efficacy or adverse effects in underrepresented populations due to differences in genomic characteristics and drug responses (Ramamoorthy, 2015; Popejoy and Fullerton, 2016; Gross, 2022). This issue emphasizes the urgent need for more inclusive datasets to ensure equitable health outcomes and more effective treatments for all populations (Hindorff, 2018; Landry, 2018).

6.1.2 Molecular bias in target selection

A substantial challenge in AI-powered drug discovery lies in the molecular bias associated with target selection. ffood and drug administration (FDA) -approved drugs tend to focus on certain protein classes, overrepresenting those with structural or functional similarities. This bias can influence AI models to prioritize well-explored targets, overlooking potentially novel or less conventional ones (Finan, 2017; Wood, 2019; Oprea, 2018). Furthermore, the lack of data on vast portions of the genome, including the "unknome," creates significant gaps in our understanding of all possible drug targets (Rocha, 2023). This incomplete knowledge impedes comprehensive target validation, making it challenging to identify truly novel drug targets, particularly in underexplored or emerging disease areas.

6.1.3 Dynamic nature of druggable targets

The idea of a "druggable" target is not stagnant, particularly in diseases such as cancer, where the rapid evolution of resistance mechanisms can render initially effective targets ineffective over time. This dynamic nature of diseases means that a "one disease, one target" approach may not be sufficient for long-term therapeutic success. AI models must account for the evolving nature of drug targets and their resistance mechanisms to maintain relevance and effectiveness in treatment strategies (Shabani and Hojjat-Farsangi, 2016). This requires continuous adaptation and refinement of AI models to stay ahead of emerging resistance patterns.

6.1.4 Experimental validation

While AI-based methods hold great promise for identifying potential drug targets, experimental validation is essential to ensure both the accuracy and clinical applicability of *in silico* calculations. Predictions made by AI models must be substantiated through experimental studies to ensure they align with real-world biological and clinical data. Without such validation, there is a risk of relying on inaccurate predictions, which could result in ineffective treatments and wasted resources (Finan, 2017; Oprea, 2018). To overcome the disparity between computational predictions and practical clinical applications, it is essential to integrate AI models with experimental research, ensuring the efficacy and safety of proposed drug targets (Shabani and Hojjat-Farsangi, 2016).

6.2 Opportunities in AI-based target identification

6.2.1 Integration of multiomics data

AI-based drug target discovery has the potential to leverage multiomics data. By assimilating these diverse datasets, AI can provide a more holistic insight into disease mechanisms, uncovering novel drug targets that traditional methods may miss. This holistic tactic permits for the identification of complex biological pathways and networks involved in diseases, enabling the discovery of more precise and efficient treatment approaches (Huang et al., 2024; Zhang et al., 2022).

6.2.2 DL and predictive modeling

Recent advancements in DL algorithms offer significant promise for improving drug target identification. These algorithms excel at handling complex, nonlinear data and can be applied to predict three-dimensional structures of target proteins, drug-target binding affinities, and interactions. AI models like AlphaFold have already revolutionized protein structure prediction, offering new insights into how proteins interact with drug molecules. As AI continues to evolve, incorporating dynamic protein structures and molecular interactions, it will enhance our ability to predict more accurate drug-target interactions and improve drug discovery outcomes (Jumper et al., 2021).

6.2.3 Expansion of the druggable genome

AI methods hold the potential to expand the boundaries of what is considered "druggable" by uncovering targets in previously unexplored regions of the genome, including the "unknome." The ability to identify and evaluate the relevance of these targets could significantly expand the range of potential drug candidates, ultimately contributing to the discovery of new therapeutic targets for diseases that are currently underserved by existing treatments (Rocha, 2023).

6.2.4 Accelerating the drug discovery pipeline

AI's capacity to model biological systems in *silico* presents a prospect to revolutionize the drug discovery process (Nayarisseri et al., 2021). By predicting protein structures, molecular docking, and gene perturbations, AI can accelerate the identification of latent drug candidates and their interactions with target proteins. This could significantly decrease both the duration and cost of developing new drugs, allowing for faster and more efficient treatments to reach the market. This acceleration of the drug discovery process benefits both pharmaceutical industries and patients, enabling the rapid development of new therapies (Jumper et al., 2021).

6.2.5 Personalized medicine

AI's competence in evaluating massive datasets, including genetic and clinical information, offers significant potential for personalized drug target identification. By tailoring drug targets to specific patient populations, AI can help ensure that treatments are more potent with reduced adverse effects. Personalized approaches can address inequalities in treatment outcomes, particularly for underrepresented populations, by considering genomic, environmental effects, and social factors that influence health. AI-driven personalized medicine could help create more equitable healthcare systems, ensuring that therapies are optimized for diverse populations and improving overall treatment outcomes (Krittanawong et al., 2022; Liu et al., 2023).

In summary, AI-driven approaches have the potential to transfigure drug discovery by aiding faster and more precise identification of novel therapeutic targets. However, several challenges must be addressed, including issues related to AI model transparency, data reliability, and the high computational costs involved in complex analyses. In addition, biases in data, limited population diversity, and gaps in genomic knowledge further complicate the identification of viable drug targets. Despite these challenges, assimilating AI with multiomics data, advanced predictive models, and DL techniques offers substantial opportunities to overcome these barriers. Moving forward, the success of AI in drug target identification hinges on addressing these obstacles while leveraging innovative technologies aimed at improving precision and performance. In conclusion, while AI presents challenges, particularly with data biases, the dynamic nature of diseases, and the necessity for experimental validation, it also holds immense promise. Through the incorporation of multiomics data, personalized medicine, and progressive computational models, AI could uncover novel drug targets, accelerate the drug discovery pipeline, and enable more effective and equitable healthcare solutions.

7 Future perspectives and emerging trends of AI in drug discovery

AI is poised to transform the future of drug discovery by speeding up development timelines, lowering costs, and enhancing the likelihood of success in the pharmaceutical industry. Emerging trends emphasize the incorporation of AI with omics data, enabling personalized medicine through comprehensive analysis of genetic, transcriptomic, and proteomic profiles. Advanced ML techniques, such as DL, are increasingly used to envisage drug-target interactions, optimize molecular structures, and identify off-target effects, thereby streamlining both preclinical and clinical research processes. Generative AI models, including generative adversarial networks and transformers, are driving the precise de novo drug design. In addition, the convergence of AI with quantum computing and molecular simulations is unlocking insights into complex biological systems, paving the way for breakthroughs in rare diseases and multitarget therapies. As AI continues to evolve, addressing ethical concerns, ensuring data quality, and refining regulatory frameworks will be critical to its success.

Techniques such as DL, NLP, and network pharmacology integrate diverse biological data to uncover novel targets, elucidate their mechanisms, and prioritize them for further study. This combined application of experimental methods and AI-based approaches marks a modern era of precision, efficacy, and scalability in drug discovery. Table 4.5 summarizes various supervised and unsupervised AI models and tools utilized in pharmaceutical applications.

In the current era, researchers have observed a surge of biological and medical data extending from basic exploration of disease and its underlying mechanisms to clinical research in humans. AI algorithms have the ability to uncover patterns and relationships within data that might not be readily apparent to humans, potentially leading to in-depth exploration of disease pathophysiology and more effective treatments (Zhavoronkov et al., 2019; Yang et al., 2024). The contributions of AI in drug discovery include facilitating biomarker and target identification, prioritizing therapeutic indications, designing drug-like molecules, predicting pharmacokinetics, analyzing drug–target interactions, and optimizing clinical trial design (Rehman et al., 2024). AI is poised to make substantial contributions in addressing complex diseases. Conditions such as cancer (Wysocka et al., 2023), neurodegenerative disorders (Kashyap and Siddiqi, 2021), and auto-immune diseases often involve intricate and multifaceted molecular mechanisms that are difficult to decipher. Target discovery using AI can help identify novel targets and the molecular pathways underlying these conditions, offering valuable insights to support the development of effective and personalized treatments (Moingeon, 2023).

Discovering targets is an energetic step in modern drug design. With only a minor fraction of theoretical druggable targets in living beings currently identified, there is an urgent need for more active target discovery approaches. The increasing success of targets identified by AI, as validated through experimental studies, underscores

Table 4.5 Various supervised and unsupervised AI models and tools utilized in pharmaceutical applications.

Supervised learning		Unsupervised learning	
ML	DL	Clustering	Dimensionally reduction
SVM	GAN	K-means	ICA
KNN	RNN	Hierarchical	t-distributed stochastic neighbor embedding (t-SNE)
RF	CNN	Nonnegative matrix factorization (NMF)	Principal component analysis (PCA)
	GNN	Autoencoder	

the advantages of integrating the process of target identification with AI algorithms. This integration significantly enhances the efficiency of discovering novel undruggable targets and accelerates the development of new therapies (Xie et al., 2023). Addressing ethical considerations, ensuring the privacy of data, and establishing robust regulatory frameworks are essential to guarantee the responsible and ethical use of AI in drug-target identification and drug development (Hasan et al., 2024). AI's predictive modeling capabilities extend to drug repurposing, enabling the exploration of existing drugs for efficacy against new targets or diseases. By analyzing known drug-target interactions, AI algorithms can predict novel potential targets based on shared molecular features or biological activity (Paul et al., 2021; Han et al., 2023). This approach not only expedites the identification of new targets but also uncovers innovative applications for established drugs, streamlining the process of drug discovery and maximizing the therapeutic potential of existing compounds (Singh et al., 2024).

Effective target validation is critical in minimizing the risk of failure during later stages of drug development by confirming that the target is both biologically relevant and therapeutically viable. This process also aids in identifying potential off-target effects and evaluating the safety profile of drug candidates. However, despite its significance, target validation remains a complex and resource-intensive task, requiring extensive experimental efforts and a comprehensive understanding of disease biology (Mitta, 2021). Advanced AI models, like GNN and DL frameworks, can process complex biological networks to identify the functional relevance of a target within a disease pathway. In addition, AI can integrate diverse data types, including structural biology data and pharmacokinetic properties, to validate the druggability of targets in a more holistic manner (Jamialahmadi et al., 2024).

AI algorithms are critical for building confidence and acceptance within the scientific and medical health communities. While AI has shown great promise in accelerating drug discovery in early stages, such as the identification of targets and their validation, it cannot significantly reduce the time period for clinical trials (Blanco-Gonzalez et al., 2023). This is due to the extended periods needed for ethical and regulatory approvals, patient recruitment, treatment duration, and analysis of data—factors that remain constant regardless of whether AI was used in the development of the drug. Aside from these advantages, AI models have certain limitations, such as the need for high-quality data, challenges in interpretability, and adherence to ethical and regulatory standards. However, their integration into drug target identification is reshaping modern drug discovery, driving the development of innovative therapies and advancing precision medicine (Kokudeva et al., 2024).

Ultimately, drug target identification by using AI is not just a tool but a transformative paradigm that will redefine the way for new therapies and unlock new opportunities to combat complex diseases, improve therapeutic outcomes, and enhance global health.

8 Conclusion

AI is significantly transforming the field of bioinformatics, fundamentally enhancing our understanding of disease pathways. By examining complex biological datasets, AI algorithms are capable of identifying genes associated with various diseases, predicting both the risk and progression of these conditions, and elucidating the underlying mechanisms of disease. Furthermore, AI is enhancing the drug discovery and development process, resulting in the creation of effective and precisely targeted therapeutic interventions. Despite the promising advancements, several challenges persist, including model interpretability, ethical considerations, and issues of data quality. Nevertheless, the future of using AI in disease pathway analysis is optimistic, with substantial potential to improve human health outcomes. Progress in developing more interpretable models, the integration of multiomics data, and a sustained focus on personalized medicine will further strengthen the capabilities of AI in this field. As AI technology advances, it promises to revolutionize bioinformatics and transform methodologies for understanding and treating diseases. AI-driven drug target identification holds tremendous promise for revolutionizing drug discovery, offering the potential for faster, more efficient, and more accurate identification of therapeutic targets. However, addressing challenges such as data biases, molecular target representation, and the dynamic nature of drug targets will be vital for realizing its potential. By overcoming these hurdles and leveraging the opportunities presented by AI, the future of drug discovery can be transformed, eventually leading to better results for patients and more effective treatments for complex diseases.

References

Abbas, M.K.G., Rassam, A., Karamshahi, F., Abunora, R., Abouseada, M., 2024. The Role of AI in drug discovery. ChemBioChem. 1439-4227. 25 (14). doi:10.1002/cbic.202300816.

Alipanahi, B., Delong, A., Weirauch, M.T., Frey, B.J., 2015. Predicting the sequence specificities of DNA- and RNA-binding proteins by deep learning. Nat. Biotechnol. 1087-0156. 33 (8), 831–838. doi:10.1038/nbt.3300.

Ament, S.A., Pearl, J.R., Cantle, J.P., Bragg, R.M., Skene, P.J., Coffey, S.R., Bergey, D.E., Wheeler, V.C., MacDonald, M.E., Baliga, N.S., Rosinski, J., Hood, L.E., Carroll, J.B., Price, N.D., 2018. Transcriptional regulatory networks underlying gene expression changes in Huntington's disease. Mol. Syst. Biol. 1744-4292. 14 (3). Available from: https://onlinelibrary.wiley.com/journal/17444292. doi:10.15252/msb.20167435.

Argelaguet, R., Velten, B., Arnol, D., Dietrich, S., Zenz, T., Marioni, J.C., Stegle, O., 2018. Multi-Omics Factor Analysis—a framework for unsupervised integration of multi-omics data sets. Mol. Syst. Biol. 14 (6), e8124. doi:10.15252/msb.20178124.

Askr, H., Elgeldawi, E., Ella, H.A., Elshaier, Y.A.M.M., Gomaa, M.M., Hassanien, A.E., 2023. Deep learning in drug discovery: an integrative review and future challenges. Artif. Intell. Rev. 1573-7462. 56 (7), 5975–6037. Available from: https://www.springer.com/journal/10462. doi:10.1007/s10462-022-10306-1.

Auslander, N., Gussow, A.B., Koonin, E.V., 2021. Incorporating machine learning into established bioinformatics frameworks. Int. J. Mol. Sci. 1422-0067. 22 (6), 1–19. Available from: https://www.mdpi.com/1422-0067/22/6/2903/pdf. doi:10.3390/ijms22062903.

Ayon, N.J., 2023. High-throughput screening of natural product and synthetic molecule libraries for antibacterial drug discovery. Metabolites. 2218-1989. 13 (5). Available from: http://www.mdpi.com/journal/metabolites. doi:10.3390/metabo13050625.

Bajwa, J., Munir, U., Nori, A., Williams, B., 2021. Artificial intelligence in healthcare: transforming the practice of medicine. Future Healthc. J. 2514-6645. 8 (2), e188. doi:10.7861/fhj.2021-0095.

Bergen, V., Lange, M., Peidli, S., Wolf, F.A., Theis, F.J., 2020. Generalizing RNA velocity to transient cell states through dynamical modeling. Nat. Biotechnol. 38 (12), 1408–14149. doi:10.1038/s41587-020-0591-3.

Bernick, J.P., 2006. Pattern classification with polynomial learning machines. MLMTA. pp. 215–221.

Bharadwaj, S., Deepika, K., Kumar, A., Jaiswal, S., Miglani, S., Singh, D., Fartyal, P., Kumar, R., Singh, S., Singh, M.P., Gaidhane, A.M., Kumar, B., Jha, V., 2024. Exploring the artificial intelligence and its impact in pharmaceutical sciences: insights toward the horizons where technology meets tradition. Chem. Biol. Drug Des. 1747-0277. 104 (4). doi:10.1111/cbdd.14639.

Blair, M.W., Iriarte, G., Beebe, S., 2006. QTL analysis of yield traits in an advanced backcross population derived from a cultivated Andean × wild common bean (*Phaseolus vulgaris* L.) cross. Theor. Appl. Genet. 0040-5752. 112 (6), 1149–1163. doi:10.1007/s00122-006-0217-2.

Blanco-Gonzalez, A., Cabezon, A., Seco-Gonzalez, A., Conde-Torres, D., Antelo-Riveiro, P., Pineiro, A., Garcia-Fandino, R., 2023. The role of AI in drug discovery: challenges, opportunities, and strategies. Pharmaceuticals 16, 891.

Blockeel, H., Devos, L., Frénay, B., Nanfack, G., Nijssen, S., 2023. Decision trees: from efficient prediction to responsible AI. Front. Artif. Intell. 2624-8212. 6. doi:10.3389/frai.2023.1124553.

Bravo, À., Piñero, J., Queralt-Rosinach, N., Rautschka, M., Furlong, L.I., 2015. Extraction of relations between genes and diseases from text and large-scale data analysis: implications for translational research. BMC Bioinformatics. 1471-2105. 16 (1). Available from: http://www.biomedcentral.com/bmcbioinformatics/. doi:10.1186/s12859-015-0472-9.

Brereton, R.G., Lloyd, G.R., 2010. Support vector machines for classification and regression. Analyst. 1364-5528. 135 (2), 230–267. Available from: http://pubs.rsc.org/en/journals/journal/an. doi:10.1039/b918972f.

Chakraborty, C., Bhattacharya, M., Lee, S.S., 2023. Artificial intelligence enabled ChatGPT and large language models in drug target discovery, drug discovery, and development. Mol. Ther. Nucleic Acids. 33, 866–868.

Chauhan, H., Bernick, J., Prasad, D., Masand, V., 2016. The role of artificial neural networks on target validation in drug discovery and development. In: Artificial Neural Network for Drug Design, Delivery and Disposition. Elsevier Inc., United States, pp. 15–27. Available from: http://www.sciencedirect.com/science/book/9780128015599. doi:10.1016/B978-0-12-801559-9.00002-8.

Cheng, F., 2021. Omics data integration in cancer research: recent advances and future directions. Nat. Rev. Cancer 21 (9), 601–617.
Cook, D., 2016. Practical machine learning with H2O: powerful, scalable techniques for deep learning and AI. O'Reilly Media, Inc.
Costa, P.R., Acencio, M.L., Lemke, N., 2010. A machine learning approach for genome-wide prediction of morbid and druggable human genes based on systems-level data. BMC Genomics. 1471-2164. 11 (5). Available from: http://www.biomedcentral.com/1471-2164-11-S5. doi:10.1186/1471-2164-11-S5-S9Brazil.
Croft, D., Lodhia, P., Lourenco, S., MacKay, C., 2023. Effectively utilizing publicly available databases for cancer target evaluation. NAR Cancer. 2632-8674. 5 (3). doi:10.1093/narcan/zcad035.
Dara, S., Dhamercherla, S., Jadav, S.S., Babu, C.M., Ahsan, M.J., 2022. Machine learning in drug discovery: a review. Artif. Intell. Rev. 1573-7462. 55 (3), 1947–1999. Available from: www.springer.com/journal/10462. doi:10.1007/s10462-021-10058-4.
Deng, J., Yang, Z., Ojima, I., Samaras, D., Wang, F., 2022. Artificial intelligence in drug discovery: applications and techniques. Brief. Bioinform. 1467-5463. 23 (1). doi:10.1093/bib/bbab430.
Dhakal, A., McKay, C., Tanner, J.J., Cheng, J., 2022. Artificial intelligence in the prediction of protein-ligand interactions: recent advances and future directions. Brief. Bioinform. 1477-4054. 23 (1). Available from: http://bib.oxfordjournals.org. doi:10.1093/bib/bbab476.
Dudek, G., Sakowski, S., Brzezińska, O., Sarnik, J., Budlewski, T., Dragan, G., Poplawska, M., Poplawski, T., Bijak, M., Makowska, J., Spilianakis, C.G., 2024. Machine learning-based prediction of rheumatoid arthritis with development of ACPA autoantibodies in the presence of non-HLA genes polymorphisms. PLoS ONE. 1932-6203. 19 (3), e0300717. doi:10.1371/journal.pone.0300717.
Esteva, A., Kuprel, B., Novoa, R.A., Ko, J., Swetter, S.M., Blau, H.M., Thrun, S., 2017. Dermatologist-level classification of skin cancer with deep neural networks. Nature. 0028-0836. 542 (7639), 115–118. doi:10.1038/nature21056.
Ezike, T.C., Okpala, U.S., Onoja, U.L., Nwike, C.P., Ezeako, E.C., Okpara, O.J., Okoroafor, C.C., Eze, S.C., Kalu, O.L., Odoh, E.C., Nwadike, U.G., Ogbodo, J.O., Umeh, B.U., Ossai, E.C., Nwanguma, B.C., 2023. Advances in drug delivery systems, challenges and future directions. Heliyon. 2405-8440. 9 (6). Available from: http://www.journals.elsevier.com/heliyon/. doi:10.1016/j.heliyon.2023.e17488.
Failli, M., Paananen, J., Fortino, V., 2019. Prioritizing target-disease associations with novel safety and efficacy scoring methods. Sci. Rep. 2045-2322. 9 (1). doi:10.1038/s41598-019-46293-7.
Finan, C., 2017. The druggable genome and the importance of target class diversity. Nat. Rev. Drug Discov. 16 (1), 65–68.
Gao, F., Huang, K., Xing, Y., 2022. Artificial intelligence in omics. Genomics, Proteomics & Bioinformatics. 1672-0229. 20 (5), 811–813. doi:10.1016/j.gpb.2023.01.002.
Gross, R., 2022. Population diversity and health disparities in drug target discovery. Nat. Biotechnol. 40 (2), 167–179.
Han, R., Yoon, H., Kim, G., Lee, H., Lee, Y., 2023. Revolutionizing medicinal chemistry: the application of artificial intelligence (AI) in early drug discovery. Pharmaceuticals. 1424-8247. 16 (9), 1259. doi:10.3390/ph16091259.
Hao, T., Huang, Z., Liang, L., Weng, H., Tang, B., 2021. Health natural language processing: methodology development and applications. JMIR Med. Inform. 2291-9694. 9 (10), e23898. doi:10.2196/23898.
Hasan, H.E., Jaber, D., Khabour, O.F., Alzoubi, K.H., 2024. Ethical considerations and concerns in the implementation of AI in pharmacy practice: a cross-sectional study. BMC Med. Ethics. 1472-6939. 25 (1). Available from: https://bmcmedethics.biomedcentral.com/. doi:10.1186/s12910-024-01062-8.

Heux, S., Fuchs, T.J., Buhmann, J., Zamboni, N., Sauer, U., 2012. A high-throughput metabolomics method to predict high concentration cytotoxicity of drugs from low concentration profiles. Metabolomics. 1573-3890. 8 (3), 433–443. doi:10.1007/s11306-011-0386-0.

Hindorff, L.A., 2018. The diversity of the human genome and its implications for personalized medicine. Nat. Rev. Genet. 19 (1), 52–63.

Huang, D., Yang, M., Wen, X., Xia, S., Yuan, B., 2024. AI-driven drug discovery: accelerating the development of novel therapeutics in biopharmaceuticals. J. Knowl. Learn. Sci. Technol. 2959-6386. 3 (3), 206–224. doi:10.60087/jklst.vol3.n3.p.206-224.

Iorio, F., Knijnenburg, T.A., Vis, D.J., Bignell, G.R., Menden, M.P., Schubert, M., Aben, N., Gonçalves, E., Barthorpe, S., Lightfoot, H., Cokelaer, T., Greninger, P., van Dyk, E., Chang, H., de Silva, H., Heyn, H., Deng, X., Egan, R.K., Liu, Q., Mironenko, T., Mitropoulos, X., Richardson, L., Wang, J., Zhang, T., Moran, S., Sayols, S., Soleimani, M., Tamborero, D., Lopez-Bigas, N., Ross-Macdonald, P., Esteller, M., Gray, N.S., Haber, D.A., Stratton, M.R., Benes, C.H., Wessels, L.F.A., Saez-Rodriguez, J., McDermott, U., Garnett, M.J., 2016. A landscape of pharmacogenomic interactions in cancer. Cell. 1097-4172. 166 (3), 740–754. Available from: https://www.sciencedirect.com/journal/cell. doi:10.1016/j.cell.2016.06.017.

Jamialahmadi, H., Khalili-Tanha, G., Nazari, E., Rezaei-Tavirani, M., 2024. Artificial intelligence and bioinformatics: a journey from traditional techniques to smart approaches. Gastroenterol. Hepatol. Bed Bench. 2008-4234. 17 (3), 241–252. Available from: https://journals.sbmu.ac.ir/ghfbb/index.php/ghfbb/article/view/2978. doi:10.22037/ghfbb.v17i3.2977.

Jeon, J., Nim, S., Teyra, J., Datti, A., Wrana, J.L., Sidhu, S.S., Moffat, J., Kim, P.M., 2014. A systematic approach to identify novel cancer drug targets using machine learning, inhibitor design and high-throughput screening. Genome Med. 1756-994X. 6 (7). Available from: http://genomemedicine.com/content/6/7/57. doi:10.1186/s13073-014-0057-7.

Jim, J.R., Talukder, M.A.R., Malakar, P., Kabir, M.M., Nur, K., Mridha, M.F., 2024. Recent advancements and challenges of NLP-based sentiment analysis: a state-of-the-art review. Nat. Lang. Process. J. 2949-7191. 6, 100059. doi:10.1016/j.nlp.2024.100059.

Jumper, J., Evans, R., Pritzel, A., Green, T., Figurnov, M., Ronneberger, O., Tunyasuvunakool, K., Bates, R., Žídek, A., Potapenko, A., Bridgland, A., Meyer, C., Kohl, S.A.A., Ballard, A.J., Cowie, A., Romera-Paredes, B., Nikolov, S., Jain, R., Adler, J., Back, T., Petersen, S., Reiman, D., Clancy, E., Zielinski, M., Steinegger, M., Pacholska, M., Berghammer, T., Bodenstein, S., Silver, D., Vinyals, O., Senior, A.W., Kavukcuoglu, K., Kohli, P., Hassabis, D., 2021. Highly accurate protein structure prediction with AlphaFold. Nature. 0028-0836. 596 (7873), 583–589. doi:10.1038/s41586-021-03819-2.

Kadurin, A., Aliper, A., Kazennov, A., Mamoshina, P., Vanhaelen, Q., Khrabrov, K., Zhavoronkov, A., 2016. The cornucopia of meaningful leads: Applying deep adversarial autoencoders for new molecule development in oncology. Oncotarget 8 (7), 10883.

Kashyap, K., Siddiqi, M.I., 2021. Recent trends in artificial intelligence-driven identification and development of anti-neurodegenerative therapeutic agents. Mol. Divers. 1573-501X. 25 (3), 1517–1539. Available from: www.wkap.nl/journalhome.htm/1381-1991. doi:10.1007/s11030-021-10274-8.

Khurana, N., Pulsipher, A., Ghandehari, H., Alt, J.A., 2021. Meta-analysis of global and high throughput public gene array data for robust vascular gene expression discovery in chronic rhinosinusitis: implications in controlled release. J. Control. Release. 330, 878–888.

Kim, J., Kim, J.J., Lee, H., 2017. An analysis of disease-gene relationship from medline abstracts by DigSee. Sci. Rep. 2045-2322. 7. Available from: www.nature.com/srep/index.html. doi:10.1038/srep40154.

Kokudeva, M., Vichev, M., Naseva, E., Miteva, D.G., Velikova, T., 2024. Artificial intelligence as a tool in drug discovery and development. World J. Exp. Med. 2220-315X. 14 (3). Available from: https://www.wjgnet.com/2220-315x/full/v14/i3/96042.htm. doi:10.5493/wjem.v14.i3.96042.

Koscielny, G., An, P., Carvalho-Silva, D., Cham, J.A., Fumis, L., Gasparyan, R., Dunham, I., 2017. Open Targets: a platform for therapeutic target identification and validation. Nucleic Acids Res. 45 (D1), D985–D994.

Krittanawong, C., Johnson, K.W., Wang, Z., 2022. Artificial intelligence in personalized medicine: applications and challenges. J. Am. Coll. Cardiol. 79 (3), 257–270.

Landry, M.L., 2018. Addressing health disparities in drug discovery: a call for more diverse data. Nat. Med. 24 (8), 1072–1078.

Le, M.H.N., Nguyen, P.K., Nguyen, T.P.T., Nguyen, H.Q., Tam, D.N.H., Huynh, H.H., Huynh, P.K., Le, N.Q.K., 2025. An in-depth review of AI-powered advancements in cancer drug discovery. Biochim. Biophys. Acta Mol. Basis Dis. 1879-260X. 1871 (3). Available from: https://www.sciencedirect.com/science/journal/09254439. doi:10.1016/j.bbadis.2025.167680.

Leung, M.K.K., Xiong, H.Y., Lee, L.J., Frey, B.J., 2014. Deep learning of the tissue-regulated splicing code. Bioinformatics. 1460-2059. 30 (12), I121. Available from: http://bioinformatics.oxfordjournals.org/. doi:10.1093/bioinformatics/btu277.

Li, M., Jiang, Y., Zhang, Y., Zhu, H., 2023. Medical image analysis using deep learning algorithms. Front. Public Health. 2296-2565. 11. doi:10.3389/fpubh.2023.1273253.

Liu, Z., Zhang, Y., Huang, R., 2023. Harnessing AI for the future of personalized drug discovery and therapy. Nat. Biotechnol. 41 (6), 657–671.

López-Cortés, A., Cabrera-Andrade, A., Echeverría-Garcés, G., Echeverría-Espinoza, P., Pineda-Albán, M., Elsitdie, N., Bueno-Miño, J., Cruz-Segundo, C.M., Dorado, J., Pazos, A., Gonzáles-Díaz, H., Pérez-Castillo, Y., Tejera, E., Munteanu, C.R., 2024. Unraveling druggable cancer-driving proteins and targeted drugs using artificial intelligence and multi-omics analyses. Sci. Rep. 2045-2322. 14 (1). Available from: https://www.nature.com/srep/. doi:10.1038/s41598-024-68565-7.

Lu, Q., De Silva, N., Dou, D., Nguyen, T.H., Sen, P., Reinwald, B., Li, Y., 2020.
Exploiting node content for multiview graph convolutional network and adversarial regularization. In: Proceedings of the 28th international conference on computational linguistics. pp. 545–555.

Madhukar, N.S., Khade, P.K., Huang, L., Gayvert, K., Galletti, G., Stogniew, M., Allen, J.E., Giannakakou, P., Elemento, O., 2019. A Bayesian machine learning approach for drug target identification using diverse data types. Nat. Commun. 2041-1723. 10 (1). Available from: http://www.nature.com/ncomms/index.html. doi:10.1038/s41467-019-12928-6.

Magness, A., Colliver, E., Enfield, K.S., Lee, C., Shimato, M., Daly, E., Angelova, M., 2024. Deep cell phenotyping and spatial analysis of multiplexed imaging with TRACERx-PHLEX. Nat. Commun. 15 (1), 5135.

Mamoshina, P., Volosnikova, M., Ozerov, I.V., Putin, E., Skibina, E., Cortese, F., Zhavoronkov, A., 2018. Machine learning on human muscle transcriptomic data for biomarker discovery and tissue-specific drug target identification. Front. Genet. 1664-8021. 9. Available from: https://www.frontiersin.org/articles/10.3389/fgene.2018.00242/full. doi:10.3389/fgene.2018.00242.

Mitta, N.R., 2021. AI-powered drug discovery platforms for target identification and validation: utilizing deep learning algorithms to enhance high-throughput screening and accelerate drug development processes. J. AI Assist. Sci. Discov. 1 (2), 169–211.

Moingeon, P., 2023. Artificial intelligence-driven drug development against autoimmune diseases. Trends Pharmacol. Sci. 0165-6147. 44 (7), 411–424. doi:10.1016/j.tips.2023.04.005.

Mostafavi, S., Ray, D., Warde-Farley, D., Grouios, C., Morris, Q., 2008. GeneMANIA: a real-time multiple association network integration algorithm for predicting gene function. Genome Biol. 9, 1–15. doi:10.1186/gb-2008-9-s1-s4.

Muslu, O., Hoyt, C.T., Lacerda, M., Hofmann-Apitius, M., Frohlich, H., 2022. GuiltyTargets: prioritization of novel therapeutic targets with network representation learning. IEEE/ACM Trans. Comput. Biol. Bioinform. 1557-9964. 19 (1), 491–500. Available from: http://ieeexplore.ieee.org/xpl/RecentIssue.jsp?punumber=8857. doi:10.1109/TCBB.2020.3003830.

Nayarisseri, A., Khandelwal, R., Tanwar, P., Madhavi, M., Sharma, D., Thakur, G., Speck-Planche, A., Singh, S.K., 2021. Artificial intelligence, big data and machine learning approaches in precision medicine & drug discovery. Curr. Drug Targets. 1873-5592. 22 (6), 631–655. Available from: https://www.eurekaselect.com/189908/article. doi:10.2174/1389450122999210104205732.

Nguyen, D.T., Mathias, S., Bologa, C., Brunak, S., Fernandez, N., Gaulton, A., Guha, R., 2017. Pharos: collating protein information to shed light on the druggable genome. Nucleic Acids Res. 45 (D1), D995–D1002. doi:10.1093/nar/gkw1072.

Nussinov, R., Zhang, M., Liu, Y., Jang, H., 2022. AlphaFold, artificial intelligence (AI), and allostery. J. Phys. Chem. B. 126 (34), 6372–6383. doi: 10.1021/acs.jpcb.2c04346.

Oprea, T.I., 2018. Chemical space for drug discovery: expanding the targetable proteome. Nat. Rev. Drug Discov. 17 (4), 261–271.

Paila, U., Chapman, B.A., Kirchner, R., Quinlan, A.R., 2013. GEMINI: integrative exploration of genetic variation and genome annotations. PLoS Comput. Biol. 9 (7), e1003153. doi:10.1371/journal.pcbi.1003153.

Pang, Z., Lu, Y., Zhou, G., Hui, F., Xu, L., Viau, C., Xia, J., 2024. MetaboAnalyst 6.0: towards a unified platform for metabolomics data processing, analysis and interpretation. Nucleic Acids Res. 52 (W1), W398–W406. doi:10.1093/nar/gkae253.

Paul, D., Sanap, G., Shenoy, S., Kalyane, D., Kalia, K., Tekade, R.K., 2021. Artificial intelligence in drug discovery and development. Drug Discov. Today. 1878-5832. 26 (1), 80–93. Available from: www.elsevier.com/locate/drugdiscov. doi:10.1016/j.drudis.2020.10.010.

Popejoy, A.B., Fullerton, S.M., 2016. Genomics is failing on diversity. Nature. 1476-4687. 538 (7624), 161–164. Available from: http://www.nature.com/nature/index.html. doi:10.1038/538161a.

Poplin, R., Chang, P.C., Alexander, D., Schwartz, S., Colthurst, T., Ku, A., DePristo, M.A., 2018. A universal SNP and small-indel variant caller using deep neural networks. Nat. Biotechnol. 36 (10), 983–987. doi:10.1038/nbt.4235.

Popova, M., Isayev, O., Tropsha, A., 2018. Deep reinforcement learning for de novo drug design. Sci. Adv. 2375-2548. 4 (7). Available from: http://advances.sciencemag.org/content/4/7/eaap7885/tab-pdf. doi:10.1126/sciadv.aap7885.

Pun, F.W., Liu, B.H.M., Long, X., Leung, H.W., Leung, G.H.D., Mewborne, Q.T., Gao, J., Shneyderman, A., Ozerov, I.V., Wang, J., Ren, F., Aliper, A., Bischof, E., Izumchenko, E., Guan, X., Zhang, K., Lu, B., Rothstein, J.D., Cudkowicz, M.E., Zhavoronkov, A., 2022. Identification of therapeutic targets for amyotrophic lateral sclerosis using pandaomics—An AI-enabled biological target discovery platform. Front. Aging Neurosci. 1663-4365. 14. Available from: https://www.frontiersin.org/journals/aging-neuroscience#. doi:10.3389/fnagi.2022.914017.

Pun, F.W., Ozerov, I.V., Zhavoronkov, A., 2023. AI-powered therapeutic target discovery. Trends Pharmacol. Sci. 1873-3735. 44 (9), 561–572. Available from: https://www.elsevier.com/locate/tips. doi:10.1016/j.tips.2023.06.010.

Puri, M., Solanki, A., Padawer, T., Tipparaju, S.M., Moreno, W.A., Pathak, Y., 2016. Introduction to artificial neural network (ANN) as a predictive tool for drug design, discovery, delivery, and disposition. In: Artificial Neural Network for Drug Design, Delivery and Disposition. Elsevier BV, pp. 3–13. doi:10.1016/b978-0-12-801559-9.00001-6.

Quazi, S., 2022. Artificial intelligence and machine learning in precision and genomic medicine. Med. Oncol. 1559-131X. 39 (8). Available from: http://www.springer.com/humana+press/journal/12032. doi:10.1007/s12032-022-01711-1.

Ramamoorthy, A., 2015. Pharmacogenomics in diverse populations: opportunities and challenges. Pharmacol. Res. 96 (3), 105–115.

Rehman, A.U., Li, M., Wu, B., Ali, Y., Rasheed, S., Shaheen, S., Liu, X., Luo, R., Zhang, J., 2024. Role of artificial intelligence in revolutionizing drug discovery. Fundam. Res. 2667-3258. doi:10.1016/j.fmre.2024.04.021.

Ren, F., Ding, X., Zheng, M., Korzinkin, M., Cai, X., Zhu, W., Mantsyzov, A., Aliper, A., Aladinskiy, V., Cao, Z., Kong, S., Long, X., Liu, B.H.M., Liu, Y., Naumov, V., Shneyderman, A., Ozerov, I.V., Wang, J., Pun, F.W., Polykovskiy, D.A., Sun, C., Levitt, M., Aspuru-Guzik, A., Zhavoronkov, A., 2023. AlphaFold accelerates artificial intelligence powered drug discovery: efficient discovery of a novel CDK20 small molecule inhibitor. Chem. Sci. 2041-6520. 14 (6), 1443–1452. doi:10.1039/d2sc05709c.

Rezayi, S., Kalhori, S.R.N., Saeedi, S., McClellan, D.A., 2022. Effectiveness of artificial intelligence for personalized medicine in neoplasms: a systematic review. Biomed. Res. Int. 2314-6133. 2022 (1). doi:10.1155/2022/7842566.

Rocha, J.C., 2023. Exploring the unkown druggable genome: AI's potential. Trends Pharmacol. Sci. 44 (7), 523–536.

Rojas-Carabali, W., Agrawal, R., Gutierrez-Sinisterra, L., Baxter, S.L., Cifuentes-González, C., Wei, Y.C., Abisheganaden, J., Kannapiran, P., Wong, S., Lee, B., de-la-Torre, A., Agrawal, R., 2024. Natural language processing in medicine and ophthalmology: a review for the 21st-century clinician. Asia-Pac. J. Ophthalmol. 2162-0989. 13 (4). Available from: https://www.sciencedirect.com/journal/asia-pacific-journal-of-ophthalmology. doi:10.1016/j.apjo.2024.100084.

Santos, A., Colaço, A.R., Nielsen, A.B., Niu, L., Strauss, M., Geyer, P.E., Coscia, F., Albrechtsen, N.J.W., Mundt, F., Jensen, L.J., Mann, M., 2022. A knowledge graph to interpret clinical proteomics data. Nat. Biotechnol. 1546-1696. 40 (5), 692–702. Available from: http://www.nature.com/nbt/index.html. doi:10.1038/s41587-021-01145-6.

Schenone, M., Dančík, V., Wagner, B.K., Clemons, P.A., 2013. Target identification and mechanism of action in chemical biology and drug discovery. Nat. Chem. Biol. 1552-4469. 9 (4), 232–240. doi:10.1038/nchembio.1199.

Selvaraj, Chandra, Singh, n.d. Artificial intelligence and machine learning approaches for drug design: challenges and opportunities for the pharmaceutical industries. Mol. Divers. 26 (3), 1893–1913. doi:10.3390/pharmaceutics16101328.

Shabani, M., Hojjat-Farsangi, M., 2016. Targeted therapy in cancer: the dynamic landscape of drug resistance. Cancer Res. 76 (13), 3942–3950.

Shiammala, P.N., Duraimutharasan, N.K.B., Vaseeharan, B., Alothaim, A.S., Al-Malki, E.S., Snekaa, B., Safi, S.Z., Singh, S.K., Velmurugan, D., Selvaraj, C., 2023. Exploring the artificial intelligence and machine learning models in the context of drug design difficulties and future potential for the pharmaceutical sectors. Methods. 1095-9130. 219, 82–94. Available from: http://www.elsevier.com/inca/publications/store/6/2/2/9/1/4/index.htt. doi:10.1016/j.ymeth.2023.09.010.

Singh, A., 2021. DeepChem and its importance in Drug Discovery and Biology. Int. J. Eng. Dev. Res. 9 (4), 56–60.

Singh, S., Pandey, A.K., Prajapati, V.K., 2024. From genome to clinic: the power of translational bioinformatics in improving human health. Adv. Protein Chem. Struct. Biol. 139, 1–25. Available from: https://www.sciencedirect.com/science/bookseries/18761623. doi:10.1016/bs.apcsb.2023.11.010.

Singh, S., Sarma, D.K., Verma, V., Nagpal, R., Kumar, M., 2023. Unveiling the future of metabolic medicine: omics technologies driving personalized solutions for precision treatment of metabolic disorders. Biochem. Biophys. Res. Commun. 1090-2104. 682, 1–20. Available from: http://www.sciencedirect.com/science/journal/0006291X. doi:10.1016/j.bbrc.2023.09.064.

Sonawane, A.R., Weiss, S.T., Glass, K., Sharma, A., 2019. Network medicine in the age of biomedical big data. Front. Genet. 10, 294.

Sun, D., Gao, W., Hu, H., Zhou, S., 2022. Why 90% of clinical drug development fails and how to improve it?. Acta Pharm. Sin. B. 2211-3835. 12 (7), 3049–3062. doi:10.1016/j.apsb.2022.02.002.

Sun, Y., Li, Y.Y., Leung, C.K., Hu, P., 2024. iNGNN-DTI:: prediction of drug–target interaction with interpretable nested graph neural network and pretrained molecule models. Bioinformatics 40 (3), btae135, doi:10.1093/bioinformatics/btae135.

Tunkiel, A.T., Sui, D., Wiktorski, T., 2022. Impact of data pre-processing techniques on recurrent neural network performance in context of real-time drilling logs in an automated prediction framework. J. Pet. Sci. Eng. 0920-4105. 208, 109760. doi:10.1016/j.petrol.2021.109760.

Uzoeto, H.O., Cosmas, S., Bakare, T.T., Durojaye, O.A., 2024. AlphaFold-latest: revolutionizing protein structure prediction for comprehensive biomolecular insights and therapeutic advancements. Beni-Suef Univ. J. Basic Appl. Sci. 13 (1), 46. doi:10.1186/s43088-024-00503-y.

Vaquero-Garcia, J., Barrera, A., Gazzara, M.R., Gonzalez-Vallinas, J., Lahens, N.F., Hogenesch, J.B., Lynch, K.W., Barash, Y., 2016. A new view of transcriptome complexity and regulation through the lens of local splicing variations. eLife. 2050-084X. 5. Available from: http://elifesciences.org/content/5/e11752full.pdf. doi:10.7554/eLife.11752.

Wang, S., Sim, T.B., Kim, Y.S., Chang, Y.T., 2004. Tools for target identification and validation. Curr. Opin. Chem. Biol. 8 (4), 371–377. doi:10.1016/j.cbpa.2004.06.001.

Wang, S., Zheng, H., Wen, X., Fu, S., 2024. Distributed high-performance computing methods for accelerating deep learning training. J. Knowl. Learn. Sci. Technol. 2959-6386. 3 (3), 108–126. doi:10.60087/jklst.v3.n3.p108-126.

Wang, W., 2024. AI based drug screening process: from data mining to candidate drug validation. Biosci. Methods 1925-1920. doi:10.5376/bm.2024.15.0005.

Wang, Z., 2020. DeepGraphMine: end-to-end learning of molecule graphs. Bioinformatics 36 (12), 3602–3612.

Wood, S.D., 2019. Targeting novel proteins for drug discovery: the untapped potential of the 'unknome'. J. Med. Chem. 62 (15), 7557–7569.

Wysocka, M., Wysocki, O., Zufferey, M., Landers, D., Freitas, A., 2023. A systematic review of biologically-informed deep learning models for cancer: fundamental trends for encoding and interpreting oncology data. BMC Bioinformatics. 1471-2105. 24 (1). doi:10.1186/s12859-023-05262-8.

Xie, X., Yu, T., Li, X., Zhang, N., Foster, L.J., Peng, C., Huang, W., He, G., 2023. Recent advances in targeting the "undruggable" proteins: from drug discovery to clinical trials. Signal Transduct. Target. Ther. 2059-3635. 8 (1). Available from: https://www.nature.com/sigtrans. doi:10.1038/s41392-023-01589-z.

Yadav, S., Singh, A., Singhal, R., Yadav, J.P., 2024. Revolutionizing drug discovery: the impact of artificial intelligence on advancements in pharmacology and the pharmaceutical industry. Intell. Pharm. 2949-866X. 2 (3), 367–380. Available from: https://www.keaipublishing.com/en/journals/intelligent-pharmacy/. doi:10.1016/j.ipha.2024.02.009.

Yan, J., Zhang, Z., Zhu, J., Zhang, K., Pei, J., Liu, Q., 2024. Deltadock: A unified framework for accurate, efficient, and physically reliable molecular docking. arXiv preprint arXiv:2410.11224.

Yang, J., Grafton, F., Ranjbarvaziri, S., Budan, A., Farshidfar, F., Cho, M., Xu, E., Ho, J., Maddah, M., Loewke, K.E., Medina, J., Sperandio, D., Patel, S., Hoey, T., Mandegar, M.A., 2022. Phenotypic screening with deep learning identifies HDAC6 inhibitors as cardioprotective in a BAG3 mouse model of dilated cardiomyopathy. Sci. Transl. Med. 1946-6242. 14 (652). Available from: https://www.science.org/doi/10.1126/scitranslmed.abl5654. doi:10.1126/scitranslmed.abl5654.

Yang, X., Huang, K., Yang, D., Zhao, W., Zhou, X., 2024. Biomedical big data technologies, applications, and challenges for precision medicine: a review. Glob. Challenges. 2056-6646. 8 (1). doi:10.1002/gch2.202300163.

Yoo, J., Kim, T.Y., Joung, I.S., Song, S.O., 2023. Industrializing AI/ML during the end-to-end drug discovery process. Curr. Opin. Struct. Biol. 1879-033X. 79. Available from: http://www.elsevier.com/locate/sbi. doi:10.1016/j.sbi.2023.102528.

Zeng, H., Gifford, D.K., 2019. DeepLigand: accurate prediction of MHC class I ligands using peptide embedding. Bioinformatics 35 (14), i278–i283. doi:10.1093/bioinformatics/btz330.

Zeng, X., Zhu, S., Lu, W., Liu, Z., Huang, J., Zhou, Y., Fang, J., Huang, Y., Guo, H., Li, L., Trapp, B.D., Nussinov, R., Eng, C., Loscalzo, J., Cheng, F., 2020. Target identification among known drugs by deep learning from heterogeneous networks. Chem. Sci. 2041-6520. 11 (7), 1775–1797. doi:10.1039/c9sc04336e.

Zhang, S., Cooper-Knock, J., Weimer, A.K., Shi, M., Moll, T., Marshall, J.N.G., Harvey, C., Nezhad, H.G., Franklin, J., Souza, C.D.S., Ning, K., Wang, C., Li, J., Dilliott, A.A., Farhan, S., Elhaik, E., Pasniceanu, I., Livesey, M.R., Eitan, C., Hornstein, E., Kenna, K.P., Blair, I., Wray, N.R., Kiernan, M., Neto, M.M., Chio, A., Cauchi, R., Robberecht, W., van Damme, P., Corcia, P., Couratier, P., Hardiman, O., McLaughin, R., Gotkine, M., Drory, V., Ticozzi, N., Silani, V., Veldink, J.H., van den Berg, L.H., de Carvalho, M., Pardina, J.S.M., Povedano, M., Andersen, P., Weber, M., Başak, N.A., Al-Chalabi, A., Shaw, C., Shaw, P.J., Morrison, K.E., Landers, J.E., Glass, J.D., Ferraiuolo, L., Snyder, M.P., 2022. Genome-wide identification of the genetic basis of amyotrophic lateral sclerosis. Neuron. 1097-4199. 110 (6), 992. Available from: http://www.cell.com/neuron/home. doi:10.1016/j.neuron.2021.12.019.

Zhavoronkov, A., Li, R., Ma, C., Mamoshina, P., 2019. Deep biomarkers of aging and longevity: from research to applications. Aging. 1945-4589. 11 (22), 10771–10780. doi:10.18632/aging.102475.

Zhou, G., Xia, J., 2018. OmicsNet: a web-based tool for creation and visual analysis of biological networks in 3D space. Nucleic Acids Res. 46 (W1), W514–W522. doi:10.1093/nar/gky510.

Zhou, S., Yuan, B., Xu, K., Zhang, M., Zheng, W., 2024. The impact of pricing schemes on cloud computing and distributed systems. J. Knowl. Learn. Sci. Technol. 2959-6386. 3 (3), 193–205. doi:10.60087/jklst.v3.n3.p206-224.

Zhou, Y., Zhang, Y., Lian, X., Li, F., Wang, C., Zhu, F., Qiu, Y., Chen, Y., 2022. Therapeutic target database update 2022: facilitating drug discovery with enriched comparative data of targeted agents. Nucleic Acids Res. 0305-1048. 50 (D1), D1398. doi:10.1093/nar/gkab953.

Zhou, Y., Zhou, B., Pache, L., Chang, M., Khodabakhshi, A.H., Tanaseichuk, O., Chanda, S.K., 2019. Metascape provides a biologist-oriented resource for the analysis of systems-level datasets. Nat. Commun. 10 (1), 1523. doi:10.1038/s41467-019-09234-6.

5

AI based target-ligand binding methods

Muthuraja Arun Pravin*, Saravanan Priyadharshini*, Mohammad Aqueel Khan, Rajaram Abhirami, and Sanjeev Kumar Singh

Computer Aided Drug Design and Molecular Modelling Lab, Department of Bioinformatics, Alagappa University, Karaikudi, Tamil Nadu, India

1 Introduction

Drug discovery is a very time-consuming (around 12–15 years), risk-driven (highest failure rate), and expensive process (around $2.8 billion) (Hughes et al., 2011) to discover a novel drug and bring it to the market with prior approval from the Food and Drug Administration (FDA), USA. (Hinkson et al., 2020; Dominguez and Willis, 2020). Thus, pharmaceutical companies need cutting-edge technology to decrease the time, expenses, and failure rates of clinical trials in the drug discovery and development processes. Artificial intelligence (AI) is one such widely recognized technique which gives machines the ability to replicate human intelligence in problem-solving and knowledge. Currently, AI is extensively used at several stages of the drug discovery and development processes, including drug screening, drug designing, repurposing of drugs, drug safety, and poly-pharmacology to classify a promising drug molecule (Blanco-Gonzalez et al., 2023). The first compound designed using AI is DSP-1181, an agonist acting on the 5-HT_{1A} receptor developed by Exscientia, and currently in Phase I clinical trial studies for obsessive-compulsive disorder (Yoshinaga et al., 2020). The journey of a drug from small-scale scientific discovery and hypothesis to large-scale market-approved therapeutics is still a highly complex endeavor. For the past few decades, the pharmaceutical industry has been constructed under the umbrella of several scientific domains, such as next-generation sequencing, multiomics analysis, proteomics, experimental validations, and clinical trials (Ferreira and

* Authors contributed equally.

The AI Frontier in Molecular Modelling and Drug Designing. https://doi.org/10.1016/B978-0-443-40338-5.00006-8

Carneiro, 2025). These scientific domains work in tandem to produce large-scale therapeutics for various diseases. However, the pharmaceutical industry has now undergone tremendous reforms with the advancement of AI. The abundance of biological datasets has allowed computational scientists to develop AI-based tools which can learn from the vast amount of biological data and predict the molecular interactions, dynamics, and pharmacological outcomes of newer drug molecules with significantly reduced time and cost.

In this chapter, we will comprehensively explore the fundamentals of drug discovery and the latest advancements in this field. The primary focus will be on the application of AI in predicting protein-ligand interactions and drug-drug interactions (DDIs) to transform the drug discovery pipeline.

2 Fundamentals of drug discovery

Biological interaction refers to the interaction of a small molecule to the protein at specific site, inducing a conformational change and resulting in cascade of downstream biological events. The activation of biological events depends on nature of interaction which is broadly classified into intra and intermolecular interaction (covalent and noncovalent interaction). The intermolecular interaction plays a crucial role in protein-ligand interaction. The strength of interaction is based on the percentage of complementarity the ligand brings for a successful interaction. The major intermolecular interactions include hydrogen bonds, π-cation interactions, salt bridges, hydrophobic interactions, and van der Waals forces. Based on the above features, several models have been introduced and have evolved over time. These models work based on the principal of binding affinity of ligand towards the protein (Wang, 2024). The two major metrics which quantify the binding affinity include dissociation constant (Kd) and inhibition constant (Ki). These metrics helps in distinguishing the strength of binding and specificity of interaction, thus minimizing off-target complications and side effects. The early-stage drug discovery involves identification of plausible drug targets in disease causing pathogen and genes responsible for the disease. The identified drug targets will be comprehensively study for their functional importance subsequently undergo experimental study. The initial phase of drug discovery and experimental validation of targets involve stringent processes such as targets' nature, druggable regions and identification of specific drug targets. Identification of drug targets and developing a specific drug target with favorable absorption, distribution, metabolism, excretion, and toxicity (ADMET) properties, has been foundational challenge in drug discovery. The above technique is a kind of linear process that requires several billions of dollars and eventually only 1% of drug molecule enters the clinical trial and approved by US FDA. As the traditional drug development pipeline has become slow and ineffective comparatively at some point, a near era of AI based drug discovery has emerged transforming the healthcare system altogether.

3 Traditional methods in computational drug design

The traditional experimental methods, along with computational techniques, were used for the identification of drug-targets, and for decades, their interactions were governed at the residue level using computational tools known as molecular docking (Eberhardt et al., 2021). Molecular docking is a widely used *in silico* technique to identify the ligands' preferred orientation within the binding cavity of macromolecules (proteins). Molecular docking tools use robust methods such as random sampling, algorithms, and scoring functions to rank the best-binding compounds for the protein's active site (Arun Pravin et al., 2024). Traditional computational drug design methods are broadly classified into structure-based drug design (SBDD) and ligand-based drug design (LBDD).

3.1 Structure-based drug design

SBDD is a widely used technique in computational drug design, where the macromolecular structure or receptor is known and the inhibitor is identified based on the binding site of the protein. In general, only the high-resolution structures that have been determined from X-ray crystallography and nuclear magnetic resonance (NMR) spectroscopy are utilized for SBDD. The high-resolution structure of the receptor is retrieved from the Protein Data Bank (PDB) (Berman et al., 2000) and is subjected to further *in silico* studies involving protein preparation, active site prediction, and molecular docking with a set of ligand molecules. Molecular docking, as discussed above, is a computational technique used to study the crucial interaction between protein and ligand. The molecular docking tool uses poses of the ligand to determine the affinity of the ligand. The ligands are sampled based on good poses and are further ranked using scoring functions (Gu et al., 2025). There are primarily three scoring functions that are widely used in molecular docking (Table 5.1).

a) **Knowledge-based scoring functions**
b) **Empirical scoring functions**
c) **Physics-based scoring functions**

Table 5.1 Comparison of different types of scoring functions.

S. No.	Scoring function	Analytical method	Advantages	Constraints	Examples of tools/ software.
1.	Knowledge-based	A data-driven approach uses a knowledge-based potential derived from known protein-ligand interactions	Good scoring method due to the use of prior knowledge of protein-ligand interaction	The reliability of scoring depends on the quality of structural data	DrugScore, GOLD, Surflex-Dock
2.	Empirical scoring	Uses a Weighted sum approach learned from experimental data	Reliable due to a calculation based on experimental data.	Requires better tuning of parameters, as the scoring can be inaccurate for unseen protein-ligand interactions	AutoDock, AutoDock Vina, and Glide
3	Physics-based	It uses physics-based calculations (force fields) to measure the distance and bonding of atoms	It is accurate due to the use of physics laws to measure the individual energy components. Contributing to the protein-ligand interaction	It is computationally demanding and takes longer to run	GROMACS, AMBER, CHARMM, MMGBSA

3.1.1 Knowledge-based scoring functions

As the name suggests, the scoring function uses the interatomic contacts from a known protein-ligand interaction database. Based on the frequency of correlation between the known database and newly docked complexes, a score will be allotted for the best pose (Gohlke et al., 2000). The knowledge-based scoring uses a statistical potential, Potential of Mean Force, to estimate the binding free energy between the interacting molecules based on knowledge of preexisting experimental structures.

3.1.2 Empirical scoring functions

The empirical scoring function works on a similar principle to known experimental binding data but includes a mathematical model, which calculates the total binding affinity of the protein-ligand complex by the summation of individual physical contributions (hydrogen bonds, van der Waals interactions, hydrophobic interactions, electrostatic interactions) (Guedes et al., 2018).

3.1.3 Physics-based scoring functions

The physics-based scoring uses fundamental physics, such as molecular mechanics, to estimate the binding energies of protein-ligand interactions. The potential energy is calculated based on the physical interactions, such as electrostatic interactions and other bonded and nonbonded interactions. A physics-based approach uses a mathematical model, which contains the parameters of atoms in a system. It calculates the potential energy of atoms based on the atomic positions and their bonds, intra and inter molecular interactions (Guedes et al., 2021). The physics-based approach provides an accurate analysis of protein-ligand interactions and has been successful in most protein-ligand docking studies.

3.2 Ligand-based drug design

LBDD is a computational technique which involves the identification of suitable drug targets for the known inhibitors. Here, the receptor structure is unavailable, and a set of inhibitors with known biological properties is available. The LBDD consists of several domains, but the primary techniques include pharmacophore modeling and quantitative structure-activity relationship (QSAR) analysis.

3.2.1 Pharmacophore modeling

Pharmacophore modeling involves the identification of key pharmacophoric features in active ligands and screening for compounds with similar biological properties (Yang, 2010). The pharmacophore model is validated and screened against a vast number of chemical libraries in a protocol known as ligand-based virtual screening. The pharmacophoric features include hydrogen-bond donors/acceptors, aromatic rings, and hydrophobic regions. These 3D descriptors play a crucial role in pharmacophore-based screening.

3.2.2 Quantitative structure–activity relationship

The QSAR is a widely used computational method for predicting the effectiveness of a compound based on its structure. QSAR is based on classical machine learning (ML) methods such as linear regression, decision trees (DTs), support vector machines (SVMs), and random forests (RFs) (Khan and Singh, 2023). These models understand the patterns of chemical descriptors and correlate them with observed biological activity. At first, the molecular descriptors are converted into numerical values and used to train the ML models. The trained model is validated and tested against new untested molecules (Fig. 5.1). There are primarily four types of QSAR prediction methods: Linear QSAR, Nonlinear QSAR, 2D-QSAR, and 3D-QSAR (Selvaraj et al., 2023). All four QSAR types have a similar principle, but differ in input features and mathematical models. The LBDD has been effective in identifying similar sets of chemical libraries, but has shown major limitations in identifying novel scaffolds along with heavily relying on the quality of active molecules used for training and human-defined descriptors which need stronger expertise to curate appropriate descriptors and select an appropriate model for training and validation.

The traditional approach has been accurate for known protein-ligand interactions and has been used for decades, but it has certain limitations, such as slow screening, lack of accuracy for flexible proteins, and the neglect of solvation effects. Despite being slow and having some limitations, the traditional molecular docking technique has been highly successful in most protein-ligand interactions. The ligand-based approaches, such as QSAR, have been the first pioneers of machine learning in computational drug design. It was effectively used over decades, with several improvisations at regular intervals of time. However, the emergence of newer computational technologies, such as AI, has proven to be instrumental in reshaping the drug

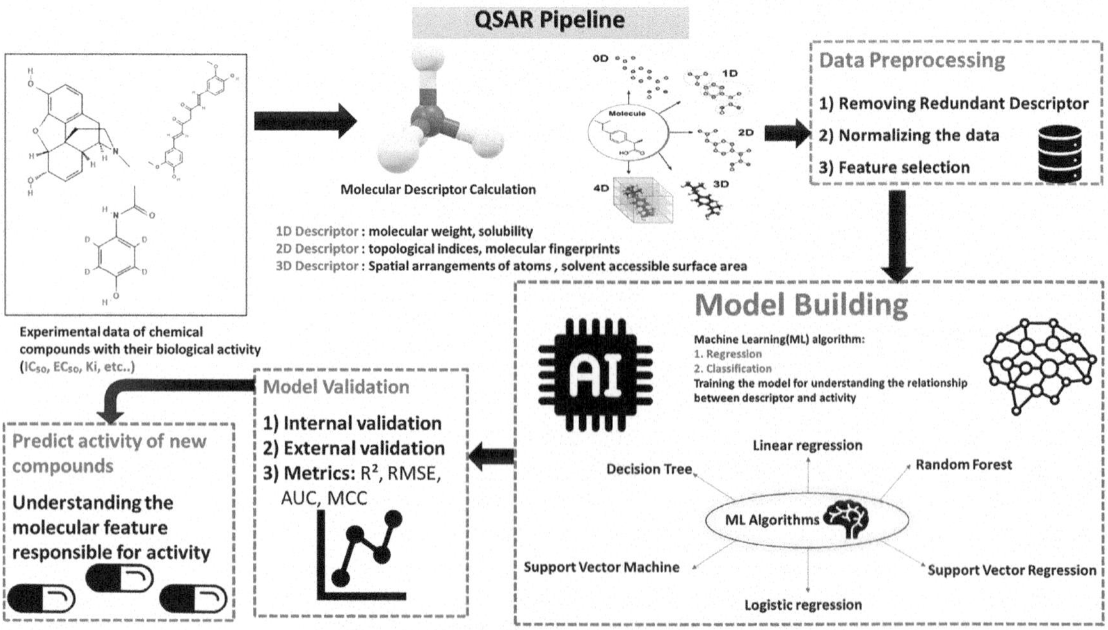

Fig. 5.1 Illustration of QSAR pipeline.

discovery landscape. The fields, particularly ML/ deep learning (DL) and large language models (LLMs), have been pivotal in transforming healthcare. The current iteration of AI has the ability to learn, analyze, and recognize patterns from large amounts of high-dimensional data, which were not possible with previous statistical models. Hence, this new revolution in computational technology can significantly enhance and improve traditional drug discovery methods.

4 The emergence of artificial intelligence in drug development

Over the past six years, the drug discovery pipeline has undergone a paradigm shift, transforming the health care industry rapidly. After the emergence of DL, LLMs and generative AI have significantly transformed the drug discovery landscape. The earlier versions of AI, such as classical ML—RF, SVM, and linear regression models, have been accurate for small quantities of data but possessed limitations when applied to larger, high-dimensional data sets. Hence, the newer iteration of AI has evolved beyond the previous ML models, with an ability to learn from a vast amount of biological data (Shiammala et al., 2023). As a result, it has significantly improved various stages of drug design. Therefore, major pharma industries have been incorporating AI in various stages of drug development such as Research and Development (R&D), target identification, lead identification, and clinical trials.

4.1 The AI-driven approaches in drug design

AI-driven drug design provides a significant enhancement over traditional computational methods. The traditional computational tools, such as QSAR, use statistical models or ML models (RF, SVM), where the data are fitted into a predefined model. Here, the molecular descriptor is selected manually, and the model is tested against a new dataset. However, in the case of DL and newer AI models, they can learn from vast libraries of raw chemical and biological data without human intervention. For instance, a DL model can automatically extract features from compound libraries and learn from raw data. Similarly, a convolutional neural network (CNN) can learn from 3D spatial patterns of protein–ligand complexes and assess the best-binding compound. A graph neural network (GNN) can operate on biologically active compounds and identify the 2D molecular graphs, recognizing important molecular features such as scaffolds and R groups for searching similar sets of compounds. These models capture novel features of compounds and complex patterns in protein-ligand interactions, which were not possible to identify using previous statistical models or tools. AI models can learn from vast, heterogeneous, and extremely diverse datasets such as protein sequences, gene expression data, and clinical outcomes. Thus, the current era of modern machine intelligence is proving to be instrumental in discovering novel drug molecules for deadly diseases.

4.1.1 A comparison of traditional versus AI drug design

The traditional computational tools, such as Genetic Optimisation for Ligand Docking (GOLD), Molecular Operating Environment (MOE), Schrödinger Grid-based Ligand Docking with Energetics (GLIDE), and AutoDock Vina, use an empirical or physics-based scoring with a random sampling approach to determine the best binding poses of screened chemical compounds. However, the newer iterations of docking and virtual screening tools have made a lot of progress by incorporating AI models such as DL, which have been consistent and shown superior performance across all sets of chemical and biological data. The workflow of traditional and AI-based drug design was depicted in Fig. 5.2. However, the increase in predictive power led to an increase in computational cost. A DL model requires a high-performance Graphics Processing Unit (GPU) system and expertise in AI algorithms. As AI algorithms such as DL are complex, it can be hard to understand the basis of prediction in any particular drug development scenario. The traditional methods use physics-based and empirical methods which are transparent and are easy to understand, as the underlying model uses physical information about two individual interacting molecules; the researcher can easily understand the basis of prediction. In contrast, a DL model has numerous parameters and intricate layers that are difficult for non-expert researchers to understand and calibrate. Below (Table 5.2) is the comprehensive comparison table of traditional computational approaches and AI-driven approaches.

5 AI in Structure Based Drug Design (SBDD)

The application of AI has been evident in diverse fields of drug design. The modern evolution of AI has been used to develop specialized algorithm and tools that can tackle specific drug discovery challenges. This section provides a comprehensive analysis of AI-driven tools and their technical details, examining the capabilities of AI in protein structure prediction, molecular interaction and novel drug identification

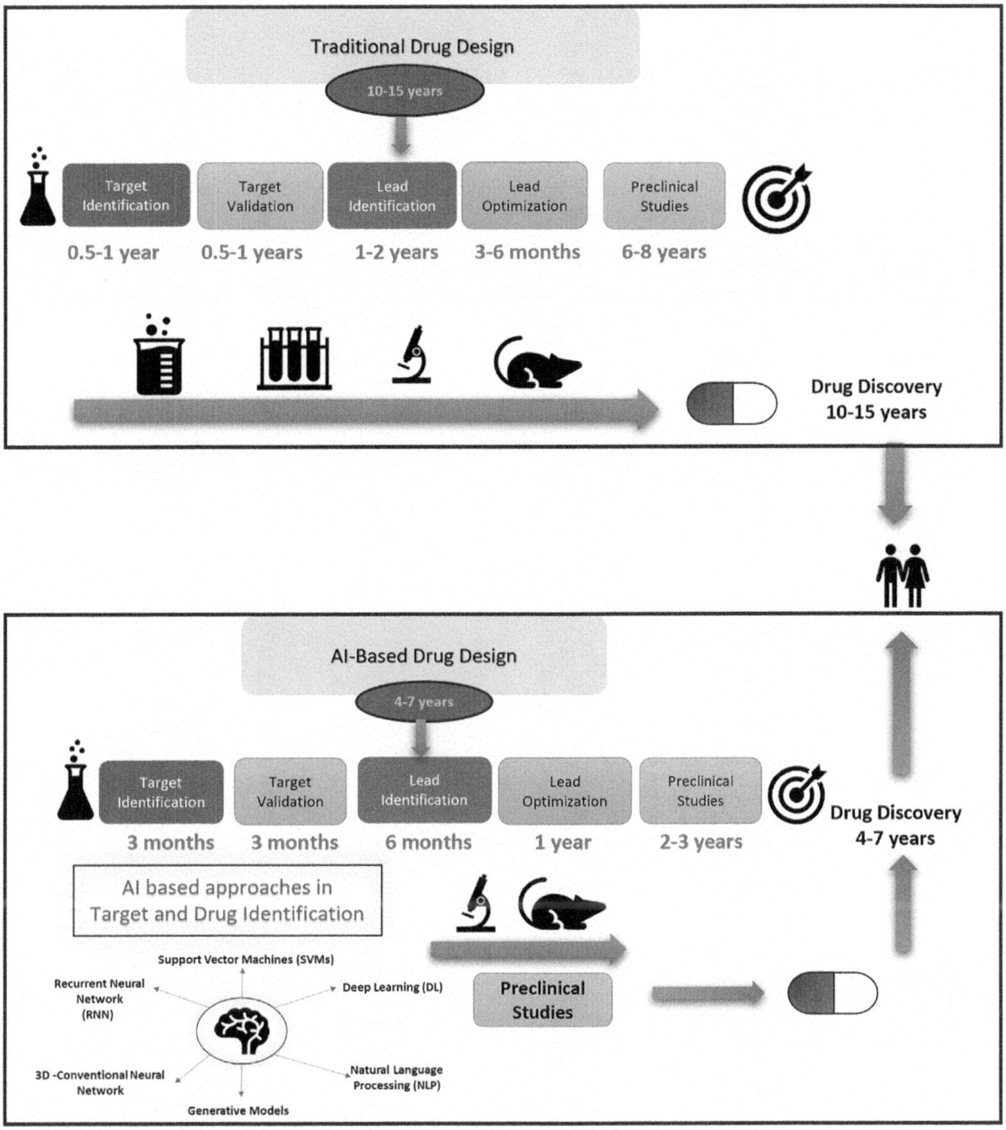

Fig. 5.2 Graphical representation of traditional and AI-based drug discovery workflows.

5.1 AI in protein structure prediction

The genomes of various organisms like pathogens, human and parasites are going through translation to produce protein, which is the building block of an organism. Proteins play an indispensable role in the growth and function of an organism. A malfunctioning protein directly influences the function of the organism. Thus,

Table 5.2 Molecular docking and screening tools with their algorithms.

	Tools name	Pose sampling method	Scoring function type	Binding accuracy	Performance
Traditional methods	GOLD	Genetic algorithm	Empirically based	Moderate	Moderate
	Schrödinger Glide (SP/XP)	Grid-based sampling + torsional sampling	Empirical-based and Physics-based	Medium to high	Faster
	AutoDock	Monte Carlo simulated annealing + Lamarckian Genetic Algorithm	Empirical + Physics-based	High	Slow
	AutoDock Vina	Iterative sampling + gradient-based optimization	Empirical	Medium to high	Faster
AI-based approaches	GNINA https://github.com/gnina/gnina	CNN-guided pose generation and scoring	Deep CNN (3D grid-based)	High	Fast
	DiffDock https://github.com/gcorso/DiffDock	Diffusion-based probabilistic pose generation	Transformer + diffusion scoring	Medium to high	Fast
	DeepDock: https://github.com/OptiMaL-PSE-Lab/DeepDock	Ligand conformation optimization using deep learning	ML-based scoring with 3D ligand-context awareness	Medium	Fast
	EquiBind: https://github.com/HannesStark/EquiBind	Direct pose-prediction equivariant GNN	GNN with coordinate regression	Medium	Very fast

protein structure prediction is the first step in drug development protocol. For decades, protein structures have been determined and studied using experimental techniques such as X-ray crystallography, NMR spectroscopy, and cryo-electron microscopy. But due to the complexity and diverse nature of proteins and experimental techniques, the protein structures of all the biologically relevant species have not been analysed. The rise of AI powered structure prediction has revolutionized the pharmaceutical industry. The advent of AlphaFold by Google's DeepMind in 2020 marked a significant leap in structural biology (Jumper et al., 2021). The accuracy of 3D structure predication was on par with the experimental method. This enhances the identification of 3D structures of diverse, experimentally unsolvable proteins. AlphaFold has a significant contribution on protein structure prediction, marking a paradigm shift in the drug discovery landscape. The AlphaFold core architecture consist of Evoformer, a deep neural network (DNN), which learns from input primary sequence and performs a multiple sequence alignment, evolutionary pattern analysis to predict spatial relationship and structural interaction between primary amino acid sequence. The AlphaFold achieved near experimental accuracy and it outperformed all methods in 14th Critical Assessment of Structure Prediction (CASP14). The AlphaFold version (AF2 & AF3) marked a significant improvement over initial model and AlphaFold3 (AF3) can predict structures of nearly all the biomolecules with unprecedented accuracy (Table 5.3). The AF3 can predict structures

Table 5.3 Comparison of different AlphaFold1, AlphaFold2, and AlphaFold3.

Features	AlphaFold1	AlphaFold2	AlphaFold3
Year	2018	2020	2024
Primary function	Protein structure prediction	Highly improved protein structure prediction	Protein structure prediction and biomolecular interaction prediction
Input molecules	Single protein sequence	Single and Multiple Protein Chains	Proteins, DNA, RNA, Ligands, Ions, and Modified Residues
Architecture	Deep convolutional neural network	Evoformer, a Transformer	Diffusion-based generative model
Accuracy (CASP performance)	Major breakthrough but had moderate accuracy	Near-experimental accuracy for monomers	Native support for complexes and improved accuracy for protein structure prediction
Availability	Not public	Open source via AlphaFold2 code and ColabFold	Limited access via a web server and no open-source code

of DNA, RNA, protein and small molecules. The critical assessments showed remarkable accuracy of AF3 in predicting protein ligand interaction, surpassing the traditional docking tools.

5.2 AI enhancements in large-scale virtual screening and de novo drug design

As AI has revolutionized structure prediction, a further challenge involves the prediction of small-molecule interaction or protein-ligand interaction. The conventional docking tool accurately predicts binding strength and ligand poses inside the protein binding site; however, the accuracy declines for complex, flexible proteins and larger compounds such as hybrid molecules. AI-based docking tools have emerged as superior contenders in both speed and accuracy of prediction. The AI-based tools use a data-driven approach for predicting protein-ligand interaction. The section below provides a detailed note on the architecture of AI-based docking tools.

5.2.1 Convolutional neural network and geometric deep learning in molecular docking studies

a) **3D-CNNs:** A 3D CNN treats the protein-ligand interaction as a 3D image, with intra and intermolecular interactions as a grid of voxels. Voxels are like 3D pixels with x, y, and z coordinates; they hold key values of atomic charge or interactions. It uses a hierarchical layer to learn the spatial arrangements of interactions, such as atomic contacts, distances, and various other features. These models do not require re-defined equations or manual selection of descriptors. The model learns from the spatial patterns and provides accurate estimates of binding energy, outperforming traditional methods.
b) **Geometric deep learning (GDL):** GDL is a highly advanced AI model, which works directly on real molecules' natural geometry. Unlike the CNN model, which treats molecule and atom positions as a grid, the GDL treats the atoms and interactions as a graph (atoms as points and bonds as connections). This allows the model to naturally predict complex, irregular molecules. GDL can predict the atoms' arrangement, rotation and translation of the input molecule. The model predicts accurately even during molecules' movement and rotation, which is essential in complex integration studies. One such example of an application is IPBind, which uses GDL for molecular interaction study of complex proteins.

5.2.2 Application of AI in virtual screening of large-scale chemical libraries

High-throughput screening is an experimental method to screen a large number of chemical libraries. A similar contemporary technique, high-throughput virtual screening (HTVS), is used to screen a diverse set of compounds. These conventional approaches are time-consuming and have major limitations such as accuracy and speed. The newer iteration of the HTVS approach has introduced several AI strategies and models which can efficiently screen billions or even trillions of molecules effortlessly. The AI is an intelligent filter that can accelerate hit finding at an exponential scale. These fast predictive models can be used to rapidly filter the best-binding compounds, reducing the time and cost of screening. Some of the core architectures used in HTVS involve 3D CNN, 3D GNN, Gradient Boosting Machine (GBM), Diffusion, and Transformer models. The architectures of AI-based virtual screening tools, including GNINA, DeepDock, DeepAffinity, DiffDock, TankBind, and AtomNet, are described in Table 5.4.

Table 5.4 The popular AI-powered docking tools with their core architecture have been described below.

Names of tools	Type	Architecture	Features
DeepDock https://github.com/OptiMaL-PSE-Lab/DeepDock	Deep learning-based molecular docking	Graph convolutional networks (GCNs)	Pose prediction and scoring
GNINA https://github.com/gnina/gnina	Convolutional neural network (CNN)-based virtual screening	3D convolutional neural network (3D-CNN)	Rescoring the conventional docking method
DeepChem: https://github.com/OptiMaL-PSE-Lab/DeepDock	Toolkit with multiple AI models for molecular docking and QSAR	Graph convolutional network (GCN) and message passing neural network (MPNN) RNN—recurrent neural network (RNN)	QSAR, ADMET, and binding prediction
AutoDock-GPU + ML filter: https://github.com/ccsb-scripps/AutoDock-GPU	Conventional docking + machine learning-based filtering	Deep learning (DL), random forest (RF)	ML filter + molecular docking

5.2.3 AI-powered de novo drug design

De Novo drug design is a novel approach in drug design that involves developing a molecule from scratch with a unique pipeline. The AI models can now use their generative capabilities to generate a novel compound based on the binding site and desired chemical properties. Such AI models play a pivotal role in the advancement of drug development. These models can generate accurate chemical compounds for rare and deadly diseases within a fraction of the time in comparison to traditional approaches. Several classes of generative models have been explored and used for De Novo Drug Design.

a) **Variational autoencoders and generative adversarial networks (GANs):** These models learn from a compressed, continuous numerical representation of known drugs called a latent space. Novel molecules are generated by sampling new points in the latent space. The generated molecules are further correlated with drug-like properties.
b) **Reinforcement learning (RL):** RL is a novel method that uses a molecular builder to create a new molecule with desired properties and has a separate reward function that checks binding affinity and ADMET properties. The AI model learns from the reward to improve molecular generation.
c) **Diffusion models:** These models have been widely used for image generation and molecule generation, and these models are very efficient in generating physically plausible 3D structures. Tools such as DiffDock use a diffusion model to generate novel molecules based on the active site of a protein structure. This enhances the binding affinity of a compound toward a particular protein. Hence, this reduces the off-target effects seen in the majority of drugs.

These generative models will be pivotal in the future of drug development to prevent pathogenic outbreaks and develop rapid therapeutics in a short period of time. Several leaders in the pharmaceutical industry are utilizing generative models to design drugs for nondruggable targets. Pharma companies like Exscientia (Centaur AI) and MilliporeSigma (AIDDISON software) use newer generative AI models to design inhibitors for complex diseases.

5.2.4 Brief overview of GNINA: AI-based tool for protein–ligand interaction study

GNINA is an open-source molecular docking and screening tool which uses the core traditional method for docking and enhances its accuracy by integrating deep learning techniques such as CNNs.

GNINA is a modified version of Smina, which itself is a derivative of AutoDock Vina. Hence, GNINA is an appropriate tool which combines traditional docking methods and a modern AI technique for accurate prediction of protein-ligand interaction (Pravin et al., 2026). It uses the traditional Monte Carlo method for sampling the ligand conformation and further scores the best binding pose using DL methods like CNNs (McNutt et al., 2021). The CNN models are trained using PyTorch, which is currently the most efficient framework for building and training neural networks. GNINA is a very simple tool with a user-friendly workflow (Fig. 5.3) similar to AutoDock Vina.

- **Molecular docking and screening workflow in GNINA**

1. **Input**: The receptor structure in Protein Data Bank (PDB)/Protein Data Bank, Partial Charge (Q), and Atom Type (T) (PDBQT) format and ligand molecules in SDF/PDBQT format.
2. **Ligand sampling:** GNINA uses Monte Carlo sampling to generate diverse ligand conformations within the binding site of the receptor.
3. **Scoring**: Each pose is ranked for the best fit based on a CNN scoring function.
4. **Output:** The compounds are ranked on the basis of CNN score, CNN affinity, CNN variance, and Binding Affinity. The output provides the top-binding ligand based on robust scoring functions.

- **Hardware requirements**

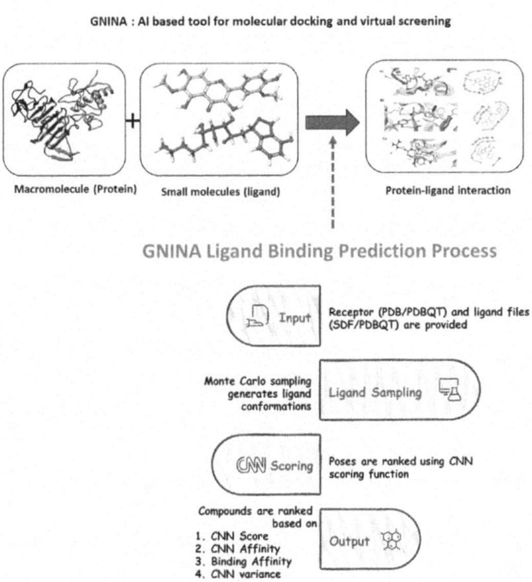

Fig. 5.3 Flowchart of the GNINA molecular docking and screening tool.

1 **CPU/GPU and RAM**: GNINA can run on both Central Processing Unit (CPU) and GPU environments. A dedicated GPU and higher Random Access Memory (RAM) can accelerate the screening of large libraries.

6 AI in pharmacokinetics and pharmacodynamic

Pharmacokinetics (PK) and pharmacodynamics (PD) are the fundamentals of drug discovery. A drug's success in clinical trials is highly dependent on these two properties. Even with good drug-like properties and binding affinity toward the desired target, most drugs fail in clinical trials due to poor PK/PD properties. Figure 5.4 displays the PK/PD pathway of a drug.

a) **PK:** It describes what the body does to the drug. The ADME properties are the crucial parameters of a drug necessary for causing pharmacological changes in the body. The majority of identified drugs fail due to poor absorption and metabolism. The advancement in AI models has enhanced the prediction of PK/PD properties before going for extensive experimental validation.
b) **PD:** It describes what a drug does to the body. It studies the interplay between concentration and physiological effects. The effective concentration of a drug required to produce

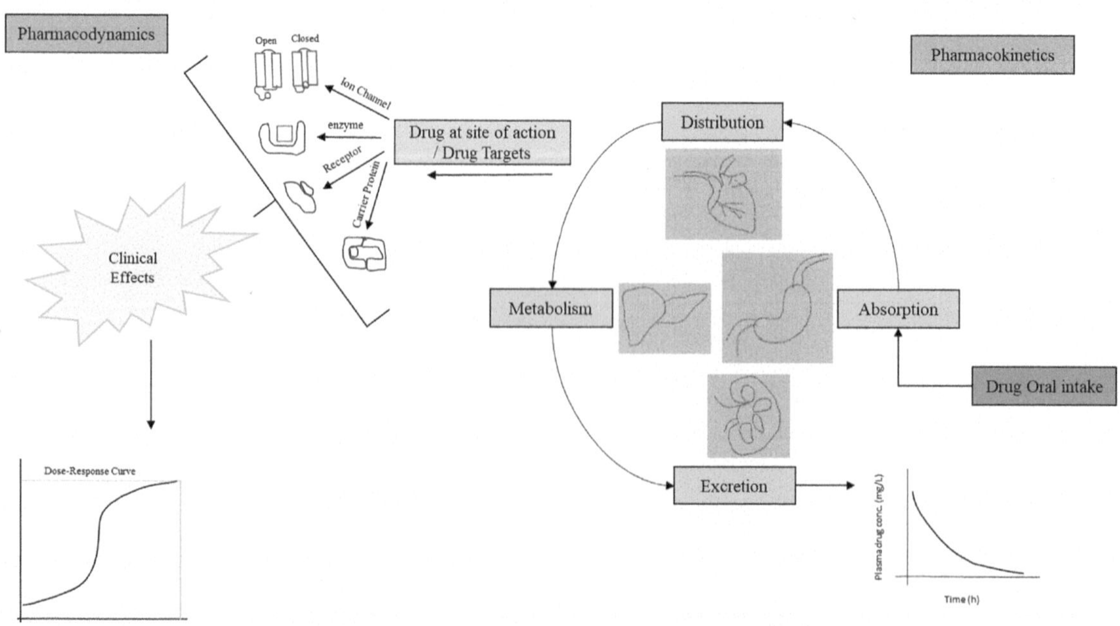

Fig. 5.4 Schematic diagram of the PK/PD pathway of a drug.

inhibitory action is determined by PD properties. The concepts include Kd, Ki, inhibitory concentration (IC50), and intrinsic activity. The interplay between PK and PD determines a drug's affinity, its agonist or antagonist activity, and ADME properties. Overall, these properties determine the success of a drug in clinical trials. Some of the currently available AI-based tools for PK and PD analysis include ADMETlab 2.0, DeepADMET, ADMETBoost, PreADMET, DeepDTA, DeepAffinity, and BindingDB ML models.

7 Real-life applications of AI in drug development

The theoretical practice of AI in drug development has produced translational results with successful experimental validation. Several drug developments through AI-based pipelines have entered clinical trials. The duration of drug development has been compressed with the advent of AI, thus marking a significant achievement in the field of therapeutic development. The following are the case studies of drugs developed through AI strategies.

a) **Exscientia and Sumitomo Pharma:** A well-known compound was successfully developed through an AI drug discovery pipeline. Exscientia and Sumitomo Pharma collaborated to develop a potent agonist of the serotonin 5-HT1A receptor. This drug was developed to treat obsessive-compulsive disorder. From initial development to the clinical trial, it took just 12 months, compared to the traditional approach of 7–12 years. Using the Centaur AI platform's generative model, the compound was modeled and optimized with several parameters. Thus, the multiproperty-optimized compound was feasible to enter a clinical trial within a year. This case study provides evidence of AI-based drug design and its ability to navigate the complex drug discovery landscape to produce translational results.
b) **In silico medicine**: In silico medicine used AI to tackle one of the lethal diseases, idiopathic pulmonary fibrosis (IPF). The AI model was used to predict the novel drug targets responsible for the disease. The TNIK protein was identified as a novel drug target, as, till now, TNIK was not reported as a drug target in IPF disease. Further, the AI-powered generative tool was used to generate a new small molecule based on the binding site of the IPF. The predicted small molecule showed significant affinity toward the identified drug target. The advanced AI models, such as DL, generative models, transformer models, and

reinforcement learning-based tools, were used for drug target identification. The entire process of drug target identification and lead identification will take 18 months for completion and validation. The drug Rentosertib has successfully transitioned into clinical phase II trials. This case study depicts flexibility, adaptability, and power of AI models in drug design.

c) **Novel antibiotic development:** Several bacterial species have caused detrimental effects in human society. Drugs have been ineffective toward the antimicrobial-resistant bacteria. AI has enabled the development of several antibiotics with novel mechanisms of inhibition. The following are a few examples of successful antimicrobial resistant bacteria.

d) **Halicin:** Massachusetts Institute of Technology (MIT) researchers have developed a supremely effective antibiotic against *Escherichia coli* using deep learning models. The model identified a novel chemical entity from existing databases. The compound Halicin acted by a novel mechanism—disrupting the electrochemical gradient within the cell membrane of bacteria. The identified drug also showed broad-spectrum antibiotic activity, killing many bacterial pathogens such as *Acinetobacter baumannii* and *Clostridium difficile.*

e) **Abaucin:** With the success of Halicin, the MIT researcher identified Abaucin, an antibiotic against A. *baumannii.* The novel mechanism of inhibition is similar to that of Halicin, targeting lipoprotein trafficking. *A. baumannii* is mainly known for hospital-borne infections. The identification of Abaucin has provided a significant leap toward bacterial antimicrobial resistance.

8 Impact of AI in understanding drug–drug interaction

In terms of drug development, the interactions between protein-protein (PPI), target (mostly protein)-ligand (TLI), and drug-drug (DD) are acquiring more attention (Fig. 5.5). PPIs are crucial for most of the biological processes like cellular organization, immune response, signal passing, cell–cell communication, and molecular functions like kinetic enzyme modification, regulation of metabolic processes, alterations in protein specificity, and transportation of molecules. An unusual PPI could cause diseases like cancer, infectious diseases, and neurological disorders (Akbarzadeh et al., 2024) at the same time, the understanding of functions and druggability of the protein supports the identification of drugs. The TLI is an event encompassing the induction of biological processes, biochemical reactions, signal passing, molecular recognition, and conformational changes (Zhao et al.,

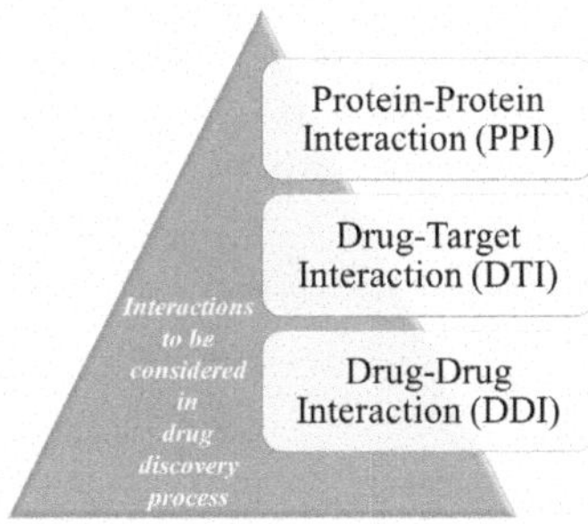

Fig. 5.5 The three important interactions considered during drug discovery.

2024). In relation to this, the specificity and affinity are two factors to be considered while studying TLI, standing for binding specifically to a particular target and the binding strength between the protein and ligand, respectively (Du et al., 2016).

DDIs are defined as an influence/disturbance in the natural behavior of one drug by another, resulting in either adverse side effects or inhibition/modification in the drug's mechanism (Palleria et al., 2013; Chen et al., 2017; Rakshith et al., 2024; Sumayli et al., 2024). DDIs are the result of an interruption in the PK/PD activity of a drug (Palleria et al., 2013) (Fig. 5.6). The PK (ADME) interaction of a drug could interrupt the pathway of one drug by another throughout the body. This interaction causes the affected drug to be present at low or high levels in one's body, making the drug ineffective. The factors that need attention here are the altered gastrointestinal motility, gastric pH, and the behavior of drug carriers in the stomach wall. The distribution of a drug is solely dependent on the concentration of plasma proteins or tissues. Most of the clinically vital DDIs occur due to the activation or inhibition of CYP enzymes. The excretion of drugs takes place through either renal tubular secretion or biliary excretion (Palleria et al., 2013; Lee et al., 2024; Rakshith et al., 2024; Sumayli et al., 2024). The PD interaction of a drug could be illustrated as similar/opposite kinds of effects of one drug on the respective interacted drug, which changes the pharmacological response that reflects at the receptor/target's site, and some of the interactions related to this are receptor interactions, enzyme inhibition/activation, ion channel interactions, and transporter interactions (Palleria et al., 2013; Rakshith et al., 2024).

The factors responsible for the occurrence of DDI are polypharmacy, genetic variation, age and physiological changes, and disease status. Polypharmacy is one of the notable factors of DDI as it is associated with the prescription of multiple combinations of

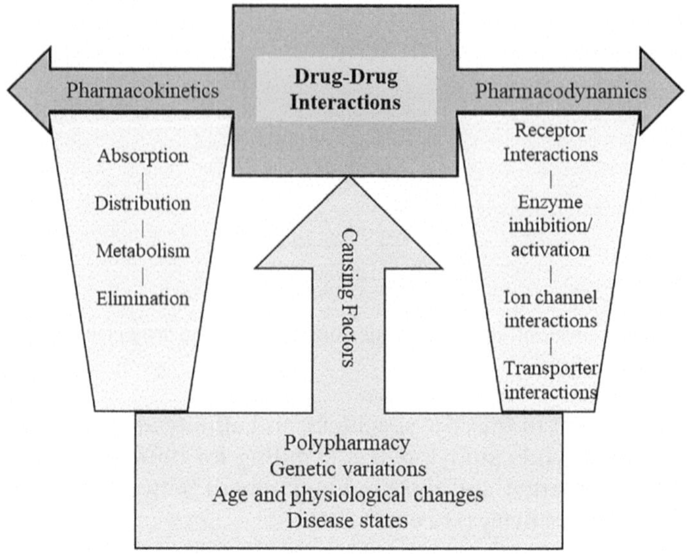

Fig. 5.6 Illustration of the two types of DDI mechanisms and their causing factors.

drugs to treat multifaceted diseases like cancer, diabetes, and so on. The patients taking multiple medications are the common cohort affected by DDIs. Polypharmacy has increased the chances of the occurrence of DDIs that reflect in incompetence, high hazard ratio, side effects (Palleria et al., 2013; Liu et al., 2023; Chen et al., 2024; Rakshith et al., 2024; Sumayli et al., 2024; Yadav et al., 2025). Even genetic variations among individuals, including disturbances in the mode of action of drug-processing catalysts and drug carriers, are also among the significant traits affecting drug PK/PD pathways. The age-associated physiological modification affects the distribution and metabolism of drugs. Hence, a clear understanding of PK/PD interactions could improve the identification and development of potential drugs with assured safety and effective treatment (Rakshith et al., 2024).

9 Traditional methods and AI-driven approaches for drug–drug interaction studies

In the drug development pipeline, identification and evaluation of DDIs prior to the marketing phase have been accounted as one of the important processes to overcome the shortcomings of the medication, like adverse reactions and drug efficacy alterations that resulted in drug failure, as the drugs named terfenadine, mibefradil, cisapride, and nefazodone were banned from the market because of their adverse activity caused by DDIs (Liu et al., 2023; Chen et al., 2024; Lee et al., 2024; Rakshith et al., 2024; Yadav et al., 2025).

The methods followed for the DDI assessment include in vitro and in vivo experiments, clinical trials, and AI-based ML/DL models that are trained based on the data reported from experimental analyses (Fig. 5.7). These methods have been classified into traditional experimental methods and AI-driven methods (Table 5.5).

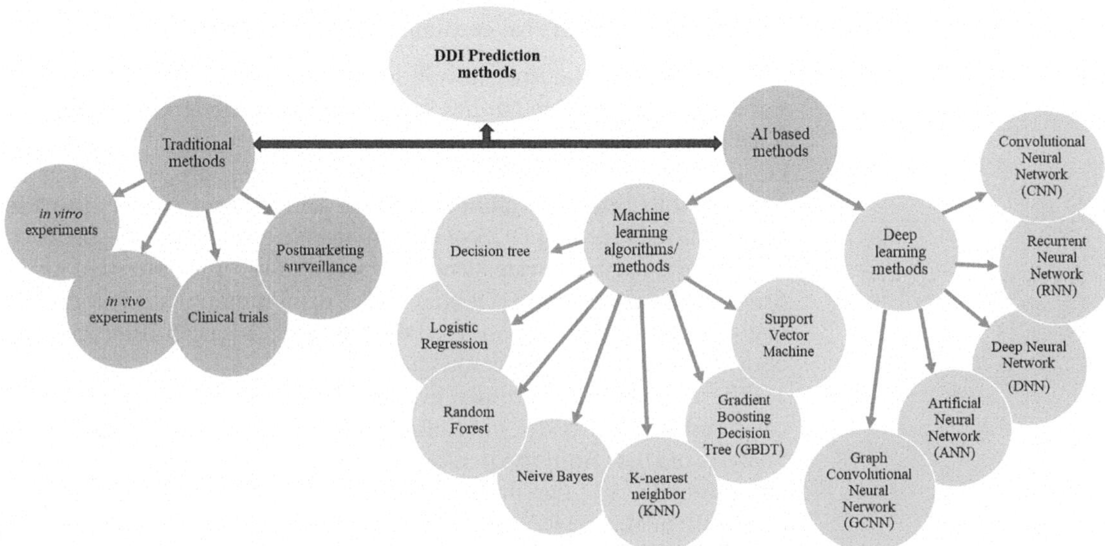

Fig. 5.7 Currently available traditional and AI-driven methods for the identification of DDIs.

Table 5.5 Methods and their respective study models used in the identification of DDI.

Methods	Study models
Traditional experimental methods	
In vitro studies	Human cell lines and tissues
In vivo studies	Animal models
Clinical studies	Human
AI methods	
Machine learning	Computationally trained models
Deep learning	Artificial neural networks

9.1 Traditional experimental methods in DDI identification

Studies involving in vitro and in vivo experiments, clinical trials, and postmarketing surveillance are the traditional ways of DDI identification. However, these techniques necessitate more manpower/human resources, are time-consuming, and, importantly, fail to recognize composite interactions (Vo et al., 2022; Liu et al., 2023; Sumayli et al., 2024; Zhu et al., 2024; Yadav et al., 2025).

a) In vitro **and** in vivo **studies in DDI identification**

In the flow of the drug development pipeline, the outcomes from the in vitro and in vivo studies stating an assessment of drug efficacy have been utilized as prior information on the PK/PD of the particular identified drug, and its interaction with other drugs and targets, before subjecting it to clinical studies. The in vitro studies provide information regarding DDIs at the subatomic level or cell/tissue level, like the action of catalysts, drug passage, and receptor interactions. A drug's interaction with CYP enzyme(s)/drug metabolism is a crucial factor for the identification of DDIs that offers a basic understanding of drug interactions (Lee et al., 2024).

The in vivo studies utilize live animal models to study drug efficacy and toxicity at the physiological level. These studies aid in the analysis of DDIs from the perspective of PK/PD interactions by evaluating the effects of two drug molecules collectively on explicit targets (Rakshith et al., 2024).

a) Clinical studies in DDI identification

Clinical investigations observe the mechanisms of drug and relative reactions occurring inside the human body that help to concentrate on the domineering complex interactions of drugs and their effects. These studies enable the assessment of the interaction of one drug in the presence or absence of another. In other words, they identify the occurrence of unfavorable and unknown DDIs in individuals. From the PD perspective, it is a kind of evaluation of alterations in biomarkers and physiological limits (Rakshith et al., 2024).

9.2 AI-driven approaches in DDI studies

The application of Bioinformatics has given a new dimension to drug discovery by the utilization of various computational techniques/approaches for the identification of small molecules and their targets (macromolecules), interaction (PPI, drug-target, DD)-related studies, PK/PD properties of the drug, and clinical data analysis. Nowadays, with the advent of knowledge and technologies, this ensures the identification of personalized medicines.

The implementation of AI/ML/DL models in fields like structural biology and pharmacology has enriched the advantages in drug development. It facilitates the identification of drug targets, drug-target interaction studies, analysis of drug ADMET properties, and DDIs in a faster and more accurate manner. The incorporation of AI with bioinformatics enables the identification of DDIs by observing the patterns from the bulk datasets. AI facilitates ML/DL models in predicting DDIs by analyzing their chemical structures, mode of action, metabolic pathway, and the patients' actual data (Zhu et al., 2024; Yadav et al., 2025). AI utilizes methods such as literature extraction, matrix factorization, similarity searches, interaction networks, and deep learning neural networks to predict significant DDIs (Chen et al., 2022; Liu et al., 2023; Chen et al., 2024; Zhu et al., 2024).

Some of the AI models are capable of identifying novel/unknown DDIs from datasets obtained from various sources. ML and DL are the branches of AI which are providing enormous support in identifying significant DDIs in order to improve the accuracy and efficacy of the drugs, as they affect the normal action of the drug involved in the interaction with the other, by processing both structured and unstructured data (Chen et al., 2022). For example, in order to enhance the safety and effectiveness in the prescription of drugs, Qin et al. (2024) recommended an ML/DL approach which utilizes an ML algorithm to hone scaling limits and behavior of the antibiotic combinations, and a feedforward neural network algorithm to build the model to predict antibiotic combination. Similarly, the Molecular Structure and Knowledge Graph (MSKG)-DDI is based on two modules: one is based on the chemical structure graph, and another is based on a knowledge graph, and it utilizes a multimodel fusion neural layer. It works well under transductive and inductive settings, and its real-world utility has been verified through ablation analysis (Chen et al., 2024). Table 5.6 describes the utility of various AI models in DDI prediction, and the following are some of the approaches available for the prediction of DDIs.

9.2.1 ML models in DDI prediction

ML models are trained on vast datasets containing drug properties, actual patient reports, and already studied drug interactions in order to learn the patterns to predict significant DDIs. ML models are efficient at managing a large amount of multifaceted data, like drug PK, genomics, and molecular structures. These models enhance the prediction quality of DDIs as the quantity of data increases and also predict DDIs across various drug classes, which is a significant feature beneficial while dealing with patients taking multiple medications (Yadav et al., 2025). The general protocol of ML consists of

Table 5.6 Comparison of various AI models in DDI Prediction.

Model	Type	Input features	Output features	Application
KNN	Supervised learning	Drug molecule descriptor in numerical form	Numerical data on interaction and confidence-level score	Similarity-based drug interaction study
SVM	Supervised learning on linear and nonlinear data	Chemical features of a drug in the form of linear and nonlinear data	Information on interaction in the form of a numerical value, a decision score, and a probability of interaction	Used for nonlinear data and for a small number of datasets
DT	Tree-based Supervised learning approach	Numerical and nominal data of drugs	A similar set of numerical data containing interaction information	Basic information on drug interactions, used for a small number of datasets
RF	Ensemble Tree-based approach	Large number of chemical data in numerical form	Class label, probability score	Widely used in bioinformatics for large datasets.
NB	Supervised probabilistic approach	Molecular fingerprint and molecular descriptor data of chemical structure	Prediction of interaction and probability score for possible interaction	It is a baseline model, giving a simple yet efficient prediction
LR	Statistical classification approach	Binary features of drugs and details of interaction	Simple and interpretable values of drug features	It is widely used in studying the drug features
GBDT	Ensemble-based approach using a regression tree	Heterogeneous features of drug molecules	A simpler set of information, such as prediction of drug interaction, probability of interaction, and drug features	It is widely used for capturing the relationships of drug-drug interaction

data collection and processing, algorithm selection and training, evaluation of the test set/model validation, parameter adjustments, and model utility. In this context, the selection of a suitable algorithm for our data is a crucial point in developing a model that could make accurate predictions of DDIs (Chen et al., 2022). Recently, two ML models were developed to predict the in vivo results from the in vitro results obtained through experiments and they provide useful insights into drug metabolism/drug clearance and to the evaluation of DDIs in clinical trials (Lee et al., 2024).

The applications of some of the commonly used ML algorithms in DDI prediction are listed below:

a) *K-nearest neighbor (KNN):* KNN is one of the supervised learning classification algorithms suitable for data with small quantities and unknown dispersion. This algorithm does not require much information or time to process the data. Although this classifier takes less time to train the model, it is a slow-learning algorithm that produces unstandardized classifications, is hard to interpret the outcome, and performs more calculations (Chen et al., 2022). A model developed based on this algorithm, which utilizes the DDIs from the STITCH database and was evaluated by DrugBank, has shown a good capability to predict novel DDIs (Chen et al., 2017).

b) *SVM:* In the SVM-based models, the hyperplane is drawn utilizing the features of the drugs to classify them into interacting and noninteracting drugs. It is capable of handling both nonlinear and linear problems. For nonlinear problems, it utilizes a suitable kernel function to map the training data to a higher dimension, and for linear problems, it classifies the data based on its chemical features (Chen et al., 2022; Vo et al., 2022; Yadav et al., 2025).

c) *DT:* It is a tree-like structure that compares the test data to the feature nodes, and based on the results, it selects a branch to be compared next, and this will continue until reaching a leaf node as the end of the decision output. This method can be applied to both numerical and nominal data and does not require data normalization, and the outcomes are interpretable and viewable. By utilizing DT, the wholeness of DDI-associated information regarding drug specifications has been studied by Ng et al. (2017), performing fundamental processes as an evaluation tool to review drug instructions and DDI resources (Chen et al., 2022).

d) *RF:* DT is the base for RF, which incorporates multitrees through ensemble learning. It validates the significance of every feature given in classification problems (Chen et al., 2022). This method classifies drug interactions by generating multiple DTs and enables the model to manage huge datasets and to recognize difficult patterns among drugs (Yadav et al., 2025).

e) *Naïve Bayes (NB):* It is a supervised classification algorithm that uses the standard NB algorithm to classify the dataset features. It takes the features as conditionally independent events to solve and ease computations. It is not suitable for datasets having features with strong connections. This algorithm is utilized to develop models predicting molecular targets, toxicity of drugs, and DDIs (Chen et al., 2022).

f) *Logistic regression (LR):* It is suitable for classification problems with dependent variables and is understandable and easily interpretable. Wang et al. (2019) utilized this in the investigation of similarity between anticancer and nonanticancer drug interactions and related features of these interactions (Chen et al., 2022; Sumayli et al., 2024). The Russell-Rao approach, which predicts 250,000 clinically relevant DDIs, has been devised by Ferdousi et al. (2017) and integrates biological factors like transporters, proteins, and targets.

g) *Gradient boosting DT:* Models based on this algorithm fit a regression tree by performing the first-order Taylor expansion of the loss function. It is useful for problems with no prior/clear information, and it provides results with high accuracy (Chen et al., 2022).

9.2.2 Deep learning methods in DDI prediction

DL algorithms rely on sequence features and structure graphs of drug molecules to train a DNN for the accurate classification and prediction of the dispersed data. This method has been applied to target prediction, protein position point prediction, and drug interaction prediction. The most commonly used neural networks, namely CNNs, recurrent neural networks (RNNs), and DNNs, detect nonlinear relationships among drugs and their related interaction profiles. These neural networks are even capable of predicting interactions without manually curated data (Vo et al., 2022; Chen et al., 2022; Yadav et al., 2025).

a) *CNN:* This network is capable of observing the vast association between input and output by detecting grid patterns of the reliable features of the given data without applying any complex calculations, and these features are obtained by convolutional kernels (Chen et al., 2022; Vo et al., 2022). Liu et al. (2016) devised a DDI mining method based on CNN and found it performed better on the available DDI extraction 2013 corpus.

Another method using a stacked bidirectional gated recurrent unit (GRU-CNN/SGRU-CNN) model was proposed to retrieve DDI etymological data (Wu et al., 2020). The hybrid CNN proposed by Sun et al. (2019) aids in extracting DDIs from biomedical literature.

b) *RNN:* This network has wide application in NLP. The layers in this network are connected to each other in the order of input layer-hidden layer-output layer. It functions by recalling the available information to compute the output. Simple RNN, bidirectional RNN, deep RNN, GRURNN, clockwork RNN, and long short-term memory (LSTM) are some of the extensions of RNN (Chen et al., 2022; Vo et al., 2022). The TM-RNN model (transfer matrix and RNN) proposed by Liu et al. (2019) extracts DDIs with more accuracy and consistency by combining multilayer bidirectional LSTM and transfer matrix methods (Chen et al., 2022).

c) *DNN:* DNN models are greatly applied in the prediction of pharmacological properties, DDIs and drug repurposing. A DNN model trained to predict DDIs based on their Simplified Molecular-Input Line-Entry System taken from DrugBank had resulted in 13,155,885 DD pairs connected by 5130 drugs (Hou et al., 2019). Liu et al. (2023) proposed a Deep Attention Neural Network-based DDI prediction that employs the graph embedding method to predict unknown DDIs by generating networks according to the drug features and drug patterns. They then conjugated the observed drug embeddings. The performance of this model has been validated through experimental methods, and it has been concluded that this model is useful for predicting DDIs and DDI-associated incidents.

d) *Artificial neural network (ANN)*: ANN utilizes the hidden functional dataset to solve linear/nonlinear problems. A model proposed by Shtar et al. (2019) combines ANN and a propagation approach to create a DDI interaction network and utilizes the XGBoost classifier for DDI classification to identify DDI (Vo et al., 2022).

e) *Graph CNN (GCNN):* GCNN supports the prediction of DDI by illustrating the mutual relationship between drugs' structures. The data structure of GCNN is represented with nodes as drugs and edges as connections between drugs (Vo et al., 2022). The SC-DDIS model developed by Liu et al. (2021) observes the ending insertions of drugs through a CNN spectral graph. GoGNN is a model based on GCNN that retrieves features from a structured entity graph and an entity interaction graph with dual-attention to handle control in DDI prediction. In addition, a wide analysis with actual clinical data states that GGNN works well on both chemical-chemical interaction prediction and DDI prediction tasks (Wang et al., 2020).

9.2.3 Natural language processing

The approach of natural language processing (NLP) toward DDI prediction is like the retrieval of associations between drugs (Liu et al., 2016). NLP is able to process bulk unstructured data obtained from research papers, case reports, and electronic health records (EHRs), and it automates the extraction of data from scientific literature, clinical guidelines, and reports regarding adverse incidents. NLP-integrated AI systems encourage the identification of different/rare drug interactions that have not been reported in clinical studies (Yadav et al., 2025). The authors Javed et al. (2015) proposed a method as an integration of bioinformatics and NLP that utilizes a pattern recognition approach to analyze patterns in NLP models to retrieve DDIs. This method used a minimum feature set, low computational power, and produced comparatively good results. They validated this with three classification models, such as Naïve Bayes, J48 (DT), and RT, and the performance of RT was found to have the best rate of accuracy. Liu et al. (2016) proposed a CNN-based DDI prediction method that also exhibits better performance comparatively.

10 Databases facilitating DDI interaction studies

It is obvious that AI-implied analyses necessitate a large amount of data in order to train and validate the model to predict clinically significant DDIs. There are numerous databases (Table 5.7) that allow us to retrieve data related to drug interactions, pharmacological profiles, and reports of adverse incidents. For instance, the clinical studies concentrating on DDI identification rely on data sources like Micromedex, UpToDate, Drugs.com, and Medscape.com, but these databases are limited to data with inconsistencies that lead to uncertain decisions, and this insists on the utility of actual clinical reports of patients in order to find clinically relevant DDIs (Sumayli et al., 2024; Ji et al., 2025).

One of the studies has incorporated clinically relevant DDIs related to Torsades de pointes from various sources, such as databases (*FDA Adverse Event Reporting System* [FAERS]) and literature, in order to develop four statistical models—Ω shrinkage measure, combination risk ratio, chi-square statistic, and additive model—which were evaluated using databases such as Lexicomp and Drugs.com. This study predicts amiodarone, citalopram,

Table 5.7 List of databases/resources offering data to predict DDI and the various ML/DL methods applied.

Category of data	Databases/ Resources	Available Data	ML/DL algorithms
Structure	PubChem, DrugBank, ChEMBL	Molecular descriptors, drug substructure/chemical structure, drug target, drug-drug interaction	Boosted Tree, Multilayer feedforward resilient backpropagation network, CNN, SVM, DNN, RF, KNN, NN, LR, Neighbor recommender method, Random-walk method, Matrix perturbation method, Siamese self-attention multimodel neural network, Node-based drug network diffusion method.
Sequences and functional annotations	eggNOG, UniProt, Zenodo, PharmVar	Orthologs' data, protein sequence	
Interaction	OSCAR EMR, DrugRef	Drug information, interaction data.	
Pathway	KEGG	Gene and Genome Pathway-related data	
PK/PD	BindingDB and Lilly in-house CYP phenotyping assays.	Activity endpoints, enzymes, ion channels, transporters, Analysis of CYP substrate loss, CYP fingerprint, and recombinant CYP phenotype	
Adverse-event reports (ADEs)	FAERS, TWOSIDES, SIDER, OFFSIDES, OSCAR, VA NDF-RT	Drug information, Mechanism of action, Drug adverse reactions.	
Patient health records.	EHRs, Drug Communication Datasets, Electronic medical records.	Patients' health-related information	

quetiapine, ondansetron, ciprofloxacin, methadone, escitalopram, sotalol, and voriconazole as the most frequently interacting drugs, and citalopram-quetiapine, amiodarone-ciprofloxacin, amiodarone-escitalopram, amiodarone-fluoxetine, ciprofloxacin-sotalol, and amiodarone-citalopram as commonly occurring interacting drug combinations (Ji et al., 2025).

The following are the databases and libraries providing DDI data:

a) *DrugBank* (https://go.drugbank.com): It provides a platform to explore drug molecules, their interactions with other drugs, chemical structures, their reactions, classifications, drug targets, pharmaco-omics-related information (Zhang et al., 2023; Sumayli et al., 2024; Yadav et al., 2025).

b) *PubChem* (https://pubchem.ncbi.nlm.nih.gov/docs/about): It is an open chemistry database maintained by the National Institutes of Health (NIH) that provides information on the structures, physico-chemical properties, biological activities, patents, health, safety, toxicity of small molecules and macromolecules, namely, nucleotides, carbohydrates, lipids, peptides, and chemically-modified macromolecules (Zhang et al., 2023).
c) *ChEMBL* (https://www.ebi.ac.uk/chembl/): It contains 25,00,000 compounds, 17,00,000 assays, 15,500 drugs, 6900 drug mechanisms, 1400 drug warnings, 48,800 drug indications, 782 tissues, 16,000 targets, 2100 cell lines, and 92,100 documents that are manually curated (Zhang et al., 2023).
d) *Kyoto Encyclopedia of Genes and Genomes* (KEGG, https://www.genome.jp/kegg/): It stores data about 12,000 medicines and 2,000 interactions based on medication packaging from Japan (Sumayli et al., 2024). It gives three search options (KEGG, DBGET, and MEDICUS to facilitate the smooth search environment and to aid to understand the biological systems at molecular-level (Zhang et al., 2023).
e) *Pharmacogenomics library* (PharmGKB; https://www.pharmgkb.org): It has 209 clinical guideline annotations, 1188 drug label annotations, 481 FDA drug label annotations, and 263 curated pathways. These data provide a platform to explore the impacts of mutations on clinically relevant drug response (Zhang et al., 2023; Sumayli et al., 2024).
f) *Therapeutic Target Database* (https://db.idrblab.net/ttd/): It offers molecular-interaction, human-system-profile, and cell-based expression-variation-related data, and it compiles the druggability of 426 successful targets, 1014 clinical-study targets, 212 preclinical-study and patented targets, and 1479 literature-reported targets (Zhang et al., 2023; Zhou et al., 2024; Sumayli et al., 2024).
g) *DailyMed* (https://www.dailymed.nlm.nih.gov/dailymed/index.cfm): It is a database containing 1,186 labelings for prescription and nonprescription drugs that are submitted by companies to the FDA (Zhang et al., 2023; Sumayli et al., 2024).
h) *Side effect resource* (http://sideeffects.embl.de) stores information on drugs available on the market and their reported adverse drug effects that are mined from public documents and medication package inserts, and allows us to obtain information such as side-effect frequency and drug and side-effect classifications from the collection of 1439 drugs, 5868 adverse reactions, and 1,756 combinations of drug-adverse events (Zhang et al., 2023; Sumayli et al., 2024; Yadav et al., 2025).

i) *TWOSIDES* (http://tatonettilab.org/resources/tatonetti-stm.HTML): It has been maintained by the Tatonetti Lab at Columbia University Medical Center and provides data related to the side effects of polypharmacy. It contains 59,220 drug pairs, 8,221 associated links, 1301 adverse events, and 37,82,910 significant relationships of drug pairs having a higher side-effect association score (Zhang et al., 2023; Sumayli et al., 2024).
j) *DDInter 2.0* (http://ddinter2.scbdd.com/server/search/) is an enhanced and curated drug interactions database. It contains 3,516 DDIs of 2290 drugs, taken from scientific literature and pharmaceutical labels, that allow users to easily identify the drugs, associated diseases, and their interactions with other drugs (Zhang et al., 2023; Sumayli et al., 2024).
k) *Systematic mechanistic clarifications of DDIs* (MecDDI, https://mecddi.idrblab.net): They assist medical scientists, algorithm scientists, and healthcare professionals to understand the DDI mechanisms, to predict clinically significant DDIs, and to enhance drug efficacy (Zhang et al., 2023; Sumayli et al., 2024).
l) *FAERS database* (https://www.fda.gov/drugs/drug-approvals-and-databases/fda-adverse-event-reporting-system-faers-database): This database consists of reports of adverse events that the FDA received from manufacturers, consumers, and healthcare professionals, and is utilized to develop AI models to identify crucial DDIs based on the actual evidence obtained from patient reports. This database recommends a new perception to ensure postmarketing drug safety. It provides useful information related to the interaction between two or more drugs (Ji et al., 2025; Yadav et al., 2025).
m) *EHRs:* The medical data in EHRs include patient details, treatment regimens, and clinical results. These data help build AI models to predict DDIs in different patient cohorts using similar patterns that include factors like genetic predispositions and existing conditions that influence drug metabolism to filter for specific DDIs, thereby encouraging the identification of personalized medicines (Sumayli et al., 2024; Yadav et al., 2025; Mandal, 2019; Moore, 2019).
n) *Drug communication datasets:* They are a collection of (pre) clinical investigations and case studies from various sources, such as healthcare services. These datasets support the determination of favorable interactions and suggest prescription routines for patients treated with polypharmacy (Tatonetti et al., 2012).
o) *Adverse drug events (ADEs):* There is a reporting system for the collection of ADEs relating to complex drug combinations (Tatonetti et al., 2012).

11 Some of the AI-based tools for DDI prediction

a) *IBM Watson for drug discovery:* It supports the analysis of large datasets of DDIs from scientific literature and clinical trial reports (Yadav et al., 2025).
b) *Medi-Span Clinical:* It was developed to screen DDIs and to provide assistance while making clinical decisions (Yadav et al., 2025).
c) *DDInter (Deep Drug Interaction Predictor):* It is a DL-based tool that predicts DDIs based on the molecular structure and pharmacological data (Yadav et al., 2025).
d) *Model-informed drug development:* It utilizes the data reported from in vivo as well as clinical studies to train AI models to predict the interaction mode of drugs with enzymes and proteins to lessen adverse reactions (Yadav et al., 2025).
e) *Caster:* It utilizes the substructures of the drugs to predict DDIs and to identify drugs effectively (Yadav et al., 2025).

12 Impact of AI in enhancing DDI studies and advancing pharmaceutical research for drug development

As already discussed, DDIs with significant clinical impact on the body may become a threat, particularly to patients following polypharmacy. As experiment-based DDI identification methods are a tedious task for researchers, the integration of AI techniques with Bioinformatics empowers the prediction of personalized DDIs through understanding various DDIs and recognizing patterns from real-time data in order to develop personalized medicines with increased efficacy by taking advantage of the facility to analyze real-time patient data (Vo et al., 2022; Blanco-Gonzalez et al., 2023).

In addition, AI with pharmacogenomics helps to understand the impact of drug-enzyme interactions in patients with genetic variations and to incorporate it into the models that are designed to recommend dosage levels and therapeutics according to the patients' genetics, and this also helps to overcome complexities due to polypharmacy (Yadav et al., 2025) by ensuring drug safety, channelizing treatment routines, and reducing the incidence of DDIs (Rakshith et al., 2024). The application of ML and DL-based traditional and advanced techniques supports the evaluation of drug interactions and augments the prediction of DDIs from a variety of data, such as clinical reports, literature findings, DDIs retrieved from chemical databases, and pharmacokinetic data (Vo et al., 2022; Sumayli et al., 2024).

Out of all the remarkable advantages of AI techniques/models, some of the drawbacks have been experienced till now, like their black-box feature that can be overcome with the development of explainable AI, and the prediction of true negative DDIs by the ML-models that can be overcome by training the model to predict positive data out of an unlabeled dataset, and biased sampling that could be rectified by random negative sampling (Vo et al., 2022).

13 Challenges and future prospects

Despite all the advantages of AI in drug discovery, data interpretability, data labelling, disproportion of labels, sample size, nature of data, data privacy, ethical issues, learning architypes, and model elucidations are some of the areas which can lead to unfavourable/unrelatable outcomes if we fail to provide more attention. The dimensionality of the biological data greatly influences various stages of ML/DL pipeline like featuring/labelling, learning and training datasets. For example, in the process of experimental validation the description of the toxicity of a compound depends on its dose and the biological system, but in clinics it depends the age, sex, race, and medical history of the patients. Likewise, the nature of protein-compound complex is also varying in patients, cells, and tissues. The black box nature of DL methods, i.e., we could not interpret the background process of how it is making a decision. This unexplainable nature leads false conclusion upon the biological targets, compounds and their interactions. Thus, these methods require the thorough understanding on the biological processes and chemical interactions as well as the utility of optimization methods like Bayesian optimization. The Bayesian method tends to identify the global optimum state (minima and maxima) of the function, that may enhance the identification of augment chemical compounds. Most importantly, the data which utilized to train the ML/ DL model should not be biased or illusory. It is essential to ensure the ethical clearance and fairness of the data (Blanco-Gonzalez et al., 2023; Qureshi et al., 2023).

14 Conclusion

The new era of AI has drastically changed the landscape of drug discovery. The novel AI approaches have enhanced traditional methods such as molecular docking, virtual screening, and de novo drug design. The introduction of generative AI in the computational field has revolutionized several fields including drug discovery, as traditional approaches lack accuracy and scalability and exhibit inefficiency in handling larger datasets. The notable improvements over the traditional methods include the use of AI models for molecular docking and screening. AI models such as DL, GANs, GNNs and tools such as DiffDock, GNINA, DeepChem, and DeepDock have been used for accurate protein–ligand interaction studies. Further, AI has been used in the field of DDIs, one of the noticeable reasons for adverse reactions to drugs, which are a result of impotent drug selection. It is essential to select a drug that forms very few interactions, in addition to acceptable pharmacokinetic and pharmacodynamic nature. The recent advancements in drug discovery have enabled the identification of more reliable drugs. Even though the drugs have passed all the stages of the drug discovery pipeline, it is obvious that some of the drugs have failed at the stage of clinical trials, and even some drugs have been banned due to their harmful effects. In these kinds of cases, most of the time it is caused by DDIs, which seek attention here. In order to overcome the shortcomings, the researchers moved on to AI to predict DDIs based on various data extracted from various sources. These models produce promising outcomes since they are capable of dealing with real-time data. But still, it is essential to ensure the reliability of the ML/DL-based models that have been developed to predict DDIs. The real-world success of AI models has been visible through the molecules' progress in clinical trials. Despite the complex drug discovery landscape and challenges, AI will transform therapeutic development by reducing the time and cost of drug development.

Acknowledgment

The authors are pleased to acknowledge the research facility provided by Alagappa University. SKS thankfully acknowledges DST-FIST, New Delhi [(SR/FST/LSI – 667/2016)]; DST-PURSE Second Phase program [Order No. SR/PURSE Phase 2/38 (G) dated 21.02.2017], Tamil Nadu State for Higher Education (TANSCHE) (Au/S.O. (P&D): TANSCHE Projects: 117/2021), MHRD-RUSA-Phase 2.0 grant sanctioned vide Letter No. [F.24-51/2014-U, Policy (TNmulti-Gen)], Department of Biotechnology, Bioinformatics Center (BIC) [No. BT/PR40154/BTIS/137/34/2021] and Department of Biotechnology, National Network Project (NNP) [No. BT/PR40156/BTIS/137/54/2023]. Ms. S. Priyadharshini would like to thank TANSCHE for the Fellowship support. RA thanks the Indian Council of Medical Research [No. BMI/11/(65)/2022, Dt. 16.06.2022] for providing a Senior Research Fellowship. AP would also like to thank DBT-NNP for providing the Fellowship.

Conflict of interest

The authors declare no conflict of interest.

References

Akbarzadeh, S., Coskun, O., Guncer, B., 2024. Studying protein-protein interactions: latest and most popular approaches. J. Struct. Biol. 216, 108118.

Arun Pravin, M., Selvaraj, C., Singh, S.K., 2024. A multiscale in silico approach to impede the interaction between Dengue NS1 and Human RPL18, aiming to suppress the Dengue viral translation and proliferation. Mol. Simul. 50 (17-18), 1642–1665. doi:10.1080/08927022.2024.2426587.

Berman, H.M., Westbrook, J., Feng, Z., Gilliland, G., Bhat, T.N., Weissig, H., et al., 2000. The protein data bank. Nucleic Acids Res. 28 (1), 235–242.

Blanco-Gonzalez, A., Cabezon, A., Seco-Gonzalez, A., Conde-Torres, D., Antelo-Riveiro, P., Pineiro, A., Garcia-Fandino, R., 2023. The role of AI in drug discovery: challenges, opportunities, and strategies. Pharmaceuticals 16 (6), 891.

Chen, L., Chu, C., Zhang, Y.-H., Zheng, M., Zhu, L., Kong, X., Huang, T., 2017. Identification of drug-drug interactions using chemical interactions. Curr. Bioinform. 12 (6), 526–534.

Chen, S., Li, T., Yang, L., Zhai, F., Jiang, X., Xiang, R., Ling, G., 2022. Artificial intelligence-driven prediction of multiple drug interaction. Brief. Bioinform. 23 (6), 1-16.

Chen, S., Semenov, I., Zhang, F., Yang, Y., Geng, J., Feng, X., Meng, Q., Lei, K., 2024. An effective framework for predicting drug-drug interactions based on molecular substructures and knowledge graph neural network. Comput. Biol. Med. 169, 107900.

Dominguez, L.W., Willis, J.S., 2020. Research and development costs of new drugs. JAMA 324 (5), 516.

Du, X., Li, Y., Xia, Y.L., Ai, S.M., Liang, J., Sang, P., Ji, X.L., Liu, S.Q., 2016. Insights into protein-ligand interactions: mechanisms, models, and methods. Int. J. Mol. Sci. 17 (2), 144.

Eberhardt, J., Santos-Martins, D., Tillack, A.F., Forli, S., 2021. AutoDock Vina 1.2. 0: new docking methods, expanded force field, and python bindings. J. Chem. Inf. Model. 61 (8), 3891–3898.

Ferdousi, R., Safdari, R., Omidi, Y., 2017. Computational prediction of drug-drug interactions based on drugs functional similarities. J. Biomed. Inform. 70, 54–64.

Ferreira, F.J., Carneiro, A.S., 2025. AI-driven drug discovery: a comprehensive review. ACS Omega 10 (23), 23889–23903.

Gohlke, H., Hendlich, M., Klebe, G., 2000. Knowledge-based scoring function to predict protein-ligand interactions. J. Mol. Biol. 295 (2), 337–356.

Gu, S., Shen, C., Zhang, X., Sun, H., Cai, H., Luo, H., et al., 2025.Benchmarking AI-powered docking methods from the perspective of virtual screening. Nat. Mach. Intell. 7 (3), 509–520.

Guedes, I.A., Barreto, A.M., Marinho, D., Krempser, E., Kuenemann, M.A., Sperandio, O., et al., 2021. New machine learning and physics-based scoring functions for drug discovery. Sci. Rep. 11 (1), 3198.

Guedes, I.A., Pereira, F.S., Dardenne, L.E., 2018. Empirical scoring functions for structure-based virtual screening: applications, critical aspects, and challenges. Front. Pharmacol. 9, 1089.

Hinkson, I.V., Madej, B., Stahlberg, E.A., 2020. Accelerating therapeutics for opportunities in medicine: a paradigm shifts in drug discovery. Front. Pharmacol. 11, 770.

Hou, X., You, J., Hu, P. (2019). Predicting drug-drug interactions using deep neural network. In: Proceedings of the 2019 11th International Conference on Machine Learning and Computing (ICMLC '19), Association for computing Machinery. New York, NY, USA, pp. 168–172.

Hughes, J., Rees, S., Kalindjian, S., Philpott, K., 2011. Principles of early drug discovery. British J. Pharmacology 162 (6), 1239–1249. doi:10.1111/j.1476-5381.2010.01127.x.

Javed, R., Farhan, S., Humdullah, S., 2015. A hybrid approach based on pattern recognition and BioNLP for investigating drug-drug interaction. Curr. Bioinform. 10 (3), 315–322.

Ji, H., Gong, M., Gong, L., Zhang, N., Zhou, R., Deng, D., Yang, Y., Song, L., Jia, Y., 2025. Detection of clinically significant drug-drug interactions in fatal torsades de pointes: disproportionally analysis of the food and drug administration adverse event reporting system. J. Med. Internet Res. 27, e65872. 1–15.

Jumper, J., Evans, R., Pritzel, A., Green, T., Figurnov, M., Ronneberger, O., et al., 2021. Highly accurate protein structure prediction with AlphaFold. Nature 596 (7873), 583–589.

Khan, M.A., Singh, S.K., 2023. Atom-based 3D-QSAR and DFT analysis of 5-substituted 2-acylaminothiazole derivatives as HIV-1 latency-reversing agents. J. Biomol. Struct. Dyn. 41 (14), 6759–6774.

Lee, J., Beers, J.L., Geffert, R.M., Jackson, K.D., 2024. A review of CYP-mediated drug interactions: mechanisms and in vitro drug-drug interaction assessment. Biomolecules 14, 99.

Liu, J., Huang, Z., Ren, F., Hua, L., 2019. Drug-drug interaction extraction based on transfer weight matrix and memory network. IEEE Access 7, 101260–101268.

Liu, S., Tank, B., Chen, Q., Wang, X., 2016. Drug-drug interaction extraction via convolutional neural networks. Comput. Math. Methods Med. 2016 (1), 6918381.

Liu, S., Zhang, Y., Cui, Y., Qiu, Y., Deng, Y., Zhang, Z., Zhang, W., 2023. Enhancing drug-drug interaction prediction using deep attention neural networks. IEEE/ACM Trans. Comput. Biol. Bioinform. 20 (2), 976–985.

Liu, T., Cui, J., Zhuang, H., Wang, H., 2021. Modeling polypharmacy effects with heterogeneous signed graph convolutional networks. Appl. Intell. 51, 8316–8333.

Mandal, L.J.N., 2019. Prediction of active drug molecule using back propagation neural network. In: Proceedings of the 8th. International Conference System Modeling and Advancement in Research Trends, pp. 22–26.

McNutt, A.T., Francoeur, P., Aggarwal, R., Masuda, T., Meli, R., Ragoza, M., et al., 2021. GNINA 1.0: molecular docking with deep learning. J. Cheminform. 13 (1), 43.

Moore, K.L., 2019. Automated radiotherapy treatment planning. Semin. Radiat. Oncol. 29 (3), 209–218.

Ng, G., Sklar, G., Chng, H., 2017. An evaluation of the completeness of drug-drug interaction-related information in package inserts. Eur. J. Clin. Pharmacol. 73 (2), 165–174.

Palleria, C., Di Paolo, A., Giofre, C., Caglioti, C., Leuzzi, G., Siniscalchi, A., De Sarro, G., Gallelli, L., 2013. Pharmacokinetic drug-drug interaction and their implication in clinical management. J. Res. Med. Sci. 18 (7), 601–610.

Pravin, M.A., Khan, M.A., Singh, S.K., 2026. Identification of potent inhibitors targeting the pre-fusion DENV envelope protein: A consensus physics-and AI-based in silico multi-tier screening approach. Biochem. Biophys. Res. Commun. 818, 153722. doi:10.1016/j.bbrc.2026.153722.

Qin, J., Yang, Y., Ai, C., Ji, Z., Chen, W., Song, Y., Zeng, J., Duan, M., Qi, W., Zhang, S., An, Z., Lin, Y., Xu, S., Deng, K., Lin, H., Yan, D., 2024. Antibiotic combinations prediction based on machine learning to multicentre clinical data and drug interaction correlation. Int. J. Antimicrob. Agents 63(5), 107122.

Qureshi, R., Irfan, M., Gondal, T.M., Khan, S., Wu, J., Hadi, M.U., Heymach, J., Le, X., Yan, H., Alam, T., 2023. AI in drug discovery and its clinical relevance. Heliyon 9, e17575.

Rakshith, U.R., Nair, S.P., Ranganath, A.H., Halagali, P., 2024. Drug interactions: mechanisms, assessment and management strategies. J. Young Pharm. 16 (3), 447–455.

Selvaraj, C., Elakkiya, E., Prabhu, P., Velmurugan, D., Singh, S.K., 2023. Advances in QSAR through artificial intelligence and machine learning methods. In: Hong, H. (Ed.), QSAR in Safety Evaluation and Risk Assessment. Academic Press. pp. 101–116.

Shiammala, P.N., Duraimutharasan, N.K.B., Vaseeharan, B., Alothaim, A.S., Al-Malki, E.S., Snekaa, B., et al., 2023. Exploring the artificial intelligence and machine learning models in the context of drug design difficulties and future potential for the pharmaceutical sectors. Methods 219, 82–94.

Shtar, G., Rokach, L., Shapira, B., 2019. Detecting drug-drug interactions using artificial neural networks and classic graph similarity measures. PLoS One 14, 8.

Sumayli, A.A., Daghriry, A.I., Sharahili, M.A., Alanazi, A.A., Alanazi, A.A., Alharbi, I.F., Alghamdi, F.N., Alqarni, K.A., Aljohani, N.M., Alfaqir, A.M., Shajiri, I.M., Albalawi, A.R., Alatwi, F.M., Alrashdi, M.S., Altaymani, K.A., Alsharari, M.B., Albalawi, M.A., Alanazi, S.R., Alanazi, A.S., 2024. An in-depth examination of drug-drug interaction databases: enhancing patient safety through advanced predictive models and artificial intelligence techniques. J. Med. Life Sci. 6 (4), 553–565.

Sun, X., Dong, K., Ma, L., Sutcliffe, R., He, F., Chen, S., Feng, J., 2019. Drug-drug interaction extraction via recurrent hybrid convolutional neural networks with an improved focal loss. Entropy 21 (1), 37.

Tatonetti, N.P., Fernald, G.H., Altman, R.B., 2012. A novel signal detection algorithm for identifying hidden drug-drug interactions in adverse event reports. J. Am. Med. Inform. Assoc. 19 (1), 79–85.

Vo, T.H., Nguyen, N.T.K., Kha, Q.H., Le, N.Q.K., 2022. On the road to explainable AI in drug-drug interactions prediction: a systematic review. Comput. Struct. Biotechnol. J. 20, 2112–2123.

Wang, H., 2024. Prediction of protein–ligand binding affinity via deep learning models. Brief. Bioinform. 25(2), bbae081.

Wang, H., Lian, D., Zhang, Y., Qin, L., Lin, X., 2020. GoGNN: graph of graphs neural network for predicting structured entity interactions. In: Proceeding of the Twenty-Ninth International Joint Conference on Artificial Intelligence, pp. 1317–1323.

Wang, W., Xiao, B., Liu, Z., Wang, D., Zhu, M., 2019. The prevalence of the potential drug-drug interactions involving anticancer drugs in China: a retrospective study. Iranian J. Public Health 48 (3), 435–443.

Wu, H., Xing, Y., Ge, W., Liu, X., Zou, J., Zhou, C., Liao, J., 2020. drug-drug interaction extraction via hybrid neural networks on biomedical literature. J. Biomed. Inform. 106, 103432.

Yadav, A., Mishra, S., Gupta, A.K., 2025. The role of artificial intelligence in predicting drug-drug interaction: a new frontier in patient safety. Int. J. Pharm. Sci. 3 (1), 2625–2631.

Yang, S.Y., 2010. Pharmacophore modeling and applications in drug discovery: challenges and recent advances. Drug Discov. Today 15 (11-12), 444–450.

Yoshinaga, H., Uemachi, H., Ohno, T., Besnard, J., 2020. U.S. Patent No. 10,800,755. Washington, DC: u.S. Patent and Trademark Office.

Zhang, Y., Deng, Z., Xu, X., Feng, Y., Junliang, S., 2023. Application of artificial intelligence in drug-drug interactions prediction: a review. J. Chem. Inf. Model. 64, 7.

Zhao, Z., Zhao, L., Kong, C., Zhou, J., Zhou, F., 2024. A review of biophysical strategies to investigate protein-ligand binding: what have we employed? Int. J. Biol. Macromol. 276, 133973.

Zhou, Y., Zhang, Y., Zhao, D., Yu, X., Shen, X., Zhou, Y., Wang, S., Qiu, Y., Chen, Y., Zhu, F., 2024. TTD: therapeutic target database describing target druggability information. Nucleic Acids Res. 52 (D1), D1465–D1477.

Zhu, J., Che, C., Jiang, H., Xu, J., Yin, J., Zhong, Z., 2024. SSF-DDI: a deep learning method utilizing drug sequence and substructure features for drug-drug interaction prediction. BMC Bioinformatics 25, 39.

6

Generative models for molecule generation

Sapna Pandey[a], Himanshu Avashthi[b], and Dev Bukhsh Singh[c]

[a]INSACOG Genomics & Molecular Epidemiology Unit, NCDC, Delhi, India

[b]Department of Bioinformatics, Marwadi University, Rajkot, Gujarat, India

[c]Department of Biotechnology, Siddharth University, Siddharth Nagar, India

1 Introduction

We aim to discover novel molecules and materials that address significant challenges in chemistry, such as disease treatment and combating climate change. Typically, this procedure relies on the expertise of human professionals who propose, design, and evaluate new molecules. Although numerous significant scientific discoveries have been achieved in this way, the extensive time and financial resources required confine the number of molecules that can be discovered. Experts estimate that only approximately 10 (Schwalbe-Koda and Gómez-Bombarelli, 2020) compounds have been synthesized to date, while the potential range of compounds that could be produced may lie between 1023 and 1060 (Reymond and Awale, 2012; Polishchuk et al., 2013). This implies that current techniques for identifying new compounds consider only a small segment of what could potentially be developed. It is essential to develop improved methods for navigating the extensive options available to identify molecules that can address significant challenges in chemistry and engineering.

Generative models offer an optimistic approach to designing novel molecules. Rather than depending on human knowledge, these models utilize the latest breakthroughs in deep learning to confront the task of engineering molecules with particular traits. They figure out which molecules can meet these traits by finding a connection between the desired properties and the structures of the molecules. This tool enables users to swiftly discover a variety of molecules that are ideal for particular applications. After being introduced, generative models for designing molecules have experienced remarkable growth in both variety and quantity. These models have different approaches to representing molecules and the kinds of issues they handle. In an effort to assess the growing number of models, several

The AI Frontier in Molecular Modelling and Drug Designing. https://doi.org/10.1016/B978-0-443-40338-5.00017-2

standard tests have been developed recently. These evaluations gauge the models according to elements such as how they learn distribution, as well as the diversity and innovation of the chemicals involved (Polykovskiy et al., 2020; Brown et al., 2019).

Although there have been substantial technological improvements, there is a scarcity of cases where generative models have been employed to search for new molecules tailored for particular uses. Research predominantly emphasizes the refinement of molecules through computational indicators such as logP, which measures a molecule's mobility across varying environments, and quantum electrodynamics, which predicts a molecule's chances of functioning as a successful drug. Very few studies actually test the promising molecules they find. This shows that gaps still exist, preventing generative models from being entirely effective in discovering new molecules. In this chapter, the newest developments in generative molecular design are outlined, and how these models can be utilized in practical research projects is explained. The essential challenges that must be considered for these models to extend their complete potential are also discussed in this chapter. The objective of this chapter is to offer readers practical information that will enable them to successfully implement generative modeling in their endeavors (Bilodeau et al., 2022).

2 Generative models

A unique and remarkable aspect of human cognition is our capacity to envision things that are not physically present. This skill may have emerged for a number of reasons. One reason is that it assists us in strategizing by imagining the potential outcomes of our actions on the future. Moreover, by picturing possible outcomes, we can experiment with our understanding of how the world operates and acquire insights without the guidance of an instructor. Generative modeling is the aspect of machine learning (ML) that strives to enable machines to replicate the ability to conceive and invent new concepts or items. In addition to achieving significant objectives, there are also practical advantages to utilizing generative models. A notable feature is that humans can employ these models to derive insights from examples while needing less labeled data. Contemplate the ways in which young learners pick up a new language.

The main advantages of employing generative models are that they allow for a more accurate evaluation of the performance of ML models. Classifiers often yield identical outcomes across a variety of inputs, which complicates the understanding of what they have truly learned from the data. Evaluating the performance of a model that generates text captions for images can be challenging when working with a dataset. It remains unclear whether the model has a true understanding of images or if it is only providing accurate predictions by relying on typical image patterns (Lamb, 2021).

The neural networks used for generative modeling began in the 1980s. They autonomously acquire knowledge from data, making the process simpler and more cost-effective than collecting labeled information. Utilizing this strategy can yield significant insights, highlighting the effectiveness of generative models in numerous domains. Generative modeling is directly applied in various ways, such as creating and enhancing images, converting text to visuals, editing various image attributes, estimating poses, generating video content, producing audio like speech and music, summarizing and translating text, reinforcing learning algorithms, rendering graphics, generating textures, animating characters, simulating liquid dynamics, discovering new medicinal compounds, switching between data formats, and detecting outlier data. Often, generative models negotiate a trade-off between their operational speed and structural design, or they optimize various performance measures. The decisions made regarding what to enhance impact the caliber of the samples created. In most cases, prioritizing direct likelihood optimization tends to produce samples that are not as high in quality as those created using different methods (Fig. 6.1). A key aspect of generative models is self-supervised learning, which focuses on acquiring valuable intermediate representations that can be utilized in various tasks without the requirement of labeled data (Jolicoeur-Martineau, 2018). While generative models are typically classified as self-supervised, not every self-supervised model falls into the generative category. There are several categories of self-supervised tasks. Auxiliary classification tasks encompass activities such as estimating the degree of rotation in an image, performing masked predictions where the model must fill in absent data, and engaging in contrastive tasks that assist the model in learning to group similar items while distancing dissimilar ones in its comprehension (Bond-Taylor et al., 2022).

2.1 Benchmarks in generative modeling

Several generative models featuring different configurations have been developed for the generation of molecules. To accurately evaluate and compare these models to see which performs better, it is essential to have testing methodologies that work with models trained on publicly sourced data. Since there are various types of problems in generating molecules, it is important to use testing methods that reflect these different goals. MOSES3 and Guacamol, two recent testing frameworks, provide techniques for generating

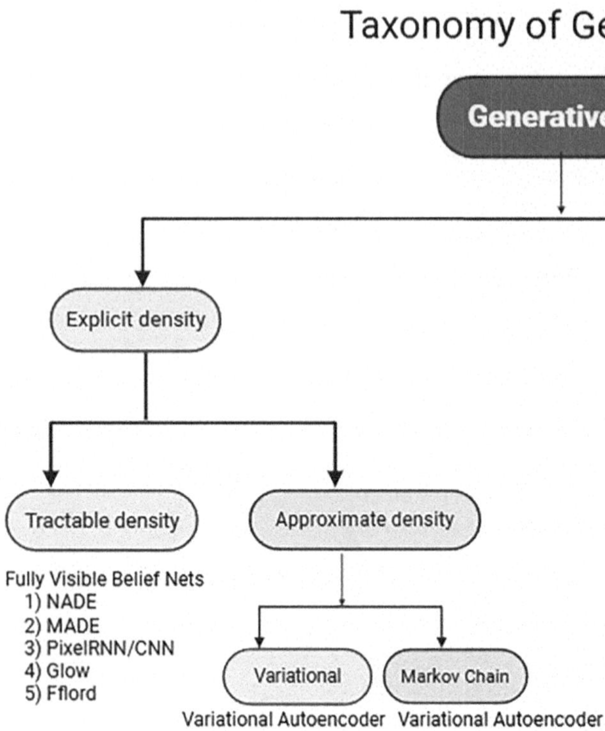

Fig. 6.1 Taxonomy of generative models.

both generic and targeted molecules, including scenarios that require certain characteristics or designs. These tests are useful for evaluating various modeling techniques, although they do not cover all the crucial aspects of identifying new molecules. Table 6.1 illustrates the common benchmarks in generative modeling along with their definitions.

3 Molecules representation

Neural networks possess significant capabilities because they can transform complicated information into simpler representations, which facilitate the execution of specific functions. The presentation of input data significantly influences how effectively the model acquires knowledge about the molecule. Typically, there are three distinct forms of input representations: (1) One-dimensional, like strings of text; (2) two-dimensional, like molecular graphs; and (3) three-dimensional, like coordinates (Bilodeau et al., 2022).

Table 6.1 Benchmarks in generative modeling (Bilodeau et al., 2022).

S. No	Definition	Benchmark	Goal type	Benchmark set
1.	Generate molecules that have optimal calculated values for characteristics such as LogP or QED.	Calculated property optimization	Goal-oriented	Guacamol Brown et al. (2019)
2.	Generate molecules that resemble a particular molecule that wasn't included in the training dataset.	Similarity	Goal-oriented	Guacamol Brown et al. (2019)
3.	Method to analyze the BRICS fragments' distribution between the generative and training sets.	Similar Fragment	Unconstrained	MOSES Polykovskiy et al. (2020)
4.	Generate molecules that closely resemble a number of existing molecules.	Median molecule discovery	Goal-oriented	Guacamol Brown et al. (2019)
5.	Unique molecules percent.	Uniqueness	Unconstrained	Guacamol Brown et al. (2019)
6.	The proportion of molecules that conform to specific criteria.	Filters	Unconstrained	Guacamol Brown et al. (2019)
7.	Removed molecules from training data are rediscovered.	Rediscovery	Goal-oriented	Guacamol Brown et al. (2019)
8.	Generated molecules that track a simple (unidentified) array.	Isomer identification	Goal-oriented	Guacamol Brown et al. (2019)
9.	Valid molecules percent with respect to valency/bond, calculated by RDKit's molecular structure analyzer.	Validity	Unconstrained	Guacamol Brown et al. (2019)
10.	Statistics show the variance among the distribution of the training set and the generated molecules.	KL divergence	Unconstrained	Guacamol Brown et al. (2019)
11.	From the training set, the percentage of molecules is missing.	Novelty	Unconstrained	Guacamol, Brown et al. (2019)
12.	Bemis-Murcko scaffolds distribution metrics comparing the training and generated sets.	Scaffold similarity	Unconstrained	MOSES Polykovskiya et al. (2020)
13.	To what extent do the produced molecules align with the GDB13 dataset, which represents chemical space?	Chemical spacecoverage	Unconstrained	Zhang et al. (2021)
14.	Compare the characteristics, such as logP/molecular weight, of the generated data with the training data.	Molecular properties distributions	Unconstrained	MOSES Polykovskiy et al. (2020)

3.1 One-dimensional representation

The standard approach to expressing a molecule using a simplified line notation is referred to as Simplified Molecular Input Line-Entry System (SMILES) (Weininger, 1988). It translates a molecule into an array of letters and symbols based on established criteria. This technique is beneficial, as it enables researchers to apply preexisting computational tools for language analysis to molecular structures (Arús-Pous et al., 2020). Through this strategy, scientists have utilized unique computer models, referred to as recurrent neural networks, to produce SMILES strings for diverse molecular structures (Chung et al., 2014; Hochreiter and Schmidhuber, 1997). Nonetheless, these models can occasionally generate erroneous SMILES that fail to correspond to actual molecular configurations due to their neglect of the intricate rules governing SMILES notation. Researchers, including Kusner and Dai, refined the models by incorporating SMILES grammar rules. However, their techniques frequently do not guarantee that the generated SMILES represent valid chemical structures (Dai et al., 2018). Krenn and his team proposed a new molecular representation approach known as Self-Referencing Embedded Strings (SELFIES) (Krenn et al., 2020) in order to overcome the difficulties posed by SMILES notation. Researchers can utilize SELFIES to train a model capable of generating molecules that comply with established guidelines, including valency rules. Yet, even if a molecule is valid, that doesn't imply it will be stable.

3.2 Two-dimensional representation

Molecules in neural networks are represented as graphs, in which nodes signify atoms and edges indicate the connections between them. This form of representation is impactful since it reveals the direct connections among atoms. On the other hand, forming these graphs poses a greater challenge than assembling sequences of data. Consequently, a variety of researchers are focused on designing neural networks that can produce authentic molecular graphs. The technique entails simultaneously creating molecular graphs by specifying both the atoms and their interconnections (Ma et al., 2018). Other researchers have developed models that construct molecules by adding one atom at a time (Samanta et al., 2020a, 2020b). Jin et al. (2018) adopted an analogous strategy by dividing atoms into smaller sections and formulating a model that assembles molecules piece by piece. The smaller units could comprise either a pair of atoms bonded together or a fully formed atomic ring, similar to a phenyl ring. Their approach begins by assembling a structure from these smaller segments, followed by a decision on how to interconnect them. Later, they improved this idea by allowing the model to work with even bigger parts (Jin et al., 2020). Their strategy proved to be superior to atom-by-atom methods across various tasks, such as the production of polymers and the optimization of drug-like features and specificity for a particular receptor.

3.3 Three-dimensional representations

Lastly, it is possible to visualize 3D molecules with point clouds, where every atom is represented as a distinct space point. This rephrasing aids in comprehending the connections between atoms and the potential changes in the molecule's shape. For instance, Gebauer and his team-built molecules progressively by positioning atoms in an organized coordinate system (Gebauer et al., 2019). Utilizing a similar approach, Simm and coworkers crafted molecules incrementally by measuring internally, atom by atom (Simm et al., 2020). Still, there are some disadvantages associated with using these methods to locate new molecules. Understanding the physical properties of a molecule involves analyzing more than just one of its possible shapes (conformers). In addition, these techniques can be time-consuming since they involve intricate calculations to optimize the shapes of molecules within the training set, a process that tends to be slow, particularly for larger and more flexible molecules. In recent times, scientists have been investigating novel techniques to form molecular shapes (Riniker, 2017). By leveraging three-dimensional generative models that have been trained on large volumes of conformer data, they can significantly lessen the time and resources needed for gathering three-dimensional training data (Xu et al., 2021).

4 Architectures of model

A deep neural network's performance is significantly influenced by its structure, which encompasses the various layers it incorporates and their configuration. The main types of neural network architectures for discovering new molecules using deep generative models include Variational Autoencoders (VAEs), Generative Adversarial Networks (GANs), and normalizing flow models (Fig. 6.2). Every category has a unique approach to how it learns to depict molecules. The goal of normalizing flow models and VAEs is to refine the model's fit to the data of the training set. Variational inference is the method employed by VAEs to roughly maximize likelihood, in contrast to normalizing flow models, which seek the closest match by ensuring the model has an invertible structure. In the GANs framework, molecule generation is handled through a rivalry between two models: a generator, which produces synthetic samples, and a discriminator, which aims to distinguish real data from counterfeit (Bilodeau et al., 2022).

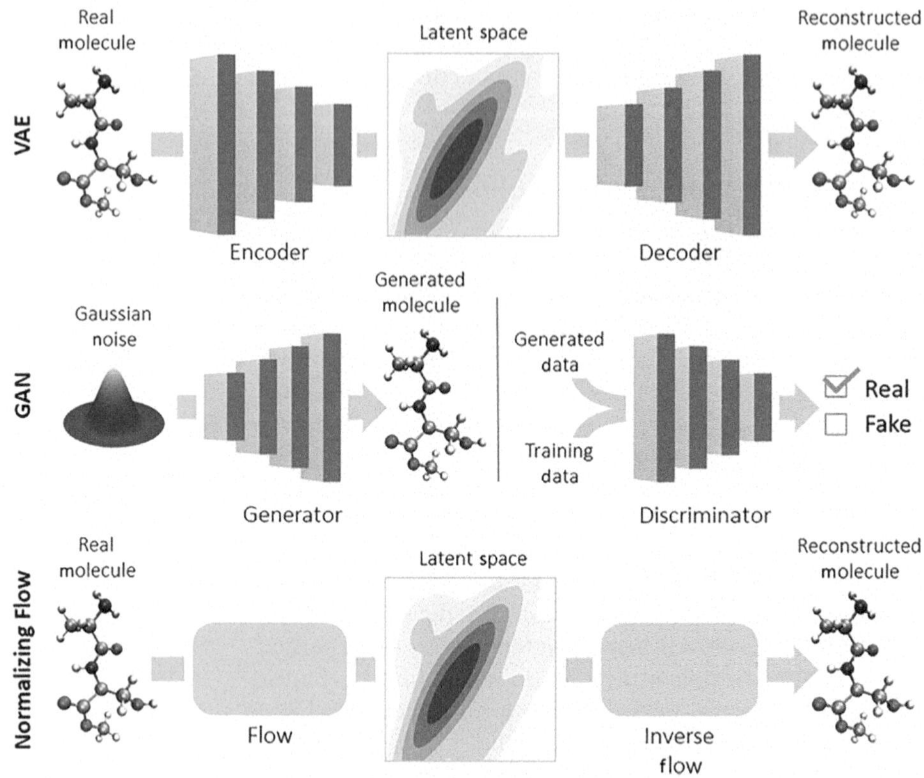

Fig. 6.2 Comparative study of the three main neural network architectures used in generative modeling (Bilodeau et al., 2022).

5 Variational autoencoders

In ML, VAEs are commonly employed for generating novel data and comprehending data representations. They enable us to discover concealed characteristics of the data, which can be advantageous for processes like image generation and working with a limited number of labeled examples. The appeal of VAEs lies in their incorporation of probabilistic modeling alongside the versatility offered by deep neural networks.

VAEs are models that generate novel data through the understanding of existing patterns. There are two essential sections in VAEs: the decoder and the encoder. The encoder receives input data and converts it to symbols situated in the area known as latent space. Following this, the decoder extracts samples from the representation and reverts them to their original data structure. The objective of training a VAE is to fine-tune these two components so that the output data closely mirrors the original dataset. Variational inference, an essential feature of VAEs, aids in simplifying the process of uncovering the underlying structures in the data. This approach employs a more straightforward distribution, such as a Gaussian (bell curve), to simplify the calculations. The VAE training objective is to enhance the Evidence Lower Bound (ELBO), a metric that evaluates the model's performance. There are two key elements in the ELBO: the reconstruction loss, which assesses to what extent the decoder can replicate the input data, and the Kullback-Leibler divergence, which maintains the similarity of the Gaussian distribution in latent space. VAEs offer the significant benefit of allowing the creation of new data points through sampling that establishes the latent space. VAEs generate novel data that mimics their training dataset by taking latent variables as samples, applying a prior distribution, and running the decoder (Sanchez, 2024).

Various types of VAEs have enhanced the quality and diversity of the images they generate. Certain VAEs, for example, InfoVAE (Zhao et al., 2017) and beta-VAE (Higgins et al., 2017) employ techniques designed to differentiate various features within the data. Similar to variation deep embedding (Jiang et al., 2016) and Gaussian mixture variational autoencoder (Dilokthanakul et al., 2016), other methods assist VAEs in categorizing data into distinct groups without requiring labeled information. Following that, feature generating VAE (Xian et al., 2019) and Zero-VAE-GAN (Gao et al., 2020) were introduced to combine VAEs with GANs to enhance image generation. While hyperspherical VAE (Davidson et al., 2018) implements a distinct kind of VAE suitable for different data forms, vector quantized VAE (Van Den Oord and Vinyals, 2017) adopts a separate method for structuring data. The model VAE-GAN (Larsen et al., 2016) combines the strengths of VAEs and GANs for generating superior images, while S3VAE (Zhu et al., 2020) focuses on processing data in sequences. In addition to their proficiency in generating new data, VAEs also inspire innovative research concepts and applications, particularly within the field of bioinformatics. As a result of these strengths, current investigations into VAEs within the field of bioinformatics are largely centered on two main areas: firstly, creating new data, and secondly, learning better representations of data. The role of VAEs in different fields of bioinformatics has been listed in Table 6.2 (Wei and Mahmood, 2020).

It is very important that VAE is not just seen as a strong tool for creating new data, but also recognized for its ability to learn complex patterns, which can lead to new research areas and diverse applications in health data studies.

Table 6.2 VAE research in molecular designing (Wei and Mahmood, 2020).

S. No.	Data Type	Dataset	Description	References
1.	ZINC	string	Molecular similarity calculation.	Samanta et al. (2020a, 2020b)
2.	ZINC	string	3D topological structure of molecules using a novel method in the latent space.	Schiff et al. (2020)
3.	ZINC	string	Improve the design of the molecules by using grammar.	Kusner et al. (2017)
4.	ZINC	string	Uses SMILES molecules in latent space to build an energy-based prior model.	Pang et al. (2020)
5.	QM9 & ZINC	string	Capable of generating representations of new molecules.	Gomez-Bombarelli et al. (2018)
6.	ZINC	string	Readjusting the loss of the VAE to produce other legitimate molecules in SMILES.	Yan et al. (2020)
7.	ZINC	graph	The graph representation is implemented using a tree structure.	Jin et al. (2018)
8.	PCBA & ZINC	graph	Adding a penalty term to the VAE's decoder improves the latent space quality.	Mohammadi et al. (2019)
9.	ZINC & QM9	graph	Graph VAE is used to represent molecules continuously.	Tavakoli and Baldi (2020)
10.	QM9, ZINC & CEPDB	graph	Able to produce sequential graph representations.	Liu et al. (2018)
11.	QM9 & ZINC	graph	Creating graphs in the latent space from a continuous representation.	Simonovsky and Komodakis (2018)
12.	ChEMBL &QM9	graph	A masked graph model for molecular graphs based on VAE.	Mahmood et al. (2021)
13.	MolPort	graph	Using VAE to model 3D molecular structures.	Ragoza et al. (2020)
14.	QM9	graph	Calculating molecular property statistics with a short training data set.	Shervani-Taber and Zabaras (2020)
15.	QM9	graph	Metric learning and VAEs are combined in molecular embedding learning.	Koge et al. (2021)
16.	QM9	graph	Exploring molecular domains inside a constant low-dimensional molecule's depiction and creating 3D chemical structures.	Nesterov et al. (2020)
17.	ChEMBL	graph	Provides scalable molecular graphs with a reduced-graph representation.	Kwon et al. (2020)
18.	Materials project	electron-density maps	A pipeline using deep learning to create 3D crystal formations and forecast their characteristics.	Court et al. (2020)

6 Generative adversarial network

Ian Goodfellow, in 2014, along with a group of researchers, developed GAN, a ground breaking learning model (Goodfellow et al., 2014). This GAN model operates through two components that compete: a generator that produces novel data and a discriminator that tries to distinguish between authentic data and the generated data from the generator. The generator takes stochastic input and learns to convert it into seemingly authentic data. The discriminator's training objective is to recognize authentic samples as opposed to fake ones. The goal of the generator is to differentiate inaccurate, falsely labeled samples as real, while the discriminator's role is to identify and separate them correctly. When the discriminator cannot recognize the difference between authentic samples and generated ones, training comes to a stop. GANs were developed based on the concept behind deep Boltzmann machines, which utilized a related method of learning. There were two phases in these machines: one that increased the likelihood of certain data and another that decreased the likelihood of different data. With continued training, the generated samples increasingly resemble the actual data. On the other hand, deep Boltzmann machines faced challenges when processing complex data like colorful images, as their negative phase couldn't synchronize with the positive phase. This hindered their ability to generate valuable outcomes efficiently.

GAN is gaining attention in ML and artificial intelligence due to recent improvements in deep learning technology. There is immense potential for GAN to be utilized across different fields, such as innovating new drugs, examining images and videos, and translating languages. The GAN application in drug design and discovery has shown promising results. For instance, scientists have employed frameworks based on GANs, like the deep adversarial autoencoder, to innovate and identify new cancer therapies by integrating chemical and biological information. The deep adversarial variational autoencoder has magnificently minimized the data volume for single-cell RNA sequencing during drug development in its initial phases. This is interesting as it demonstrates the potential usefulness of these technologies. Current research is centered on three key domains in the area of drug development and design. These domains encompass the development of novel molecules, streamlining single-cell data during preliminary studies, and the design of innovative peptides and proteins. Each of these studies utilizes frameworks that are grounded in GANs. There is currently little research in drug design that utilizes frameworks based on GANs, which is why researchers are concentrating on these three domains along with different GAN models (Table 6.3). Research outcomes from these areas have the potential to stimulate fresh investigations into drug formulation using GAN technology (Tripathi et al., 2022).

Table 6.3 Overview of common GAN variants, methodology, and network architecture (Tripathi et al., 2022).

Criteria	GAN	CGAN	LAPGAN	DCGAN	AAE	INFOGAN
Learning	Supervised	Supervised	Unsupervised	Unsupervised	Supervised, semisupervised & unsupervised	Unsupervised
Network Architecture	Multilayer perceptrons	Multilayer perceptrons	Laplacian pyramid of convolutional networks	Convolutional networks with constraints	Autoencoders	Multilayer perceptrons
Gradient updates	SGD using k steps for D and a single step for G	SGD using k steps for D and a single step for G	No updates	SGD for both G and D using the Adam optimizer	Regularization and reconstruction phases in SGD.	Improvements to G and D using SGD
Methodology	Decrease the value function for G and increase it for D.	Decrease the value function for G and increase it for D, depending on additional information.	Images creation in coarse-to-fine fashion	In both G and D, discover the hierarchy of representations from object fragments to scenes	Finding the posterior of the autoencoder's hidden code vector by comparing it to the prior distribution	Maximize mutual information to learn disentangled representations
Performance metrics	Log-likelihood	Log-likelihood	Log-likelihood and human evaluation	Accuracy and error rate	Log-likelihood and error-rate	Information metric and representation learning

7 Applications of GAN

7.1 Drug candidate searching

Drug discovery using GANs in drug research presents a notable strength in their potential to uncover new molecular candidates for medication. The conventional approach to drug discovery encounters difficulties because the sheer volume of potential chemical compounds makes comprehensive exploration complex. It creates challenges for researchers in selecting the optimal choices from among comparable compounds, which could exhibit slight differences in their drug effects. Even though GANs have their limitations, they excel compared to other approaches in probing chemical spaces, representing all conceivable chemical compounds that follow certain guidelines (Blanchard et al., 2021). Through the application of many biological models, including population trends, diversity algorithms, and evolutionary data, GANs can be trained to pinpoint compounds that produce the desired effects. Training GANs with this kind of data leads to two significant outputs. Initially, they create multiple new drug variations to evaluate their efficacy and minimize adverse effects. Further, this method allows GANs to progressively adjust and improve their generated alternatives based on the specific chemical effects targeted by the researcher. A challenge with GANs is that they may excessively fixate on a narrow range of training data, leading to mode collapse, where the generated variations are overly similar to the initial samples. In response to this problem, researchers like Blanchard have been dedicated to the continuous revision and integration of training data throughout their work (Blanchard et al., 2021). This approach mitigates the limitations of GANs in drug discovery, positioning it as a valuable resource for accelerating the process of finding new medications.

7.2 Artificial DNA sequences generation

Biomolecular GANs are utilized to produce artificial DNA sequences capable of generating proteins with varying lengths. A research project employed a feedback mechanism to design synthetic genes that generate antimicrobial peptides, tailoring these genes for the peptides' specific shapes. A significant number of tests reveal that the proteins synthesized by GANs have the desired physical and chemical traits (Gupta and Zou, 2018). By examining large datasets, deep learning models uncover sophisticated connections between chemical structures and their drug-related and biological attributes, which allows computers to synthesize new molecules that exhibit targeted properties in a lab environment (Chen et al., 2018) Utilizing ML or statistical methods, a quantitative structure-activity relationship (QSAR) framework seeks to uncover relationships among the molecule's biological activity and its characteristics. In addition, it's significant to understand that VAEs and Adversarial Autoencoders (AAEs) perform well with different types of chemical structures. Multiple models of generative AAEs were applied, in contrast to QSAR, to design novel chemical structures.

7.3 Drug-target interactions

Drug development GANs are designed to improve the effectiveness of research in drug discovery. GANs offer insights into the necessary interactions between a drug and its target, an important aspect in predicting the drug's effectiveness (Zhao et al., 2020). The deep learning models' applications allow the rapid identification of drugs that tightly bind to specific proteins linked to diseases, thus expediting the research process. One of the main reasons GANs are considered powerful is that they operate more quickly and at a lower cost than many other ML models. Although other models have made comparable predictions, GANs require less manual intervention and are more economical in generating training data by leveraging components of their networks.

7.4 Targeted drug delivery analysis

Targeting a key challenge with conventional drug delivery is that it typically necessitates a large dosage to achieve proper efficacy at the desired site. Nevertheless, consuming a high quantity can produce negative side effects. To address this issue, researchers are working on methods to target drug delivery precisely to the affected area, potentially reducing the required dosage. Simple strategies include applying the drug directly to the problem area, while more advanced options may utilize normal body temperature, pH, or magnetic fields. Using specific molecules referred to as vector molecules, which have enhanced sticking properties, is among the most effective means of targeting drugs to the desired regions. This strategy can be adapted for diverse drug dosages, sizes, and their ease of passing through other barriers (Torchilin, 2000). Currently, determining the drug-targeting interactions (DTIs) remains a challenge. A large number of DTIs are based on ML, which involves analyzing vast amounts of known data to generate predictions, often resulting in high costs and extended timeframes. Utilizing a semisupervised strategy with GANs could be an effective way to estimate the drug's binding effectiveness to its target. The implementation of sophisticated computer techniques and ML can accelerate drug development processes and reduce costs (Tripathi et al., 2022).

8 Quantitative structure-activity relationship modeling

In 1962, Corwin Hansch and his team first created QSAR, a methodology that blends chemistry with the assessment of drugs in a virtual environment (Hansch et al., 1962). Over the course of the last five decades, it has transformed from using simple statistical comparisons of similar compounds to leveraging advanced ML technologies that can assess large volumes of data regarding molecular structures. The application of QSAR models has gained popularity for examining the properties of diverse chemicals and for evaluating how drugs and materials could impact both human health and the environment (Shin et al., 2017, 2018). Lee et al. (2013) developed a QSAR system named Management system of high energy molecules (MSHEMs), specifically designed to study molecules with high-energy. Now in the field of CADD (Computer-Aided Drug Design), QSAR is an esteemed approach that aids in drug development and optimization by analyzing molecular structures and pertinent insights (Mao et al., 2021). By examining the structure of new chemicals, a QSAR model can forecast their effects on living organisms. This approach is quicker than the more time-consuming process known as molecular docking. The inclusion of amino acid sequences in the QSAR model enables the effective use of protein information. By applying this method, the predictions can be made more reliable. In general, QSAR proves valuable in drug development as it allows for the rapid analysis of numerous compounds while maintaining a high level of accuracy. Recently, there has been a rise in its usage within domains like drug formulation, predicting the toxicity of medications (Wu and Wang, 2018), researching enzymes, and comprehending chemical interactions in biological environments (Mao et al., 2021).

8.1 Molecular descriptor based QSAR

QSAR focuses on obtaining numerical information from chemical structures, referred to as molecular descriptors (Park et al., 2013). Over the last 50 years, many kinds of these descriptors have been developed, such as quantitative descriptors and qualitative descriptors. Vector, Boolean, integer, real, tensor, vector field, and scalar field are the different molecular categories of descriptors based on the type of data. Based on their definitions and structural characteristics, molecular descriptors can be organized into different classes.

The descriptors are of various types and can be categorized into four groups: property descriptors, composition descriptors, geometric descriptors, and topological descriptors. Depending on their structure, molecular descriptors may range from one to six dimensions (1D to 6D). These various kinds of molecular descriptors are commonly used in studying the variety of compounds and predicting how compounds will behave (Mao et al., 2021).

8.2 QSAR model construction approaches

Current QSAR methodologies utilize multiple measurements and encompass both straightforward and intricate modeling techniques, concentrating on comprehensive testing to ensure the creation of reliable and predictive QSAR models. The overview of the QSAR modeling process is described briefly in the following steps:

8.2.1 Preparation of dataset & data curation

A major challenge in QSAR analysis is gathering data with a specific objective in mind. It's essential to clearly define your prediction goals, as these can be influenced by the design of the experiments and the circumstances in which they are conducted. Effective data organization is a vital and laborious step in the formation of QSAR models. To ensure accurate predictive modeling, it is crucial to meticulously scrutinize any erroneous data related to chemical structures or biological information obtained online (Ambure and Cordeiro, 2020).

8.2.2 Molecular descriptors calculation

In QSAR modeling, it's essential to transform molecular structures into numerical values known as molecular descriptors. Based on the chemical composition, these descriptors convey essential information about a chemical compound in a numerical format (Table 6.4). The methodology facilitates the relationship between a chemical's structure and its physical attributes, chemical behaviors, or biological consequences (Consonni et al., 2010). QSAR models consist of descriptors that highlight particular molecular characteristics and serve as predictors (X) for an outcome variable (Y). A QSAR investigation involves various descriptors that are organized into different groups (De et al., 2022).

8.2.3 Dataset division

In order to consider the efficiency of a predictive model, it is essential to split the data into two segments: a testing set and a training set. A selection of chemicals forms our training set, which we employ to generate QSAR models. Next, we evaluate the accuracy of these

Table 6.4 Various software used for molecular descriptor calculations (Peter et al., 2019).

S. No.	Package	Specification	Access
1.	PaDEL Descriptors (yapcwsoft.com/dd/padeldescriptor/)	2D & 3D descriptors calculation	Free
2.	MOLGEN (MolGen—Global DNA & RNA Extraction Solutions)	Topological, constitutional, & geometrical descriptors calculation	Free
3.	ACD/LogP Freeware (Free Chemical Drawing Software for Students: ChemSketch, ACD/Labs)	Fragment-based algorithm for prediction of logP prediction	Free
4.	Dragon (Molecular descriptors calculation—Dragon—Talete srl)	Topological, constitutional, & geometrical descriptors calculation	Commercial

models by testing their predictions on a separate dataset comprised of different chemicals. It's essential to incorporate a diverse range of chemicals when selecting the training set. It is also essential for the test set to include chemicals that are similar to those in the training set. There are various techniques available for dividing the dataset, including Kennard-Stone (Kennard and Stone, 1969), sorted response (Roy, 2018), Euclidean distance (Golmohammadi et al., 2012), and k-means clustering (Likas et al., 2003).

8.2.4 Selection of feature

Identifying key variables through trait selection is a significant phase in understanding the main response variable. By utilizing this method, the model becomes less complex, the likelihood of overfitting or overtraining diminishes, and it highlights the most relevant features among numerous alternatives. This approach diminishes the total number of input variables while preserving all the important information (Goodarzi et al., 2012). A mathematical model is constructed from the chosen features to demonstrate the biological activity of the compounds. Several approaches for feature selection, like Genetic Function Approximation (GFA), Genetic Algorithms (GA), backward elimination, forward selection, simulated annealing, and stepwise regression, have been applied.

8.2.5 Algorithms for model constructions

It is essential to develop a QSAR model utilizing a well-defined algorithm. The goal of this guideline is to ensure that the model is understandable, allowing others to replicate it and achieve identical outcomes. It involves several stages, including data preparation, splitting the dataset, identifying key features, and constructing the model. Various linear modeling methods employed include partial least squares and ordinary least squares (Wold et al., 2001), multiple linear regression (De and Roy, 2018), principal component analysis (Abdi and Williams, 2010) among several others.

8.2.6 Domain applicability determination

Identifying the model's "applicability domain" (AD) is an important stage in QSAR modeling. The AD indicates the specific scope of chemical properties and structures suitable for making dependable predictions with the QSAR model (Roy et al., 2015a, Roy et al. (2015b)). The characteristics of the compounds from the training set are the main focus of this section, which emphasizes the necessity of determining how reliable the model's predictions are for novel compounds in the test set. The concept of an AD aids in avoiding predictions that lack data support.

8.2.7 Validation of QSAR model

Validation of the QSAR model is necessary before it can be used to forecast how untested compounds will interact biologically. This involves assessing its ability to forecast and align with the actual functions of these substances. Statistically validating a model is a critical phase in its development process. Validation of this model is crucial if it is intended for use in virtual screening. Validation evaluates the accuracy of the predictions, focusing on the proximity of the model's estimated values to the real experimental outcomes. The accuracy of the model is measured through metrics like the determination coefficient and correlation coefficient, based on the training data, to illustrate the degree of alignment between predicted and actual values. Simply fitting the model to the data does not confirm its capacity to predict future results. Both regression and classification models utilize distinct methods of internal and external validation to determine their effectiveness in making predictions.

8.2.8 Interpretation of mechanistic

It's crucial to comprehend the various elements that could clarify the reaction under investigation. To produce chemicals that operate effectively, one must utilize structures that are comparable. Yet, it is apparent that there are times when offering this level of detail is impossible. According to the guideline, individuals constructing the model should provide any relevant information they have, as it will contribute to future investigations in that area. Incorporating insights from prior research can enhance the comprehension of the modeled reaction.

8.3 Metrics of regression validation & classification validation

The process of validation is used to assess the reliability of QSAR models. This involves confirming the integrity of the input data, utilizing a range of data types, accurately forecasting outcomes with novel data, clarifying the model's scope of application, and gaining insights into the underlying dynamics using different validation metrics. There are two primary forms of validation for QSAR models: first, internal validation, which checks how well the model predicts the activity of the same molecules that were used to create it. It focuses on determining the correctness of the predictions. Techniques like cross-validation (Konovalov et al., 2008) utilize internal validation effectively, as they involve segregating the data into different sections for model training and testing its forecast results. The component used for model development is termed the calibration set, in contrast to the component used for evaluation, which is labeled the validation set. Second, external validation assesses how well the model can predict new or untested molecules. External validation metrics are employed to assess the model's applicability to novel designs. In many cases, when adequate external data isn't accessible, a few compounds from the real dataset are employed for validation (De et al., 2022).

8.4 Machine learning-based QSAR models

The ML-based QSAR model is being used extensively in drug design and screening, property prediction, category prediction, and other applications. Since the 1990s, ML techniques such as support vector machines and random forests have been frequently employed to identify or create new treatments. This approach has also been applied to a molecular docking-based scoring function (Lima et al., 2016). In a variety of ML models and prediction tasks, a set of two- or three-dimensional chemical descriptors can be extracted through data mining based on chemical graphs and packed into chemical fingerprints. A key innovation in this field is the combination of big data and ML, which includes the mining of gene sequences and protein structures, single-cell sequences, multiomics interaction data, and protein-gene interactions, enabling the QSAR model to learn and predict a wider range of biological laws.

Previously, QSAR models focused solely on the predictive abilities of candidate compounds; consequently, discriminative prediction models are the most widely used ML models. Generative and discriminative prediction models are the two primary categories of ML techniques (Jebara, 2001). The essence of the discriminative model is to learn the mapping relationship between the properties of the characterizing sample and the prediction target from the data, which is connected to pattern recognition; thus, the model can only discriminate and predict. The generative model learns the sample's data distribution directly. In addition to being integrated with the discriminative model, the generative model can directly produce fresh samples based on the learned distribution and is therefore used to generate candidate compounds.The four primary categories of techniques for discovering patterns concealed in data are self-supervised learning, unsupervised learning, semisupervised learning, and supervised learning. Since the QSAR model solely considers a model's capacity to predict candidate compounds, discriminative models are frequently employed in supervised learning. The key to this type of model is feature selection, algorithm selection, and training set quality.

Molecular dynamics simulations, quantum chemistry, and semiempirical techniques can all be used to perform conformational calculations for isomers. The QSAR has also taken into consideration conformation-related indications. Because the relative stability of conformational isomerism is relevant to toxicity detection, the compound's conformation may change when the solvent environment changes, affecting the 3D correlation properties and ultimately influencing the final screening result. Thus, it is possible to forecast whether the relative stability of the conformation will have an impact on the experimental results using techniques for computing isomer conformations. It is also possible to use the ML-based QSAR method to forecast the link between conformational changes and molecular energy, analyze the energy changes between conformational changes, and ascertain how the solvent environment affects the conformation (Lokuge et al., 2010; Singh et al., 2016).

Different structure-activity or characteristic prediction tasks assign different values to these features; however, ML may learn from the data which features are more significant. To learn from the training set, we must thus use the conventional ML technique and exhaust as many of the attributes associated with the nature of QSAR jobs as possible. Under the typical circumstance where the system being studied is too complicated to be physically modeled, ML-based QSAR techniques are successful. Theoretical approaches like density functional theory or MD can be used to calculate many physical and chemical properties, but cheminformatics models can often calculate them. This is particularly relevant for water solubility and logP (the logarithm of the octanol:water partition coefficient), which are directly related to drug activity. The melting point, solubility, and sublimation energy are among the characteristics that may be computed using cheminformatics and are indirectly linked to pharmacological activity. The QSAR techniques might not be appropriate, of course, if the underlying mechanisms are sufficiently well understood. Quantum chemistry can be used to directly calculate, for instance, dipole moment, polarizability, and vibration frequency.

According to the conventional QSAR model, a compound's properties are created in the perfect setting. But in practice, the solvent environment is not optimal. For instance, in an acidic atmosphere, acidic compounds are readily absorbed. Therefore, a drug's hydrophilicity and lipophilicity must be taken into account in order to provide the intended effect in a real-world context (Ditzinger et al., 2019). Studies have identified the primary environmental parameters of a solvent (Bruno et al., 2021).

The next phase, after the preparation indicated above, is to create a QSAR model using ML, which mostly entails the following actions:

- Through "molecular coding," which represents complex molecules with a vector of different attributes, the chemical qualities and characteristics can be inferred from experimental data or the chemical structure. To prevent excessive association, molecular features should be as distinct as possible. The best way to obtain the solvent environmental coefficients and biological activity data is through standard experiments, which should be as precise and comprehensive as feasible.
- To create the training and testing sets, the right amount of compounds must be selected. In order to increase the quality of the data, it is ideal to perform conformation optimization using Molecular Mechanism/Quantum Mechanics (MM/QM) first. Reducing the dimensionality of the feature vector and identifying the most pertinent features are accomplished through unsupervised learning. An empirical function, either explicit or implicit, that can achieve the best possible mapping between the input feature vector and the biological activity is determined using a supervised ML model.
- The model's predictability and applicability are assessed through internal and external verification. Upon producing exhaustive feature sets, the algorithm identifies the largest difference between positive and negative samples in the training set to determine which feature combinations can be used for new predictions; as a result, the training and testing sets ought to have comparable data distributions. Studies have been conducted to detect out-of-distribution samples (Hendrycks and Gimpel, 2017). Until the optimal model is achieved, it is crucial to continuously add and experiment with new feature combinations, alter the training set's divisions, and modify the algorithm's parameters.

The most recent ML techniques are increasing adaptability, yet ML models trained on particular target sets are not general. In addition,

QSAR models have been enhanced by improvements in software performance and processing power. It is possible to continuously optimize the model by incorporating new algorithms and descriptive features. The ML-based QSAR's general concept is the same, although various targets may have distinct input characteristics. GANs, AutoEncoders, self-learning, multitask learning, and Bidirectional Encoder Representations from Transformers are examples of recent advancements in general representation learning (Mao et al., 2021).

9 Future perspective and limitations

Moreover, the expanding tendency to share research data and scripts is expected to foster improvements in the field of computational drug development. This effort will lead to a growing and useful compilation of information that builds upon past contributions, similar to a snowball that gathers mass as it rolls. Funding agencies and publishers have recently adopted policies that encourage the dissemination of data and code. Platforms such as Authorea, Code Ocean, Jupyter Notebook, and Manuscripts.io facilitate this process by enabling the editing and execution of online documents and code in real-time, rather than merely providing static downloadable files. The field of predictive modeling encounters several obstacles while striving to develop efficient and dependable computer tools for the pharmaceutical sector (Nissan et al., 2024). Studies highlight the significance of strong cooperation between researchers in drug development, data modeling, and their support teams. Improving collaboration among these groups requires a greater mutual understanding and consistent terminology, yet they struggle with distinct challenges rooted in the wide array of disciplines involved.

It's important for modelers of data, developers of tools, and administrators to take into account that their tools will be utilized by technologists operating in an ever-evolving landscape. Due to the constantly changing nature of this environment, it might not always align with the suggestions from the community of data science. Such circumstances might result in differing opinions among model developers about the optimal course of action. User-generated data, such as observational findings or distinctive 3D models, can provide valuable insights, but integrating them into specific models can be challenging and time-consuming (Soliman et al., 2024). Occasionally, understanding the model's framework is more valuable than simply evaluating its ability to predict results. Frequently, models are selected based on statistical data rather than actual user requirements, leading to the absence of some valuable models in today's automated tools.

The advantage of open-source tools lies in their transparent processes and user-friendly options for evaluating results. Keeping track of the various tools and configurations when handling data can be quite complex. Consequently, there is an increasing trend in the adoption of drug discovery workflow solutions. They assist in producing accurate calculations, making it easier to reproduce results. The Common Workflow Language exemplifies an initiative to standardize these processes by promoting compatibility between diverse workflow languages. As massive amounts of data are generated, the use of shared computing resources, such as High Performance Computing (HPC)/Cloud, becomes vital, but this increases the difficulty of achieving reproducible outcomes. The use of virtual machines and software containers facilitates the compatibility of data analysis tools with different systems (Piane et al., 2024). The integration of workflow systems with this technology enhances automation and improves the consistency of outcomes. With this virtual configuration, employing networked services guarantees reliable service delivery that can be easily duplicated.

10 Conclusion

The use of sophisticated ML techniques, including GANs, can facilitate the search for beneficial chemical compounds. It is not easy to determine how effectively a drug will perform against its target when developing new medications. The process of obtaining labeled data for supervised systems is not only costly but also hard to scale, which limits the feasibility of these methods for general use. Useful representations can be extracted from raw data on proteins and drugs using GANs, and convolutional regression can assist in estimating the strength of their binding affinity. Developments in various branches of science have produced a wealth of data that is valuable for the discovery of new pharmaceuticals. Although this extensive array of information has the potential to significantly advance healthcare, it simultaneously raises questions about the validity and trustworthiness of the conclusions drawn. Understanding the current benchmarks for research reproducibility in computer-based drug discovery is essential for avoiding possible complications. This understanding will help to uphold the quality of the research and allow fellow researchers to duplicate the techniques employed.

References

Abdi, H., Williams, L.J., 2010. Principal component analysis. Wiley Interdiscip. Rev. Comput. Stat. 1939-0068. 2 (4), 433–459. Available from http://www3.interscience.wiley.com/cgi-bin/fulltext/123569814/PDFSTART. doi:10.1002/wics.101.

Ambure, P., Cordeiro, M.N.D.S., 2020. Importance of data curation in QSAR studies especially while modeling large-size datasets. In: Methods in Pharmacology and

Toxicology. Humana Press Inc., Portugal, pp. 97–109. Available from: http://www.springer.com/series/7653 http://www.springer.com/humana+press/book/978-1-934115-23-7?cm_mmc=AD-_-enews-_-HUM1627-_-0&. doi:10.1007/978-1-0716-0150-1_5.

Arús-Pous, J., Patronov, A., Bjerrum, E.J., Tyrchan, C., Reymond, J.L., Chen, H., Engkvist, O., 2020. SMILES-based deep generative scaffold decorator for de-novo drug design. J. Cheminform. 1758-2946. 12 (1). Available from: https://jcheminf.biomedcentral.com/. doi:10.1186/s13321-020-00441-8.

Bilodeau, C., Jin, W., Jaakkola, T., Barzilay, R., Jensen, K.F., 2022. Generative models for molecular discovery: recent advances and challenges. Wiley Interdiscip. Rev. Comput. Mol. Sci. 1759-0884. 12 (5). Available from: http://onlinelibrary.wiley.com/journal/10.1111/(ISSN)1759-0884. doi:10.1002/wcms.1608.

Blanchard, A.E., Stanley, C., Bhowmik, D., 2021. Using GANs with adaptive training data to search for new molecules. J. Cheminform. 13, 1–8.

Bond-Taylor, S., Leach, A., Long, Y., Willcocks, C.G., 2022. Deep generative modelling: a comparative review of VAEs, GANs, normalizing flows, energy-based and autoregressive models. IEEE Trans. Pattern Anal. Mach. Intell. 0162-8828. 44 (11), 7327–7347. doi:10.1109/tpami.2021.3116668.

Brown, N., Fiscato, M., Segler, M.H.S., Vaucher, A.C., 2019. GuacaMol: benchmarking models for de novo molecular design. J. Chem. Inf. Model. 1549-960X. 59 (3), 1096–1108. Available from: http://pubs.acs.org/journal/jcisd8. doi:10.1021/acs.jcim.8b00839.

Bruno, C.D., Harmatz, J.S., Duan, S.X., Zhang, Q., Chow, C.R., Greenblatt, D.J., 2021. Effect of lipophilicity on drug distribution and elimination: influence of obesity. Br. J. Clin. Pharmacol. 1365-2125. 87 (8), 3197–3205. Available from: http://onlinelibrary.wiley.com/journal/10.1111/(ISSN)1365-2125. doi:10.1111/bcp.14735.

Chen, N., Klushyn, A., Kurle, R., Jiang, X., Bayer, J., Smagt, P., 2018. Metrics for deep generative models. In International Conference on Artificial Intelligence and Statistics. PMLR, pp. 1540-1550.

Chung, J., Gulcehre, C., Cho, K., Bengio, Y., 2014. Empirical evaluation of gated recurrent neural networks on sequence modeling. arXiv preprint arXiv:1412.3555 .

Consonni, V., Todeschini, R., Puzyn, T., Leszczynski, J., Cronin, M.T., 2010. Recent Advances in QSAR Studies . Challenges and Advances in Computational Chemistry and Physics, Vol. 8. Dordrecht: Springer, pp. 29–48. doi:10.1007/978-1-4020-9783-6_3.

Court, C.J., Yildirim, B., Jain, A., Cole, J.M., 2020. 3-D inorganic crystal structure generation and property prediction via representation learning. J. Chem. Inf. Model. 1549-960X. 60 (10), 4518–4535. Available from: http://pubs.acs.org/journal/jcisd8. doi:10.1021/acs.jcim.0c00464.

Dai, H., Tian, Y., Dai, B., Skiena, S., Song, L., 2018. Syntax-directed variational autoencoder for structured data. In: 6th International Conference on Learning Representations, ICLR 2018 - Conference Track Proceedings. International Conference on Learning Representations, ICLR, Singapore. https://dblp.org/db/conf/iclr/iclr2018.html.

Davidson, T.R., Falorsi, L., De, C.N., Kipf, T., Tomczak, J.M., 2018. Hyperspherical variational auto-encoders 2. In: 34th Conference on Uncertainty in Artificial Intelligence 2018, UAI 2018. 9781510871601. Association For Uncertainty in Artificial Intelligence (AUAI), Netherlands. pp. 856–865.

De, P., Kar, S., Ambure, P., Roy, K., 2022. Prediction reliability of QSAR models: an overview of various validation tools. Arch. Toxicol. 0340-5761. 96 (5), 1279–1295. doi:10.1007/s00204-022-03252-y.

De, P., Roy, K., 2018. Greener chemicals for the future: QSAR modelling of the PBT index using ETA descriptors. SAR QSAR Environ. Res. 1062-936X. 29 (4), 319–337. doi:10.1080/1062936x.2018.1436086.

Dilokthanakul, N., Mediano, P.A., Garnelo, M., Lee, M.C., Salimbeni, H., Arulkumaran, K., Shanahan, M., 2016. Deep unsupervised clustering with Gaussian mixture variational autoencoders. ArXiv, abs/1611.02648 .

Ditzinger, F., Price, D.J., Ilie, A.R., Köhl, N.J., Jankovic, S., Tsakiridou, G., Aleandri, S., Kalantzi, L., Holm, R., Nair, A., Saal, C., Griffin, B., Kuentz, M., 2019. Lipophilicity and hydrophobicity considerations in bio-enabling oral formulations approaches—a PEARRL review. J. Pharm. Pharmacol. 2042-7158. 71 (4), 464–482. Available from: http://onlinelibrary.wiley.com/journal/10.1111/(ISSN)2042-7158. doi:10.1111/jphp.12984.

Gao, R., Hou, X., Qin, J., Chen, J., Liu, L., Zhu, F., Zhang, Z., Shao, L., 2020. Zero-VAE-GAN: generating unseen features for generalized and transductive zero-shot learning. IEEE Trans. Image Process. 1057-7149. 29, 3665–3680. doi:10.1109/tip.2020.2964429.

Gebauer, N., Gastegger, M., Schütt, K., 2019. Symmetry-adapted generation of 3d point sets for the targeted discovery of molecules. ArXiv, abs/1906.00957 .

Golmohammadi, H., Dashtbozorgi, Z., Acree Jr, W.E., 2012. Quantitative structure-activity relationship prediction of blood-to-brain partitioning behavior using support vector machine. Eur. J. Pharm. Sci. 47 (2), 421–429.

Gómez-Bombarelli, R., Wei, J.N., Duvenaud, D., Hernández-Lobato, J.M., Sánchez-Lengeling, B., Sheberla, D., Aspuru-Guzik, A., 2018. Automatic chemical design using a data-driven continuous representation of molecules. ACS Cent. Sci. 4 (2), 268–276.

Goodarzi, M., Dejaegher, B., Heyden, Y.V., 2012. Feature selection methods in QSAR studies. J. AOAC Int. 95 (3), 636–651.

Goodfellow, I.J., Pouget-Abadie, J., Mirza, M., Xu, B., Warde-Farley, D., Ozair, S., Bengio, 2014. Generative adversarial networks. Communications of the ACM, 63, 139-144.

Gupta, A., Zou, J. (2018). Feedback GAN (FBGAN) for DNA: a novel feedback-loop architecture for optimizing protein functions. arXiv preprint arXiv:1804.01694.

Hansch, C., Maloney, P.P., Fujita, T., Muir, R.M., 1962. Correlation of biological activity of phenoxyacetic acids with Hammett substituent constants and partition coefficients. Nature. 0028-0836. 194 (4824), 178–180. doi:10.1038/194178b0.

Hendrycks, D., Gimpel, K., 2017. A baseline for detecting misclassified and out-of-distribution examples in neural networks. In: 5th International Conference on Learning Representations, ICLR 2017 - Conference Track Proceedings. International Conference on Learning Representations, ICLR, United States. https://dblp.org/db/conf/iclr/iclr2017.html.

Higgins, I., Matthey, L., Pal, A., Burgess, C., Glorot, X., Botvinick, M., Lerchner, A., 2017. Beta-vae: learning basic visual concepts with a constrained variational framework. In: International conference on learning representations.

Hochreiter, S., Schmidhuber, J., 1997. Long short-term memory. Neural Comput. 9 (8), 1735–1780.

Jebara, T., 2001. Discriminative, generative and imitative learning (Doctoral dissertation, PhD thesis, Media laboratory, MIT).

Jiang, Z., Zheng, Y., Tan, H., Tang, B., Zhou, H., 2016. Variational deep embedding: an unsupervised and generative approach to clustering. arXiv preprint arXiv:1611.05148.

Jin, W., Barzilay, R., Jaakkola, T., 2018. Junction tree variational autoencoder for molecular graph generation. In: International conference on machine learning. PMLR. pp. 2323–2332.

Jin, W., Barzilay, R., Jaakkola, T., 2020. Hierarchical generation of molecular graphs using structural motifs. In: International conference on machine learning. PMLR. pp. 4839–4848.

Jolicoeur-Martineau, A., 2018. The relativistic discriminator: a key element missing from standard GAN. arXiv. 2331-8422. Available from: https://arxiv.org. doi:10.48550/arxiv.1807.00734.

Kennard, R.W., Stone, L.A., 1969. Computer aided design of experiments. Technometrics. 0040-1706. 11 (1), 137–148. doi:10.1080/00401706.1969.10490666.

Koge, D., Ono, N., Huang, M., Altaf-Ul-Amin, M., Kanaya, S., 2021. Embedding of molecular structure using molecular hypergraph variational autoencoder with metric learning. Mol. Inform. 40(2), 2000203.

Konovalov, D.A., Llewellyn, L.E., Heyden, Y.V., Coomans, D., 2008. Robust cross-validation of linear regression QSAR models. J. Chem. Inf. Model. 1549-960X. 48 (10), 2081–2094. Available from: http://pubs.acs.org/journal/jcisd8. doi:10.1021/ci800209k.

Krenn, M., Häse, F., Nigam, A., Friederich, P., Aspuru-Guzik, A., 2020. Self-referencing embedded strings (SELFIES): a 100% robust molecular string representation. Mach. Learn. Sci. Technol. 2632-2153. 1 (4), 045024. doi:10.1088/2632-2153/aba947.

Kusner, M.J., Paige, B., Hernández-Lobato, J.M., 2017. Grammar variational autoencoder. In: International conference on machine learning. PMLR. pp. 1945–1954.

Kwon, Y., Lee, D., Choi, Y.S., Shin, K., Kang, S., 2020. Compressed graph representation for scalable molecular graph generation. J. Cheminform. 1758-2946. 12 (1). Available from: https://jcheminf.biomedcentral.com/. doi:10.1186/s13321-020-00463-2.

Lamb, A., 2021. A brief introduction to generative models. arXiv. 2331-8422. Available from: https://arxiv.org. doi:10.48550/arxiv.2103.00265.

Larsen, A.B.L., Sønderby, S.K., Larochelle, H., Winther, O., 2016. Autoencoding beyond pixels using a learned similarity metric. In: International conference on machine learning. PMLR. pp. 1558–1566.

Lee, S., Kang, Y.M., Park, H., Dong, M.S., Shin, J.M., No, K.T., 2013. Human nephrotoxicity prediction models for three types of kidney injury based on data sets of pharmacological compounds and their metabolites. Chem. Res. Toxicol. 26 (11), 1652–1659.

Likas, A., Vlassis, N., Verbeek, J.J., 2003. The global k-means clustering algorithm. Pattern Recognit. 36 (2), 451–461.

Lima, A.N., Philot, E.A., Trossini, G.H.G., Scott, L.P.B., Maltarollo, V.G., Honorio, K.M., 2016. Use of machine learning approaches for novel drug discovery. Expert Opin. Drug Discov. 1746-045X. 11 (3), 225–239. doi:10.1517/17460441.2016.1146250.

Liu, Q., Allamanis, M., Brockschmidt, M., Gaunt, A.L., 2018. Constrained graph variational autoencoders for molecule design. In: Advances in Neural Information Processing Systems. 10495258. Neural information processing systems foundation, United States. pp. 7795–7804. https://papers.nips.cc/.

Lokuge, S., Hewavitarne, H., Wimalaratne, P., Ranawana, R., 2010. Machine learning based QSAR for discovering potential drug candidate from endemic plants of Sri Lanka- case study: HIV-1 RT. In: Proceedings - 2nd Vaagdevi International Conference on Information Technology for Real World Problems, VCON 2010. Sri Lanka. pp. 12–17 doi:10.1109/VCON.2010.10.

Ma, T., Chen, J., Xiao, C., 2018. Constrained generation of semantically valid graphs via regularizing variational autoencoders. ArXiv, abs/1809.02630 .

Mahmood, O., Mansimov, E., Bonneau, R., Cho, K., 2021. Masked graph modeling for molecule generation. Nat. Commun. 12 (1), 3156.

Mao, J., Akhtar, J., Zhang, X., Sun, L., Guan, S., Xinyu, L., Chen, G., Liu, J., Jeon, H.-N., Kim, M.S., Kyoung Tai, N., Wang, G., 2021. Comprehensive strategies of machine-learning-based quantitative structure-activity relationship models. iScience. 2589-0042. 24 (9), 103052. doi:10.1016/j.isci.2021.103052.

Mohammadi, S., O'Dowd, B., Paulitz-Erdmann, C., Görlitz, L., 2019. Penalized variational autoencoder for molecular design. ChemRxiv. 2573-2293. Available from: https://chemrxiv.org. doi:10.26434/chemrxiv.7977131.v2.

Nesterov, V., Wieser, M., Roth, V., 2020. 3DMolNet: a generative network for molecular structures. arXiv preprint arXiv:2010.06477.

Nissan, N., Allen, M.C., Sabatino, D., Biggar, K.K., 2024. Future perspective: harnessing the power of artificial intelligence in the generation of new peptide drugs. Biomolecules. 2218-273X. 14 (10). Available from: http://www.mdpi.com/journal/biomolecules. doi:10.3390/biom14101303.

Pang, B., Han, T., Nijkamp, E., Zhu, S.C., Wu, Y.N., 2020. Learning latent space energy-based prior model. In: Advances in Neural Information Processing Systems. 10495258. Neural information processing systems foundation, United States. https://papers.nips.cc/

Park, H., Kim, K.K., Kim, C.H., Shin, J.M., No, K.T., 2013. Descriptor-based profile analysis of kinase inhibitors to predict inhibitory activity and to grasp kinase selectivity. Bull. Korean Chem. Soc. 1229-5949. 34 (9), 2680–2684. Available from: http://journal.kcsnet.or.kr/main/j_search/j_download.htm?code=B130925. doi:10.5012/bkcs.2013.34.9.2680.

Peter, S.C., Dhanjal, J.K., Malik, V., Radhakrishnan, N., Jayakanthan, M., Sundar, D., 2019. Quantitative structure-activity relationship (QSAR): modeling approaches to biological applications. In: Encyclopedia of Bioinformatics and Computational Biology: ABC of Bioinformatics. Elsevier, India, pp. 661–676. Available from: https://www.sciencedirect.com/book/9780128114148. doi:10.1016/B978-0-12-809633-8.20197-0.

Piane, F.L., Vozza, M., Baldoni, M., Mercuri, F., 2024. Integrating high-performance computing, machine learning, data management workflows, and infrastructures for multiscale simulations and nanomaterials technologies. Beilstein J. Nanotechnol. 2190-4286. 15, 1498–1521. doi:10.3762/bjnano.15.119.

Polishchuk, P.G., Madzhidov, T.I., Varnek, A., 2013. Estimation of the size of drug-like chemical space based on GDB-17 data. J. Comput.-Aided Mol. Des. 27 (8), 675–679.

Polykovskiy, D., Zhebrak, A., Sanchez-Lengeling, B., Golovanov, S., Tatanov, O., Belyaev, S., Kurbanov, R., Artamonov, A., Aladinskiy, V., Veselov, M., Kadurin, A., Johansson, S., Chen, H., Nikolenko, S., Aspuru-Guzik, A., Zhavoronkov, A., 2020. Molecular sets (MOSES): a benchmarking platform for molecular generation models. Front. Pharmacol. 1663-9812. 11. doi:10.3389/fphar.2020.565644.

Ragoza, M., Masuda, T., Koes, D.R., 2020. Learning a continuous representation of 3D molecular structures with deep generative models. arXiv preprint arXiv:2010.08687.

Reymond, J.L., Awale, M., 2012. Exploring chemical space for drug discovery using the chemical universe database. ACS Chem. Neurosci. 3 (9), 649–657.

Riniker, S., 2017. Molecular dynamics fingerprints (MDFP): machine learning from MD data to predict free-energy differences. J. Chem. Inf. Model. 1549-9596. 57 (4), 726–741. doi:10.1021/acs.jcim.6b00778.

Roy, K., 2018. Quantitative structure-activity relationships (QSARs): a few validation methods and software tools developed at the DTC laboratory. J. Indian Chem. Soc. 0019-4522. 95 (12), 1497–1502. Available from: http://indianchemicalsociety.com/journal/new_rjournal.

Roy, K., Kar, S., Ambure, P., 2015a. On a simple approach for determining applicability domain of QSAR models. Chemom. Intell. Lab. Syst. 145, 22–29.

Roy, K., Kar, S., Das, R.N., 2015b. Statistical methods in QSAR/QSPR. In: A Primer on QSAR/QSPR Modeling. SpringerBriefs in Molecular Science, Springer, Cham. doi:10.1007/978-3-319-17281-1_2.

Samanta, B., De, A., Jana, G., Gomez, V., Chattaraj, P.K., Ganguly, N., Gomez-Rodriguez, M., 2020a. NEVAE: a deep generative model for molecular graphs*. J. Mach. Learn. Res. 1533-7928. 21. Available from: http://jmlr.csail.mit.edu/papers/volume21/19-671/19-671.pdf.

Samanta, S., O'Hagan, S., Swainston, N., Roberts, T.J., Kell, D.B., 2020b. VAE-Sim: a novel molecular similarity measure based on a variational autoencoder. Molecules 25 (15), 3446.

Sanchez, D.M., 2024. Variational autoencoders - theory and applications: exploring variational autoencoder models and their applications in generative modeling, representation learning, and beyond. Adv. Deep Learn. Tech. 4 (1), 18–32.
Schiff, Y., Chenthamarakshan, V., Ramamurthy, K.N., Das, P., 2020. Characterizing the latent space of molecular deep generative models with persistent homology metrics. arXiv. 2331-8422. Available from: https://arxiv.org. doi:10.48550/arxiv.2010.08548.
Schwalbe-Koda, D., Gómez-Bombarelli, R., 2020. Generative models for automatic chemical design. In: Schütt, K.T., Chmiela, S., von Lilienfeld, O.A., Tkatchenko, A., Tsuda, K., Müller, K.R. (Eds.), Machine Learning Meets Quantum Physics. Lecture Notes in Physics, Vol. 968 . Springer: Cham, pp. 445–467. doi:10.1007/978-3-030-40245-7_21.
Shervani-Tabar, N., Zabaras, N. (2020). Physics-constrained predictive molecular latent space discovery with graph scattering variational autoencoder. arXiv preprint arXiv:2009.13878.
Shin, H.K., Kim, K.Y., Park, J.W., No, K.T., 2017. Use of metal/metal oxide spherical cluster and hydroxyl metal coordination complex for descriptor calculation in development of nanoparticle cytotoxicity classification model. SAR QSAR Environ. Res. 1062-936X. 28 (11), 875–888. doi:10.1080/1062936x.2017.1400998.
Shin, H.K., Seo, M., Shin, S.E., Kim, K.Y., Park, J.W., No, K.T., 2018. Meta-analysis of Daphnia magna nanotoxicity experiments in accordance with test guidelines. Environ. Sci. Nano 5 (3), 765–775.
Simm, G., Pinsler, R., Hernández-Lobato, J.M., 2020. Reinforcement learning for molecular design guided by quantum mechanics. In: International Conference on Machine Learning. PMLR. pp. 8959–8969.
Simonovsky, M., Komodakis, N., 2018. Graphvae: towards generation of small graphs using variational autoencoders. In: International conference on artificial neural networks. Springer International Publishing, Cham. pp. 412–422.
Singh, N., Shah, P., Dwivedi, H., Mishra, S., Tripathi, R., Sahasrabuddhe, A.A., Siddiqi, M.I., 2016. Integrated machine learning, molecular docking and 3D-QSAR based approach for identification of potential inhibitors of trypanosomal N-myristoyltransferase. Mol. Biosyst. 1742-2051. 12 (12), 3711–3723. Available from: http://www.rsc.org/is/journals/current/mbs/mbspub.htm. doi:10.1039/C6MB00574H.
Soliman, M.M., Ahmed, E., Darwish, A., Hassanien, A.E., 2024. Artificial intelligence powered Metaverse: analysis, challenges and future perspectives. Artif. Intell. Rev. 1573-7462. 57 (2). Available from: https://www.springer.com/journal/10462. doi:10.1007/s10462-023-10641-x.
Tavakoli, M., Baldi, P., 2020. Continuous representation of molecules using graph variational autoencoder. arXiv preprint arXiv:2004.08152.
Torchilin, V.P., 2000. Drug targeting. Eur. J. Pharm. Sci. 0928-0987. 11 (2), S81–S91. doi:10.1016/S0928-0987(00)00166-4.
Tripathi, S., Augustin, A.I., Dunlop, A., Sukumaran, R., Dheer, S., Zavalny, A., Haslam, O., Austin, T., Donchez, J., Tripathi, P.K., Kim, E., 2022. Recent advances and application of generative adversarial networks in drug discovery, development, and targeting. Artif. Intell. Life Sci. 2667-3185. 2, 100045. doi:10.1016/j.ailsci.2022.100045.
Van Den Oord, A., Vinyals, O., 2017. Neural discrete representation learning. arXiv preprint arXiv:1711.00937. doi:10.48550/arXiv.1711.00937.
Wei, R., Mahmood, A., 2020. Recent advances in variational autoencoders with representation learning for biomedical informatics: a survey. IEEE Access 9, 4939–4956.
Weininger, D., 1988. SMILES, a chemical language and information system. 1. Introduction to methodology and encoding rules. J. Chem. Inf. Comput. Sci. 0095-2338. 28 (1), 31–36. doi:10.1021/ci00057a005.
Wold, S., Sjöström, M., Eriksson, L., 2001. PLS-regression: a basic tool of chemometrics. Chemom. Intell. Lab. Syst. 58 (2), 109–130.

Wu, Y., Wang, G., 2018. Machine learning based toxicity prediction: from chemical structural description to transcriptome analysis. Int. J. Mol. Sci. 1422-0067. 19 (8), 2358. doi:10.3390/ijms19082358.

Xian, Y., Sharma, S., Schiele, B., Akata, Z., 2019. F-VAEGAN-D2: a feature generating framework for any-shot learning. In: Proceedings of the IEEE Computer Society Conference on Computer Vision and Pattern Recognition. 9781728132938. IEEE Computer Society, Netherlands. pp. 10267–10276. doi:10.1109/CVPR.2019.01052.

Xu, M., Luo, S., Bengio, Y., Peng, J., Tang, J., 2021. Learning neural generative dynamics for molecular conformation generation. In: ICLR 2021 - 9th International Conference on Learning. Representations International Conference on Learning Representations, ICLR, Canada. https://iclr.cc/virtual/2021/papers.html?filter=titles.

Yan, C., Wang, S., Yang, J., Xu, T., Huang, J., 2020. Re-balancing variational autoencoder loss for molecule sequence generation. In: Proceedings of the 11th ACM international conference on bioinformatics, computational biology and health informatics. pp. 1–7.

Zhang, J., Mercado, R., Engkvist, O., Chen, H., 2021. Comparative study of deep generative models on chemical space coverage. J. Chem. Inf. Model. 61 (6), 2572–2581.

Zhao, L., Wang, J., Pang, L., Liu, Y., Zhang, J., 2020. GANsDTA: predicting drug-target binding affinity using GANs. Front. Genet. 1664-8021. 10. doi:10.3389/fgene.2019.01243.

Zhao, S., Song, J., Ermon, S. (2017). Infovae: information maximizing variational autoencoders. arXiv preprint arXiv:1706.02262.

Zhu, Y., Min, M.R., Kadav, A., Graf, H.P., 2020. S3VAE: self-supervised sequential VAE for representation disentanglement and data generation. In: Proceedings of the IEEE Computer Society Conference on Computer Vision and Pattern Recognition. 1063-6919. IEEE Computer Society, United States. pp. 6537–6546. doi:10.1109/CVPR42600.2020.00657.

7

Artificial intelligence enabled virtual screening

Sanjay Kumar[a] and Manish Kumar Gupta[b]

[a]*Department of Structural & Molecular Biology, City College of New York, New York, NY, United States*

[b]*Department of Biotechnology, Faculty of Science, Veer Bahadur Singh Purvanchal University, Jaunpur, Uttar Pradesh, India*

1 Introduction

Humans are still in a constant battle with numerous diseases and infections. In 2019, the COVID-19 outbreak and subsequent pandemic awakened researchers to the importance of quickly finding effective drugs (World Health Organization (WHO), 2020). To help in this fight, computer-aided drug design serves as a cornerstone of modern drug discovery. It uses computers to design and improve drug molecules. By simulating how a drug might interact with a receptor, researchers can predict if the drug will work and how strong its effect might be (Zhou and Zhong, 2017). This makes it easier to find new and better medications faster, which can help drug development save considerable time and money (Waring et al., 2015). drug design includes a variety of computational tools and techniques used in drug research, such as computational chemistry, virtual docking simulations, pharmacophoric pattern identification, and structure–activity prediction modeling (Muegge et al., 2017; Kumar and Acharya, 2024). In recent drug developments, new methods have been introduced to search for new molecules by employing artificial intelligence (AI) learning methods (Zhang et al., 2017). The virtual screening (VS) method is widely used to search for new molecules; it identifies potential drug-like molecules from chemical libraries through computational tools. With the exponential growth of chemical libraries and drug targets, big data has emerged (Marx, 2013). Traditional VS methods based on structure and ligand-based similarity have been performed, but these methods are expected to be replaced soon by AI approaches (Scheeder et al., 2018; Chan et al., 2019). AI-VS combines the power of learning models—machine

The AI Frontier in Molecular Modelling and Drug Designing. https://doi.org/10.1016/B978-0-443-40338-5.00010-X

learning (ML) and deep learning (DL)—with molecular modeling to accelerate discovery pipelines, reduce costs, and improve prediction accuracy (Gorgulla et al., 2020).

1.1 Evolution of virtual screening

VS came about in the early 1990s as a way to quickly search through vast chemical libraries and find the compounds that are most likely to bind to certain specific receptors. VS has emerged as a critical component of contemporary molecular discovery pipelines, encompassing domains such as drug development (Stahl et al., 2006). The Walters group first described VS as the process of automatically analyzing large collections of chemical compounds with the help of computer software (Patrick Walters et al., 1998). As a computational strategy, VS enables the computational identification of biologically active molecules from chemical compound libraries, bypassing exhaustive and cost-intensive experiments (Burns, 1995). Traditional approaches, including ligand and structure-based strategies, have made a substantial contribution to the identification of early-stage hits over the past two decades (Fig. 7.1). However, the inherent limitations of these approaches in terms of scalability, precision, and adaptability have made way for a new era: AI-VS. In its essence, AI-VS integrates computational intelligence with cheminformatics and bioinformatics

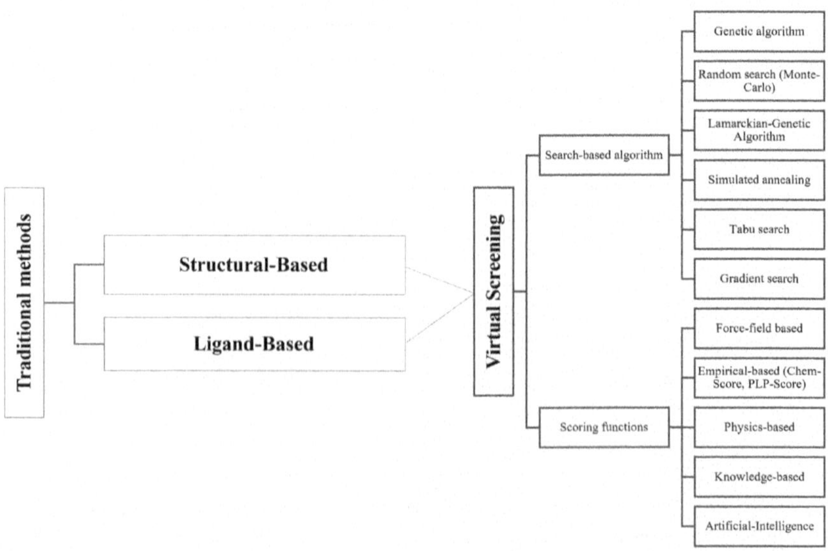

Fig. 7.1 Overview of traditional virtual screening methods and algorithms. A comprehensive summary of classical virtual screening strategies, including structure-based, ligand-based, and hybrid approaches, highlights their underlying algorithms, computational workflows, and applications in early-stage drug discovery.

to intelligently predict molecular activities, interactions, and functional properties. This paradigm shift allows researchers not only to accelerate molecular discovery but also to gain deeper insights into structure-activity relationships (SAR), bioavailability, toxicity profiles, and synthetic feasibility—areas often constrained by classical methods. Muegge I and Oloff S define the following key points that must be followed in the VS setup (Muegge and Oloff, 2006):

- This must be powerful enough to analyze approximately a million compounds.
- Only a tiny fraction ($\leq 0.1\%$) of compounds in traditional screening is usually active; VS needs to be much better. It should find at least 10 times more active compounds than random guessing to be useful.
- For difficult drug targets, where active compounds are very rare, this enrichment rate might need to be even higher.
- The compounds selected as "hits" by VS should be both high-ranking (likely active) and structurally different from each other. This increases the chances of discovering new types of drug molecules.

Once promising hits are found, researchers should conduct a second round of testing by trying similar molecules (called analogs) to optimize the best candidates.

1.2 Traditional VS

It represents a cornerstone of modern computational drug development, allowing experts to characterize the expected bioactivity of diverse chemical repositories against a particular target. The overarching objective is to prioritize small-molecule candidates that are best suited to interact with a receptor, such as a protein or nucleic acid, and therefore warrant additional experimental evaluation. Identification of active compounds, early-stage optimization, and advanced lead development have all incorporated VS as a standard practice (Fig. 7.1). In the past, VS has been classified into two main categories according to the availability of data: ligand-based and structure-based VS (SBVS). Each method has its own assets, limitations, and areas of application. It is imperative to investigate the fundamental principles and methodologies that characterize classical VS techniques before discussing AI-driven transformations in screening.

1.3 Ligand-based VS

Ligand-based VS (LBVS) is a way to find compounds that are chemically or structurally related to known active molecules (ligands) that work against a certain target. In the absence of experimentally determined receptor structures, LBVS methods remain effective, as they rely solely on known ligand information. In LBVS, various 2D chemical descriptors are combined with ML models that learn from previously identified active compounds (Muegge and Mukherjee, 2016). Researchers can use more complex ligand-based methods, including pharmacophore modeling, to find new compounds that match specific pharmacophoric patterns. These methods help researchers identify the important chemical properties that are responsible for biological activity. Quantitative SAR (QSAR) modeling employs statistical ML methods to correlate descriptors with experimentally observed pharmacological activity (Cherkasov et al., 2014). Subsequently, models facilitate LBVS by forecasting the biological effects of unknown molecules. While LBVS is highly effective when a robust set of known actives is available, it can be limited in novelty and diversity, often identifying compounds closely related to the existing ligands (Lusci et al., 2013).

1.4 Molecular descriptors and similarity metrics

In LBVS, molecular descriptors are often used to measure molecular similarity; they encode the structural or physicochemical attributes of substances. They can be broadly classified into:

- **1D descriptors:** 1D molecular descriptors are simple, single numbers that come from the basic structure and elemental makeup of a molecule. These descriptors provide important details such as molecular mass, total atom count, and concentrations of selected molecular features like carbon, nitrogen, and oxygen. They also include structural properties such as the quantity of heavy atoms, rotatable bonds, rings (aromatic or aliphatic), and hydrogen bond donors and acceptors, which are very important for determining how molecules interact. Log and molar refractivity.
- **2D descriptors:** 2D molecular descriptors gather information on the shape and connections of molecules from their 2D structures. These descriptors show how atoms are linked without using 3D locations. Some common 2D descriptors are topological indices (such as the Wiener, Zagreb, and Balaban indices), molecular fingerprints like the Extended-Connectivity Fingerprints (ECFP) and Molecular ACCess System (MACCS), adjacency matrices, and counts of different types of atoms (Rogers and Hahn, 2010). They also include features such as molecular connections, branching, ring systems, and patterns of substructures.
- **3D descriptors:** 3D molecular descriptors show how molecules are shaped, how much space they take up, and how their electrons are spread out in three dimensions. They examine the molecule's shape, conformation, and atom locations in 3D space, which is different from 1D descriptors. Molecular surface area,

molecular volume, polarizability, dipole moment, and 3D pharmacophore characteristics are all common 3D descriptors. These characteristics are very important for predicting how drugs interact with biological targets, especially when designing drugs based on their structure.

These descriptors are widely utilized in QSAR and VS as they provide extensive structural information at a low cost. Programs like RDKit, PaDEL, Dragon, and ChemDes are among the most frequently used tools for calculating these descriptors.

1.5 Pharmacophore modeling

It outlines the required chemical characteristics and their spatial orientation that lead to high-affinity binding with a certain biological receptor. LBVS can use pharmacophore hypotheses based on active ligands to find compounds in large libraries that share the same compound's three-dimensional shape (Wolber and Langer, 2005). Recent advancements include ML-assisted pharmacophore modeling, which can handle noisy datasets and ambiguous binding modes more robustly (Cieślak et al., 2024).

1.6 Structure–activity relationship modeling

SAR models find statistical links between molecular features and biological activity (Cherkasov et al., 2014). There are many different ways to do this, ranging from simple linear regression to more advanced supervised ML algorithms. QSAR is especially effective at predicting the potency, selectivity, and Absorption, Distribution, Metabolism, Excretion, and Toxicity (ADMET) profiles of compounds. DeepAutoQSAR and DeepChem are examples of tools that provide semiautomated pipelines for QSAR modeling.

1.7 Applications and strengths of LBVs

It works best when only ligand information is available. This makes it a useful tool when the target structure is unknown or poorly characterized. It is quite good at quickly screening very large chemical libraries, like ZINC15 and Enamine REAL Space, which makes it easy to find interesting bioactive molecules. LBVS also makes it easier to bounce across scaffolds and look into a wider range of chemical space, which helps researchers find new chemotypes that have similar biological activity. This method can be used in a lot of different situations, including an early discovery pipeline encompassing hit identification through optimization. A recent example of how useful it is was during the COVID-19 pandemic, when LBVS pipelines were used to find new uses for existing medications, such as antihistamines and antidepressants, as possible antiviral agents. This sped up the search for therapeutic interventions (Ton et al., 2020).

1.8 Structure-based VS

It utilizes the 3D conformation of the receptor to predict how candidate compounds might interact with it. Molecular docking is the most important part of SBVS. In this process, tiny molecules are "fitted" into the binding region of the receptor. Scoring functions are then used to assess the binding conformation and the strength of the interaction (Kitchen et al., 2004). By analyzing covalent and noncovalent interactions, scoring functions determine how strongly the compound binds to the protein. One benefit of SBVS is that it might find new chemical scaffolds, especially if the protein's binding site is well-known. However, this method can require a lot of computing resources. The results are only as good as the protein structure they are based on. It also depends on how accurate the scoring systems are. Despite their utility, these methods encounter substantial drawbacks. LBVS may fail when few known ligands exist, limiting the predictive model's robustness. SBVS, while mechanistically insightful, is computationally intensive and often inaccurate due to rigid receptor assumptions, solvent effects, and entropic contributions. Moreover, both methods are vulnerable to high false-positive rates, leading to attrition in experimental validation.

1.9 Molecular docking

The most important part of SBVS is molecular docking, which occurs when ligands are placed into a specific binding site on the target macromolecule. The goal is to predict both the binding position and the binding affinity (Pagadala et al., 2017). A typical docking pipeline includes:

- **Step 1: Ligand preparation** (conformer generation, protonation states)
- **Step 2: Protein preparation** (energy minimization, side-chain optimization)
- **Step 3: Docking algorithm**: Whether they are rigid or flexible, they usually involve scoring functions (based on empirical data, force fields, or knowledge) and optimization approaches. For example, genetic algorithms, simulated annealing, and Monte Carlo are used to explore conformational space. Scoring functions, which assess the binding free energy (ΔG) between ligand and receptor, are very important for the accuracy of SBVS. To enhance their accuracy, modern scoring functions are combined with ML or DL. For instance, RF-Score uses random forests (RFs) that have been trained on experimental binding affinities (Ballester and Mitchell,

2010), and DL approaches use graph-based DL models to predict ΔG (Nguyen et al., 2021).

The following tools are commonly used for docking: AutoDock (autodock.scripps.edu), Glide, part of the commercial Schrödinger suite (schrodinger.com/glide), DOCK, developed by UCSF (dock.compbio.ucsf.edu), GOLD (ccdc.cam.ac.uk), and web-based solutions like SwissDock (swissdock.ch), LeDock (lephar.com), FlexX, part of the SeeSAR platform from BioSolveIT (biosolveit.de), rDock (github.com/rddock), and MOE (Molecular Operating Environment) Group (chemcomp.com), which integrates docking with QSAR, pharmacophore modeling, and visualization tools, as well as RosettaLigand (rosettacommons.org).

1.10 Applications and strengths of SBVS

It applies experimental and predicted model structures of the receptor to provide us with useful information about how ligands and targets interact. It works best when you have access to quality models from experimental methods or AI tools such as AlphaFold. Researchers can use SBVS to analyze and improve how molecules interact in the binding site, which helps them develop selective inhibitors in a logical way. It also enables more advanced screening methods, like fragment-based and covalent inhibitor discovery, increasing the likelihood of finding strong lead compounds. One recent use of SBVS that stands out is the docking of millions of molecules to the cryo-EM-derived M^{pro} structure (Gorgulla et al., 2021).

1.11 Limitations of traditional VS

Despite their widespread use, both LBVS and SBVS face significant challenges. Among the most critical are:

- Classical scoring functions may not be able to reliably forecast the correct binding position and classification of substances. They might yield false positives and false negatives, meaning that some compounds thought to be active may not be active experimentally, while some genuinely active compounds might be missed.
- Classical scoring algorithms frequently use linear functions, which may not completely capture complex, nonlinear interactions crucial for accurate binding affinity predictions.
- Some classical VS tools are optimized for specific types of molecules or targets, limiting their performance in more general applications.
- Accurate prediction requires considering the ligand and receptor's conformational flexibility. Classical approaches may struggle to adequately model the various conformational states that molecules can adopt, which could lead to inaccurate predictions.

- Some VS methods may yield unreliable results due to biased training datasets. For example, some decoys (nonbinding compounds) may contain structural biases that allow ML scoring systems to pick up on fake variations between actives and decoys instead of real binding patterns (Cantrell et al., 2022).
- Generating high-energy conformations that are unlikely to occur at room temperature can be misleading and may contribute to false-positive results.
- As the size of chemical libraries increases, classical VS methods may become computationally intensive and require significant resources.
- The majority of VS studies rely heavily on *in-vitro* bioassays for validation, which might not always reflect the compound's overall behavior as a drug.
- Choosing potential compounds based on their apparent binding characteristics might be subjective and may not always be reproducible.
- Many compounds predicted to be active fail in experimental validation due to limitations in scoring accuracy or model assumptions.
- LBVS requires well-characterized actives; SBVS depends on accurate 3D structures.
- Traditional VS methods often ignore dynamic phenomena, such as induced fit, allosteric modulation, and multitarget effects.

Moreover, the ever-expanding size of chemical libraries (now reaching tens of billions of synthetically accessible compounds) and the growing biological complexity of therapeutic targets demand more robust, flexible, and intelligent computational tools. These factors have underscored the limitations of traditional rule-based and physics-based approaches and have accelerated the adoption of AI as a transformative solution in VS workflows.

1.12 Need for AI integration in drug discovery

Advances in technology and the increased complexity of biological systems are two main reasons why AI is becoming increasingly important in drug discovery. From a business point of view, AI-driven drug development is becoming more and more valuable. According to industry forecasts, by 2025, the sector is estimated to be valued at around $800 million and is anticipated to grow by 15% from 2025 to 2033. Leading companies such as Schrödinger (https://www.schrodinger.com/), OpenEye (https://www.eyesopen.com/), BioSolveIT (https://www.biosolveit.de/), Certara (https://www.certara.com/), and Cresset (https://cresset-group.com/) already generate over $500 million annually, collectively accounting for nearly 40% of the current $1.25 billion market. Meanwhile, smaller startups, academic labs, and open-source platforms continue to shape the remaining landscape, highlighting the widespread interest and investment in this field. This commercial expansion is matched by a surge in academic research. By 2025, more 4500 scientific publications focusing on AI-VS have been published, garnering over 64,000 citations, a clear indicator of the field's growing scientific credibility (Fig. 7.2). This momentum is not just about popularity; it's rooted in the real limitations of traditional approaches. Classical methods often struggle with false positives, where predicted "hits" fail in experimental validation. AI helps with this by using DL models, especially graph neural networks (GNNs), which are better at identifying true binders by learning complex molecular patterns directly from data. Another major hurdle in conventional screening is structural rigidity. Traditional docking tools typically use static representations of proteins, thereby missing critical details like side-chain movements or ligand flexibility. AI models, however, can incorporate these flexible dynamics and predict more biologically relevant poses. This is especially important when dealing with modern drug targets that involve intrinsically disordered regions, multidomain proteins, or allosteric sites, which are inherently dynamic and not well-captured by rigid-receptor assumptions (Visan and Negut, 2024). AI doesn't just improve predictions; it enables entirely new capabilities. For instance, Deep Neural Networks (DNNs) trained on diverse protein-ligand complexes can still make accurate predictions

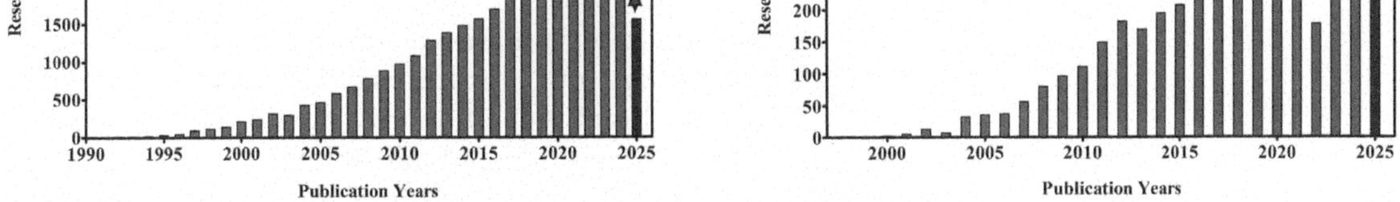

Fig. 7.2 The rising significance of AI in the domain of virtual screening. We conducted a comparative analysis of research publications related to traditional VS and AI-based virtual screening. On April 22, 2025, we searched the PubMed database using the keywords "Virtual Screening" and "AI-based Virtual Screening" to assess publication trends. This allowed us to observe the use of AI applications. We wanted to show how AI is playing a bigger role in speeding up drug development processes and finding new bioactive chemicals by looking at the quantity and scope of publications in each category.

even when structural data is incomplete or noisy. AI can also perform multitask learning, which means it can predict a molecule's binding affinity, toxicity, and selectivity qualities simultaneously. Traditional techniques can't do this. The vast quantity of digital biological data is driving this change. There are millions of molecular structures, bioactivities, and chemical descriptors in chemical databases. While this data explosion opens up unprecedented opportunities, it also creates challenges in data curation, integration, and feature extraction. This is precisely where AI excels. Unlike traditional rule-based models that rely on predefined scoring functions, AI learns directly from raw data. DL models, in particular, can uncover complex, nonlinear relationships that humans may overlook, using tools like graph-based embeddings, Simplified Molecular Input Line Entry System (SMILES) language models, and molecular fingerprints to represent and learn from chemical space. Speed is another driving factor. Traditional SBVS methods are computationally intensive and time-consuming. When dealing with libraries of millions or even billions of molecules, these methods can become a bottleneck. AI dramatically accelerates this process by predicting binding potential in milliseconds. Furthermore, active, reinforcement learning (RL), and generative model frameworks are now enabling machines to design new compounds, select the best candidates for lab testing, and learn from experimental feedback, making drug discoveries not just faster but smarter (Vamathevan et al., 2019). Altogether, these advancements mark a paradigm shift from static, manually tuned methods to adaptive, intelligent systems that evolve with data. This convergence of technological progress, commercial momentum, and scientific innovation underscores why AI is not just an optional add-on but a central force shaping the future of molecular discovery and therapeutic development.

2 Artificial intelligence in VS

Historically, VS has relied on traditional computational approaches like molecular docking and ligand-based similarity models. However, these classical methods often fall short in handling complex biological systems and large datasets. This is where AI is reshaping the landscape. The integration of AI into virtual screening began gaining momentum in the early 2010s, with supervised learning models such as RFs and support vector machines (SVMs) being used to predict descriptors (Ramsundar et al., 2017). These models showed early promise, especially when trained on curated datasets like ChEMBL or PubChem. As biological data became more abundant and complex, the need for more advanced models led to the rise of DL in this domain (Fig. 7.3). In recent years, particularly between 2020 and 2025, DL has significantly accelerated

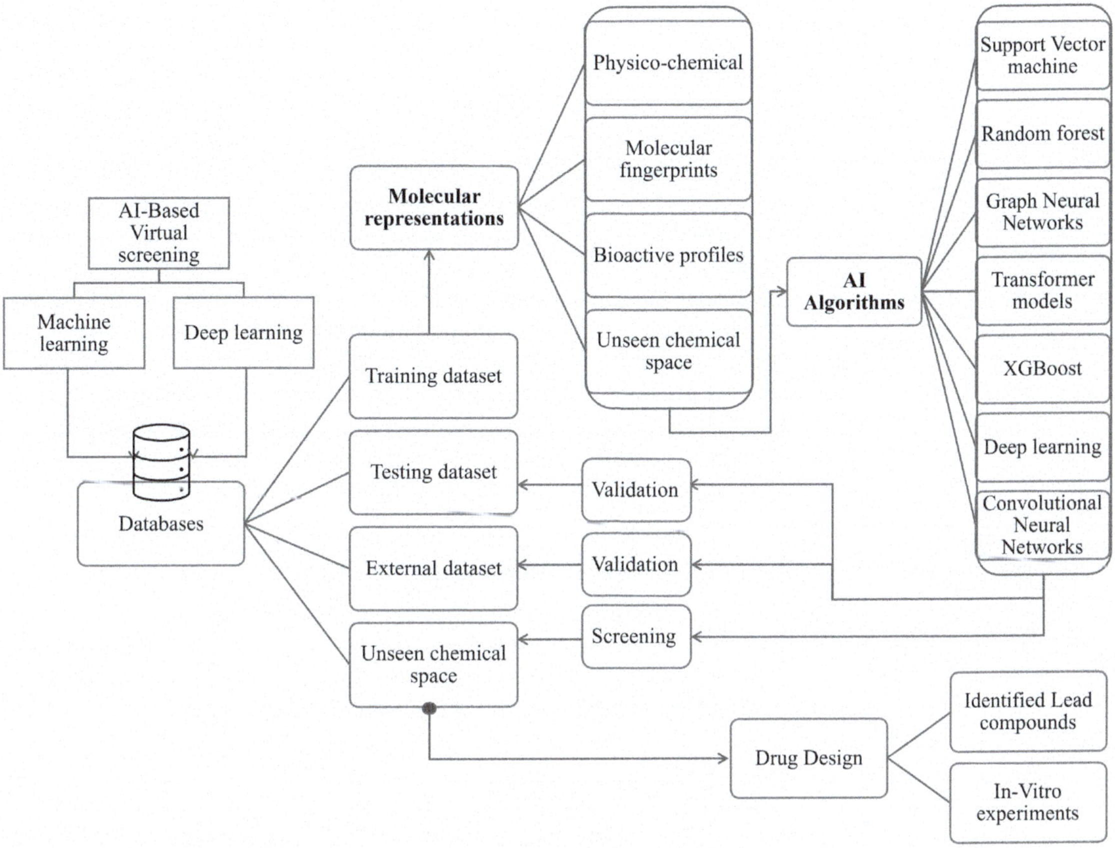

Fig. 7.3 Flowchart showing how AI-based virtual screening works in drug discovery. It begins with databases and molecular representations, feeds into ML and DL models, and uses algorithms to screen and validate new compounds. The process helps identify lead drug candidates, which are then tested in laboratory experiments.

the capabilities of VS. DNNs, GNNs, and transformer-based models like AlphaFold have demonstrated that they can describe molecular interactions quite well, even when the input data is restricted or noisy (https://alphafold.ebi.ac.uk/). Notably, MIT's implementation of AI systems in discovering Halicin (Stokes et al., 2020) stands out as one of the earliest examples of AI-driven discovery. From early discovery to lead optimization and toxicity prediction, AI models are now widely deployed in both academia and industry (Ramsundar et al., 2017). screening commonly draws upon two major branches of AI: ML and DL. These approaches rely on large collections of data stored in biological and chemical databases (Fig. 7.3). These databases include various types of chemical and biological information that are used to create training, testing, and external datasets, as well as data from unexplored chemical spaces (new compounds not previously explored). To work with this data, researchers convert molecules into understandable formats called molecular representations. These may include properties such as physicochemical features, molecular fingerprints (digital codes that describe molecules), bioactive profiles, or representations of entirely new chemical spaces. Next, AI algorithms use this information to find patterns and make predictions. These algorithms include well-known models such as SVM, RF, GNN, transformer models, XGBoost, and convolutional neural networks (CNN). These tools help in validating the data and running screening tests to identify which molecules might work as potential drugs (Fig. 7.3). Once the promising compounds are identified through AI screening, they are used in drug design. The most promising candidates, known as lead compounds, move forward into *in-vitro* experiments—lab tests that help confirm whether the predictions made by the AI were correct.

2.1 Learning-based algorithms

ML is the use of algorithms that allow machines to learn from given user data and predict their own choices. In VS, ML is predominantly used for regression (predicting binding affinities) or classification (predicting active vs. inactive compounds) (Fig. 7.4).

2.2 Random forests

RFs are a powerful ML method that has found wide application in cheminformatics, especially for tasks like predicting chemical properties and classifying compounds. These models are particularly popular for QSAR modeling, where the goal is to link a compound's structure to its biological or chemical behavior (Svetnik et al., 2003). RF is a type of model that belongs to a larger group of models called ensemble learning approaches. Instead of using a single decision tree to make predictions, RF generates a large number of decision trees, each trained on a unique collection of data points and feature sets. The model combines the outputs of all the trees to provide prediction results by using the average for regression tasks and majority voting for classification tasks (Table 7.1). This method helps lower the chance of overfitting, which is a typical problem in ML when models don't function well on new data and are overly particular to the training set. The outcome is a model that is both accurate and robust. RF stands out for several reasons. First, they consistently deliver strong performance on various predictive tasks, often matching or even outperforming more complex models like neural networks or SVMs. Second, they offer a useful feature: they can highlight which molecular features or descriptors (like size, polarity, or shape of molecules) are most important for a given prediction. This insight can

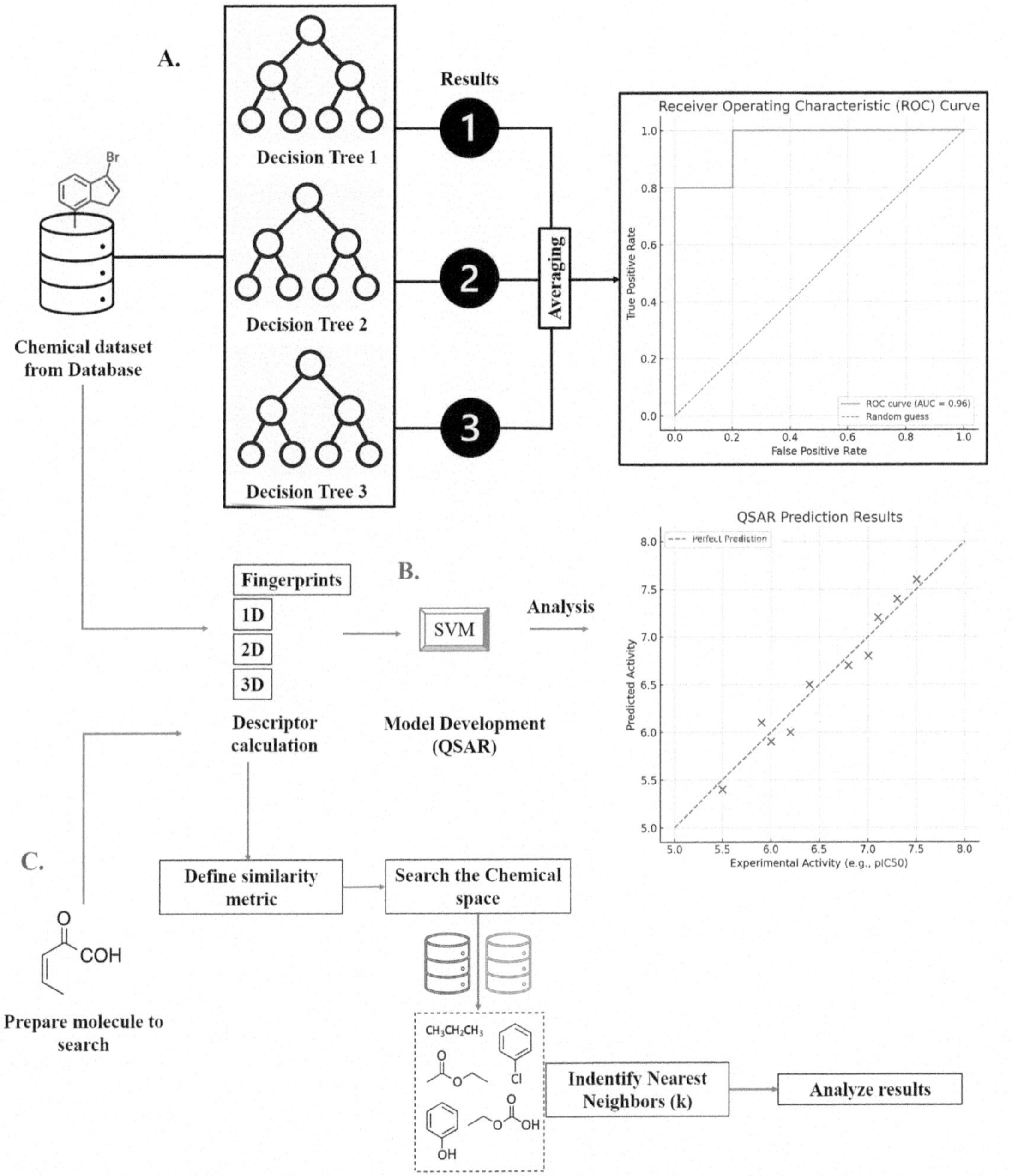

Fig. 7.4 Workflow of machine learning algorithms. A *Black arrows*. Random Forest uses a group of models to identify compounds with potential biological activity and predict their toxicity. The method generates numerous decision trees and combines their outputs to enhance accuracy and reliability, especially when working with QSAR datasets that are often imbalanced or noisy. B *Orange arrows* (dark gray in print version): A standard QSAR pipeline using a Support Vector Machine (SVM). It includes data collection, molecular descriptor generation, dataset splitting, model training, cross-validation, and external testing. C *Cyan arrows* (light gray in print version): The k-Nearest Neighbors (kNN) approach is used to classify compounds based on their chemical similarities. It identifies the closest neighbors in the training dataset and assigns a class (e.g., active or inactive) based on the majority vote.

Table 7.1 List of tools, databases, and web servers that use ML algorithms to search for molecules in chemical libraries.

Tool name	Functions	Uses	Web address
admetSAR 2.0	Predict ADMET properties (e.g., toxicity, metabolism)	RF and SVM are used for the classification and regression of ADMET endpoints	https://lmmd.ecust.edu.cn/admetsar2/
SwissTargetPrediction	Predict protein targets for bioactive molecules	RF model trained in bioactivity fingerprints	http://www.swisstargetprediction.ch/
ProTox-II	Predict toxicity and LD_{50} class, as well as organ effects	RF and SVM models are used to predict toxicity outcomes	https://tox-new.charite.de/protox_II/
PreADMET	Predict ADME & toxicity properties	RF and SVM models were implemented for backend computation	https://preadmet.bmdrc.kr/
eTOXlab	Predict toxicity endpoints (liver injury, mutagenicity)	RF-based models for regulatory safety endpoints	https://etoxlab.univie.ac.at/
Toxtree	Predict toxicological hazards using rule-based + ML tools	Some plugins use RF for chemical toxicity prediction	https://toxtree.sourceforge.net/
TargetNet	Predict drug-target interaction profiles	Uses both RF and SVM models in ensemble classification	http://targetnet.scbdd.com/
Mordred + scikit-learn (Local)	Compute descriptors and train RF models	Community pipeline for local QSAR with RF using Python	https://github.com/mordred-descriptor/mordred
ChemDes	Online descriptor calculation for ML models	Supports RF as one of the available classifiers	http://www.scbdd.com/chemdes/
SwissADME	Predict drug-likeness and ADME properties	SVM is used for the classification of pharmacokinetics	http://www.swissadme.ch/
PASS Online	Predict biological activity spectra of molecules	Part of ensemble models with SVM-based classification	http://www.way2drug.com/passonline/
Pred-hERG	Predict hERG channel blockage (cardiotoxicity)	Main model for binary classification using SVM	http://predherg.labmol.com.br/
KNIME	Visual ML workflow platform for data analysis	Offers built-in SVM module for classification tasks	https://www.knime.com/
Orange	Visual ML and bioinformatics toolkit	SVM integrated as a classification widget	orangedatamining.com
PubChem Similarity Search	Search for compounds similar to a query molecule	Uses Tanimoto + k-NN for fast similarity comparison	https://pubchem.ncbi.nlm.nih.gov
SwissSimilarity	Ligand-based virtual screening & similarity	Employs k-NN search with fingerprint-based similarity	https://www.swisssimilarity.ch
ChemSpider	Explore similar chemical structures	k-NN and clustering-based structure comparison	http://www.chemspider.com
ZINC Search	Search purchasable compounds by similarity	Uses k-NN on molecular fingerprints	https://zinc15.docking.org
ChEMBL Similarity Search	Search compounds in the ChEMBL database	k-NN and Tanimoto methods on bioactivity data	https://www.ebi.ac.uk/chembl
ChemMine Tools	Chemical clustering and similarity computation	Offers k-NN using various descriptors	https://chemminetools.ucr.edu
RDKit (Local)	Python toolkit for cheminformatics	Built-in support for k-NN chemical similarity search	https://www.rdkit.org

help researchers better understand what structural components are influencing a molecule's activity. In addition, RF can be adapted to measure similarity between compounds, considering the importance of different features. While the model is more complex than a single decision tree, it is generally more interpretable than DL models, providing some transparency into how it arrives at its predictions. Their versatility is another big advantage; they can be used for both classification (e.g., is a compound active or inactive?) and regression (e.g., what is the solubility of a compound?) (Table 7.1). There are many practical uses for RF. For instance, they are widely used in QSAR modeling to predict properties such as blood-brain barrier permeability, toxicity, and solubility (Stéen et al., 2022). They're also helpful in compound classification, identifying whether a molecule targets a specific protein or falls into a particular chemical category. RF has been used to predict how much of a reaction will happen and how molecules interact with a receptor, while also helping prioritize the most promising features. This helps scientists focus on the molecular descriptors that will give them the most useful information for a certain problem. But, like any model, RF has certain considerations. How well parameters are set, such as how many trees are used or how many features are considered at each decision split, might affect how effectively they work. If the training data lacks consistency or accuracy, the resulting predictions may be unreliable or incorrect. Lastly, there is always a trade-off between how easy it is to describe a model and how accurate it is, especially when working with complicated chemical datasets.

This technique helps reduce the risk of overfitting, which is a common issue in ML when models become too tailored to the training data and perform poorly on new data. The result is a model that is not only accurate but also robust. RF stands out for several reasons. First, they consistently deliver strong performance on various predictive tasks, often matching or even outperforming more complex models like neural networks or SVMs. Second, they offer a useful feature: they can highlight which molecular features or descriptors (like size, polarity, or shape of molecules) are most important for a given prediction. This insight can help researchers better understand what structural components are influencing a molecule's activity. In addition, RFs can be adapted to measure similarity between compounds, considering the importance of different features (Sobral et al., 2025). While the model is more complex than a single decision tree, it is generally more interpretable than DL models, providing some transparency into how it arrives at its predictions. Their versatility is another big advantage; they can be used for both classification (e.g., is a compound active or inactive?) and regression (e.g., what is the solubility of a compound?). There are many practical uses for RF.

For instance, they are widely used in QSAR modeling to predict properties like blood-brain barrier permeability, toxicity, and solubility (Stéen et al., 2022). They're also helpful in compound classification, identifying whether a molecule targets a specific protein or falls into a particular chemical category. RFs have been used to predict reaction yields, drug–target interactions, and even assist with feature selection, helping scientists focus on the most informative molecular descriptors for a specific problem.

2.3 Support vector machines

This algorithm identifies separating hyperplanes that maximize the margin between classes in a multidimensional feature space, enabling accurate classification. Functions like the radial basis function and polynomial kernels take data input and project it into higher-dimensional spaces. This allows linear classifiers to separate data that cannot be separated in a straight line. SVMs are especially effective with small to medium-sized datasets, providing high accuracy and robustness against overfitting (Cichonska et al., 2018). SVMs can be used for VS, including classifying ligands as active/inactive, predicting toxicity endpoints, and screening drug-like compounds based on physicochemical profiles (Fig. 7.4B). The following properties are considered for classification and ADMET predictions:

1. A multidimensional feature space is defined by molecular descriptors, where each compound is represented as a data point. In this hyperspace, SVMs identify an optimal hyperplane (a decision boundary) that is most effective in distinguishing between active and inactive compounds.
2. It was learned from a set of known active and inactive compounds; it may be used to predict how new hits are active. The compounds on one side of the hyperplane are called active, and the ones on the other side are called inactive. Another way to rank compounds, according to their drug-likeness, is to use their distance from the hyperplane.

In VS, molecular descriptors are used to describe molecules. These descriptors capture important physical features. Some of these include molecular weight, lipophilicity (e.g., LogP), solubility, pKa, polarity, and the number of hydrogen bonding profiles. These features aid in the development of models by predicting how molecules will bind to receptors and help us create models for QSAR and AI-based screening. SVMs face challenges such as high computational cost with large datasets, sensitivity to parameter tuning (e.g., C and kernel settings), and limited interpretability with complex kernels. They also struggle with imbalanced data, where class distribution is uneven. Careful optimization and preprocessing are needed to ensure effective SVM performance in predictive modeling (Zhao et al., 2025).

2.4 k-nearest neighbors

kNN is a distribution-free learning algorithm that sorts compounds into groups using a majority vote from the *k* closest instances in the feature representation. Similarity is typically computed using Euclidean distance or Tanimoto similarity (for binary molecular fingerprints) (Fig. 7.4C). Though simplistic, kNN remains relevant for VS tasks like chemical similarity searches, scaffold hopping, library clustering, and annotation (Halder et al., 2024). Its limitations include sensitivity to feature scaling and poor performance with high-dimensional data, which has led to reduced use in favor of more sophisticated ensemble or deep models (Nayarisseri et al., 2021).

2.5 Deep learning algorithm

It uses multilayered neural networks to extract hierarchical models from input data (LeCun et al., 2015). DL differs from typical ML methods in that it doesn't require human feature engineering because it extracts latent features directly from raw input. This makes it especially useful for complicated, high-dimensional datasets like chemical graphs or 3D conformations (Fig. 7.5) (Martínez Mora et al., 2022).

2.6 Convolutional neural networks

Originally developed for visual recognition tasks, CNNs are becoming increasingly useful in drug development, especially in VS, as they are capable of modeling complex spatial relationships from input features (Martínez Mora et al., 2022). CNNs are often used in VS to predict molecular characteristics and sort molecules. CNNs do not usually work with pixel data from images; instead, they work with molecular graphs, 2D/3D grid representations, or even image-analogous molecular fingerprints (Fig. 7.5A). For example, a CNN can learn to tell the difference between active and inactive substances by looking at visual-like input representations such as chemical interaction fields, electrostatic potential maps, or even 2D structural diagrams. The DeepChem framework is a well-known example of this. It uses CNNs on chemical grids to estimate binding likelihood or toxicity. In receptor-based docking, CNNs can predict docking scores by voxelizing the 3D shape and charge distribution around a ligand–protein complex and feeding it into a CNN model. AtomNet (https://www.atomwise.com/) is a famous example of a deep CNN trained on 3D molecular grids to accurately predict how proteins and ligands will interact (Table 7.2). CNNs have also been combined with docking outputs to improve scoring functions. They work better than other ML algorithms and traditional docking methods, especially when it comes to finding active chemicals with

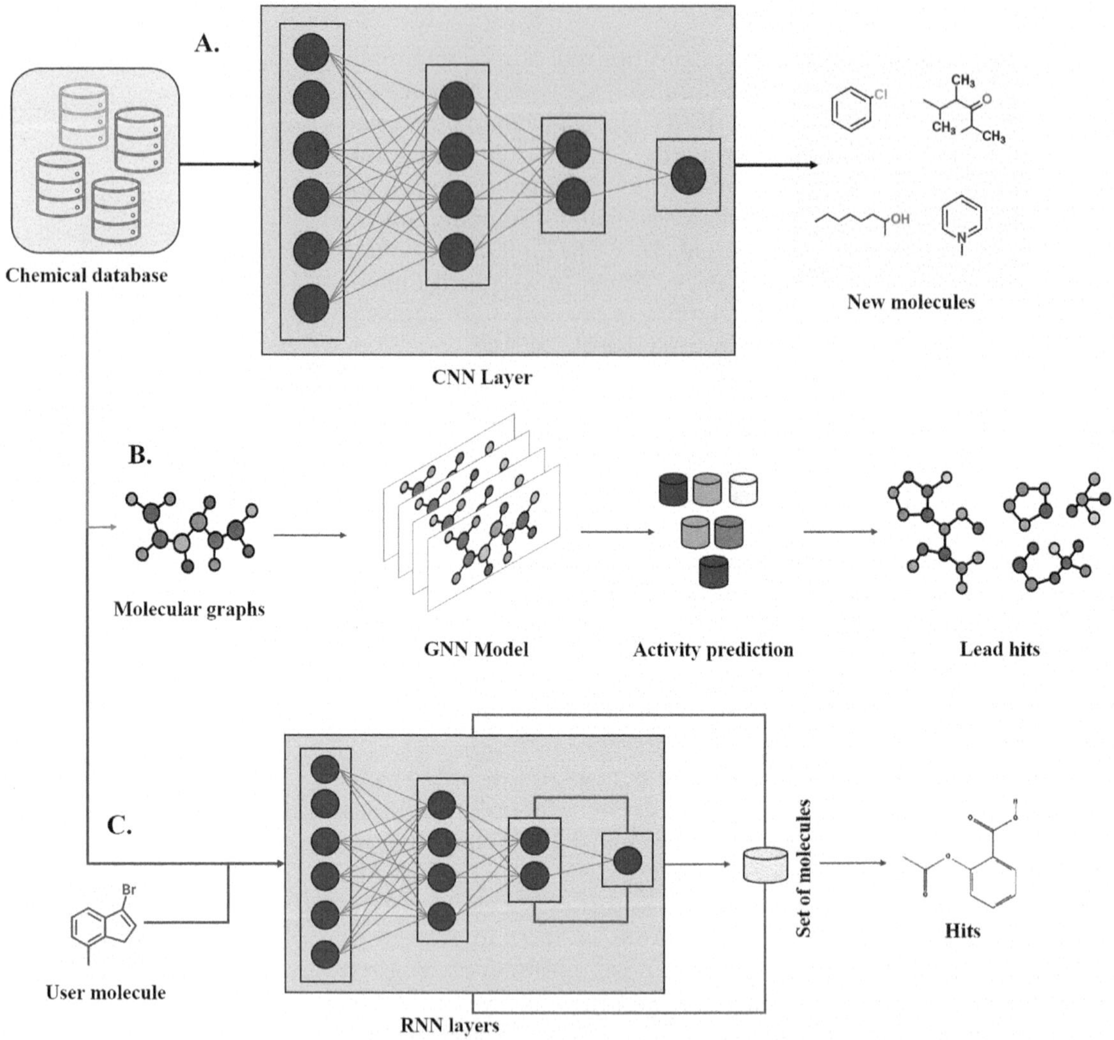

Fig. 7.5 Workflow of DL algorithms. A. Flowchart of CNN algorithms that includes preprocessing, feature extraction, model training, validation, and prediction. B. Shows the GNN model used for VS. This represents molecules as graphs (nodes as atoms, edges as bonds), enabling more accurate compound screening by capturing topological and spatial features. C. Workflow of the RNN model and its ability to model sequential data (e.g., SMILES strings). It emphasizes the feedback loop from the output layer to the hidden state through backpropagation through time, enabling the learning of long-range dependencies in chemical sequences.

high accuracy. CNNs make it easier to choose good drug candidates by improving the accuracy of protein-ligand interactions and binding affinities (Chen et al., 2023). They can quickly screen large molecular libraries as they are capable of handling large datasets

Table 7.2 List of tools and platforms that use DL algorithms.

Tool/Platform	Purpose	Use	Web address
DeepChem	ML framework for chemistry/biology	CNNs and GNNs for property prediction, protein–ligand modeling	https://deepchem.io
AtomNet (Atomwise)	Structure-based drug screening	CNNs analyze 3D ligand–target voxel grids	https://www.atomwise.com
Chemception	Molecule classification from images	Uses CNNs on 2D molecule images without engineered features	https://github.com/deepchem/chemception
Pafnucy	Binding affinity prediction	CNNs trained on 3D protein–ligand complexes	https://github.com/oddt/pafnucy
GNINA	Deep learning-enhanced docking	3D CNNs predict pose scoring and binding affinity	https://gnina.github.io/
DeepTox	Toxicity prediction	CNNs on molecular descriptors and bioactivity profiles	https://github.com/EBjerrum/DeepTox
DGL-LifeSci	GNN library for life sciences (built on DGL)	Prebuilt models for molecule and protein interaction prediction	https://github.com/awslabs/dgl-lifesci
Open Graph Benchmark	GNN benchmarking datasets & models	Includes molecular datasets for evaluating GNNs	https://ogb.stanford.edu
Chemprop	Molecular property prediction	Uses message-passing neural networks (a GNN type)	https://github.com/chemprop/chemprop
TorchDrug	Drug discovery toolkit using PyTorch	Supports GNNs for DTI, property prediction, molecule generation	https://torchdrug.ai
MolGNet	AI platform for virtual screening	GNNs used for ligand–target prediction and QSAR	https://github.com/BioPharmMolGraph/molGNet
GraphDTA	Predict binding affinity between drug and protein	Uses GNNs to encode both drugs and protein sequences	https://github.com/thinng/GraphDTA
GDL4Mol	Research project	Develop scalable GNN-based drug design pipelines	https://gdl4mol.github.io
REINVENT	AI-VS	Uses RNNs (LSTM) to generate valid SMILES strings	https://github.com/MolecularAI/Reinvent
ChemTS	Molecular generator based on reinforcement learning	RNN + Monte Carlo Tree Search for exploring chemical space	https://github.com/tsudalab/ChemTS
SmilesLSTM	Trainable molecular generator using SMILES format	LSTM (RNN variant) for molecule generation from SMILES	https://github.com/aspuru-guzik-group/chemical_vae
Molecule Chef	Commercial drug design engine	SMILES generation using RNNs and reinforcement learning	https://polarisqb.com
DeepSMILES	SMILES-based sequence modeling	Supports RNN models trained on modified SMILES	https://deepsmiles.readthedocs.io
MolRNN	Drug-like molecule generation tool	RNNs with scaffolding for controlled generation	https://github.com/nyu-dl/dl4chem-molrnn
TDC	AI benchmarking and tools	Supports RNNs for sequence-based generation and prediction	https://tdcommons.ai

efficiently. This significantly speeds up the discovery process. In addition, CNNs are highly flexible and can work with different chemical representations and target proteins.

2.7 Graph neural networks

It models molecules as graphs, comprising atoms as vertices and bonds as connecting edges. This is different from traditional approaches that use fixed descriptors or rule-based characteristics. This method enables GNNs to learn complex structural relationships between different regions of a molecule. It can find both local patterns, like functional groups, and global aspects, like the shape of the molecule (St John et al., 2019). This makes GNNs especially effective for predicting biological properties such as binding affinity and critical ADMET (Yang et al., 2019; Haneczok and Delijewski, 2021). In VS, GNNs are often used to quickly look through large libraries of chemical compounds and predict how likely they are to interact with a biological target (Fig. 7.5B). This speeds up the process of finding hits and also helps with lead optimization by recommending changes to molecules that could make them better at what they do. One of the biggest strengths of GNNs is their ability to learn task-specific molecular representations. GNNs autonomously learn representations from compound topology that are optimized for the specific task at hand, whether that is forecasting toxicity or binding strength. This is different from previous methods that use preset features. Another major advantage is their capacity to generalize to molecules that weren't seen during training. Because GNNs learn underlying patterns in molecular structures, they can predict how new or novel compounds might behave, which is particularly valuable when exploring uncharted areas of chemical space. In addition, since GNNs avoid computationally heavy steps like molecular docking, they can significantly increase screening efficiency, making them suitable for high-throughput applications. However, there are also challenges to using GNNs effectively. First, they usually need big, varied datasets to work at their best. If the training data is too small or not a good sample, the model may not be able to generalize. GNNs can also have trouble accurately modeling some molecular properties that aren't additive and don't follow simple compositional laws. Another worry is scalability, because it can be expensive to handle particularly big or complicated molecular graphs. In addition, while GNNs are powerful, it can be hard to comprehend why certain predictions are made with these models because they aren't always easy to interpret. This is an issue of growing concern in fields such as drug development, where explainability is key. To overcome these limitations, ongoing research is focusing on integrating domain knowledge, such as expert-defined descriptors, into GNN models, which can enhance accuracy and improve interpretability. Despite the current hurdles, GNNs represent a significant advancement in VS, and more available tools are discussed in Table 7.2. Researchers are pushing the limits of drug development by using ML, which enables computers to understand complex, data-driven chemical representations and make quick, accurate predictions (Qiu et al., 2024). This makes the process smarter, faster, and cheaper.

2.8 Recurrent neural networks

It is designed to handle sequential data, called a recurrent neural network (RNN). This makes them very effective in cheminformatics, as molecular representations like SMILES strings follow a linear style (Segler et al., 2018). Because they can learn patterns across sequences, RNNs are becoming more and more popular in VS (Fig. 7.5C). One of the key uses of RNNs in this space is generating focused molecule libraries. By training RNNs on databases of active compounds, researchers can generate novel molecules that are structurally similar to known bioactive compounds. These generative models are very helpful for adding drug-like candidates to virtual libraries. They can even be fine-tuned using a narrower selection of compounds that target a specific protein (Segler et al., 2018). RNNs are also employed for predicting molecular properties. Once new molecules are generated, the model can estimate attributes like toxicity, solubility, or drug-likeness, helping prioritize compounds for further testing. Another powerful application of RNNs is in exploring chemical space. Unlike rule-based approaches, RNNs can venture into unexplored chemical territories, identifying novel scaffolds with promising bioactivity profiles. RNNs are employed in iterative cycles for de novo drug design: they generate new molecules, rank them based on desired properties (such as binding affinity and ADME profiles), and re-train on the top candidates, gradually improving the quality of generated compounds (Gómez-Bombarelli et al., 2018). Moreover, RNNs have proven effective in LBVS, where they analyze the SAR of known inhibitors and extrapolate this knowledge to screen large compound libraries (Table 7.2). For example, RNN-based models have been applied to develop virtual screens for protein kinase inhibitors, where sequence data plays a crucial role in predicting activity against diverse targets. The main advantage of RNNs in this context is that their native handling of sequential input is a perfect fit for SMILES strings and reaction sequences. They also enable de novo molecular generation, allowing the discovery of novel compounds that might not exist in traditional databases. Furthermore, by exploring regions of chemical space previously overlooked by human intuition or rule-based methods, RNNs expand the frontiers of drug design (Krishnan et al., 2022). However, RNNs are not without limitations. The disappearing or exploding gradient problem is a well-known issue that can make learning harder when sequences are excessively long. Standard RNNs may also struggle with capturing long-term dependencies, a critical feature when key molecular substructures are spaced far apart in the sequence. While models like LSTM and GRU offer partial solutions, training still demands significant computational resources (Hochreiter and Schmidhuber, 1997). In comparison with other architectures, RNNs are highly suited to sequential data, but not necessarily to spatial or compound topology. For example, CNNs perform better when analyzing grid-based inputs like 3D voxelized images or chemical fingerprints. Meanwhile, GNNs have become increasingly favored for modeling molecular graphs, capturing atomic connectivity and spatial structure more effectively than sequence-based models (Gilmer et al., 2017).

2.9 Advanced AI strategies

Beyond supervised learning, several novel AI strategies have been adopted to address challenges in molecular screening, such as limited labeled data, the exploration of large chemical spaces, and continuous learning from new experiments.

2.10 Transfer learning

It allows a model to be trained for a specific job or a dataset to be adapted to a related task, typically with fewer labeled examples (https://aws.amazon.com/what-is/transfer-learning/). In VS, models pretrained on large databases (ChEMBL, ZINC) can be fine-tuned for specific targets or endpoints. It is revolutionizing how models predict molecular activity, particularly when data is limited (https://github.com/seyonechithrananda/bert-loves-chemistry). Transfer learning is applied to fine-tuning a GNN for a rare disease target and adapting general ADMET models to a new compound class. In a 2021 study, Altae-Tran et al. demonstrated the effectiveness of transfer learning by using GNNs pretrained on ChEMBL data. These models were then fine-tuned on limited-label bioassays like the Tox21 toxicity panel (https://tox21.gov/) and achieved higher accuracy than traditional QSAR models trained from scratch (Altae-Tran et al., 2017). In the same vein, the Chemprop platform facilitates property prediction through transfer learning by utilizing Message Passing Neural Networks (MPNNs). Researchers often pretrain on large-scale public datasets (MoleculeNet - https://moleculenet.org/) and fine-tune on target-specific assays like kinase inhibition or antiviral activity, drastically reducing the need for massive experimental datasets.

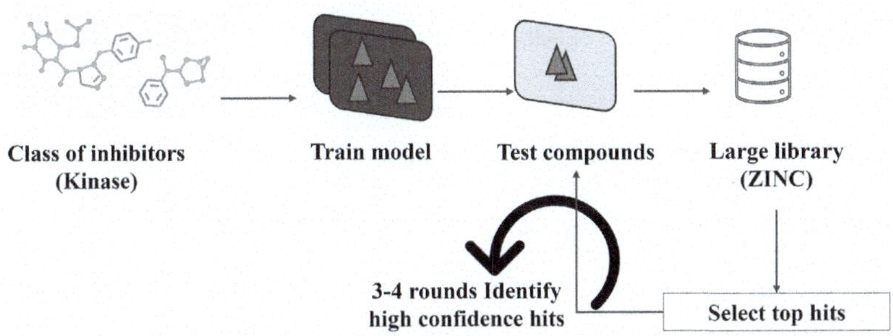

Fig. 7.6 Active learning flowchart: A schematic representation of the active learning workflow, illustrating the iterative cycle of model training, uncertainty sampling, data labeling, and retraining to progressively enhance prediction performance.

2.11 Active learning

In active learning, models don't just passively learn from a fixed dataset; they actively pick the compounds that will teach them the most. This strategy is particularly useful in VS and drug discovery, where labeled data (biological assay results) are expensive and time-consuming to obtain (Fig. 7.6). Instead of randomly selecting molecules to test or train on, active learning helps the model decide which compounds will provide the most value if labeled (i.e., experimentally tested). Researchers employed active learning to find compounds that inhibit the protein kinase PIM1 (Smith et al., 2018). The researchers started with only 100 labeled compounds and iteratively selected new compounds for experimental testing based on model uncertainty. By the third round, they had improved the hit rate by over threefold while testing fewer compounds than a random screening strategy.

Steps:

- Train a model using Chemprop or any tool from Table 7.3
- Select the top 20 most uncertain compounds from a ZINC library
- Test them experimentally (or via docking from AutoDock)
- Retrain the model and repeat
- In 3–4 rounds, identify high-confidence hits with ~ 80% fewer experiments

Active learning makes the process of gathering data smarter and more efficient, which is a big plus for drug discovery. One of its main benefits is that it lowers the cost of conducting experiments. Active learning models don't test hundreds of compounds at random; rather, they identify and select only the most instructive ones that, if labeled, can best teach the model. This reduces the number of expensive lab tests that need to be conducted. It also integrates well with real-time experimental settings, allowing scientists to use model feedback after each round of data acquisition, thereby supporting

Table 7.3 List of tools supporting active and reinforcement learning in virtual screening.

Tool/Platform	Use case	Web address
MODAL	Bayesian active learning for molecular design	https://github.com/nyu-dl/modal
Chemprop	Active learning-enabled property prediction	https://github.com/chemprop/chemprop
DeepChem	Uncertainty sampling + QSAR + retraining loop	https://deepchem.io
MoleculeNet + AL	Benchmarks using active learning on MoleculeNet datasets	https://moleculenet.org
ALiPy (Python lib)	General-purpose active learning framework	https://github.com/NUAA-AL/ALiPy
AMPL (Atomwise)	Active learning + molecular modeling	https://www.atomwise.com
REINVENT	De novo drug design & SMILES generation	https://github.com/MolecularAI/Reinvent
MolDQN	Molecular optimization via Q-learning	https://github.com/microsoft/molecule-generation
GraphAF	Flow-based generative model + RL	https://github.com/DeepGraphLearning/GraphAF
GENTRL	Generative Tensorial RL framework	https://github.com/insilicomedicine/GENTRL
MERMAID	Molecular design using memory-augmented policy networks	https://github.com/synergetics-research/MERMAID
ORGANIC	Objective-Reinforced Generative Adversarial Network	https://github.com/gablg1/ORGANIC
MUBDsyn	Multiobjective unbiased dataset synthesis	https://github.com/xiaoyuan1996/MUBDsyn
RationaleRL	Molecule generation via fragment-based reinforcement learning	https://github.com/bowenliu16/RationaleRL

iterative and adaptive workflows in the lab. Despite its strengths, active learning also comes with some challenges. Even though it reduces the total number of labeled compounds required, each selected compound still needs to undergo experimental validation, which can be resource-intensive.

2.12 Reinforcement learning

It works well when other computational methods don't work well. By learning through trial and error, RL-based models can make informed decisions about which compounds to explore or generate, making the process of drug discovery more efficient and adaptive (Atance et al., 2022). One notable application of RL in VS is in the development of benchmarking datasets, steps discussed in detail. Traditional datasets often suffer from biases, such as unrealistic decoy compounds that can mislead ML evaluations. To address this, deep RL (DRL) has been applied to create improved benchmarking sets like MUBDsyn (https://github.com/taoshen99/MUBDsyn) and others (Table 7.4) which generate more realistic and controlled

Table 7.4 RL step-by-step process.

Step	What happens	Example
Define the environment	The environment is a virtual chemical space containing millions of molecules or fragments.	A database like ZINC15 or ChEMBL containing chemical compounds
Define the agent	The RL agent is an AI model trying to learn how to pick or generate the best molecules.	A model like REINVENT or MolDQN
Define actions	Actions are things the agent can do, like adding a chemical group, changing a bond, or choosing a molecule to test.	Add a hydroxyl group to a molecule
Define rewards	The agent gets a reward score after each action based on how "good" the new molecule is, which can depend on how similar it is to a medicine, how toxic it is, or how well it binds.	+1 if the molecule is predicted to bind well to the target; – 1 if it's toxic
Train the agent	The agent tries many actions, receives feedback, and learns which types of moves create better molecules.	The AI improves after generating and scoring thousands of molecules
Generate Optimized compounds	Eventually, the agent learns how to design or select molecules that have a high chance of being effective drugs.	The model outputs 100 drug-like candidates with good docking scores

decoys. These synthetic datasets provide a better testing ground for emerging ML-based VS models, making evaluation more reliable and fairer. The RL approach sees building molecules as a series of decisions, learning the ideal order of activities, like adding atoms or changing bonds, to make molecules that fulfill certain requirements. By continuously analyzing the relationship between actions (chemical modifications) and their outcomes (predicted efficacy or ADMET profiles), RL models can learn strategies for navigating chemical space more effectively than random or brute-force search methods. During the COVID-19 pandemic, researchers combined RL with a transformer model to generate inhibitors for the viral Mpro protein (Hazemann et al., 2024). The RL agent was rewarded based on binding affinity, synthetic accessibility, and drug-likeness, leading to promising candidates in just a few cycles. There are several benefits to using RL in VS. One is enhanced bias control, especially in dataset generation, which leads to more accurate evaluations of ML-based screening methods. Another is the acceleration of drug discovery, as RL can guide the generation of promising compounds more quickly when combined with powerful generative models like transformers or variational autoencoders (VAEs). The REINVENT framework is a prominent example that uses RL for SMILES-based generation of bioactive molecules (Olivecrona et al., 2017).

2.13 Generative AI models

They figure out how the data is spread out and then use that knowledge to make new, comparable data samples (Gómez-Bombarelli et al., 2018). These models can build new molecular structures that have certain chemical or biological properties. The two most common categories employed in medication design are:

- **VAEs**: They are neural networks that encode chemical information into a hidden space with fewer dimensions and then decode that information to reconstruct it. You can explore the hidden space to create new compounds with the qualities you desire. The first step is to transform molecular representations, such as SMILES strings, into a compressed form that is difficult to interpret. New points within this space can then be sampled and decoded to generate previously unseen compounds. They can learn from a set of known inhibitors that target a specific protein. After training, the model can design molecules that are structurally comparable and still possess the requisite bioactivity, demonstrating that a VAE could be used to produce new small compounds with drug-like properties (Gómez-Bombarelli et al., 2018).
- **Generative adversarial networks (GANs)**: They consist of a discriminator and a generator, two neural networks that compete with one another. The generator creates new structures, and the discriminator checks to see if these molecules are real or made up. The generator improves over time through this adversarial process, producing molecules that are more realistic and chemically sound. A key application of GANs is in drug design, where they can be trained to generate molecules with specific properties. For instance, Objective-Reinforced GAN uses a reward function to make the molecules it generates more drug-like and easier to synthesize, which leads to a wide range of potent compounds. This method demonstrates that GANs could help accelerate the search for new drugs. However, it also faces numerous challenges in molecule generation. Mode collapse is a significant issue because it means that the generator only produces a small number of different molecules, often repeating the same structures instead of exploring the entire chemical space. Currently, two advanced autoencoders are also used, which are:
- **Junction tree VAE (JT-VAE):** It was made expressly to solve a significant problem in molecular generation—making sure that the molecules it generates are chemically correct (Jin et al., 2020). Traditional VAEs often struggle with creating valid molecules when decoding directly from SMILES strings. JT-VAE solves this by generating molecules in a more structured and interpretable manner. It decomposes a molecule into a junction tree of molecular

substructures (like rings, bonds, and functional groups). It then separately learns how to generate the tree structure and how to assemble the actual molecule. The VAE first encodes the molecule into a latent space using its tree representation and then decodes it in two steps: first generating the tree and then assembling atoms around the tree to form a valid molecule. It is particularly useful in lead optimization, where small changes in structure can greatly affect activity. Jin et al. optimized molecules for logP (a measure of solubility and lipophilicity), and the model successfully produced valid molecules with improved properties over the original compounds (https://github.com/wengong-jin/icml18-jtnn).

2.14 Molecular generative adversarial network (MolGAN)

It uses GANs and GNNs to make molecular graphs directly, sans SMILES strings. MolGAN is different from other GANs since it works with graph-structured data (De Cao and Kipf, 2018). The generator in MolGAN makes molecular graphs, and the discriminator checks to see if the graphs look like genuine molecules from the training data. It can quickly and easily make molecular graphs, which makes it useful for exploring new chemical spaces or building compounds with many optimal features. One problem with it, though, is that it can sometimes make graphs that aren't connected or molecules that aren't chemically acceptable. This has led to the creation of better versions of MolGAN (https://github.com/nicola-decao/molgan).

3 AI-enabled virtual screening workflow

Using data science, cheminformatics, and AI, the AI-enabled VS pipeline transforms raw molecular data into actionable insights through a series of iterative steps (Fig. 7.7) (Vamathevan et al., 2019). Each module works together to make molecular discovery faster and more accurate, from data curation to candidate prioritization to feedback integration. AI-based VS has the potential to change not just drug discovery but also materials research, agrochemical development, and personalized medicine by systematically using advanced feature extraction methods, strong ML models, and dynamic feedback systems.

3.1 Step 1: Data collection and preprocessing

AI-driven VS can only work if it has access to high-quality, varied datasets. Key sources include ChEMBL (bioactivity data), ZINC (purchasable compounds), PubChem BioAssay (HTS results),

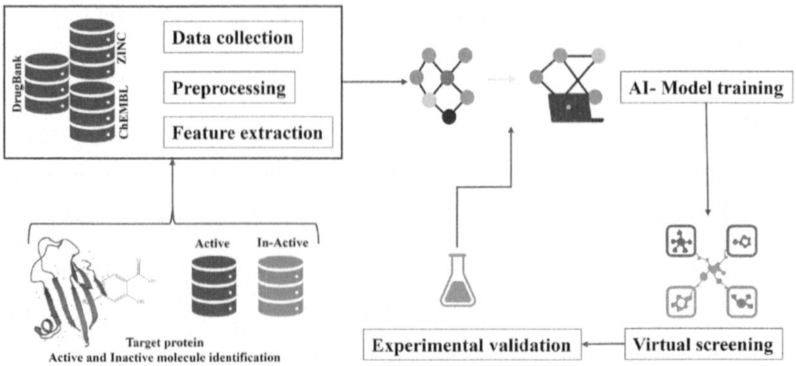

Fig. 7.7 AI-enabled virtual screening flowchart using both ligand and target receptor. A conceptual flowchart depicting the AI-driven virtual screening pipeline that integrates both ligand features and target receptor information, combining data preprocessing, model training, binding prediction, and iterative refinement for improved drug discovery outcomes.

BindingDB (binding affinities), and DrugBank (known drugs). Preprocessing involves structure standardization, duplicate removal, error filtering, and normalization (e.g., converting IC_{50} to pIC_{50}). Class balancing techniques like SMOTE may be applied to address imbalanced datasets. For example, download bioactivity data by selecting a target such as BACE1 (CHEMBL234) and downloading IC50 data from ChEMBL.

3.2 Step 2: Molecular feature extraction

Molecules must be converted into numerical representations. Fingerprints (ECFP, MACCS, Daylight) encode substructures, while descriptors (1D, 2D, 3D) capture physicochemical properties. SMILES strings enable sequence-based models, and graph representations facilitate GNNs such as MPNN and Graph Attention Networks (GAT) for learning molecular connectivity. Example: Clean and preprocess the dataset by removing missing SMILES or activity values. Convert IC50 to [–log10(IC50 in molar)] and define a binary activity label (active if IC50 ≥ 6).

3.3 Step 3: Model building and training

Once feature vectors are available, models can be created that learn to connect input characteristics to output labels or scores. The task type determines which type of models are chosen from the following:

- Classification models: Used when labels are binary (active/inactive)
- Regression models: Predict continuous outcomes (e.g., binding affinity)
- Multitask models: Learn across multiple targets or endpoints simultaneously
- Generative models: Produce novel molecular structures satisfying learned objectives

Common architectures include RF, XGBoost, DNNs, GNNs, and Transformers. Hyperparameter optimization (grid search, Bayesian optimization, AutoML platforms (e.g., AutoKeras, H2O.ai)) and cross-validation (k-fold, leave-one-out) ensure model robustness.

3.4 Step 4: Performance assessment

Classification performance is often measured using metrics like overall accuracy, how well positive cases are identified (precision and recall), a balanced score (F1), and area under the curve (AUC) values from receiver operating characteristic (ROC) and precision-recall curves. Measurements like R^2, the average error size, the typical squared error, and Spearman's rank correlation are used to evaluate how well regression models perform. To determine if the model can work with data that hasn't been seen before, it has to be tested on external datasets.

3.5 Step 5: Screening and candidate prioritization

Once the model has been trained and thoroughly evaluated, it is used to search through chemical libraries; ZINC and Mcule are just a few of the libraries that contain billions of compounds. AI models can predict how much a target will favor a compound, sort by ADMET qualities, and ensure that the compound can be synthesized. We use composite scoring systems to rank candidate compounds. These include predicting binding affinity, adhering to drug-likeness guidelines (Lipinski's Rule of Five), avoiding toxicity, and selecting for variety (maximizing chemical diversity).

3.6 Step 6: Feedback loop and model refinement

Unlike static models, AI-VS can incorporate feedback from wet-lab experiments to refine its predictive capabilities. Active learning can identify uncertain predictions for experimental validation. Results from assays are fed back into the dataset to retrain models. Model confidence improves through iterative learning cycles. This loop ensures the model remains relevant and improves over time, making it more aligned with dynamic drug discovery pipelines.

4 AI-case studies

4.1 Case study 1

Researchers at MIT used DL models to find Halicin (Stokes et al., 2020). Researchers trained DL models on a set of over 2500 compounds that are known to have antibacterial activity to study Halicin. The model architecture, which was built on an MPNN, was designed to predict the antibacterial efficacy of compounds in different chemical spaces. After training, the program looked through the ZINC15 database of over 100 million chemicals, focusing on molecules that were structurally different from antibiotics already available. Candidates with the highest scores were chosen based on their low toxicity and new scaffolds. Halicin was first developed to treat diabetes, but it turned out to be a strong antibiotic that acted through a novel mechanism. *In vitro* tests against *Clostridium difficile, Mycobacterium tuberculosis,* and in vivo mice infection models showed that it worked (Brown and Wright, 2016).

4.2 Case study 2

Exscientia used a human-AI hybrid design loop for DSP-1181 (https://www.exscientia.com/). At first, a DRL algorithm created molecular candidates that were optimal for binding to certain serotonin receptors and exhibited good pharmacokinetics. Medicinal chemists reviewed the chemicals generated by AI and provided feedback on them in a series of iterative steps, helping the algorithm improve subsequent generations. ADMET forecasts, synthetic feasibility, and target selectivity were all incorporated into each design cycle. This method produced the final optimized molecule, DSP-1181, which entered Phase I clinical trials within a year. This demonstrates that AI can accelerate the process of bringing medicine from the lab to the clinic without compromising regulatory standards.

4.3 Case study 3

Atomwise employed its AtomNet model, which is a structure-based CNN, to test millions of molecules against 3D target structures in a virtual environment. AtomNet learned how to estimate binding affinity based on molecular docking poses by being trained on a collection of drug complexes. This was done for Ebola and other viral targets. The trained algorithm looked through large chemical libraries for high-affinity binders and created a sorted list of virtual hits. They synthesized and tested some of the selected chemicals in the lab, and some of them showed promise (https://www.atomwise.com/).

5 AI applications in VS

AI improves VS by predicting which compounds are most likely to bind to a receptor. Traditional docking methods can take a long time and may be inaccurate, but AI models, especially DL and GNNs, can learn from existing bioactivity data and quickly screen millions of compounds for activity, binding affinity, or toxicity. This enables them to select the most promising hits for experimental testing. The Zhou et al. (2024) group comprehensively explained how AI can be used in drug design. The following AI applications are widely used:

- AI-driven generative models (VAEs and GANs) and RL frameworks can create entirely new chemical structures from scratch. Tools like REINVENT and MolGAN have demonstrated the ability to produce novel candidates with desired pharmacological profiles.
- Once promising hits are identified, AI helps improve these leads by predicting how chemical changes will influence their ADMET, selectivity, and effectiveness features. By learning from SAR, AI can suggest optimized analogs faster and more cost-effectively than traditional medicinal chemistry.
- AI can analyze massive biological datasets (genomic, transcriptomic, proteomic) to discover novel disease-associated targets. ML models can identify patterns of gene expression or protein–protein interactions linked to disease, supporting the selection of viable and druggable targets.
- Predicting pharmacokinetic and toxicity properties is critical in early-stage drug development. AI models can predict solubility, bioavailability, hERG inhibition, and liver toxicity, among other properties, minimizing late-stage failures and improving safety profiles. Tools such as admetSAR, pkCSM, and ProTox-II use ML to automate this process.
- AI excels at identifying new uses for existing drugs by discovering hidden connections between diseases, targets, and compounds. By integrating clinical, genomic, and pharmacological data, AI models can predict alternative indications, reducing development time and cost. During the COVID-19 pandemic, AI helped identify antivirals and antiinflammatory agents for repurposing.
- AI allows the design of compounds that interact with multiple targets simultaneously (polypharmacology), which is useful for treating complex diseases like cancer, neurodegeneration, or multidrug-resistant infections. ML can optimize compounds for multiple endpoints, improving therapeutic efficacy while minimizing side effects.
- AI-based models predict whether a compound will interact with a particular protein target, even when structural data is limited. Techniques include using graph-based molecular encodings and DL architectures to predict interactions across large biological networks.

- AI helps chemists in predicting synthetic routes for designed molecules. Tools such as IBM RXN (Reaction) or ASKCOS use neural networks trained on reaction data to suggest feasible and efficient synthesis pathways, closing the loop between molecular design and lab synthesis.
- AI models can use genetic and clinical data from individual patients to predict how they will react to medications. This makes it possible to build or choose medications that are specific to their genetic profiles.

6 Advantages of AI-driven VS

- AI can screen millions to billions of compounds within minutes, far faster than traditional docking methods. Pipelines like Deep Docking screened 1.3 billion molecules against COVID-19 targets in less than a week (Gentile et al., 2020). AI also benefits from GPU acceleration and cloud scalability, significantly shortening timelines.
- In clinical settings, AI models can rapidly analyze patient-specific data and suggest drug candidates in real-time, aiding personalized therapy design. Tools like OncoKB (https://www.oncokb.org/) and DeepTarget exemplify this potential.
- DL models outperform traditional QSAR and are effective at capturing complicated patterns. They predict bioactivity, binding affinity, and ADMET properties with higher precision (Chithrananda et al., 2020).
- AI can combine molecular structures, protein sequences, omics data, and clinical outcomes into unified models. Multimodal tools like DeepDTA and MolTrans (https://github.com/kexinhuang12345/MolTrans) leverage this to better model drug-target interactions.
- Pretrained models (MolBERT -https://github.com/BenevolentAI/MolBERT, and GENTRL- https://github.com/insilicomedicine/GENTRL) can be adjusted for new goals, even with limited data. This makes AI particularly valuable in early-stage or rare disease research.
- Generative models can create entirely new molecular scaffolds, going beyond existing libraries. This enables scaffold hopping and the discovery of structurally novel drug candidates.
- AI systems can incorporate new experimental data, retrain models, and refine predictions.
- AI can flag undesirable properties (toxicity, poor solubility) at an early stage, reducing late-stage failures. Models also predict off-target effects, like hERG inhibition, improving candidate safety profiles.

- By prioritizing only the most promising compounds, AI reduces the cost of synthesis and biological testing. Estimates show up to 30%–50% cost savings and 1–2 years' time reduction in drug discovery cycles (Mak and Pichika, 2019).

7 Challenges and limitations

AI has undoubtedly enhanced the power and efficiency of VS; however, the approach is not without its limitations. The promise of accelerated discovery, precision in molecular design, and reduced attrition rates often depends on overcoming several scientific, technical, and infrastructural challenges (Paul et al., 2021). The quality of the incoming data is directly related to how well AI-VS works, the robustness of ML algorithms, integration with laboratory workflows, and, ultimately, the ability to generate reproducible and actionable biological insights. A fundamental principle in ML, "garbage in, garbage out," holds particularly true in drug discovery, where models trained on noisy, incomplete, or biased datasets tend to produce unreliable predictions. For instance, many bioactivity datasets lack comprehensive annotations, such as missing IC_{50} or Ki values, leading to sparse data matrices that hinder learning. In addition, variations in assay conditions (e.g., pH, buffer composition, temperature) across laboratories introduce systematic noise. Simplified binary labels (active/inactive) may also fail to capture the full spectrum of biological activity, reducing model resolution. Another significant limitation arises from data bias. AI models often overfit chemical scaffolds or targets that are overrepresented in the training data. As a result, they may generalize poorly to novel chemical classes or underexplored targets. This is especially problematic in imbalanced datasets, such as those used in toxicology, where inactive compounds vastly outnumber active ones. Models trained on such datasets may exhibit class imbalance bias. To overcome this challenge, researchers have proposed techniques like Synthetic Minority Over-sampling Technique (SMOTE), adjusting class weights in loss functions, and implementing stratified sampling (Kokudeva et al., 2024). Moreover, high-throughput screening (HTS) results, commonly used as input for AI-VS, can produce both false positives and negatives. The reproducibility of bioassays remains a concern; even interlaboratory comparisons often reveal significant variation in hit rates for the same compound-target pairs (Arrowsmith, 2011). Models trained on data that is noisy and inconsistent may learn incorrect patterns, leading to a reduction in predictive accuracy.

In terms of model architecture, DL methods like CNNs and GNNs are powerful but often function as "black boxes." While they may provide accurate predictions, they lack interpretability, which is a critical requirement in regulated fields such as pharmaceuticals. Regulatory agencies like the Food and Drug Administration (FDA) and European Medicines Agency (EMA) often require mechanistic transparency for drug approvals and intellectual property protection. Explainable AI (XAI) has emerged, with tools like SHapley Additive exPlanations (SHAP), Local Interpretable Model Agnostic Explanations (LIME), and integrated gradients helping identify key features influencing model predictions. However, these tools often yield localized explanations that may not generalize across different molecules, targets, or prediction tasks. Simpler models like decision trees or RFs are easier to interpret but may underperform on large, high-dimensional datasets compared to DL architectures. The correct balance between accuracy and explainability is still a topic of research in AI-driven drug discovery.

Another common problem is overfitting, which happens when a model learns not just the patterns in the training set but also the random "ghost" patterns. This means that the model works well on training sets but not so well on new or outside datasets. Contributing factors include small sample sizes (especially for rare targets), excessive numbers of molecular descriptors, and data leakage due to improper validation splits. In addition, many models lack generalizability across target classes or molecular representations. For example, a model trained on kinase inhibitors may perform poorly when applied to GPCR ligands, and a SMILES-based RNN may not transfer effectively to graph-based or 3D input formats. These issues are compounded when crossing species or assay types, where biological contexts differ significantly.

To mitigate these limitations, various strategies are employed: cross-assessment approaches, regularization, ensemble learning, transfer learning, and multitask learning. Public benchmarks like MoleculeNet (https://moleculenet.org/) and the Therapeutics Data Commons (https://tdcommons.ai/) provide standardized platforms for assessing model generalizability across diverse datasets and tasks. Despite advances in model architecture and evaluation, a persistent bottleneck in AI-VS remains the disconnect between computational predictions and experimental validation. Even high-scoring in silico candidates frequently fail in wet-lab assays due to real-world liabilities such as poor solubility, low synthetic accessibility, unstable conformations, or off-target effects. This gap arises because most AI models optimize for a single objective, often binding affinity, without accounting for the multifaceted constraints of medicinal chemistry and biology. For instance, many AI-generated molecules are theoretically potent but synthetically inaccessible, as they lack integration with retrosynthetic logic. As a result, the proposed molecules may be impractical to synthesize using known reagents or reaction pathways. To address this, AI tools are increasingly being paired with retrosynthesis planners such as ASKCOS (https://askcos.mit.edu/) and AiZynthFinder (https://github.com/MolecularAI/aizynthfinder), though this integration is still in its early stages. To bridge the gap between computational output and experimental utility, an active learning loop can be implemented. In this iterative strategy, AI models propose a subset of high-confidence candidates, which are then synthesized and tested in the lab. The model is retrained, and its predictions are refined by incorporating the resulting assay data. Over time, this cycle improves both model precision and recall. However, operationalizing such feedback loops requires close collaboration between computational chemists, medicinal chemists, and biologists—something that is often hindered by siloed workflows and institutional boundaries.

8 Recent trends and future perspectives

Another barrier is the lack of standardized pipelines for reproducible AI workflows. While software like DeepChem, Chemprop, and KNIME helps automate pipelines, inconsistencies in data formats, modeling assumptions, and evaluation metrics continue to impede reproducibility. Reproducibility is especially critical for regulatory acceptance, where agencies require transparent documentation of both computational and experimental workflows. AI-VS has the potential to change drug discovery procedures in a big way, yet its broad use is limited by significant problems. These include inconsistencies in data quality, difficulties in interpreting complex model outputs, issues of overfitting and poor generalization, and disconnects between computational predictions and real-world validation. As DL models grow in complexity, so does the need for transparency. Regulatory frameworks, clinical applicability, and scientific credibility all demand an understanding of why a model makes certain predictions. This has fueled the emergence of XAI, a suite of methodologies designed to interpret, rationalize, and visualize AI decision-making (Karim et al., 2023). Recent tools have made significant strides:

- **SHAP**: It figures out how much each molecular property contributes to a certain prediction. It has been used by AstraZeneca and Novartis for internal drug prioritization pipelines (https://shap.readthedocs.io/en/latest/).
- **GNNExplainer**: Provides subgraph-level explanations for GNNs, making it ideal for highlighting molecular fragments that influence bioactivity or toxicity predictions (Ying et al., 2019).
- **ChempropX**: An extension of the Chemprop platform that integrates SHAP and Integrated Gradients directly into GNN-based models, allowing researchers to map attention scores to atomic positions. (https://github.com/chemprop/chemprop)

8.1 Hybrid docking-AI models

Hybrid models that combine traditional physics-based simulations (molecular docking, molecular dynamics) with AI-based learning are emerging as a powerful paradigm. These AI-augmented docking approaches leverage the best of both worlds: the mechanistic insights of physics and the scalability of ML.

- **DeepDock:** A deep neural network that learns molecular binding poses directly from docking simulation outputs, then refines them using a GNN-based attention model. (https://github.com/OptiMaL-PSE-Lab/DeepDock)
- **TANKBind**: A structure-aware transformer model developed by Stanford that integrates protein pocket representations with ligand structures, achieving state-of-the-art accuracy in pose prediction and affinity estimation. (https://github.com/luwei0917/TankBind)
- **EquiBind**: A GNN-based model that predicts binding poses without traditional sampling, reducing computational costs by 100x compared to AutoDock Vina while achieving comparable accuracy (https://github.com/HannesStark/EquiBind).
- **GNINA 1**: Integrated CNNs into AutoDock for rescoring docking poses. It demonstrated improvements in ranking accuracy across DUD-E benchmark datasets (https://github.com/gnina/gnina).

8.2 Industrial adoption

Pfizer and Genentech have piloted hybrid pipelines, where initial docking scores are re-ranked using ML models trained on historical binding data. This two-stage screening reduces false positives and improves hit rates in HTS campaigns.

8.3 Future outlook

Hybrid modeling is expected to evolve toward tight coupling, where AI models directly predict pose, energy, and even downstream effects like conformational entropy. The integration of quantum mechanics-informed neural networks, like OrbNet, is already showing promise in capturing nuanced electronic effects in protein-ligand interactions (Qiao et al., 2020).

8.4 Cloud-based and open-source AI platforms

The barrier to entry for AI-based drug discovery has been substantially reduced by the availability of cloud infrastructure and open-source tools. Researchers, startups, and academic labs now have access to industrial-grade tools without proprietary licenses or expensive hardware.

- **DeepChem**: Offers standardized APIs for training and deploying models on molecular datasets. Its 2023 update added pretrained GNNs and support for large-scale multitask learning.
- **Chemprop**: Built on PyTorch, it is widely adopted for regression and classification tasks involving drug-likeness, ADMET, and binding affinity.
- **MolBERT and ChemBERTa**: Transformer-based models trained on billions of SMILES strings.
- **RxRx3**: Open-cell imaging dataset from Recursion Pharmaceuticals for AI-driven phenotypic screening using cellular morphology (https://www.rxrx.ai/rxrx3).
- **BioNeMo**: Cloud-hosted models for biomolecular simulation, accessible through a GUI or API, facilitating ML-based protein folding, reaction prediction, and sequence generation (https://github.com/NVIDIA/bionemo-framework).
- Startups like Insilico Medicine (https://insilico.com/) and Valence Labs (https://www.valencelabs.com/) use these platforms to run full AI discovery pipelines remotely, enhancing speed and flexibility.

8.5 Future of autonomous drug design

The next frontier in AI-based molecular discovery is autonomous drug design, where AI agents not only screen compounds but also generate, evaluate, and iterate on novel candidates with minimal human intervention. This “closed-loop” or “self-driving lab” approach promises to reduce time-to-clinic from years to months (Schneider, 2018). Autonomous discovery systems are built on Design-Make-Test-Analyze loops that integrate generative design using VAEs, GANs, or diffusion models to generate compounds, synthetic route planning via AI retrosynthesis tools (ASKCOS, AiZynthFinder), VS and scoring using hybrid or multitask models, and automated synthesis and bioassay using robotic labs [Strateos (https://strateos.com/), Eli Lilly’s Lilly LifeLab (https://www.lilly.com/)].

Examples:

- **Insilico Medicine’s PandaOmics and Chemistry42**: Fully automated platforms for target identification, molecule generation, and optimization. In 2021, they identified a novel antifibrotic compound (ISM001-055), now in Phase I trials (https://insilico.com/chemistry42_fr).
- **Exscientia**: Delivered a compound to Phase I trials in under 12 months using AI-designed multiobjective optimization and virtual HTS. (https://www.exscientia.com/)
- **PostEra’s Manifold** Integrates ML with retrosynthesis and experimental feedback to optimize antiviral lead compounds collaboratively under the COVID Moonshot initiative (https://app.postera.ai/).

9 Conclusion

VS has been boosted because of AI. Traditional VS methods often struggle to handle large datasets and make accurate predictions. AI addresses these gaps by introducing ML and DL models that enhance prediction, expedite screening, and efficiently explore immense chemical spaces. This chapter delves into a diverse selection of AI tools, including RF, SVMs, advanced GNNs, and transformers. It also delves into the methods by which these tools process molecular data through learning methods. The discovery of Halicin and its use in environmental toxicology and catalyst design showed us how AI is helpful in drug discovery. Improvements in speed, accuracy, scalability, and early risk reduction are among the benefits of AI-VS.

References

Altae-Tran, H., Ramsundar, B., Pappu, A.S., Pande, V., 2017. Low data drug discovery with one-shot learning. ACS Cent. Sci. 2374-7951. 3 (4), 283–293. Available from: http://pubs.acs.org/journal/acscii. doi:10.1021/acscentsci.6b00367.

Arrowsmith, J., 2011. Phase II failures: 2008–2010. Nat. Rev. Drug Discov. 1474-1776. 10 (5), 328–329. doi:10.1038/nrd3439.

Atance, S.R., Diez, J.V., Engkvist, O., Olsson, S., Mercado, R., 2022. De novo drug design using reinforcement learning with graph-based deep generative models. J. Chem. Inf. Model. 1549-960X. 62 (20), 4863–4872. Available from: http://pubs.acs.org/journal/jcisd8. doi:10.1021/acs.jcim.2c00838.

Ballester, P.J., Mitchell, J.B.O., 2010. A machine learning approach to predicting protein-ligand binding affinity with applications to molecular docking. Bioinformatics. 1460-2059. 26 (9), 1169–1175. doi:10.1093/bioinformatics/btq112.

Brown, E.D., Wright, G.D., 2016. Antibacterial drug discovery in the resistance era. Nature. 1476-4687. 529 (7586), 336–343. Available from: http://www.nature.com/nature/index.html. doi:10.1038/nature17042.

Burns, R.F., 1995. Exploiting Molecular Diversity: Symposium Proceedings 2. Cambridge Healthtech Institute (CHI), Waltham, MA, USA.

Cantrell, J.M., Chung, C.H., Chandrasekaran, S., 2022. Machine learning to design antimicrobial combination therapies: promises and pitfalls. Drug Discov. Today. 1878-5832. 27 (6), 1639–1651. Available from: https://www.elsevier.com/locate/drugdiscov. doi:10.1016/j.drudis.2022.04.006.

Chan, H.C.S., Shan, H., Dahoun, T., Vogel, H., Yuan, S., 2019. Advancing drug discovery via artificial intelligence. Trends Pharmacol. Sci. 0165-6147. 40 (8), 592–604. doi:10.1016/j.tips.2019.06.004.

Chen, J., Bolhuis, D.L., Laggner, C., Kong, D., Yu, L., Wang, X., Emanuele, M.J., Brown, N.G., Liu, P., 2023. AtomNet-aided OTUD7B inhibitor discovery and validation. Cancers. 2072-6694. 15 (2). Available from: http://www.mdpi.com/journal/cancers/. doi:10.3390/cancers15020517.

Cherkasov, A., Muratov, E.N., Fourches, D., Varnek, A., Baskin, I.I., Cronin, M., Dearden, J., Gramatica, P., Martin, Y.C., Todeschini, R., Consonni, V., Kuz'Min, V.E., Cramer, R., Benigni, R., Yang, C., Rathman, J., Terfloth, L., Gasteiger, J., Richard, A., Tropsha, A., 2014. QSAR modeling: where have you been? Where are you going to?. J. Med. Chem. 1520-4804. 57 (12), 4977–5010. Available from: http://pubs.acs.org/jmc. doi:10.1021/jm4004285.

Chithrananda, S., Grand, G., Ramsundar, B., 2020. ChemBERTa: large-scale self-supervised pretraining for molecular property prediction. arXiv preprint arXiv:2010.09885.

Cichonska, A., Pahikkala, T., Szedmak, S., Julkunen, H., Airola, A., Heinonen, M., Aittokallio, T., Rousu, J., 2018. Learning with multiple pairwise kernels for drug bioactivity prediction. Bioinformatics. 1367-4803. 34 (13), i509. doi:10.1093/bioinformatics/bty277.

Cieślak, M., Danel, T., Krzysztyńska-Kuleta, O., Kalinowska-Tłuścik, J., 2024. Machine learning accelerates pharmacophore-based virtual screening of MAO inhibitors. Sci. Rep. 2045-2322. 14 (1). doi:10.1038/s41598-024-58122-7.

De Cao, N., Kipf, T., 2018. MolGAN: an implicit generative model for small molecular graphs. arXiv. 2331-8422. Available from: https://arxiv.org. doi:10.48550/arxiv.1805.11973.

Gentile, F., Agrawal, V., Hsing, M., Ton, A.T., Ban, F., Norinder, U., Gleave, M.E., Cherkasov, A., 2020. Deep Docking: A Deep Learning Platform for Augmentation of Structure Based Drug Discovery. ACS central science 6 (6), 939–949. doi:10.1021/acscentsci.0c00229.

Gilmer, J., Schoenholz, S.S., Riley, P.F., Vinyals, O., Dahl, G.E., 2017. Neural message passing for quantum chemistry. In: 34th International Conference on Machine Learning, ICML 2017, Vol. 3. 9781510855144. International Machine Learning Society (IMLS), United States. pp. 2053–2070.

Gómez-Bombarelli, R., Wei, J.N., Duvenaud, D., Hernández-Lobato, J.M., Sánchez-Lengeling, B., Sheberla, D., Aguilera-Iparraguirre, J., Hirzel, T.D., Adams, R.P., Aspuru-Guzik, A., 2018. Automatic chemical design using a data-driven continuous representation of molecules. ACS Cent. Sci. 2374-7951. 4 (2), 268–276. Available from: http://pubs.acs.org/journal/acscii. doi:10.1021/acscentsci.7b00572.

Gorgulla, C., Boeszoermenyi, A., Wang, Z.F., Fischer, P.D., Coote, P.W., Das, K.M.P., Malets, Y.S., Radchenko, D.S., Moroz, Y.S., Scott, D.A., Fackeldey, K., Hoffmann, M., Iavniuk, I., Wagner, G., Arthanari, H., 2020. An open-source drug discovery platform enables ultra-large virtual screens. Nature. 1476-4687. 580 (7805), 663–668. Available from: http://www.nature.com/nature/index.html. doi:10.1038/s41586-020-2117-z.

Gorgulla, C., Das, K.M.P., Leigh, K.E., Cespugli, M., Fischer, P.D., Wang, Z.F., Tesseyre, G., Pandita, S., Shnapir, A., Calderaio, A., Gechev, M., Rose, A., Lewis, N., Hutcheson, C., Yaffe, E., Luxenburg, R., Herce, H.D., Durmaz, V., Halazonetis, T.D., Fackeldey, K., Patten, J.J., Chuprina, A., Dziuba, I., Plekhova, A., Moroz, Y., Radchenko, D., Tarkhanova, O., Yavnyuk, I., Gruber, C., Yust, R., Payne, D., Näär, A.M., Namchuk, M.N., Davey, R.A., Wagner, G., Kinney, J., Arthanari, H., 2021. A multi-pronged approach targeting SARS-CoV-2 proteins using ultra-large virtual screening. iScience. 2589-0042. 24 (2). Available from: www.cell.com/iscience. doi:10.1016/j.isci.2020.102021.

Halder, R.K., Uddin, M.N., Uddin, M.A., Aryal, S., Khraisat, A., 2024. Enhancing K-nearest neighbor algorithm: a comprehensive review and performance analysis of modifications. J. Big Data. 2196-1115. 11 (1). Available from: https://journalofbigdata.springeropen.com. doi:10.1186/s40537-024-00973-y.

Haneczok, J., Delijewski, M., 2021. Machine learning enabled identification of potential SARS-CoV-2 3CLpro inhibitors based on fixed molecular fingerprints and graph-CNN neural representations. J. Biomed. Inform. 1532-0464. 119, 103821. doi:10.1016/j.jbi.2021.103821.

Hazemann, J., Kimmerlin, T., Lange, R., Sweeney, A.M., Bourquin, G., Ritz, D., Czodrowski, P., 2024. Identification of SARS-CoV-2 Mpro inhibitors through deep reinforcement learning for de novo drug design and computational chemistry approaches. RSC Med. Chem. 2632-8682. 15 (6), 2146–2159. Available from: https://www.rsc.org/journals-books-databases/about-journals/medchemcomm/. doi:10.1039/d4md00106k.

Hochreiter, S., Schmidhuber, J., 1997. Long short-term memory. Neural Comput. 0899-7667. 9 (8), 1735–1780. doi:10.1162/neco.1997.9.8.1735.

Jin, W., Barzilay, R., Jaakkola, T., 2020. Chapter 11. Junction tree variational autoencoder for molecular graph generation. In: Drug Discovery.Royal Society of Chemistry (RSC), pp. 228–249. 2021. doi:10.1039/9781788016841-00228.

Karim, M.R., Islam, T., Shajalal, M., Beyan, O., Lange, C., Cochez, M., Rebholz-Schuhmann, D., Decker, S., 2023. Explainable AI for bioinformatics: methods, tools and applications. Brief. Bioinform. 1477-4054. 24 (5). Available from: http://bib.oxfordjournals.org. doi:10.1093/bib/bbad236.

Kitchen, D.B., Decornez, H., Furr, J.R., Bajorath, J., 2004. Docking and scoring in virtual screening for drug discovery: methods and applications. Nat. Rev. Drug Discov. 3 (11), 935–949. doi:10.1038/nrd1549.

Kokudeva, M., Vichev, M., Naseva, E., Miteva, D.G., Velikova, T., 2024. Artificial intelligence as a tool in drug discovery and development. World J. Exp. Med. 2220-315X. 14 (3). Available from: https://www.wjgnet.com/2220-315x/full/v14/i3/96042.htm. doi:10.5493/wjem.v14.i3.96042.

Krishnan, S.R., Bung, N., Vangala, S.R., Srinivasan, R., Bulusu, G., Roy, A., 2022. De novo structure-based drug design using deep learning. J. Chem. Inf. Model. 1549-960X. 62 (21), 5100–5109. Available from: http://pubs.acs.org/journal/jcisd8. doi:10.1021/acs.jcim.1c01319.

Kumar, N., Acharya, V., 2024. Advances in machine intelligence-driven virtual screening approaches for big-data. Med. Res. Rev. 0198-6325. 44 (3), 939–974. doi:10.1002/med.21995.

LeCun, Y., Bengio, Y., Hinton, G., 2015. Deep learning. Nature. 0028-0836. 521 (7553), 436–444. doi:10.1038/nature14539.

Lusci, A., Pollastri, G., Baldi, P., 2013. Deep architectures and deep learning in chemoinformatics: the prediction of aqueous solubility for drug-like molecules. J. Chem. Inf. Model. 1549-9596. 53 (7), 1563–1575. doi:10.1021/ci400187y.

Mak, K.K., Pichika, M.R., 2019. Artificial intelligence in drug development: present status and future prospects. Drug Discov. Today. 1878-5832. 24 (3), 773–780. Available from: www.elsevier.com/locate/drugdiscov. doi:10.1016/j.drudis.2018.11.014.

Martínez Mora, A., Subramanian, V., Miljković, F., 2022. Multi-task convolutional neural networks for predicting in vitro clearance endpoints from molecular images. J. Comput. Aided Mol. Des. 0920-654X. 36 (6), 443–457. doi:10.1007/s10822-022-00458-1.

Marx, V., 2013. The big challenges of big data. Nature. 0028-0836. 498 (7453), 255–260. doi:10.1038/498255a.

Muegge, I., Bergner, A., Kriegl, J.M., 2017. Computer-aided drug design at Boehringer Ingelheim. J. Comput. Aided Mol. Des. 1573-4951. 31 (3), 275–285. Available from: https://www.springer.com/journal/10822. doi:10.1007/s10822-016-9975-3.

Muegge, I., Mukherjee, P., 2016. An overview of molecular fingerprint similarity search in virtual screening. Expert Opin. Drug Discov. 1746-045X. 11 (2), 137–148. doi:10.1517/17460441.2016.1117070.

Muegge, I., Oloff, S., 2006. Advances in virtual screening. Drug Discov. Today Technol. 1740-6749. 3 (4), 405–411. doi:10.1016/j.ddtec.2006.12.002.

Nayarisseri, A., Khandelwal, R., Tanwar, P., Madhavi, M., Sharma, D., Thakur, G., Speck-Planche, A., Singh, S.K., 2021. Artificial intelligence, big data and machine learning approaches in precision medicine & drug discovery. Curr. Drug Targets. 1873-5592. 22 (6), 631–655. Available from: https://www.eurekaselect.com/189908/article. doi:10.2174/1389450122999210104205732.

Nguyen, T., Le, H., Quinn, T.P., Nguyen, T., Le, T.D., Venkatesh, S., 2021. GraphDTA: predicting drug target binding affinity with graph neural networks. Bioinformatics. 1460-2059. 37 (8), 1140–1147. Available from: http://bioinformatics.oxfordjournals.org/. doi:10.1093/bioinformatics/btaa921.

Olivecrona, M., Blaschke, T., Engkvist, O., Chen, H., 2017. Molecular de-novo design through deep reinforcement learning. J. Cheminform. 1758-2946. 9 (1). doi:10.1186/s13321-017-0235-x.

Pagadala, N.S., Syed, K., Tuszynski, J., 2017. Software for molecular docking: a review. Biophys. Rev. 1867-2469. 9 (2), 91–102. Available from: http://www.springer.com/life+sciences/biochemistry+%26+biophysics/journal/12551. doi:10.1007/s12551-016-0247-1.

Patrick Walters, W., Stahl, M.T., Murcko, M.A., 1998. Virtual screening—An overview. Drug Discov. Today. 1359-6446. 3 (4), 160–178. Available from: www.elsevier.com/locate/drugdiscov. doi:10.1016/s1359-6446(97)01163-x.

Paul, D., Sanap, G., Shenoy, S., Kalyane, D., Kalia, K., Tekade, R.K., 2021. Artificial intelligence in drug discovery and development. Drug Discov. Today. 1878-5832. 26 (1), 80–93. Available from: www.elsevier.com/locate/drugdiscov. doi:10.1016/j.drudis.2020.10.010.

Qiao, Z., Welborn, M., Anandkumar, A., Manby, F.R., Miller, T.F., 2020. OrbNet: deep learning for quantum chemistry using symmetry-adapted atomic-orbital features. J. Chem. Phys. 1089-7690. 153 (12). Available from: http://scitation.aip.org/content/aip/journal/jcp. doi:10.1063/5.0021955.

Qiu, X., Wang, H., Tan, X., Fang, Z., 2024. G-K BertDTA: a graph representation learning and semantic embedding-based framework for drug-target affinity prediction. Comput. Biol. Med. 0010-4825. 173, 108376. doi:10.1016/j.compbiomed.2024.108376.

Ramsundar, B., Liu, B., Wu, Z., Verras, A., Tudor, M., Sheridan, R.P., Pande, V., 2017. Is multitask deep learning practical for pharma?. J. Chem. Inf. Model. 1549-960X. 57 (8), 2068–2076. Available from: http://pubs.acs.org/journal/jcisd8. doi:10.1021/acs.jcim.7b00146.

Rogers, D., Hahn, M., 2010. Extended-connectivity fingerprints. J. Chem. Inf. Model. 1549-9596. 50 (5), 742–754. doi:10.1021/ci100050t.

Scheeder, C., Heigwer, F., Boutros, M., 2018. Machine learning and image-based profiling in drug discovery. Curr. Opin. Syst. Biol. 2452-3100. 10, 43–52. doi:10.1016/j.coisb.2018.05.004.

Schneider, G., 2018. Automating drug discovery. Nat. Rev. Drug Discov. 1474-1776. 17 (2), 97–113. doi:10.1038/nrd.2017.232.

Segler, M.H.S., Kogej, T., Tyrchan, C., Waller, M.P., 2018. Generating focused molecule libraries for drug discovery with recurrent neural networks. ACS Cent. Sci. 2374-7951. 4 (1), 120–131. Available from: http://pubs.acs.org/journal/acscii. doi:10.1021/acscentsci.7b00512.

Smith, J.S., Nebgen, B., Lubbers, N., Isayev, O., Roitberg, A.E., 2018. Less is more: sampling chemical space with active learning. J. Chem. Phys. 0021-9606. 148 (24). Available from: http://scitation.aip.org/content/aip/journal/jcp. doi:10.1063/1.5023802.

Sobral, P.S., Carvalho, T., Izadi, S., Castilho, A., Silva, Z., Videira, P.A., Pereira, F., 2025. Advancements in drug discovery: integrating CADD tools and drug repurposing for PD-1/PD-L1 axis inhibition. RSC Adv. 2046-2069. 15 (4), 2298–2316. Available from: http://pubs.rsc.org/en/journals/journal/ra. doi:10.1039/d4ra08245a.

St John, P.C., Phillips, C., Kemper, T.W., Wilson, A.N., Guan, Y., Crowley, M.F., Nimlos, M.R., Larsen, R.E., 2019. Message-passing neural networks for high-throughput polymer screening. J. Chem. Phys. 0021-9606. 150 (23). Available from: http://scitation.aip.org/content/aip/journal/jcp. doi:10.1063/1.5099132.

Stahl, M., Guba, W., Kansy, M., 2006. Integrating molecular design resources within modern drug discovery research: the Roche experience. Drug Discov. Today. 1359-6446. 11 (7-8), 326–333. doi:10.1016/j.drudis.2006.02.008.

Stéen, E.J.L., Vugts, D.J., Windhorst, A.D., 2022. The application of in silico methods for prediction of blood-brain barrier permeability of small molecule PET tracers. Front. Nucl. Med. 2673-8880. 2. Available from: https://www.frontiersin.org/journals/nuclear-medicine/about. doi:10.3389/fnume.2022.853475.

Stokes, J.M., Yang, K., Swanson, K., Jin, W., Cubillos-Ruiz, A., Donghia, N.M., MacNair, C.R., French, S., Carfrae, L.A., Bloom-Ackerman, Z., Tran, V.M., Chiappino-Pepe, A., Badran, A.H., Andrews, I.W., Chory, E.J., Church, G.M., Brown, E.D., Jaakkola, T.S., Barzilay, R., Collins, J.J., 2020. A deep learning approach to antibiotic discovery. Cell. 1097-4172. 180 (4), 688. Available from: https://www.sciencedirect.com/journal/cell. doi:10.1016/j.cell.2020.01.021.

Svetnik, V., Liaw, A., Tong, C., Culberson, J.C., Sheridan, R.P., Feuston, B.P., 2003. Random forest: a classification and regression tool for compound classification and QSAR modeling. J. Chem. Inf. Comput. Sci. 0095-2338. 43 (6), 1947–1958. doi:10.1021/ci034160g.

Ton, A.T., Gentile, F., Hsing, M., Ban, F., Cherkasov, A., 2020. Rapid identification of potential inhibitors of SARS-CoV-2 main protease by deep docking of 1.3 billion compounds. Mol. Inform. 1868-1751. 39 (8). Available from: http://onlinelibrary.wiley.com/journal/10.1002/(ISSN)1868-1751. doi:10.1002/minf.202000028.

Vamathevan, J., Clark, D., Czodrowski, P., Dunham, I., Ferran, E., Lee, G., Li, B., Madabhushi, A., Shah, P., Spitzer, M., Zhao, S., 2019. Applications of machine learning in drug discovery and development. Nat. Rev. Drug Discov. 1474-1776. 18 (6), 463–477. doi:10.1038/s41573-019-0024-5.

Visan, A.I., Negut, I., 2024. Integrating artificial intelligence for drug discovery in the context of revolutionizing drug delivery. Romania Life. 2075-1729. 14 (2). Available from: www.mdpi.com/journal/life/. doi:10.3390/life14020233.

Waring, M.J., Arrowsmith, J., Leach, A.R., Leeson, P.D., Mandrell, S., Owen, R.M., Pairaudeau, G., Pennie, W.D., Pickett, S.D., Wang, J., Wallace, O., Weir, A., 2015. An analysis of the attrition of drug candidates from four major pharmaceutical companies. Nat. Rev. Drug Discov. 1474-1784. 14 (7), 475–486. Available from: http://www.nature.com/nrd/index.html. doi:10.1038/nrd4609.

Wolber, G., Langer, T., 2005. LigandScout: 3-D pharmacophores derived from protein-bound ligands and their use as virtual screening filters. J. Chem. Inf. Model. 1549-9596. 45 (1), 160–169. doi:10.1021/ci049885e.

World Health Organization (WHO), 2020. WHO Director-General's opening remarks at the media briefing on COVID-19 - 11 March 2020. Accessed online at: www.who.int.

Yang, K., Swanson, K., Jin, W., Coley, C., Eiden, P., Gao, H., Guzman-Perez, A., Hopper, T., Kelley, B., Mathea, M., Palmer, A., Settels, V., Jaakkola, T., Jensen, K., Barzilay, R., 2019. Analyzing learned molecular representations for property prediction. J. Chem. Inf. Model. 1549-9596. 59 (8), 3370–3388. doi:10.1021/acs.jcim.9b00237.

Ying, R., Bourgeois, D., You, J., Zitnik, M., Leskovec, J., 2019. GNNExplainer: generating explanations for graph neural networks. In: Advances in Neural Information Processing Systems, Vol. 32. 1049-5258. Neural information processing systems foundation, United States. https://papers.nips.cc/.

Zhang, L., Tan, J., Han, D., Zhu, H., 2017. From machine learning to deep learning: progress in machine intelligence for rational drug discovery. Drug Discov. Today. 1359-6446. 22 (11), 1680–1685. doi:10.1016/j.drudis.2017.08.010.

Zhao, X., Tian, Y., Zheng, C., 2025. Robust one-class support vector machine. Neural Netw. 0893-6080. 188, 107416. doi:10.1016/j.neunet.2025.107416.

Zhou, G., Rusnac, D.V., Park, H., Canzani, D., Nguyen, H.M., Stewart, L., Bush, M.F., Nguyen, P.T., Wulff, H., Yarov-Yarovoy, V., Zheng, N., DiMaio, F., 2024. An artificial intelligence accelerated virtual screening platform for drug discovery. Nat. Commun. 2041-1723. 15 (1). Available from: https://www.nature.com/ncomms/. doi:10.1038/s41467-024-52061-7.

Zhou, S.F., Zhong, W.Z., 2017. Drug design and discovery: principles and applications. Molecules. 1420-3049. 22 (2). Available from: http://www.mdpi.com/1420-3049/22/2/279/pdf. doi:10.3390/molecules22020279.

8

Natural language processing for drug discovery

Pankaj Tyagi[a], Ankish Arya[b], Prabhat Tripathi[b], Nidhi Dubey[b], Uma Shanker Tiwary[a], and Pritish Kumar Varadwaj[b]

[a]*Department of Information Technology, Indian Institute of Information Technology Allahabad, Prayagraj, Uttar Pradesh, India*

[b]*Systems Biology Lab, Department of Applied Sciences, Indian Institute of Information Technology Allahabad, Prayagraj, Uttar Pradesh, India*

1 Introduction

As a branch of artificial intelligence (AI), natural language processing (NLP) facilitates computers in processing, analyzing, interpreting, and performing operations on natural text or spoken data. It analyzes text or spoken data by utilizing syntactic and semantic analysis techniques. Over the past decade, NLP has made significant progress and is now deeply integrated into daily life, powering applications such as email filtering, voice assistants, language translations, electronic phone calls, and text analysis (Khurana et al., 2023). The enormous growth of big data in healthcare is paving the way for NLP to enhance the quality of healthcare. A significant challenge in the healthcare sector is that approximately 80% of medical data, such as text, images, and signals, remains unstructured and unutilized after being generated. NLP has demonstrated great potential in addressing this issue, particularly in model-informed drug development (MIDD) and healthcare, by improving the use and management of natural language data. It has facilitated the transition from labor-intensive data curation to automated and standardized processes for analyzing text and speech data. MIDD utilizes quantitative models to guide decision-making in drug discovery (Bhatnagar et al., 2022; Wang et al., 2019). NLP can be applied to extract valuable information from both structured and unstructured data sources, such as electronic health records (EHRs) and research papers, to optimize and speed up various stages of the drug development process. These processes include identifying drug-target and drug-drug interactions, discovering biomarkers, drug repurposing,

The AI Frontier in Molecular Modelling and Drug Designing. https://doi.org/10.1016/B978-0-443-40338-5.00003-2

conducting model-based metaanalyses, and modeling disease progression (Madabushi et al., 2022). NLP applications play a critical role by analyzing large volumes of scientific literature to uncover potential relationships between drugs, target proteins, and disease-related pathways. In addition, NLP can help expedite the repurposing of approved drugs for new conditions, allowing pharmacologists to address new markets more quickly and cost-effectively. Matching patients with clinical trials using automated text mining is another crucial application of NLP and AI (Tissot et al., 2020), offering a practical solution to save time and improve trial efficiency. This chapter explores various applications of NLP in drug discovery and development, covering the technical aspects of different tools and open-source resources for developing NLP models for MIDD applications. In addition, it covers basic NLP concepts, libraries, tools, techniques, algorithms, datasets, NLP models and their technical aspects, and NLP applications across various stages of the drug discovery and development lifecycle.

2 Basic concepts of NLP

Basic concepts of NLP include text preprocessing, feature extraction, and text representation and analysis techniques.

2.1 Text preprocessing

These text preprocessing techniques are used to transform raw text into an efficiently analyzable format; these techniques include tokenization, stemming, and lemmatization. These text preprocessing techniques can be implemented using the *Natural Language Toolkit (NLTK) Python* library (Bird et al., 2009).

1. **Tokenization:** This involves splitting texts into smaller units, such as words, sentences, or phrases. For instance, the following statement, "NLP simplifies language processing," is tokenized into ["NLP," "simplifies," "language," "processing"]. Tokenization is the most fundamental concept in NLP since most of the NLP operations operate on tokens.
2. **Stemming:** This reduces the word to its root form by stripping affixes. For example, "running", "runner", and "runs" are stemmed to "run". Stemming reduces words to vocabulary size, but it can produce nondictionary forms, like "studies" stemmed to "studi".
3. **Lemmatization:** Unlike stemming, lemmatization considers a word's grammatical structure to obtain its dictionary form (lemma). For example, "better" is lemmatized to "good". Lemmatization yields better output but requires more processing power.

2.2 Text feature extraction

Feature extraction techniques convert textual data into numerical features that algorithms can leverage. These techniques can be implemented in Python using the *NLTK* library. The following are the key feature extraction techniques:

1. **Bag of words (BoW):** In NLP, BoW represents a set of distinct words or tokens found within a given text or collection of documents.
2. **N-grams:** It is a sequence of n consecutive elements taken from a text or speech sample, where n is a positive number. In NLP, n-grams are frequently used to understand the contextual connections between words within a text.
3. **Count vectorization:** Text vectorization involves converting textual information into numerical vectors suitable for input into machine learning (ML) algorithms. One of the most common approaches is the bag-of-words technique, which represents text based on the presence and frequency of words without considering grammar or word order. This method can be implemented using the *Scikit-learn Python* library (Pedregosa et al., 2011).
4. **Term frequency-inverse document frequency (TF-IDF):** This is a numerical statistic used in text mining and information retrieval to reflect the importance of a word in a document relative to a collection (corpus) of documents. In this method, two matrices, Term Frequency (TF) and Inverse Document Frequency (IDF), are calculated. TF measures how frequently a term appears in a document, and IDF measures how unique or rare a term is across the corpus. This method is commonly applied in text classification, keyword extraction, and information retrieval.
5. **Word embedding:** Techniques like Word2Vec, GloVe, and contextual embeddings (e.g., Bidirectional Encoder Representations from Transformers (BERT)) are advanced methods to create dense vector representations of words, capturing semantic relationships and context. These methods use large datasets and advanced algorithms for meaningful word association compared to BoW or TF-IDF methods. Word2Vec and GloVe generate static embeddings, where each word has a single fixed vector representation regardless of the context in which it is used. On the other hand, contextual embeddings such as BERT change the representations of words according to the context, allowing for a more nuanced understanding, especially in complex sentences. These advancements have significantly improved performance in tasks such as machine translation, sentiment analysis, and question-answering.

2.3 Text sorting

Text sorting is an important NLP task, categorizing text into predefined labels or classes. It is used in applications such as sentiment analysis and spam detection, where text is classified into specific categories. Text sorting organizes textual data based on some criteria, such as alphabetical order, relevance, or predefined rules, and plays a key role in creating efficient data retrieval systems, ranking algorithms, and organizing large datasets for analysis. In Python, text sorting can be implemented using the *scikit-learn* library (Pedregosa et al., 2011).

2.4 Stop word removal

These are common words like "and," "the," or "is," which do not contribute much meaning to a text. They are, therefore, noise, and removing them can improve the performance of the algorithm. *NLTK* and *SpaCy* (spaCy) libraries include built-in stop-word lists, which can be modified for specific applications.

2.5 Named-entity-recognition

It involves methods to extract and identify specific entities from text, such as drugs, chemicals, and genes. Entities can be considered category types found within the text, such as the name of a particular drug, a chemical compound, a protein, etc. Named-entity-recognition (NER) can be implemented using *the spaCy* Python library.

2.6 Parts of speech tagging

It is used to assign grammatical labels to words in a text, such as verb, adjective, noun, etc. It is useful in syntactic parsing and is necessary for higher-level NLP tasks such as machine translation and text generation. Fig. 8.1 illustrates the summarization of basic concepts of NLP.

3 NLP techniques for drug discovery

The applications of NLP in drug discovery transform biomedical literature for further research. Key techniques include NER, relationship extraction, text summarization, sentiment analysis, and contextual embeddings. These provide deeper insights into drug mechanisms through the faster analysis of biomedical literature as a source for automated text analysis to establish drug targets.

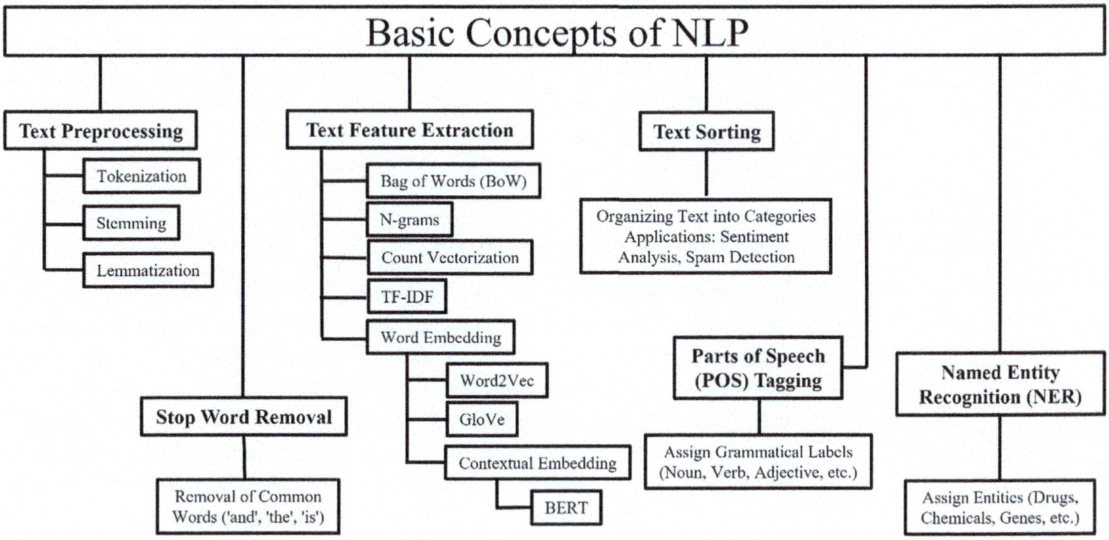

Fig. 8.1 Summarization of basic concepts of NLP.

3.1 Biomedical entity extraction

In this process, NER is used to extract biomedical entities, like drugs, genes, proteins, and diseases, from unstructured text sources, such as research papers, patents, and clinical records. Models such as SciSpacy (*https://github.com/allenai/scispacy*), BioBERT (Lee et al., 2020), PubMedBERT, and ChemNER (Wang et al., 2021) have provided very good results for specific terms. For example, BioBERT is used to extract drug names and disease entities from abstracts in PubMed. Likewise, ChemNER outperforms most of the other models in chemical compound drug design. A SciSpacy-driven case study has successfully identified gene-disease associations, helping to personalize medicine (Lee et al., 2020). The challenges are vague terminology and limited annotated data, but advanced models make drug development easier by automatically extracting key biomedical data.

3.2 Relation extraction

Relation Extraction identifies links between biomedical entities like drug-target and drug-disease relationships. Popular models for the task are BioBERT and SciBERT (Beltagy et al., 2019). In one such case, BioBERT made predictions on drug-target interactions from PubMed abstracts in a research direction on cancer therapy (Aldahdooh et al., 2022). In another case, extracting drug-drug interaction pairs from clinical trial reports aided drug repurposing efforts (KafiKang and Hendawi, 2023). Relations between drugs and diseases from EHRs have also been used to establish associations for hypertension and heart failure treatments. Relation extraction using NLP has shown great potential; however, there are some challenges, such as insufficient labeled data and ambiguous context.

3.3 Text summarization

Text summarization aims to distill complex biomedical literature into concrete conclusions. Abstractive models, such as Bidirectional and Auto-Regressive Transformers (BART) (*https://huggingface.co/docs/transformers/en/model_doc/bart*), generate concise summaries of text. SciBERT has even summarized clinical trial data, reducing manual review times. During the COVID-19 pandemic, summarization models tracked progress in vaccine development using the CORD-19 dataset. One study was successful in condensing clinical case studies, thereby supporting individual treatment decisions. Abstractive summarization is extremely difficult, especially in a domain-specific language; however, ongoing advances enable faster processing of massive scientific content in drug development and clinical trial management.

3.4 Sentiment and opinion analysis

Sentiment analysis is used to measure opinions about the efficacy, side effects, or safety of drugs from scientific reviews and patient forums. For example, RoBERTa (Liu et al., 2019) analyzes patient reviews on drugs (*https://www.drugs.com/*) to predict the levels of drug satisfaction. During the initial rollout of COVID-19 vaccines, sentiment analysis classified tweets as positive, negative, or neutral to inform public health messaging. Pharmaceutical enterprises depend on these insights for modifications in the market, whereas aspect-oriented sentiment analysis underscores apprehensions regarding adverse effects within clinical studies. Models tailored to specific domains that are trained on meticulously assembled biomedical datasets are crucial for precise sentiment assessment in healthcare settings.

3.5 Contextual embeddings in drug research

Contextual embeddings revolutionize biomedical NLP by capturing semantic meanings from vast text corpora. Models like BioBERT, ClinicalBERT (Huang et al., 2019), BioWordVec (Zhang et al., 2019), and BioSentVec (Chen et al., 2019) are remarkable in NER, relationship extraction, and literature summarization. Pretrained models, such as BioBERT, trained on abstracts of PubMed, have been applied in the extraction of drug-target interactions from DrugBank (*https://go.drugbank.com/*), while ClinicalBERT, which was fine-tuned on the patient records of the Medical Information Mart for Intensive Care (MIMIC-III) (Johnson et al., 2016), has predicted clinical outcomes and responses to treatment. BioWordVec has assisted in representing chemical compounds for drug repurposing, whereas BioSentVec supports systematic literature reviews. Transfer learning using general models like BERT strengthens these tasks by adapting them to biomedical text with minimal labeled data. A case study of therapeutic targets was found in COVID-19 studies, where BioBERT outperformed other language NLP models to identify the same (Liu et al., 2021). Despite the cost of pretraining and managing large biomedical vocabularies, models like BioBERT are being used for advancements in personalized medicine and drug discovery.

4 Tools and resources for NLP in drug discovery

In the context of drug discovery, NLP tools are designed to analyze unstructured biomedical text, including scientific literature, clinical records, and patents, to derive valuable insights. These tools utilize domain-specific ontologies, patterns, and ML models to facilitate the interpretation of complex biomedical data.

4.1 Biomedical NLP tools and pretrained models

A. PubTator: It is used to extract knowledge and curate scientific literature and annotates biomedical text with genes, diseases, and chemicals (Wei et al., 2024).

B. BioBERT: It is a pretrained transformer model for biomedical texts. It's applicable for disease-gene relationship discovery and the analysis of drug-target interactions (Lee et al., 2020). Its strength lies in text extraction and document classification.

C. NLTK: It is a general NLP library adapted for text mining in biomedical contexts and records. It is used for hypothesis generation and scientific literature analysis.

D. ChemDataExtractor: These tools extract chemical information, such as the name of a compound, its properties, and their related reactions, from text. Its primary focus is on compound discovery and reaction database development (Swain and Cole, 2016).

E. PubMedBERT: It is pretrained on PubMed abstracts and PMC articles, and it can be used for scientific literature mining for drug discovery.

F. **MolBERT:** MolBERT processes SMILES notation and molecular data to predict drug-target interactions using molecular text descriptors. It leverages chemical similarity learning for virtual screening and integrates textual and structural chemical information (Li and Jiang, 2021).

G. **AlphaFold:** AlphaFold was developed by DeepMind to predict protein 3D structures. It can be used in drug discovery to better understand the drug-target binding mechanism and to design novel therapeutics by analyzing protein conformations (Jumper et al., 2021).

Details of the above tools and other pretrained models are provided in Table 8.1.

4.2 Databases for drug discovery

A. **PubMed:** It is a database of biomedical scientific literature that acts as a primary source. It helps in text mining to discover drug-disease relationships and their therapeutic pathways.

B. **ChEMBL:** This database contains information about bioactive molecules, including molecular targets and drug-like properties (Zdrazil et al., 2024). It can be used to integrate with ML models to prioritize drug candidates.

Table 8.1 List of NLP tools and pretrained models used in drug discovery.

Models	Pretrained on	Architecture	Built-on	Reference/Source
BioBERT	PubMed	Transformer	BERT	Lee et al. (2020)
SciBERT	Semantic Scholar	Transformer	BERT	
ClinicalBERT	MIMIC III	Transformer	BERT	
BioMed-RoBERTa	Semantic scholar	Transformer	RoBERTa	Liu et al. (2019)
BioALBERT	PubMed, PMC, MIMIC III	Transformer	ALBERT	https://github.com/usmaann/BioALBERT
MolBERT	SMILES, molecular structures	Transformer	BERT	https://github.com/BenevolentAI/MolBERT
PubMedBERT	PubMed and PMC	Transformer	BERT	https://huggingface.co/NeuML/pubmedbert-base-embeddings/tree/main
AlphaFold	UniProt and PDB	Deep learning	TensorFlow	Jumper et al. (2021)

C. **DrugBank:** This database consists of drugs, which include biological, chemical, molecular, and pharmacological information (Knox et al., 2024). It can be used to extract drug interactions, discover targets, and analyze the mechanism of action, etc.
D. **ClinicalTrials:** It is a publicly available database governed by the US National Library of Medicine (NLM). It provides information about clinical studies to the public, researchers, and the healthcare sector. Clinical studies contain information about their design, status, interventions, and outcomes of a study.
E. **PubChem:** An open-access chemistry database offering detailed information on molecules, including chemical structures, identifiers, physical and chemical properties, and biological activities.
F. **Drug Target Commons (DTC)**: A crowd-sourced database stores drug-target bioactivity information and target classifications.
G. **Search Tool for Interactions of Chemicals (STITCH):** A repository of predicted and known protein and chemical interactions includes 9,643,763 proteins from 2031 different organisms.
H. **Side Effect Resource (SIDER):** A repository of available drugs and their known adverse reactions.
I. **ChemDB:** A data repository for chemicals and their physicochemical properties. It contains information on approximately 5 million small molecules.
J. **DGIdb:** Druggable Genomes and drug-target information database, compiled from over 30 trusted sources. Details of the aforementioned databases are shown in Table 8.2.

Table 8.2 List of databases for NLP-based drug discovery.

Database	Database URL
PubMed	https://pubmed.ncbi.nlm.nih.gov/
ChEMBL	https://www.ebi.ac.uk/chembl/
DrugBank	http://www.drugbank.ca
ClinicalTrials	https://clinicaltrials.gov/
PubChem	https://pubchem.ncbi.nlm.nih.gov/
DTC	http://drugtargetcommons.fimm.fi/
STITCH	http://stitch.embl.de/
SIDER	http://sideeffects.embl.de
ChemDB	http://cdb.ics.uci.edu
DGIdb	http://www.dgidb.org

5 Machine learning platforms and frameworks for NLP-driven drug discovery

ML frameworks and platforms are important in drug discovery and in facilitating NLP applications. They represent a computational backbone to build, train, and deploy ML models capable of interpreting complex biomedical literature. These models facilitate automation tasks such as literature mining, text classification, drug-drug interaction, and drug-target prediction, which can accelerate the drug discovery process.

A. **TensorFlow:** It is a widely used open-source framework designed by Google for scalable deep learning (DL) and ML applications. It supports various ML/DL algorithms, which include recurrent networks and transformers (Abadi et al., 2016). In the context of drug discovery, TensorFlow assists in fine-tuning pretrained NLP biomedical models such as BioBERT, which creates an advantage for researchers when it comes to capitalizing on domain-specific information for tasks like text classification.
B. **PyTorch:** PyTorch is a flexible, open-source DL framework developed by Meta. It offers a developer-friendly design, and its dynamic computation graph provides advantages in debugging and model customization. In addition, robust GPU and distributed training support ensure the effective processing of extensive datasets and computationally demanding tasks (Paszke et al., 2019). In drug discovery, it actively trains customized models for text summarization and relation extraction, assisting in extracting critical insights from biomedical literature.
C. **AutoNLP:** It is an automated NLP tool that simplifies the building and deploying of NLP models. Its user-friendly interface requires minimal ML expertise, which allows researchers to utilize pre-trained models such as BioBERT and SciBERT. In drug discovery, it plays a significant role by automating the extraction of drug-disease relationships from biomedical literature, classifying clinical trial results, optimizing complex data analysis, and accelerating therapeutic developments.
D. **Azure ML:** It is a cloud service developed by Microsoft to accelerate and manage ML projects. It provides a platform for building, training, and deploying ML models. It offers end-to-end pipeline management, simplifying the workflow for researchers and developers. Its excellent integration with leading frameworks like TensorFlow and PyTorch enhances its functional role and capabilities. In drug discovery, this platform effectively scales NLP models for processing vast biomedical literature and automates complex tasks via cloud-based NLP pipelines.

Table 8.3 illustrates the various ML and NLP libraries supported by these ML platforms.

Table 8.3 List of various machine learning and NLP libraries.

NLP library	programming language	Usefulness	Characteristics	Source/URL
Gensim	Python	Topic modeling, word embeddings	Unsupervised topic modeling, memory-efficient, scalable	https://github.com/RaRe-Technologies/gensim
CoreNLP	Java	Full NLP pipeline	Syntactic parsing, named entity recognition, and robust linguistic analysis	https://stanfordnlp.github.io/CoreNLP/
SciSpacy	Python	Biomedical text processing	Pretrained biomedical models integrate with SpaCy	https://allenai.github.io/scispacy/
SparkNLP	Python, Java, Scala, R	Large-scale NLP pipelines	Distributed NLP, deep learning support, scalable via Apache Spark	https://github.com/JohnSnowLabs/spark-nlp
SpaCy	Python	Industrial-strength NLP	Fast, production-ready, efficient pipelines	https://spacy.io/
NLTK	Python	Teaching and prototyping	Educational, extensive documentation, and a wide range of algorithms	https://www.nltk.org/
Scikit learn	Python	Machine learning integration	Classical ML algorithms, model evaluation, integration with NLP pipelines	https://scikit-learn.org/
Hugging Face	Python	Transformer-based NLP	Pretrained models, model hub, support BERT, GPT, etc.	https://huggingface.co/
Spacyr	R	SpaCy integration in R	Leverages SpaCy's capabilities in R	https://cran.r-project.org/web/packages/spacyr/
Flair	Python	Simple interfaces for advanced NLP	Stacked embeddings, multilingual support, sequence tagging	https://github.com/flairNLP/flair

6 Evaluation metrics for NLP in drug discovery

Evaluation metrics play an extremely key role in measuring the effectiveness of NLP models on drug discovery tasks, primarily in named entity relation extraction and information retrieval. Important metrics are:

1. **Accuracy:** It provides the ratio of correct predictions to the total predictions. However, it cannot be used when datasets are imbalanced, which is a frequent issue encountered in biomedical research (Naidu et al., 2023).

$$\text{Accuracy} = (\text{TP} + \text{TN})/(\text{TP} + \text{TN} + \text{FP} + \text{FN})$$

Where TP is True Positive, TN is True Negative, FP is False Positive, and FN is False Negative.

2. **Precision:** It provides the ratio of true positives with respect to all positive predictions, which is vital in discovering drug-target interactions, where false positives could divert the research findings.

$$\text{Precision} = \text{TP}/(\text{TP} + \text{FP})$$

3. **Recall:** It depicts the ratio of true positive classifications to the overall positives. This is crucial in exhaustive drug-disease association studies.

$$\text{Recall} = \text{TP}/(\text{TP} + \text{FN})$$

4. **F1-Score:** It combines precision and recall into a balanced metric, frequently applied in Named Entity Recognition (NER) (e.g., sentiment analysis) and classification tasks in drug discovery.

$$\text{F-score} = 2 \times (\text{precision} \times \text{recall})/(\text{precision} + \text{recall})$$

5. **Receiver operating characteristic curve (ROC curve):** It assesses binary classification models, such as the prediction of adverse drug reactions. The ROC curve is created by calculating the true positive rates (TP/(TP + FN)) and false positive rates (FP/(FP + TN)) at every possible threshold. Plotting the area under the ROC curve (AUC - Area Under the Curve) measures the ML algorithm's performance (Bradley, 1997). A perfect model has an AUC of 1. An illustration of a typical ROC curve is provided in Fig. 8.2.
6. **Mean reciprocal rank (MRR):** MRR assesses how effectively a drug discovery model ranks relevant drug candidates. It determines the position of the first relevant molecule in a ranking of predictions. If the first relevant drug is present at rank k, then: reciprocal Rank (RR) = 1/k.

$$MRR = \frac{1}{N}\sum_{i=1}^{N}\frac{1}{K_i}$$

Where, N is the number of queries (e.g., targets), and K_i is the position of the first relevant drug.

7. **BLEU score:** The BLEU score evaluates the similarity between machine-generated text and human reference translations by analyzing n-gram overlap. It is an extensively used metric for assessing the performance of machine translation models. However, it has some disadvantages, such as not capturing fluency or grammatical correctness and having a high sensitivity to the choice of reference translations.
8. **Rouge score:** The ROUGE score assesses how much machine-generated text overlaps with human-written summaries by examining n-gram precision and recall. It is commonly used to evaluate text summarization systems. However, it has limitations, such as its

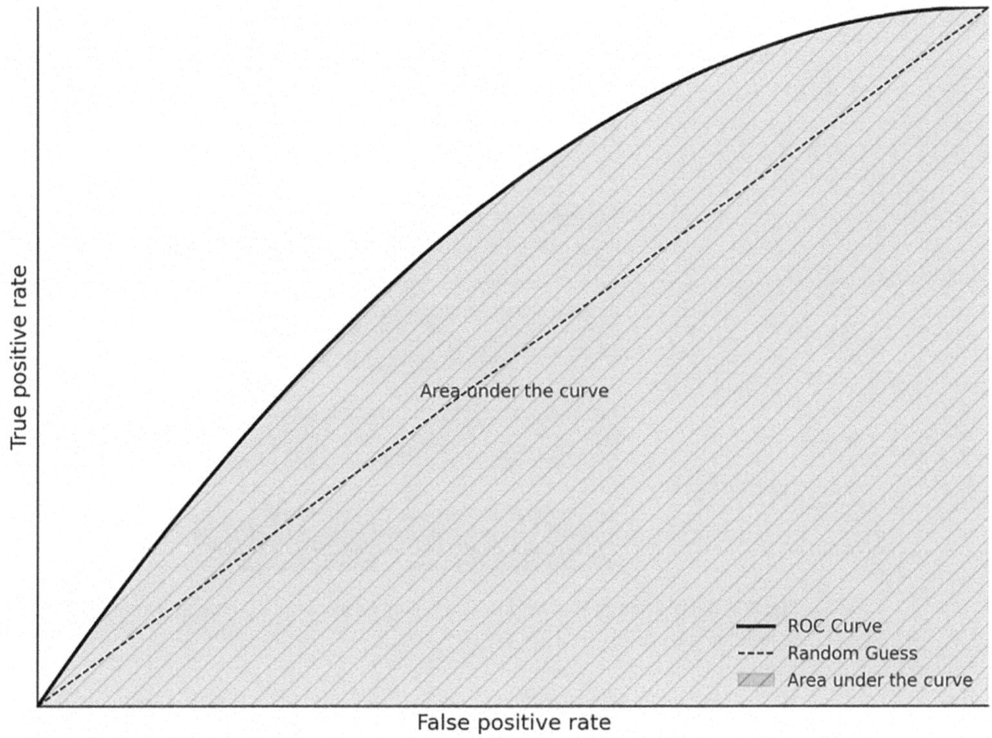

Fig. 8.2 A description of the receiver operating characteristic (ROC) curve.

lack of sensitivity to the selection of reference summaries and its failure to account for semantic similarity between texts.

9. **Perplexity:** It is the measure of how effectively a large language model predicts the next word in a given sequence. Perplexity is simple to understand and allows for comparisons between models of varying sizes. Despite its usefulness, perplexity has drawbacks, such as not directly assessing the quality of generated text and being significantly affected by infrequent words and n-grams.

7 Workflow to extract information from scientific literature

An algorithmic workflow to extract valuable information from scientific literature and patent repositories is presented in this section. Fig. 8.3 illustrates the summarized workflow.

Step 1: Data acquisition and preprocessing

- Collect data from PubMed, clinical trials, and patent repositories such as USPTO (United States Patent and Trademark Office), EPO (European Patent Office), and PubMed.

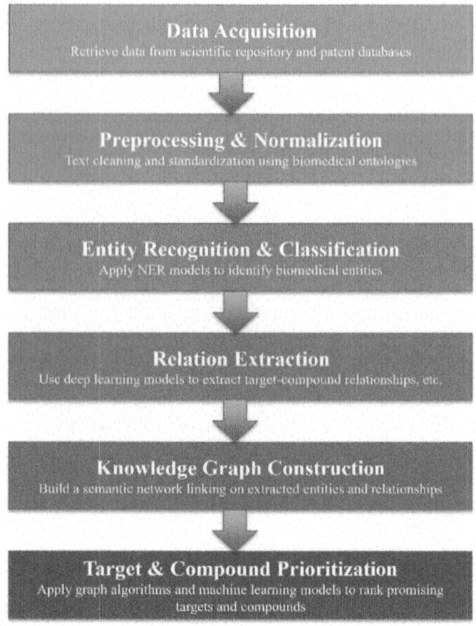

Fig. 8.3 Illustration of the workflow pipeline to extract valuable information from scientific literature.

- Perform text cleaning, such as tokenization, lemmatization, and removal of stop words and noise.
- Apply NER to identify genes, proteins, diseases, chemicals, etc.

Step 2: Information extraction

- Use dependency parsing and semantic role labeling to understand context and relationships.
- Employ relation extraction models, such as BERT-based classifiers, to detect interactions.
- Extract cooccurrence patterns and map them to biological ontologies (e.g., MeSH (Medical Subject Headings), GO (Gene Ontology).

Step 3: Knowledge graph (KG) construction

- Build a domain-specific KG to visualize and structure the relationships.
- Construct a graph network from extracted entities and relationships.
- Apply graph-based algorithms to detect novel relationships and influential nodes.

Step 4: Target compound prioritization

- Rank entities based on relevance and novelty.
- Use ML models like neural networks, random forests, and DL for predictive scoring.
- Validate top candidates through cross-referencing with experimental databases.

Step 5: Insight generation and hypothesis formation

- Generate interpretable reports highlighting new therapeutic leads.
- Suggest hypotheses for experimental validation.
- Enable iterative refinement by integrating feedback from wet-lab experiments.

8 Applications of NLP in drug discovery

NLP has emerged as a transformative tool in drug discovery and offers innovative solutions to complex challenges in biomedical and pharmaceutical research. This section explores six key applications of NLP that are revolutionizing the drug discovery process. The process of drug discovery and the use of NLP in various stages are illustrated in Fig. 8.4.

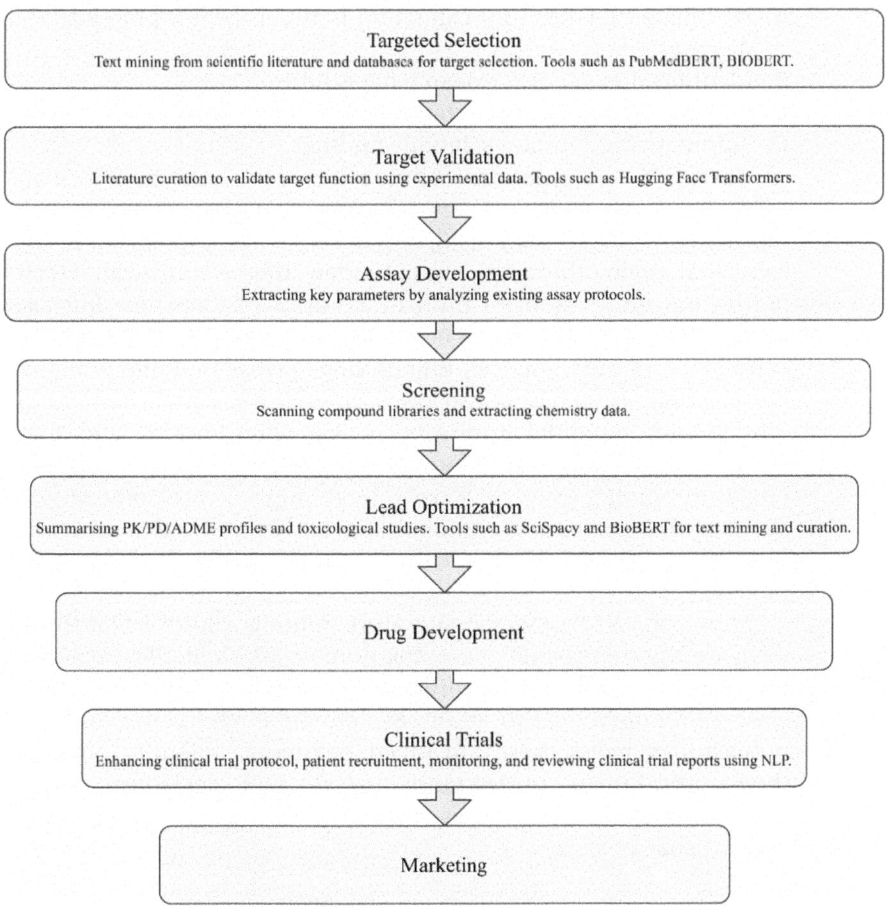

Fig. 8.4 Illustration of using NLP in various stages of drug discovery.

8.1 Literature mining for drug discovery

Literature mining is one of the key applications of NLP to speed up scientific discovery; NLP-powered literature mining reduces research time by as much as 70% and enables faster discovery of potential drug targets. In light of the exponential increase in scientific publications, the task of manual literature review becomes increasingly daunting; thus, NLP becomes a crucial tool in drug discovery research. NLP offers a variety of sophisticated automated extraction and synthesis techniques that can extract useful insights from huge biomedical literature databases, transforming how researchers identify and analyze potential drug targets. The use of NLP techniques automates the extraction of valuable information from large repositories of scientific literature for rapid knowledge synthesis (Zhang et al., 2020).

The following are the key capabilities of NLP in literature mining:

A. Automated relationship extraction between genes, proteins, and diseases
B. Identification of novel research hypotheses
C. Tracking emerging research trends
D. Summarizing complex scientific findings

Advanced computational approaches now leverage ML algorithms and semantic analysis to parse complex scientific texts, extracting nuanced relationships between genes, proteins, and diseases that might otherwise remain hidden. These sophisticated techniques not only automate the extraction of relationships but also facilitate the identification of novel research hypotheses through the connection of different scientific findings across multiple domains. For example, researchers can track emerging research trends rapidly, identify potential drug repurposing opportunities, and summarize complex scientific findings with unprecedented efficiency. Literature mining using NLP has a huge impact, with some studies showing that such computational approaches can reduce research time by up to 70%, dramatically accelerating the drug discovery process.

Moreover, NLP-powered literature mining allows scientists to navigate the increasingly complex domain of biomedical research in a way that provides comprehensive insights, which would otherwise be impractical to attain. Systematic analysis of millions of publications helps these advanced techniques identify potential therapeutic targets, understand intricate biological mechanisms, and generate innovative research hypotheses better than ever before (Zhao et al., 2021).

8.2 Drug repurposing

It offers a strategic alternative to traditional drug development, and NLP can play a critical role in this process. By analyzing medical literature, EHRs, and scientific databases, NLP can uncover hidden drug-disease connections using advanced ML algorithms and semantic analysis. These techniques enable automated hypothesis generation, identifying new therapeutic uses for existing drugs with high precision. NLP-driven approaches can reduce drug development costs by up to 60% and significantly accelerate timelines, transforming the process of drug repurposing and enabling researchers to explore novel treatment strategies with reduced risks (Steiert et al., 2024).

8.3 Clinical trial matching

Patient recruitment for clinical trials of a drug is the most time-consuming process in drug development. NLP can play a pivotal role in clinical trials by enhancing patient recruitment, protocol analysis, and data management. It helps automate the extraction and interpretation of data from unstructured sources such as EHRs or medical narratives, which assist in matching eligible participants to clinical trial criteria more effectively. NLP can analyze clinical trial protocols by identifying key requirements for eligibility, endpoints, and factors critical to compliance using semantic parsing and ML algorithms. In addition, it can make trial management efficient and synthesize huge datasets while improving insights in real-time for better decision-making in drug discovery pipelines. This can lead to speedier recruitment, cost efficiency, and better protocol compliance, thus making the clinical trial process more efficient (Ni et al., 2019).

8.4 Predicting drug-drug interactions

The prediction of drug-drug interactions is also an important task in healthcare and an issue of patient safety. NLP is a strong solution for the prediction of pharmacological interactions, utilizing ML algorithms and semantic analysis of medical literature and clinical data (Han et al., 2022). Beyond text processing, NLP combines structured and unstructured data to develop predictive models, identifying subtle relationships and contraindications while offering early warnings for risky drug combinations. Various studies have indicated that NLP can achieve over 75% accuracy in detecting interactions, thereby enhancing pharmaco-vigilance and reducing adverse drug events. This innovation in medical informatics supports the safer and more effective use of medication (Shi et al., 2024).

8.5 Biomarker discovery

Biomarker discovery is one of the important areas in precision medicine, which can revolutionize diagnostics and therapies through the identification of molecular signatures. NLP has a major role in applying advanced ML and semantic analysis to analyze complex biomedical data, mine scientific literature, integrate multiomics data, and reveal hidden relationships across genetic, proteomic, and clinical datasets. Research indicates that NLP might even increase the speed of biomarker identification by as much as 40%, accelerating drug development by analyzing unstructured data in the form of research articles and clinical trial information. The innovation enhances personalized medicine, as it delves in-depth into biological systems and allows for more focused therapeutic strategies.

8.6 Knowledge graph construction

KG construction represents a sophisticated computational approach to organizing and understanding complex scientific information (Jeynes et al., 2023). KGs in drug discovery represent information about entities and their relationships. KGs are constructed using triples of the head, relation, and tail entities (h, r, t), where entities are nodes and relations are links between entities. Basic approaches that are being used to construct KGs include translational models using distance-based scoring, semantic matching models, graph convolutional networks, attention networks, and context-based encoding approaches. NLP techniques facilitate sophisticated relationship extraction from unstructured text, semantic linking of scientific concepts, and automated ontology development, transforming how scientists comprehend and explore complex KGs. By integrating information from multiple sources, these NLP-powered KGs provide unprecedented insights into intricate biological systems, research connections, and potential scientific discoveries. Empirical research demonstrates the remarkable potential of this approach, with studies indicating that NLP-driven KGs can significantly enhance information synthesis, reduce research redundancy, and accelerate scientific understanding (Mondal et al., 2021).

9 Challenges and limitations

NLP integration in drug discovery is a novel yet challenging approach within computational biomedical research. There is the significant challenge of processing scientific and medical literature, which tends to be unstructured and very noisy, necessitating sophisticated approaches for understanding the complex terminologies at the domain level, linguistic complexities, as well as contextual nuances (Jeynes et al., 2023).

Another concern is interpretability, as the "black box" nature of many ML models undermines transparency and confidence, especially in high-stakes medical research. Furthermore, there are ethical and regulatory concerns to address, including algorithmic bias, data privacy issues, and technical challenges such as handling domain-specific terminology and semantic variations in scientific texts. In addition, representing complex relationships between biomedical concepts requires careful consideration before this technology can be adopted for clinical purposes (Wong et al., 2018). Data quality and representation are also major obstacles due to variability in terminology and reporting standards. Developing mechanisms to standardize and integrate diverse sources is essential for adopting NLP technology in drug discovery.

10 Conclusion

The use of NLP in drug discovery can revolutionize breakthroughs in scientific research and medical innovation. Hybrid models are emerging, combining NLP with advanced ML algorithms to overcome current limitations, thereby presenting a more holistic approach toward biomedical knowledge exploration, designed for near-human levels of semantic reasoning. These models can transform how researchers discover, interpret, and apply complex medical insights. Another important focus area is the development of context-aware NLP models that can capture subtle relationships and nuances in biomedical texts. With DL architectures and transformer-based models, researchers can extract, synthesize, and translate scientific information into actionable medical advancements with unprecedented accuracy. Moreover, NLP is transforming clinical trials by addressing critical challenges in patient recruitment and data analysis. It extracts key insights from unstructured data sources. This data, including trial reports and digital health records, improves patient trial matching and reduces recruitment delays, impacting 86% of all trials. In addition, NLP facilitates real-time monitoring and adverse event detection, ultimately improving safety outcomes. Regardless of challenges such as data privacy, NLP yields cost-effective solutions that enhance trial success rates and accelerate drug development timelines.

References

Abadi, M., Agarwal, A., Barham, P., Brevdo, E., Chen, Z., Citro, C., Corrado, G.S., Devis, A., Dean, J., Devin, M., Ghemawat, S. , 2016. Tensorflow: large-scale machine learning on heterogeneous distributed systems. arXiv preprint arXiv:1603.04467.

Aldahdooh, J., Vähä-Koskela, M., Tang, J., Tanoli, Z., 2022. Using BERT to identify drug-target interactions from whole PubMed. BMC Bioinform. 1471-2105. 23 (1). doi:10.1186/s12859-022-04768-x.

Beltagy, I., Lo, K., Cohan, A. 2019 SCIBERT: a pretrained language model for scientific text. In: EMNLP-IJCNLP 2019 - 2019 Conference on Empirical Methods in Natural Language Processing and 9th International Joint Conference on Natural Language Processing, Proceedings of the Conference. 9781950737901. Association for Computational Linguistics, United States, pp. 3615–3620.

Bhatnagar, R., Sardar, S., Beheshti, M., Podichetty, J.T., 2022. How can natural language processing help model informed drug development?: a review. JAMIA Open. 2574-2531. 5 (2). Available from: https://academic.oup.com/jamiaopen. doi:10.1093/jamiaopen/ooac043.

Bird, S., Klein, E., Loper, E. , 2009 . Natural Language Processing with Python: Analyzing Text with the Natural Language Toolkit. 1st edn. Sebastopol, C.A: O'Reilly Media. ISBN 978-0-596-51649-9.

Bradley, A.P., 1997. The use of the area under the ROC curve in the evaluation of machine learning algorithms. Pattern Recognit. 0031-3203. 30 (7), 1145–1159. Available from: www.elsevier.com/inca/publications/store/3/2/8/. doi:10.1016/S0031-3203(96)00142-2.

Charles, J., Jeynes, G., James, T., Corney, M., 2023. Natural language processing for drug discovery knowledge graphs: promises and Pitfalls. In: Methods in Molecular Biology, Vol. 2716. Science and Business Media LLC, pp. 223–240. doi:10.1007/978-1-0716-3449-3_10.

Chen, Q., Peng, Y., Lu, Z. 2019 BioSentVec: creating sentence embeddings for biomedical texts. IEEE International Conference on Healthcare Informatics, ICHI 2019. 9781538691380. Institute of Electrical and Electronics Engineers Inc., United States. http://ieeexplore.ieee.org/xpl/mostRecentIssue.jsp?punumber=8895688. doi:10.1109/ICHI.2019.8904728.

Han, K., Cao, P., Wang, Y., Xie, F., Ma, J., Yu, M., Wang, J., Xu, Y., Zhang, Y., Wan, J., 2022. A review of approaches for predicting drug–drug interactions based on machine learning. Front. Pharmacol. 1663-9812. 12. doi:10.3389/fphar.2021.814858.

Huang, K., Altosaar, J., Ranganath, R., 2019. ClinicalBert: modeling clinical notes and predicting hospital readmission. arXiv. 2331-8422. Available from: https://arxiv.org. doi:10.48550/arxiv.1904.05342.

Jeynes, J.C.G., Corney, M., James, T., Tayara, H., 2023. A large-scale evaluation of NLP-derived chemical-gene/protein relationships from the scientific literature: implications for knowledge graph construction. PLoS ONE. 1932-6203. 18 (9), e0291142. doi:10.1371/journal.pone.0291142.

Johnson, A.E.W., Pollard, T.J., Shen, L., Lehman, L.W.H., Feng, M., Ghassemi, M., Moody, B., Szolovits, P., Celi, L.A., Mark, R.G., 2016. MIMIC-III, a freely accessible critical care database. Sci. Data. 2052-4463. 3. Available from: https://www.nature.com/sdata/. doi:10.1038/sdata.2016.35.

Jumper, J., Evans, R., Pritzel, A., Green, T., Figurnov, M., Ronneberger, O., Tunyasuvunakool, K., Bates, R., Žídek, A., Potapenko, A., Bridgland, A., Meyer, C., Kohl, S.A.A., Ballard, A.J., Cowie, A., Romera-Paredes, B., Nikolov, S., Jain, R., Adler, J., Back, T., Petersen, S., Reiman, D., Clancy, E., Zielinski, M., Steinegger, M., Pacholska, M., Berghammer, T., Bodenstein, S., Silver, D., Vinyals, O., Senior, A.W., Kavukcuoglu, K., Kohli, P., Hassabis, D., 2021. Highly accurate protein structure prediction with AlphaFold. Nature. 0028-0836. 596 (7873), 583–589. doi:10.1038/s41586-021-03819-2.

KafiKang, M., Hendawi, A., 2023. Drug-drug interaction extraction from biomedical text using relation BioBERT with BLSTM. Mach. Learn. Knowl. Extr. 2504-4990. 5 (2), 669–683. doi:10.3390/make5020036.

Khurana, D., Koli, A., Khatter, K., Singh, S., 2023. Natural language processing: state of the art, current trends and challenges. Multimed. Tools Appl. 1380-7501. 82 (3), 3713–3744. doi:10.1007/s11042-022-13428-4.

Knox, C., Wilson, M., Klinger, C.M., Franklin, M., Oler, E., Wilson, A., Pon, A., Cox, J., Chin, N.E.L., Strawbridge, S.A., Garcia-Patino, M., Kruger, R., Sivakumaran, A.,

Sanford, S., Doshi, R., Khetarpal, N., Fatokun, O., Doucet, D., Zubkowski, A., Rayat, D.Y., Jackson, H., Harford, K., Anjum, A., Zakir, M., Wang, F., Tian, S., Lee, B., Liigand, J., Peters, H., Wang, R.Q.R., Nguyen, T., So, D., Sharp, M., da Silva, R., Gabriel, C., Scantlebury, J., Jasinski, M., Ackerman, D., Jewison, T., Sajed, T., Gautam, V., Wishart, D.S., 2024. DrugBank 6.0: the DrugBank Knowledgebase for 2024. Nucleic Acids Res. 1362-4962. 52 (1), D1265. Available from: https://academic.oup.com/nar/issue. doi:10.1093/nar/gkad976.

Lee, J., Yoon, W., Kim, S., Kim, D., Kim, S., So, C.H., Kang, J., 2020. BioBERT: a pre-trained biomedical language representation model for biomedical text mining. Bioinformatics. 1460-2059. 36 (4), 1234–1240. Available from: http://bioinformatics.oxfordjournals.org/. doi:10.1093/bioinformatics/btz682.

Li, J., Jiang, X., 2021. Mol-BERT: an effective molecular representation with BERT for molecular property prediction. Wirel. Commun. Mob. Comput. 1530-8677. 2021. Available from: https://www.hindawi.com/journals/wcmc/. doi:10.1155/2021/7181815.

Liu, Y., Ott, M., Goyal, N., Du, J., Joshi, M., Chen, D., Levy, O., Lewis, M., Zettlemoyer, L., Stoyanov, V., 2019. RoBERTa: a robustly optimized BERT pretraining approach. arXiv. 2331-8422. Available from: https://arxiv.org. doi:10.48550/arxiv.1907.11692.

Liu, Z., Roberts, R.A., Lal-Nag, M., Chen, X., Huang, R., Tong, W., 2021. AI-based language models powering drug discovery and development. Drug Discov. Today. 1878-5832. 26 (11), 2593–2607. Available from: www.elsevier.com/locate/drugdiscov. doi:10.1016/j.drudis.2021.06.009.

Madabushi, R., Seo, P., Zhao, L., Tegenge, M., Zhu, H., 2022. Review: role of model-informed drug development approaches in the lifecycle of drug development and regulatory decision-making. Pharm. Res. 0724-8741. 39 (8), 1669–1680. doi:10.1007/s11095-022-03288-w.

Mondal, I., Hou, Y., Jochim, C., 2021. End-to-end NLP knowledge graph construction. arXiv. 2331-8422. Available from: https://arxiv.org.

Naidu, G., Zuva, T., Sibanda, E.M., 2023. A Review of Evaluation Metrics in Machine Learning Algorithms. In: Lecture Notes in Networks and Systems, Vol. 724. Springer Science and Business Media Deutschland GmbH, South Africa, pp. 15–25. 23673389 https://www.springer.com/series/15179. doi:10.1007/978-3-031-35314-7_2.

Ni, Y., Bermudez, M., Kennebeck, S., Liddy-Hicks, S., Dexheimer, J., 2019. A real-time automated patient screening system for clinical trials eligibility in an emergency department: design and evaluation. JMIR Med. Inform. 2291-9694. 7 (3), e14185. doi:10.2196/14185.

Paszke, A., Gross, S., Massa, F., Lerer, A., Bradbury, J., Chanan, G., Killeen, T., Lin, Z., Gimelshein, N., Antiga, L., Desmaison, A., Köpf, A., Yang, E., DeVito, Z., Raison, M., Tejani, A., Chilamkurthy, S., Steiner, B., Fang, L., Bai, J., Chintala, S. 2019 PyTorch: an imperative style, high-performance deep learning library. Adv. Neural Inf. Process. Sys. 1049-5258. 32. https://papers.nips.cc/.

Pedregosa, F., Varoquaux, G., Gramfort, A., Michel, V., Thirion, B., Grisel, O., Blondel, M., Prettenhofer, P., Weiss, R., Dubourg, V., Vanderplas, J., Passos, A., Cournapeau, D., Brucher, M., Perrot, M., Duchesnay, E., 2011. Scikit-learn: machine learning in Python. J. Mach. Learn. Res. 1533-7928. 12, 2825–2830. Available from: http://jmlr.csail.mit.edu/papers/volume12/pedregosa11a/pedregosa11a.pdf.

Shi, Y., He, M., Chen, J., Han, F., Cai, Y., Gallo, J., 2024. SubGE-DDI: a new prediction model for drug-drug interaction established through biomedical texts and drug-pairs knowledge subgraph enhancement. PLoS Comput. Biol. 1553-7358. 20 (4), e1011989. doi:10.1371/journal.pcbi.1011989.

Steiert, D., Wittig, C., Banerjee, P., Preissner, R., Szulcek, R., Li, F., 2024. An exploration into CTEPH medications: combining natural language processing, embedding learning, in vitro models, and real-world evidence for drug repurposing. PLoS Comput. Biol. 1553-7358. 20 (9), e1012417. doi:10.1371/journal.pcbi.1012417.

Swain, M.C., Cole, J.M., 2016. ChemDataExtractor: a Toolkit for automated extraction of chemical information from the scientific literature. J. Chem. Inf. Model. 1549-960X. 56 (10), 1894–1904. Available from: http://pubs.acs.org/journal/jcisd8. doi:10.1021/acs.jcim.6b00207.

Tissot, H.C., Shah, A.D., Brealey, D., Harris, S., Agbakoba, R., Folarin, A., Romao, L., Roguski, L., Dobson, R., Asselbergs, F.W., 2020. Natural language processing for mimicking clinical trial recruitment in critical care: a semi-automated simulation based on the LeoPARDS trial. IEEE J. Biomed. Health Inform. 2168-2208. 24 (10), 2950–2959. Available from: http://ieeexplore.ieee.org/xpl/RecentIssue.jsp?punumber=6221020. doi:10.1109/JBHI.2020.2977925.

Wang, X., Hu, V., Song, X., Garg, S., Xiao, J., Han, J., 2021. CHEMNER: fine-grained chemistry named entity recognition with ontology-guided distant supervision. In: EMNLP 2021—2021 Conference on Empirical Methods in Natural Language Processing, Proceedings. 9781955917094. Association for Computational Linguistics (ACL), United States, pp. 5227–5240. doi:10.18653/v1/2021.emnlp-main.424.

Wang, Y., Zhu, H., Madabushi, R., Liu, Q., Huang, S.M., Zineh, I., 2019. Model-informed drug development: current US regulatory practice and future considerations. Clin. Pharmacol. Ther. 1532-6535. 105 (4), 899–911. Available from: http://onlinelibrary.wiley.com/journal/10.1002/(ISSN)1532-6535. doi:10.1002/cpt.1363.

Wei, C.-H., Allot, A., Lai, P.-T., Leaman, R., Tian, S., Luo, L., Jin, Q., Wang, Z., Chen, Q., Lu, Z., 2024. PubTator 3.0: an AI-powered literature resource for unlocking biomedical knowledge. Nucleic Acids Res. 0305-1048. 52 (W1), W540. doi:10.1093/nar/gkae235.

Wong, A., Plasek, J.M., Montecalvo, S.P., Zhou, L., 2018. Natural language processing and its implications for the future of medication safety: a narrative review of recent advances and challenges. Pharmacotherapy. 0277-0008. 38 (8), 822–841. doi:10.1002/phar.2151.

Zdrazil, B., Felix, E., Hunter, F., Manners, E.J., Blackshaw, J., Corbett, S., de Veij, M., Ioannidis, H., Lopez, D.M., Mosquera, J.F., Magarinos, M.P., Bosc, N., Arcila, R., Kizilören, T., Gaulton, A., Bento, A.P., Adasme, M.F., Monecke, P., Landrum, G.A., Leach, A.R., 2024. The ChEMBL Database in 2023: a drug discovery platform spanning multiple bioactivity data types and time periods. Nucleic Acids Res. 0305-1048. 52 (D1), D1180. doi:10.1093/nar/gkad1004.

Zhang, T., Leng, J., Liu, Y., 2020. Deep learning for drug–drug interaction extraction from the literature: a review. Brief. Bioinform. 1467-5463. 21 (5), 1609–1627. doi:10.1093/bib/bbz087.

Zhang, Y., Chen, Q., Yang, Z., Lin, H., Lu, Z., 2019. BioWordVec, improving biomedical word embeddings with subword information and MeSH. Sci. Data. 2052-4463. 6 (1). doi:10.1038/s41597-019-0055-0.

Zhao, S., Su, C., Lu, Z., Wang, F., 2021. Recent advances in biomedical literature mining. Brief. Bioinform. 1467-5463. 22 (3). doi:10.1093/bib/bbaa057.

Role of AI in predicting drug efficacy and toxicity

Neeraj Kumar[a], Manish Kumar Gupta[b], and Dev Brat Mishra[c]
[a]*Fish Biology Research Lab, Department of Zoology, T.D. P.G. College, Jaunpur, Uttar Pradesh, India*
[b]*Department of Biotechnology, Faculty of Science, Veer Bahadur Singh Purvanchal University, Jaunpur, Uttar Pradesh, India*
[c]*Fish Biology Research Lab, Department of Zoology, T.D.College, Jaunpur, India*

1 Introduction

The procedure for identifying and creating new drugs is extremely difficult, costly, and time-consuming; it frequently takes 10 to 15 years and costs billions of dollars. Despite significant investments, many medication candidates fail late-stage clinical trials because of unexpected toxicity or insufficient efficacy (Paul et al., 2010). By enhancing drug efficacy and toxicity prediction, decreasing failure rates, and hastening the creation of safer and more efficient treatments, artificial intelligence (AI) is revolutionizing pharmaceutical research (Ekins, 2016).

2 The need for AI in drug development

Traditional drug discovery methods rely on high-throughput screening, computational modeling, and preclinical testing, but these approaches often fail to accurately predict human responses (Mak et al., 2014). AI-driven models can analyze massive datasets, uncover hidden patterns, and make data-driven predictions about a drug's effectiveness and safety before it enters clinical trials (Vamathevan et al., 2019). AI improves drug development decision-making by combining real-world evidence, electronic health records (EHRs), and multiomics data.

2.1 AI in drug efficacy prediction

Drug-target interactions (DTI), biomarker-based therapy responses, and customized medical strategies are frequently predicted using

The AI Frontier in Molecular Modelling and Drug Designing. https://doi.org/10.1016/B978-0-443-40338-5.00014-7

AI approaches, especially machine learning (ML) and deep learning (DL) (Chen et al., 2018). DL models such as convolutional neural networks (CNNs) and recurrent neural networks (RNNs) analyze biological interactions and molecular structures to accurately determine a drug's efficacy (Zhou et al., 2020).

2.2 AI analyzes chemical structures, protein targets, and biological pathways to assess efficacy

2.2.1 Chemical structure analysis

AI uses molecular fingerprints, SMILES representations, and graph neural networks (GNNs) to learn features of drug-like molecules (Tropsha, 2010). Whether a molecule has potential therapeutic action is predicted by methods like DL (CNNs, RNNs) and Quantitative Structure-Activity Relationship (QSAR) models. Example: DeepChem and ChemProp platforms use ML models to analyze chemical structures and forecast bioactivity (Yang et al., 2019).

2.2.2 Protein target analysis

AI models assess a drug's capacity to bind to its protein target, which is necessary for therapeutic efficacy (Jumper et al., 2021). Molecular docking and AI-driven binding affinity prediction simulate interactions between ligands and proteins. Tools like AlphaFold (DeepMind) now provide accurate 3D structures of proteins, improving target-based drug design (Öztürk et al., 2018).

2.2.3 Biological pathway analysis

AI integrates omics data (genomics, proteomics, metabolomics, transcriptomics) to map how a drug influences cellular pathways. ML helps identify disease-relevant pathways and predict whether modulating them will produce therapeutic effects. Pathway-level analysis supports precision medicine, tailoring drugs to patient-specific molecular profiles (Zitnik et al., 2018; Ståhl et al., 2019).

2.3 Integrated efficacy prediction

By combining chemical structure analysis, protein-ligand interaction modeling, and pathway-level insights, AI provides a comprehensive efficacy prediction pipeline. This reduces experimental workload, accelerates drug repurposing, and improves hit-to-lead optimization in pharmaceutical R&D (Vamathevan et al., 2019).

2.4 AI in predicting drug toxicity

Since medication-induced toxicity continues to be one of the main causes of treatment failure, toxicity prediction is a crucial component of drug research. AI-based in silico toxicity screening methods analyze chemical structures, biological pathways, and preclinical data to identify potential safety risks (Xu et al., 2021). AI-driven pharmacovigilance systems further improve postmarket drug safety by detecting adverse drug reactions (ADRs) from clinical reports, social media, and also EHRs (Priya et al., 2022).

3 AI detects potential adverse drug reactions before clinical trials

3.1 Role of AI in ADR prediction

Unexpected and detrimental side effects from drugs are known as ADRs, and they frequently result in drug withdrawals or late-stage clinical trial failures (Vilar et al., 2012). AI helps identify ADR risks before clinical trials, reducing cost, time, and patient risk. To forecast possible toxicity and off-target consequences, ML algorithms (MLAs) examine chemical structures, drug–target interactions, and biological pathways (Chen and Butte, 2016).

3.2 Using AI to transform drug discovery

The addition of AI to drug examination has already yielded promising results. AI-powered platforms such as Deep Mind's Alpha Fold have revolutionized protein structure prediction, while AI-driven drug discovery companies like Benevolent AI and Insilico Medicine have successfully identified new drug candidates in record time (Jumper et al., 2021; Zhavoronkov, 2018). AI is becoming more and more important in the creation of contemporary drugs since regulatory organizations like the European Medicines Agency and the Food and Drug Administration (FDA) depend on it to evaluate the safety of drugs (Fig. 9.1).

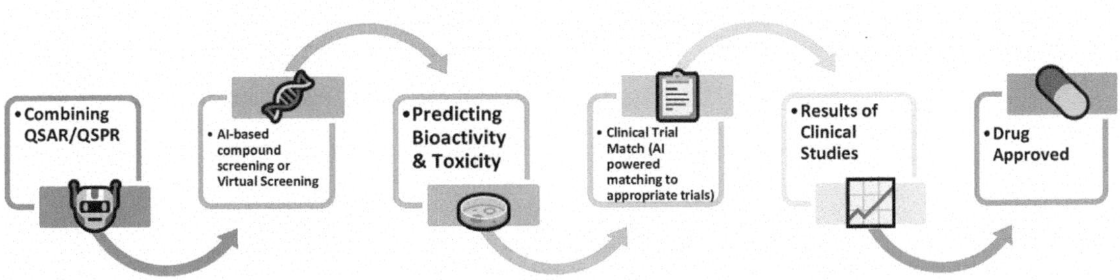

Fig. 9.1 AI-powered drug development.

3.3 Deep learning models model therapeutic response and drug receptor binding

3.3.1 Drug-receptor binding prediction

DL models such as CNNs and GNNs can be used to learn drug and protein molecular representations. These models predict binding affinity, i.e., how strongly a drug interacts with a receptor, which is a primary determinant of efficacy. Example: DeepDTA and GraphDTA are widely used DL frameworks that predict drug-target binding affinity directly from sequence/graph data (Öztürk et al., 2018; Nguyen et al., 2021).

3.3.2 Molecular docking with DL

Traditional molecular docking predicts drug-receptor binding poses, but it is computationally expensive (Wallach et al., 2015). DL improves docking accuracy by learning from experimental binding data and predicting receptor-ligand interactions rapidly. AI-based docking frameworks (e.g., AtomNet) simulate the 3D binding conformations and score drug candidates (Jiménez et al., 2018).

3.3.3 Therapeutic response simulation

To anticipate cellular and patient-level treatment responses, DL combines predictions of drug-target binding with multiomics data (genomics, transcriptomics, and proteomics) (Tang et al., 2019). Models like DeepDR and Tissue-specific Cancer Response Prediction predict how drugs affect different cell types or disease states. These models support precision medicine by identifying which patients will likely respond to a given therapy (Chang et al., 2018) (Fig 9.2).

3.3.4 Integrated applications

- DL provides a virtual laboratory to simulate drug-receptor interactions and therapeutic outcomes before in vivo testing
- Faster screening of large chemical libraries
- Lower R&D costs
- Improved hit-to-lead optimization
- Personalized therapy predictions

4 AI techniques used in drug prediction

Using ML, DL, natural language processing (NLP), and reinforcement learning (RL) to forecast pharmacological efficacy and toxicity, AI has emerged as a transformative tool in drug development. By evaluating vast biological datasets, enhancing DTI modeling, and enhancing ADR prediction, these AI techniques drastically cut down on the time and cost associated with developing traditional medications (Vamathevan et al., 2019).

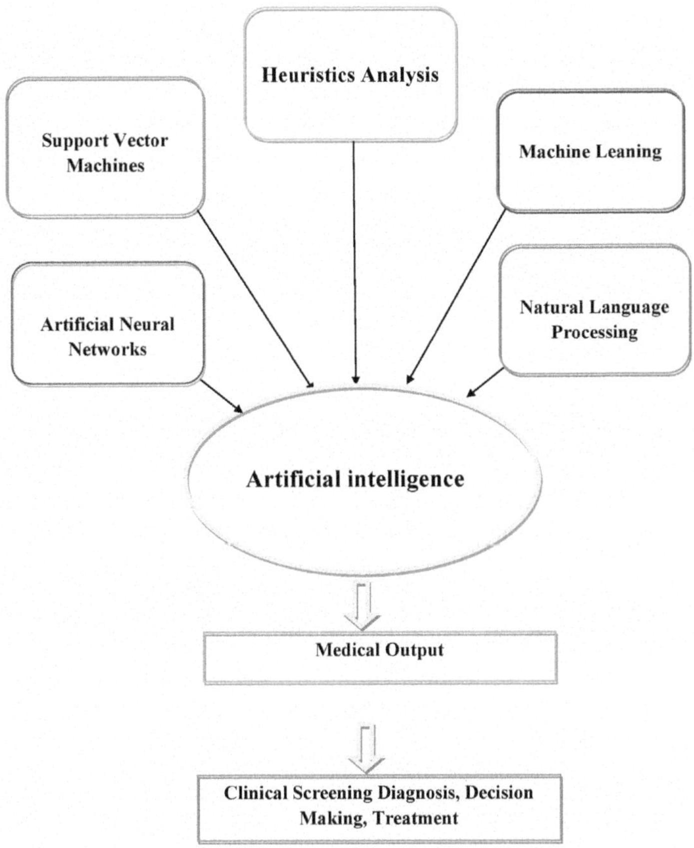

Fig. 9.2 Artificial intelligence process chats in the medical domain.

4.1 Using machine learning to predict drug use

Large-scale datasets are used by MLAs to discover pharmacokinetic characteristics, toxicity trends, and medication interactions.

4.1.1 Supervised learning

It trains models for predicting the affinity of drug–target binding using labeled data sets. Random Forest (RF) and Support Vector Machine (SVM) models have been used to forecast toxicity and perform virtual screening (Chen et al., 2018).

4.1.2 Unsupervised learning

It finds hidden patterns in biological data that aren't organized. For instance, comparable medicinal molecules have been grouped using clustering algorithms like k-means based on structural similarities (Ekins, 2016).

4.1.3 Learning by reinforcement

Through trial and error, AI agents discover the best drug design techniques. For instance, RL has been used in de novo drug design to optimize chemical structures for increased safety and efficacy (Olivecrona et al., 2017).

4.2 Using DL to predict drug use

In order to analyze complex biological and chemical data and provide extraordinarily accurate drug predictions, neural networks are employed in DL, a subset of ML (Zhou et al., 2020).

4.2.1 Convolutional neural networks

It is used for molecular property prediction by analyzing 2D and 3D drug structures. Example: CNNs have been successfully applied in toxicity prediction and protein-ligand binding analysis (Xu et al., 2021).

4.2.2 Recurrent neural networks and long short-term memory

Analyze sequential biological data for predicting drug responses. Example: LSTMs help in predicting drug–drug interactions (DDIs) and time-series toxicity assessments (Chen and Engkvist, 2019).

4.2.3 Generative adversarial networks

Make new molecular structures with the pharmacological characteristics you choose. Example: (Kadurin et al., 2017). Generative adversarial networks (GAN)-based drug design has produced potential candidates for cancer and infectious diseases.

4.3 Natural language processing for drug discovery

Clinical trial papers, EHRs, and biomedical literature are all sources of insightful information that can be extracted using NLP.

Mining biomedical texts, NLP assists in the analysis of clinical trial data and PubMed publications to find novel therapeutic possibilities (Zeng et al., 2019).

ADR prediction: AI models extract drug safety signals from social media and clinical reports (Kumar et al., 2022).

Clinical trial optimization: NLP processes patient records to improve participant selection and trial outcomes (Jagannatha and Yu, 2016).

4.4 AI in computational drug design

AI accelerates drug design through quantum mechanics-based simulations and AI-generated molecular structures.

Molecular docking simulations: AI predicts how drugs bind to targets, improving hit identification (Zhou et al., 2020).

AI-driven drug repurposing: ML models find novel medicinal uses for already-approved medications (Table 9.1).

5 Personalized efficacy predictions using patient-specific data (genomics, proteomics, clinical history)

5.1 Genomics-based predictions

AI models integrate genomic data (DNA sequencing, SNPs, mutations) to predict how an individual's genetic profile influences drug response (Relling and Evans, 2015). Example: Certain CYP450 gene variants affect drug metabolism, and AI models can predict whether a patient will metabolize a drug quickly, slowly, or be at risk of adverse effects. Pharmacogenomic databases like PharmGKB are used to train AI systems for personalized efficacy prediction (Yuan et al., 2021).

5.2 Proteomics and biomarker data

AI uses proteomic signatures (protein expression levels, posttranslational modifications) to identify predictive biomarkers of drug response (Li and Zhang, 2020). DL models can map drug-protein-pathway interactions, tailoring therapy based on proteomic patterns. This helps in predicting target engagement and therapeutic outcome (Aebersold and Mann, 2016)

Table 9.1 AI techniques used in drug prediction.

S. No	AI technique	Purpose	Example
1	Machine learning (ML)	Predict DTI and toxicity patterns	SVM, Random Forest
2	Deep learning (DL)	Process complex biological data	CNNs for molecular properties, RNNs for sequential data
3	Reinforcement learning (RL)	De novo medication development and virtual trials	Optimizing drugs through trial and error
4	Natural language processing (NLP)	Extract toxicity signals from texts	Mining EHRs, PubMed, and Social Media

5.3 Clinical history and real-world data

To forecast medication success in individual patients, AI examines medical imaging, lifestyle variables, EHRs, and past treatment results (Miotto et al., 2018). Real-world clinical data are used to build MLAs, which enhance therapeutic success prediction and reduce negative consequences. Integration of clinical notes, lab reports, and treatment history enhances precision treatment strategies (Rajkomar et al., 2019).

5.4 Integrated personalized prediction

By combining genomics + proteomics + clinical history, AI creates a holistic model of personalized efficacy prediction (Topol, 2019).

5.4.1 Applications

Oncology → Predicting patient-specific responses to chemotherapy or immunotherapy
Cardiology → AI-powered medication selection for arrhythmia or hypertension
Psychiatry → Predicting antidepressant efficacy based on genetic and clinical history

This moves toward precision medicine, reducing "trial-and-error" prescribing.

6 Helps in finding novel therapeutic applications for current drugs via drug repurposing

6.1 AI in the repurposing of drugs

When compared to creating new medications from scratch, drug repurposing, also known as repositioning, saves time and money by looking for new therapeutic indications for already-approved medications. AI accelerates this process by analyzing chemical structures, protein–drug interaction profiles, clinical data, and biomedical literature to uncover novel uses. Since repurposed drugs already have known safety and pharmacokinetic profiles, AI-guided repurposing can reach clinical application much faster (Pushpakom et al., 2019).

6.2 Data-driven repurposing

ML integrates multiomics datasets, EHRs, and pharmacovigilance databases to identify hidden associations between drugs and diseases (Jin and Wong, 2014). NLP scans scientific publications and clinical trial reports to extract evidence of potential new drug–disease links.

6.3 Advantages of AI-driven drug repurposing

Cost-effective: Avoids initial safety trials

- Time-saving Significantly reduces R&D timelines
- High success rate: Leverages existing safety and pharmacological data

Supports precision medicine by aligning drugs with patient-specific molecular profiles

7 Predicting drug toxicity

7.1 AI detects potential ADRs before clinical trials

7.1.1 Role of AI in ADR prediction

Unexpected and detrimental side effects from drugs are known as ADRs, and they frequently result in drug withdrawals or late-stage clinical trial failures (Vilar et al., 2012). AI helps identify ADR risks before clinical trials, reducing cost, time, and patient risk. To forecast possible toxicity and off-target consequences, MLAs examine chemical structures, drug–target interactions, and biological pathways (Chen, et al., 2016).

7.1.2 Databases and training data

AI leverages toxicological and pharmacovigilance databases (e.g., SIDER, FAERS, MedDRA) to train models for ADR detection (Kuhn et al., 2016). Models identify patterns linking drug chemical features or target profiles with historical side effect data (Tatonetti et al., 2012).

7.1.3 DL and systems biology

In order to anticipate ADRs, deep neural networks (DNNs) and graph convolutional networks (GCNs) model how medications interact with biological systems (Wang et al., 2016). Systems biology models integrate genomics, proteomics, and metabolomics data to anticipate toxicities in specific organ systems (e.g., hepatotoxicity, cardiotoxicity, and nephrotoxicity) (Zitnik et al., 2018).

7.1.4 Applications before clinical trials

- Screening drug candidates for toxicological red flags (e.g., cardiotoxicity via human Ether-à-go-go-related gene (hERG) channel inhibition).
- Detect possible DDIs that may increase ADR risk.
- Prioritizing safe compounds for preclinical testing thus minimizes clinical trial attrition.

8 ML models analyze toxicological databases and predict off-target effects

8.1 Role of ML in toxicology

Conventional toxicity assessment uses in vitro tests and animal studies, which are expensive, time-consuming, and might not accurately reflect human reactions. ML models overcome these limitations by analyzing toxicological databases to detect hidden patterns linking chemical structures and toxic outcomes. ML can predict off-target interactions, i.e., unintended drug binding to proteins other than the primary therapeutic target, which often cause ADRs (Cheng et al., 2011; Ekins et al., 2019).

8.2 Toxicological databases as training data

- Widely used toxicological databases include:
- Side Effect Resource (SIDER): drug–side effect associations.
- The FDA Adverse Event Reporting System, or FAERS, collects information on adverse events that occur in the real world.
- Tox21 & ToxCast → high-throughput toxicity screening datasets.
- These databases allow ML models to generalize and forecast the toxicity risks of new compounds.

9 AI in predicting drug efficacy

An essential part of drug discovery is predicting a medicine's effectiveness. Accurate predictions can help identify promising candidates early, optimize clinical trial designs, and personalize treatment plans. Because AI-driven techniques provide more accurate insights than conventional methods, they are being employed more and more to anticipate DTI, biomarker development, and patient-specific responses. To forecast how effectively a medication will function in certain patient populations, these AI algorithms examine vast amounts of data from proteomics, genomics, and clinical trials.

9.1 Drug–target interaction prediction

Understanding a drug's effectiveness requires being able to predict how it will interact with its target. ML and DL algorithms, in particular, make it easier to predict drug–target binding affinity, a crucial sign of therapeutic efficacy.

9.1.1 ML models for DTI prediction

RF and SVMs are commonly used to predict DTIs based on the chemical and biological properties of the substances (Chen et al., 2018). For instance, predicting the binding affinity of tiny molecules to protein targets using ML models can significantly enhance the drug screening process.

9.1.2 DL models for DTI prediction

To increase the precision of DTI predictions, CNNs and RNNs process chemical structures and biological data (Zhou et al., 2020). In order to predict chemical bioactivity from compound characteristics, for instance, DL models such as Deep Chem and Deep Purpose have produced remarkable results (Ramsundar et al., 2017).

9.2 Finding biomarkers and forecasting treatment outcomes

AI techniques, especially DL and RL, are being used to find new biomarkers that predict a patient's reaction to a particular treatment. A key component of customized medicine is predicting how a patient will react to a medication.

9.2.1 Multiomics integration of data

To find biomarkers that are associated with medication efficacy, AI can combine data from proteomics, transcriptomics, and genomics (Zhong et al., 2018). For instance, by linking gene expression profiles with treatment response, artificial neural networks (ANNs) and autoencoders are utilized to forecast the effectiveness of targeted medicines.

9.2.2 Personalized medicine

AI models can tailor drug treatment based on individual genetic profiles, allowing for precision medicine that predicts how a drug will affect a specific patient. Example: Companies like Tempus and Foundation Medicine use AI to integrate clinical and genomic data to predict the best treatments for cancer patients.

9.3 Clinical trial optimization

Clinical trials are costly and time-consuming, with a significant risk of failure due to ineffective drug responses in patients. By forecasting which patient groups are most likely to react to therapy, AI is improving trial designs.

9.3.1 Recruitment and stratification of patients

To identify which patients are most likely to benefit from a certain medicine, AI systems use data from previous clinical studies. To link patients with clinical trials and forecast the effectiveness of various treatments based on patient profiles, IBM Watson for Oncology, for instance, analyzes clinical data.

9.3.2 Virtual clinical trials

AI models are used to model clinical studies and forecast results, reducing the need for extensive human trials. Example: Virtual screening tools, powered by RL and Monte Carlo simulations, simulate drug interactions within a virtual environment to predict efficacy before physical trials (Vamathevan et al., 2019) Fig. 9.3).

9.4 Repurposing drugs

AI is also being used in drug repurposing, which is the process of finding new therapeutic applications for drugs that have been granted licenses. This can significantly cut down on medication

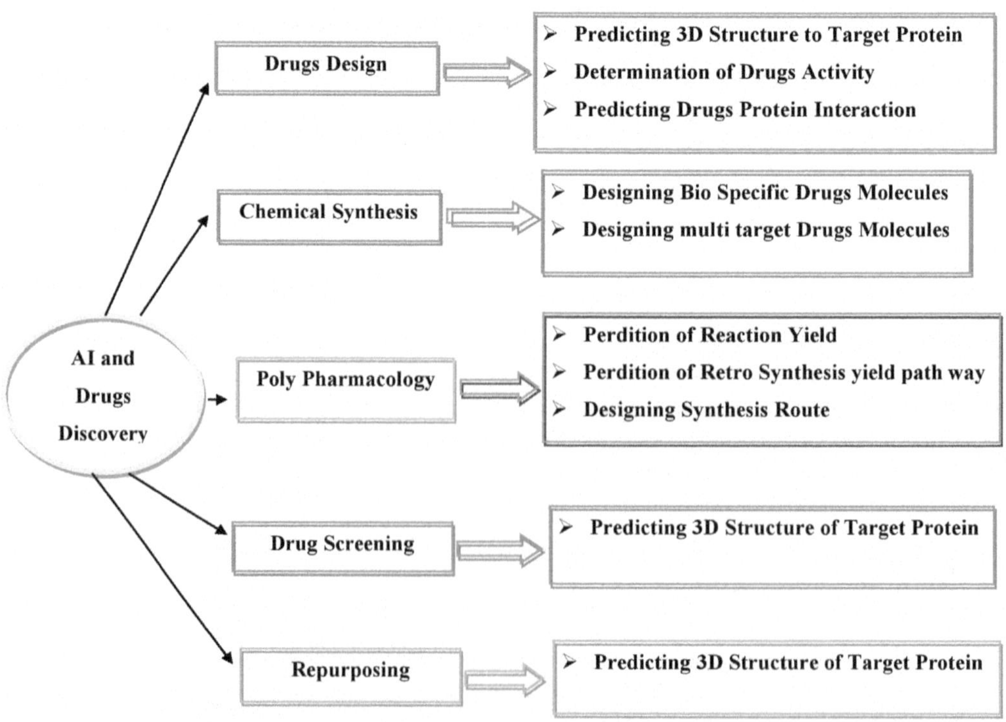

Fig. 9.3 Various uses of AI in pharmaceutical development.

development time and expense without sacrificing effectiveness. DL models predict efficacy by assessing existing drugs' effects on different diseases based on genetic, biochemical, and clinical data. For example, Benevolent AI used AI to repurpose a drug for COVID-19 by analyzing scientific literature, clinical trial data, and molecular interactions (Zhavoronkov, 2020) Table 9.2).

10 Predicting off-target effects

ML and DL models integrate chemical structure data with known protein–ligand interaction profiles to identify unintended binding partners (Bender and Cortés-Ciriano, 2021; Wang, et al., 2016). Examples of predictive methods: Molecular characteristics and toxicity outcomes are connected by QSAR models. Complex patterns in DTIs are learned by DNNs and GCNs. This helps anticipate organ-specific toxicities such as cardiotoxicity (hERG channel inhibition) or hepatotoxicity.

10.1 Applications in drug safety

Preclinical safety assessment → screening out toxic compounds early.

- DDI prediction → detection of synergistic toxic effects.
- Drug repurposing safety → ensuring safe new uses for old drugs.
- Precision medicine → tailoring treatments by predicting individual-specific off-target risks.

11 AI identifies risks of organ toxicity (liver, kidney, heart, etc.)

11.1 AI's broad function in predicting organ toxicity

One of the main reasons for drug attrition in late-stage clinical trials and postmarket removal is medication-induced organ damage. AI

Table 9.2 Role of AI in predicting drug efficacy.

S. No	Aspect	Details
1	Applications	Drug discovery, repurposing, diagnostics, clinical trial design, and pharmaceutical production
2	Methods used	Deep learning (DL), causal machine learning, and machine learning (ML)
3	Key approaches	Drug–target interaction (DTI) modeling, biomarker discovery, Personalized therapy prediction
4	Techniques	CNNs, RNNs, LSTM, GANs, reinforcement learning, multiomics integration
5	Examples	Tempus, foundation medicine, IBM Watson for oncology, Virtual Clinical Trials
6	Impact	Higher treatment efficacy, faster drug discovery, personalized medicine optimization

models integrate chemical structure data, toxicological databases, and biological assays to predict organ-specific toxic effects before human testing. This helps pharmaceutical companies screen out unsafe compounds early, improving drug safety (Vamathevan et al., 2019).

11.2 Hepatotoxicity, or liver toxicity

Since the liver is the primary site of drug processing, hepatotoxicity poses a significant safety risk. The compound's potential to cause liver injury can be predicted by AI models trained on DILI (drug-induced liver injury) datasets. ML approaches combine chemical descriptors + gene expression profiles to forecast hepatotoxic potential (Wang, et al., 2016; Chen et al., 2011)

11.3 Kidney toxicity (nephrotoxicity)

The kidney is vulnerable to toxicity because of its role in drug excretion and high blood flow. AI-based predictive models identify nephrotoxic compounds using in vitro renal cell assays, toxicogenomic data, and chemical features. Early prediction reduces the risk of renal failure during trials (Zhang et al., 2014; Howell et al., 2012).

11.4 Heart toxicity (cardiotoxicity)

Cardiotoxicity, especially related to QT prolongation and hERG channel inhibition, is a major cause of drug withdrawal. AI models simulate drug–ion channel interactions to predict cardiac safety risks. DL integrates in vitro electrophysiological data with chemical descriptors to detect arrhythmia risks (Li et al., 2019; Siramshetty et al., 2018).

11.4.1 Other organs (brain, lungs, and GI tract)

AI models are also being developed for:

- Neurotoxicity → predicting drugs that may impair CNS function or cross the blood–brain barrier in harmful ways.
- Pulmonary toxicity → e.g., interstitial lung disease caused by certain anticancer drugs.
- Gastrointestinal toxicity → predicting risks like ulcers or bleeding from NSAIDs.

12 AI predicts dose-dependent toxicity and long-term side effects

12.1 Dose-dependent toxicity prediction

- Drug toxicity is often dose-dependent, meaning that low doses may be safe while higher doses cause adverse effects.
- AI models analyze dose–response relationships by integrating:
  - In vitro bioassay data (e.g., from ToxCast and Tox21).
  - Pharmacokinetic/pharmacodynamic (PK/PD) models
  - Chemical structure descriptors
- ML can predict toxic thresholds (NOAEL, LOAEL), enabling safer dose design in preclinical and clinical studies.

12.2 Prediction of long-term side effects

- Many adverse effects appear only after chronic drug exposure (e.g., cancer risk, metabolic disorders, organ failure) (Bender and Cortés-Ciriano, 2021). AI uses longitudinal clinical data, real-world evidence, and EHRs to detect patterns of delayed toxicity (Shah et al., 2019).
- NLP algorithms mine medical literature and adverse event reporting systems (e.g., FAERS, WHO-VigiBase) to flag potential long-term risks.

12.3 Integration with simulation models

- AI enhances physiologically based pharmacokinetic models to simulate long-term accumulation of drugs and metabolites.
- DL predicts cumulative toxicity risks, such as:
  - Carcinogenicity (e.g., cancer risk from chronic drug exposure)
  - Immunotoxicity (immune suppression or overactivation)
  - Reproductive toxicity (fertility or developmental effects)

12.4 Examples

- Nonsteroidal Anti-Inflammatory Drugs (NSAIDs) (e.g., diclofenac, ibuprofen) → dose-dependent GI and renal toxicity; AI can simulate safe dosing ranges.
- Anthracyclines (e.g., doxorubicin) → cumulative cardiotoxicity predicted using ML-based cardiomyocyte toxicity assays.

Biologics (e.g., checkpoint inhibitors) → AI predicts immune-related long-term side effects from immunotherapy datasets.

13 Clinical trial optimization

AI predicts patient responses to drugs, improving trial design and participant selection.

13.1 Personalized response prediction

To forecast how various individuals will react to a medication, AI models combine clinical history and multiomics data (genomics, transcriptomics, proteomics, and metabolomics) (Kourou et al., 2015). This enables precision medicine, where therapies are tailored to patients likely to benefit while avoiding ineffective or harmful treatments (Li et al., 2021).

13.2 AI in clinical trial design

- Traditional clinical trials often fail due to heterogeneous patient responses (Waring et al., 2015).
- AI uses predictive modeling to stratify patients into subgroups (responders vs. nonresponders) before enrollment (Yu et al., 2018).
- This reduces trial size, improves statistical power, and increases the chances of success.

13.3 Biomarker discovery for patient selection

AI identifies predictive biomarkers (genetic mutations, protein expression, metabolic signatures) linked to drug efficacy or toxicity (Chaudhary et al., 2018; Poplin et al., 2018). Example: Predicting response to immunotherapy by analyzing tumor genomics and immune signatures.

13.4 Improved participant selection

AI helps avoid enrolling patients unlikely to respond or at high risk of severe side effects (Bender and Cortés-Ciriano, 2021). This leads to more efficient recruitment, reduced dropout rates, and higher trial success rates.

14 AI reduces trial failures by identifying ineffective or unsafe compounds early

14.1 Early efficacy prediction

AI analyzes chemical structures, protein interactions, and biological pathways to predict whether a compound will effectively target a disease (Zhavoronkov et al., 2019). This allows for filtering out ineffective compounds before advancing to costly preclinical or clinical trials (Vamathevan et al., 2019).

14.2 Toxicity and safety screening

Many trial failures result from toxic side effects discovered late in development (Xu et al., 2015). AI integrates toxicogenomic data, PK/PD models, and toxicological databases (e.g., Tox21, ToxCast) to predict organ-specific and systemic toxicity early (Bender and Cortés-Ciriano, 2021), helping eliminate unsafe compounds before animal testing or Phase I trials.

14.3 Virtual screening & high-throughput filtering

AI-powered virtual screening rapidly evaluates millions of molecules for binding affinity, Absorption, Distribution, Metabolism, Excretion, Toxicity, and safety profiles (Chen et al., 2018). This significantly reduces time and cost by eliminating unsuitable candidates before lab-based screening (Ekins et al., 2019).

14.4 Lowering clinical trial attrition

According to Waring et al. (2015), around 90% of medications that enter exploratory trials fail, primarily because they are ineffective (approximately 50%) or have safety concerns (30%). AI reduces attrition by selecting the most promising candidates and excluding those with high failure risks (Paul et al., 2010).

15 AI in predicting drug toxicity

Since ADRs can result in clinical trial failures, market withdrawals, and patient harm, predicting toxicity is a crucial step in the development of novel medications. Traditional experimental methods for toxicity testing, including animal models and in vitro tests, are time-consuming, expensive, and sometimes unreliable due to species differences. AI-driven models offer a faster, cost-effective, and more accurate alternative for predicting drug toxicity at various stages of development.

15.1 AI approaches for drug toxicity prediction

AI-based toxicity prediction techniques examine chemical, biological, and clinical data using ML, DL, and NLP. These models detect toxic compounds, classify their severity, and predict potential adverse effects.

15.1.1 Models for ML

SVM, RF, and Gradient Boosting Machines (GBM) are commonly used for toxicity classification. Large-scale bioactivity and toxicity screening findings are found in databases like Tox21 and ToxCast, which are used to train MLAs (Mayr et al., 2016). Example: Based on molecular descriptors, ML models have been used to forecast a chemical's cytotoxicity and genotoxicity (Huang et al., 2016).

15.1.2 DL models

In order to identify hazardous chemical substructures, CNNs examine 2D and 3D molecular structures. Time-series toxicity data are analyzed by Transformer-based models and RNNs to improve long-term effect prediction (Xu et al., 2021). For instance, in predicting toxicity, the DL-based platform DeepTox performed better than conventional QSAR models (Mayr et al., 2016).

15.1.3 Toxicity mining using NLP

NLP retrieves data about toxicity from clinical reports, scholarly publications, and adverse event databases like FAERS. Example: AI-powered NLP models have successfully identified previously unrecognized drug toxicities by analyzing social media and EHRs (Sarker et al., 2015) Fig. 9.4).

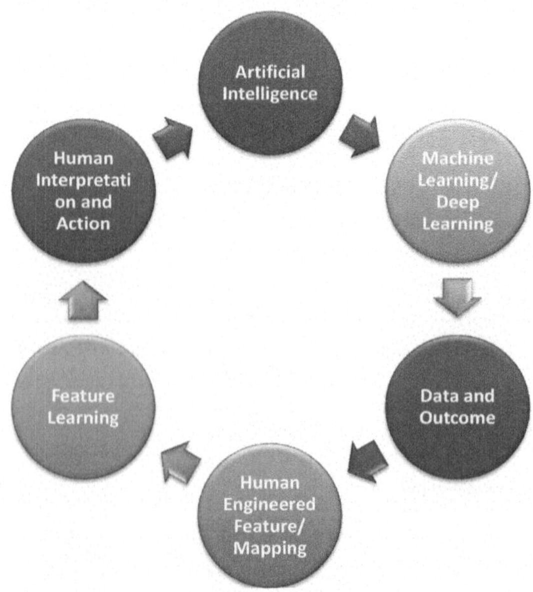

Fig. 9.4 Schematic illustration of artificial intelligence.

15.2 AI in predicting organ-specific toxicity

AI models are being applied to predict specific organ toxicities, which is critical for ensuring drug safety.

15.2.1 Hepatotoxicity (liver toxicity) prediction

AI predicts DILI by analyzing hepatic enzyme interactions and metabolic pathways. Example: DILIrank, an AI-enhanced database, classifies drugs based on their potential to cause liver toxicity (Chen et al., 2021).

15.2.2 Cardiotoxicity (heart toxicity) prediction

AI models predict hERG inhibition, which is linked to Q and T wave (QT) prolongation and arrhythmias. Example: a DL model called hERGNet uses ion channel interactions to forecast the likelihood of cardiotoxicity (Polak et al., 2019).

15.2.3 Neurotoxicity prediction

AI evaluates blood-brain barrier permeability and neuro receptor interactions to identify neurotoxic compounds. Example: NeuroToxAI, an AI-based tool, integrates multiomics data to predict neurotoxicity in drug candidates (Deng et al., 2022).

15.3 AI for predicting genotoxicity and carcinogenicity

AI-based models forecast chromosomal abnormalities associated with carcinogenicity, mutagenicity, and DNA binding affinity. A DL framework called DeepGenTox evaluates mutagenesis potential by looking at molecular characteristics (Zhang, 2020). Example: AI-powered QSAR models classify chemicals as carcinogenic or non-carcinogenic with high accuracy.

15.4 AI for ADR prediction

AI can analyze real-world patient data to predict unknown ADRs before they manifest in clinical settings. NLP and ML models extract toxicity-related signals from EHRs, scientific articles, and also social media. The FAERS has been used to train AI algorithms that have successfully found previously unreported ADRs (Kumar et al. 2022).

15.5 AI for drug repurposing and toxicity reduction

AI can also be used to redesign toxic drugs and identify safer alternatives.

De novo drug design: AI modifies molecular structures to enhance efficacy while minimizing toxicity (Stokes et al., 2020). Example: AI-powered screening identified less toxic analogs of chemotherapy drugs, reducing harmful side effects while maintaining anticancer activity (Yang et al., 2022) (Table 9.3).

16 Data sources and integration in AI models for drug toxicity prediction

AI-driven toxicity prediction relies on high-quality datasets and integrated multisource data to enhance accuracy and reliability. By combining chemical, biological, and clinical data, AI models can identify toxicity risks at early stages, reducing drug development costs and improving patient safety.

16.1 Data sources for AI-based toxicity prediction

AI models train and validate toxicity prediction algorithms using a variety of data sources. These sources can be broadly categorized into chemical databases, bioassays, clinical records, and literature sources.

16.1.1 Chemical structure and toxicity databases

PubChem: A public repository containing chemical properties, bioassay results, and toxicological profiles (Kim et al., 2019).

hERGCentral: A database of ion channel interactions for predicting cardiotoxicity (Mendez et al., 2019).

Tox21 and ToxCast: High-throughput screening programs providing bioassay data on environmental and pharmaceutical compounds (Richard et al., 2016).

Table 9.3 Role of AI in predicting drug toxicity.

S. No	Aspect	Details
1	Applications	Early detection of ADRs, toxicity screening, postmarket surveillance, organ-specific toxicity prediction
2	Methods used	Machine learning (SVM, RF, GBM), Deep Learning (CNNs, RNNs, Transformers), NLP
3	Key approaches	Toxicogenomics, Predicting DILI, hERG inhibition (cardiotoxicity), Neurotoxicity detection
4	Techniques	DeepTox platform, NLP on EHRs and social media, Knowledge Graph integration
5	Examples	DILIrank (Liver), hERGNet (Heart), NeuroToxAI (Brain)
6	Impact	Reduced animal testing, early hazard identification, safer drug development

EPA CompTox: A predictive toxicology database integrating chemical hazard data (Williams et al., 2017).

16.1.2 Bioassay and in vitro screening data

Open TG-GATEs is a large-scale transcriptomics dataset used for predicting drug-induced liver toxicity (Uehara et al., 2016).

Sequencing Quality Control project (SEQC) Provides RNA-seq data for toxicity assessment and biomarker discovery (Shi et al., 2016).

hERGCentral: An ion channel interaction database for cardiotoxicity prediction (Polak et al., 2019).

16.1.3 Clinical and postmarket monitoring information

Patient-reported ADRs are included in the FAERS.

EHRs: AI models extract toxicity signals from patient records, improving ADR detection (Sarker et al., 2015).

WHO's worldwide drug safety report database, VigiBase, is utilized for AI pharmacovigilance applications (Lindquist, 2008).

16.1.4 Biomedical literature and real-world data

PubMed and MEDLINE: Scientific publications used for AI-driven knowledge extraction. **Social Media and Patient Forums**: AI-based NLP extracts real-world toxicity reports (Yeleswarapu et al., 2014) Table 9.4).

16.2 Integration of multisource data in AI models

To improve toxicity prediction, AI models integrate data from several sources using data fusion and multiomics approaches.

16.2.1 Data fusion for toxicity modeling

Multimodal AI models combine chemical structures, bioassays, and clinical data for comprehensive toxicity assessment. Example:

Table 9.4 Data sources for AI-based drug prediction.

S. No	Data source	Description	Example use
1	Chemical databases	Molecular structures and properties	PubChem, Tox21, EPA CompTox
2	Bioassay and Screening Data	Biological activity data	Open TG-GATEs, SEQC
3	Clinical data and reports	ADRs and patient outcomes	FDA AERS, VigiBase
4	Biomedical literature & real-world data	Research papers, forums	PubMed, Social Media Mining

DeepTox, a DL model integrating Tox21 bioassay data and PubChem molecular features, outperforms traditional QSAR models (Mayr et al., 2016).

16.2.2 Multiomics integration of data

By collecting drug–biomarker interactions and data from genomics, transcriptomics, proteomics, and metabolomics, toxicity prediction is enhanced (Xu et al., 2021). Example: NeuroToxAI integrates multiomics data to predict neurotoxicity risk.

16.2.3 Knowledge graphs and ai-driven data mining

AI models use knowledge graphs to connect drug toxicity profiles across different databases. Example: The Open Predictive Data Infrastructure links chemical toxicity data with clinical outcomes (Chen et al., 2021).

16.3 Data integration difficulties for AI-based toxicology prediction

Despite advances in AI, integrating toxicity data presents challenges:

Data heterogeneity: Inconsistent formats and missing values affect model performance.

Limited labeled toxicity data: AI models rely on high-quality annotations, which are scarce for rare toxic effects.

Bias and reproducibility: Imbalanced datasets may lead to biased toxicity predictions (Hong et al., 2022).

16.4 Future directions in ai-based data integration for toxicity prediction

Federated learning is the process of training AI models across several universities while maintaining data privacy. Increasing the interpretability of AI-driven toxicity forecasts for regulatory approval is known as explainable AI.

Integration of real-world data Using wearable devices and patient monitoring for real-time toxicity detection.

16.4.1 Artificial intelligence's use in forecasting drug effectiveness and toxicity for human life

AI is having a big impact on the pharmaceutical and healthcare industries, especially in the areas of toxicity prediction and treatment efficacy. These two factors—how well a drug works (efficacy) and whether it causes harmful side effects (toxicity)—are critical in drug development and directly impact human health. By using AI, researchers can significantly improve the safety, precision, and speed of discovering and developing new medicines, which is ultimately beneficial for society.

Predicting a drug's effectiveness before it is put through human trials is one of the main ways AI may improve human lives. Historically, a number of costly and time-consuming phases of clinical trials and comprehensive laboratory testing were required to ascertain if a medication was effective. However, AI models are able to anticipate how effectively a treatment will work by analyzing large datasets, such as genetic profiles, molecular structures, clinical trial findings, and disease processes. Algorithms for ML find connections and patterns in data that human researchers would miss. By finding the most promising drug candidates early in the process, this approach can help save time and money. AI also helps with personalized medicine, which tailors medicines according to a patient's age, environment, genetic composition, and health status. By analyzing data from clinical trials, genetic databases, and electronic medical records, AI may help predict how different people might respond to a drug. By allowing doctors to choose the safest and most effective treatment plan for each patient, this approach reduces the trial-and-error approach that is commonly employed in contemporary medical practice. Another crucial application is in predicting drug toxicity, which helps to protect patients from harmful side effects. Many drugs fail in late-stage trials or are withdrawn after reaching the market because of toxic reactions. AI can predict these risks much earlier by analyzing the chemical properties of drugs and how they interact with human cells and organs. Advanced AI models simulate how drugs affect biological systems, identifying potential toxic effects like liver damage, heart problems, or allergic reactions. In addition to safeguarding human health, this approach expedites the regulatory procedure and lessens the need for animal testing.

Additionally, AI helps in drug repurposing, which finds new uses for pharmaceuticals that have already received approval. This is especially useful in urgent health crises, such as pandemics, where time is critical. Since these drugs already have known safety profiles, AI can rapidly evaluate their potential effectiveness for other conditions, speeding up treatment development and availability. AI has disadvantages despite its benefits, such as algorithmic bias, low-quality data, and the need for regulatory approval. AI systems must be educated on a range of accurate data sets in order to generate reliable predictions that are advantageous to all parties.

16.4.2 AI's role in drug efficacy and toxicity prediction in human life

By greatly improving the prediction of therapeutic efficacy and toxicity—two critical factors in ensuring the safety and effectiveness of pharmaceutical compounds—drug development and discovery are being revolutionized by AI. The development of conventional drugs is costly, time-consuming, and prone to failure, often due to unexpected toxicity or insufficient efficacy. AI offers promising solutions by leveraging large datasets, advanced algorithms, and predictive models to streamline and improve the drug evaluation process. Predicting a drug's efficacy—the capacity of a medication to achieve the intended therapeutic effect—is one ofAI's main functions. AI models analyze vast datasets from clinical trials, biomedical literature, and real-world patient data to identify patterns and biomarkers associated with positive treatment outcomes. In order to anticipate how effectively a treatment will work in particular populations or individuals, ML algorithms can correlate molecular structures, genetic information, and illness features. The ability of AI systems to extract useful insights from unstructured data, including scientific publications and medical records, through methods like DL and NLP, speeds up target identification and candidate drug selection. Equally important is the prediction of drug toxicity, which is vital for minimizing adverse effects and ensuring patient safety. AI tools can forecast potential toxicological responses by analyzing chemical structures, metabolic pathways, and gene expression profiles. In silico models simulate human biological systems to assess how drugs interact with various tissues and organs. These models help detect risks like hepatotoxicity, cardiotoxicity, and neurotoxicity before clinical trials, thereby reducing reliance on animal testing and improving early-stage screening. AI is also capable of identifying off-target effects and medication interactions that may cause adverse side effects. AI also supports precision medicine, which tailors medications to the particular genetic and environmental conditions of each patient. By merging genetic, proteomic, and metabolomic data, AI facilitates the development of tailored therapies with optimal efficacy and minimal toxicity. Pharmacogenomic models, for example, employ AI to forecast how genetic variants affect drug response, enabling safer and more efficient dosage schedules. Furthermore, by finding current medications that might work well for novel indications, AI improves drug repurposing. This not only accelerates treatment availability but also leverages already-approved safety profiles to reduce the risk of unexpected toxicity. Notwithstanding its promise, using AI to forecast a drug's toxicity and efficacy is fraught with difficulties. Data quality, algorithm transparency, and regulatory acceptance are ongoing concerns. Robust, diverse datasets are essential for accurate predictions, and AI models must be interpretable and validated through rigorous testing to gain trust from clinicians and regulators.

17 Conclusion

AI is transforming the pharmaceutical sector by enhancing therapeutic efficacy and toxicity prediction, cutting expenses, and raising success rates. AI models will play an increasingly important role in medication safety, regulatory compliance, and precision medicine as they develop further. However, if AI is to realize its full potential in drug research, issues with data quality, model interpretability, and ethical considerations must be resolved. AI-driven drug prediction techniques have revolutionized pharmaceutical research by enhancing drug-target modeling, toxicity measurement, and clinical decision-making. The combination of ML, DL, NLP, and computational chemistry has led to faster, cost-effective, and more accurate drug development pipelines. But in order to fully realize AI's promise in drug discovery, issues including model interpretability, data quality, and regulatory compliance must be resolved. AI is enabling personalized medicine, improving clinical trial design, facilitating drug repurposing, and improving the accuracy of medication efficacy forecasts from DTI models. These advancements enable a more efficient drug discovery process, which significantly boosts success rates and reduces the time and cost associated with developing new drugs. Through the use of ML, DL, NLP, and big data analytics, AI has significantly improved the prediction of pharmaceutical toxicity. AI lowers medication development costs, improves patient safety, and allows early detection of dangerous chemicals by combining chemical, biological, and real-world clinical data. These developments are revolutionizing postmarket surveillance, clinical trial optimization, and preclinical screening, leading to safer and more effective drugs. AI-driven toxicity prediction relies on diverse datasets and advanced data integration techniques to improve accuracy and reliability. By combining chemical, biological, and clinical data, AI models enhance early toxicity screening, optimize drug development, and support regulatory decision-making. Addressing challenges in data standardization, interpretability, and scalability will further advance AI applications in drug safety. AI's ability to forecast a drug's toxicity and efficacy is extremely helpful for human life. It improves the drug development process, enhances patient safety, supports personalized treatment, and helps deliver effective medicines faster. As AI develops further, its application in healthcare will result in safer, more intelligent, and more effective methods of illness prevention and treatment. AI is revolutionizing therapeutic effectiveness and toxicity prediction, providing notable benefits in excess of conventional techniques in terms of speed, cost, and accuracy. By enabling early classification of promising drug candidates and the identification of potential safety concerns, AI contributes to more efficient, personalized, and safer healthcare, ultimately improving human life and well-being. As technology and data integration advance, AI's impact on pharmacology and personalized medicine is expected to grow even more profound.

References

Aebersold, R., Mann, M., 2016. Mass-spectrometric exploration of proteome structure and function. Nature 537 (7620), 347–355.

Bender, A., Cortés-Ciriano, I., 2021. Artificial intelligence in drug discovery: what is realistic, what are illusions? Part 2: a discussion of chemical and biological data. Drug Discov. Today 26 (4), 1040–1052.

Chang, Y., Park, H., Yang, H.J., Lee, S., Lee, K.Y., Kim, T.S., Jung, J., Shin, J.M., 2018. Cancer drug response profile scan (CDRscan): a deep learning model that predicts drug effectiveness from cancer genomic signature. Sci. Rep. 8, 8857. doi:10.1038/s41598-018-27214-6.

Chaudhary, K., et al., 2018. Deep learning–based multi-omics integration for cancer survival prediction. PLoS Comput. Biol. 14 (9), e1005976.

Chen, B., Butte, A.J., 2016. Leveraging big data to transform target selection and drug discovery. Clin. Pharmacol. Ther. 99 (3), 285–297. doi:10.1002/cpt.318.

Chen, H., Engkvist, O., 2019. Has drug design augmented by artificial intelligence become a reality? Trends Pharmacol. Sci. 40 (11), 806–809. doi:10.1016/j.tips.2019.09.004.

Chen, H., Engkvist, O., Wang, Y., Olivecrona, M., Blaschke, T., 2018. The rise of deep learning in drug discovery. Drug Discov. Today 23 (6), 1241–1250.

Chen, M., Vijay, V., Shi, Q., Liu, Z., Fang, H., Tong, W., 2011. FDA-approved drug labeling for the study of drug-induced liver injury. Drug Discov. Today 16 (15–16), 697–703. doi:10.1016/j.drudis.2011.05.007.

Chen, Z., Liu, X., Hogan, W.R., Shenkman, E.A., Bian, J., 2021. Applications of artificial intelligence in drug development using real-world data. Drug Discov. Today 26 (5), 1256–1264. doi:10.1016/j.drudis.2020.12.013.

Deng, J., Yang, Z., Ojima, I., Samaras, D., Wang, F., 2022. Artificial intelligence in drug discovery: Applications and techniques. Brief. Bioinform. 23 (1), bbab430. doi:10.1093/bib/bbab430.

Ekins, S., 2016. The next era: deep learning in pharmaceutical research. Pharm. Res. 33 (11), 2595–2603. doi:10.1007/s11095-016-2029-7.

Ekins, S., et al., 2019. Exploiting machine learning for end-to-end drug discovery and development. Nat. Mater. 18 (5), 435–441.

Howell, L.A., Bowater, R.A., O'Connell, M., Reszka, A.P., Neidle, S., Searcey, M., 2012. Synthesis of small molecules targeting multiple DNA structures using click chemistry. ChemMedChem 7 (5), 792–804. doi:10.1002/cmdc.201200060.

Huang, R., Xia, M., Nguyen, D.T., Zhao, T., Sakamuru, S., Zhao, J., Shahane, S.A., Rossoshek, A., Simeonov, A., 2016. Tox21 challenge to build predictive models of nuclear receptor and stress response pathways as mediated by exposure to environmental chemicals and drugs. Front. Environ. Sci. 3, 85. doi:10.3389/fenvs.2015.00085.

Jagannatha, A.N., Yu, H., 2016. Bidirectional RNN for medical event detection in electronic health records. In: Proceedings of the Conference on Machine Learning for Healthcare, pp. 327–338.

Jiménez, J., et al., 2018. DeepSite: protein-binding site predictor using 3D-convolutional neural networks. Bioinformatics 33 (19), 3036–3042.
Jin, G., Wong, S.T.C., 2014. Toward better drug repositioning: prioritizing and integrating existing methods into efficient pipelines. Drug Discov. Today 19 (5), 637–644.
Jumper, J., Evans, R., Pritzel, A., et al., 2021. Highly accurate protein structure prediction with AlphaFold. Nature 596, 583–589.
Kadurin, A., Nikolenko, S., Khrabrov, K., Aliper, A., Zhavoronkov, A., 2017. druGAN: an advanced generative adversarial autoencoder model for de novo generation of new molecules with desired molecular properties in silico. Mol. Pharm. 14 (9), 3098–3104. doi:10.1021/acs.molpharmaceut.7b00346.
Kim, S., Thiessen, P.A., Bolton, E.E., Bryant, S.H., 2019. PubChem substance and compound databases. Nucleic Acids Res. 47 (D1), D1388–D1395.
Kourou, K., et al., 2015. Machine learning applications in cancer prognosis and prediction. Comput. Struct. Biotechnol. J. 13, 8–17.
Kuhn, M., et al., 2016. The SIDER database of drugs and side effects. Nucleic Acids Res. 44 (D1), D1075–D1079.
Li, J., Zhang, W., 2020. Integrating multi-omics data for drug response prediction using deep learning. Brief. Bioinform. 21 (4), 1169–1178.
Li, X., et al., 2021. Deep learning-based prediction of drug response in cancer. Brief. Bioinform. 22 (1), 360–379.
Li, Z., et al., 2019. Assessment of an in silico mechanistic model for proarrhythmia risk prediction under the CiPA initiative. Clin. Pharmacol. Ther. 105 (2), 466–475.
Lindquist, M., 2008. VigiBase, the WHO global ICSR database system: basic facts. Drug Inf. J. 42 (5), 409–419.
Mak, I.W., Evaniew, N., Ghert, M., 2014. Lost in translation: animal models and clinical trials in cancer treatment. Am. J. Transl. Res. 6 (2), 114–118.
Mayr, A., Klambauer, G., Unterthiner, T., Hochreiter, S., 2016. DeepTox: toxicity prediction using deep learning. Front. Environ. Sci. 4, 23.
Mendez, D., Gaulton, A., Bento, A.P., Chambers, J., Hersey, A., 2019. ChEMBL: towards direct deposition of bioassay data. Nucleic Acids Res. 47 (D1), D930–D940.
Miotto, R., Wang, F., Wang, S., Jiang, X., Dudley, J.T., 2018. Deep learning for healthcare: review, opportunities and challenges. Brief. Bioinform. 19 (6), 1236–1246.
Nguyen, T., Le, H., Venkatesh, S., 2021. GraphDTA: predicting drug–target binding affinity with graph neural networks. Bioinformatics 37 (8), 1140–1147.
Olivecrona, M., Blaschke, T., Engkvist, O., Chen, H., 2017. Molecular de novo design through deep reinforcement learning. J. Cheminform. 9 (1), 48.
Öztürk, H., et al., 2018. DeepDTA: deep drug–target binding affinity prediction. Bioinformatics 34 (17), i821–i829.
Paul, S.M., Mytelka, D.S., Dunwiddie, C.T., Persinger, C.C., Munos, B.H., Lindborg, S.R., Schacht, A.L., 2010. How to improve R&D productivity: the pharmaceutical industry's grand challenge. Nat. Rev. Drug Discov. 9 (3), 203–214.
Polak, S., Tylutki, Z., Holbrook, M., Wiśniowska, B., 2019. Better prediction of the local concentration–effect relationship: The role of physiologically based pharmacokinetics and quantitative systems pharmacology and toxicology in the evolution of model-informed drug discovery and development. Drug Discov. Today 24 (7), 1344–1354. doi:10.1016/j.drudis.2019.05.016.
Poplin, R., et al., 2018. Prediction of cardiovascular risk factors from retinal fundus photographs via deep learning. Nat. Biomed. Eng. 2 (3), 158–164.
Priya, S., Tripathi, G., Singh, D.B., Jain, P., Kumar, A., 2022. Machine learning approaches and their applications in drug discovery and design. Chem. Biol. Drug Des. 100 (1), 136–153. doi:10.1111/cbdd.14057.
Pushpakom, S., et al., 2019. Drug repurposing: progress, challenges and recommendations. Nat. Rev. Drug Discov. 18 (1), 41–58.

Rajkomar, A., et al., 2019. Machine learning in medicine. N. Engl. J. Med. 380 (14), 1347–1358.
Ramsundar, B., Eastman, R., Walters, R., 2017. DeepChem: a deep learning platform for drug discovery. J. Chem. Inf. Model. 57 (4), 1013–1017.
Relling, M.V., Evans, W.E., 2015. Pharmacogenomics in the clinic. Nature 526 (7573), 343–350.
Richard, A.M., Judson, R.S., Houck, K.A., 2016. ToxCast chemical landscape: paving the road to 21st century toxicology. Chem. Res. Toxicol. 29 (8), 1225–1251.
Sarker, A., Ginn, R., Nikfarjam, A., et al., 2015. Utilizing social media data for pharmacovigilance: a review. J. Biomed. Inform. 54, 202–212. doi:10.1016/j.jbi.2015.02.004.
Shah, P., et al., 2019. Artificial intelligence and machine learning in clinical development: a translational perspective. NPJ Digit. Med. 2 (1), 1–9.
Shi, L., et al., 2016. The sequencing quality control (SEQC) project: a comprehensive assessment of RNA-seq accuracy, reproducibility and information content. Nat. Biotechnol. 34 (3), 303–311. doi:10.1038/nbt.3519.
Siramshetty, et al., 2018. PreSS/MD: predictor of hERG-mediated cardiotoxicity using machine learning. J. Chem. Inf. Model. 58, 529–539.
Ståhl, N., Falkman, G., Karlsson, A., Mathiason, G., Boström, J., 2019. Deep learning for molecular design—A review of the state of the art. Mol. Inform. 38 (8–9), 1900082. doi:10.1002/minf.201900082.
Stokes, J.M., Yang, K., Swanson, K., Jin, W., 2020. Deep learning-based de novo design of antibiotics. Cell 180 (4), 688–702.e13.
Tang, B., Pan, Z., Yin, K., Khateeb, A., 2019. Recent advances of deep learning in bioinformatics and computational biology. Front. Genet. 10 (214). doi:10.3389/fgene.2019.00214.
Tatonetti, N.P., et al., 2012. Data-driven prediction of drug effects and interactions. Sci. Transl. Med. 4 (125), 125ra31.
Topol, E.J., 2019. High-performance medicine: the convergence of human and artificial intelligence. Nat. Med. 25 (1), 44–56.
Tropsha, A., 2010. Best practices for QSAR model development, validation, and exploitation. Mol. Inform. 29 (6-7), 476–488.
Uehara, T., Minowa, Y., Morikawa, Y., Kondo, C., 2016. Open TG-GATES: a large-scale transcriptomics database for predicting drug-induced liver toxicity. PLoS ONE 11(3), e0151066.
Vamathevan, J., Clark, D., Czodrowski, P., et al., 2019. Applications of machine learning in drug discovery and development. Nat. Rev. Drug Discov. 18 (6), 463–477.
Vilar, S., Harpaz, R., Uriarte, E., Friedman, C., 2012. Drug-drug interaction through molecular structure similarity analysis. J. Am. Med. Inform. Assoc. 19 (6), 1066–1074.
Vilar, S., Harpaz, R., Uriarte, E., Santana, L., Rabadan, R., Friedman, C., 2012. Drug-drug interaction through molecular structure similarity analysis. J. Am. Med. Inform. Assoc. 19 (6), 1066–1074. doi:10.1136/amiajnl-2012-000935.
Wallach, I., Dzamba, M., Heifets, A., 2015. AtomNet: a deep convolutional neural network for bioactivity prediction in structure-based drug discovery. arXiv. https://doi.org/10.48550/arXiv.1510.02855.
Wang, Z., et al., 2016. Predicting drug-induced liver injury by machine learning. Biochem. Pharmacol. 110, 62–72.
Waring, M.J., et al., 2015. An analysis of the attrition of drug candidates from four major pharmaceutical companies. Nat. Rev. Drug Discov. 14 (7), 475–486.
Williams, A.J., Grulke, C.M., Edwards, J., McEachran, A.D., 2017. The CompTox chemistry dashboard: a community data resource for environmental chemistry. J. Cheminform. 9 (1), 61.
Xu, Y., et al., 2015. Deep learning for toxicity prediction in drug development. J. Chem. Inf. Model. 55 (10), 2085–2093.

Xu, Y., Dai, Z., Chen, F., Gao, S., Pei, J., Lai, L., 2021. Deep learning for drug-induced toxicity prediction. Chem. Res. Toxicol. 34 (9), 1943–1956. doi:10.1021/acs.chemrestox.1c00169.

Yang, B., Li, K., Zhong, X., Zou, J., 2022. Implementation of deep learning in drug design. MedComm – Future Medicine 1, e18. doi:10.1002/mef2.18.

Yang, K., et al., 2019. Analyzing learned molecular representations for property prediction. J. Chem. Inf. Model. 59 (8), 3370–3388.

Yeleswarapu, S., Rao, A., Joseph, T., Saipradeep, V.G., Srinivasan, R., 2014. A pipeline to extract drug-adverse event pairs from multiple data sources for pharmacovigilance. BMC Med. Inform. Decis. Mak. 14 (Suppl 3), S8.

Yu, K.H., et al., 2018. Artificial intelligence in healthcare. Nat. Biomed. Eng. 2 (10), 719–731.

Yuan, H., et al., 2021. Machine learning for pharmacogenomics and precision medicine. Front. Pharmacol. 12, 682804.

Zeng, X., Zhu, S., Liu, X., Zhou, Y., Nussinov, R., Cheng, F., 2019. deepDR: A network-based deep learning approach to in silico drug repositioning. Bioinformatics 35 (24), 5191–5198. doi:10.1093/bioinformatics/btz418.

Zhang, J.D., Berntenis, N., Roth, A., Ebeling, M., 2014. Data mining reveals a network of early-response genes as a consensus signature of drug-induced in vitro and in vivo toxicity. Pharmacogenomics J. 14 (3), 208–216. doi:10.1038/tpj.2013.39.

Zhang, Y., 2020. An in-depth summary of recent artificial intelligence applications in drug design. arXiv:2110.05478.

Zhavoronkov, A., 2018. Artificial intelligence for drug discovery, biomarker development, and generation of novel chemistry. Mol. Pharm. 15 (10), 4311–4313. doi:10.1021/acs.molpharmaceut.8b00930.

Zhavoronkov, A., Ivanenkov, Y.A., Aliper, A., et al., 2019. Deep learning enables rapid identification of potent DDR1 kinase inhibitors. Nat. Biotechnol. 37 (9), 1038–1040.

Zhong, F., Xing, J., Li, X., Liu, X., Fu, Z., Xiong, Z., et al., 2018. Artificial intelligence in drug design. Sci. China Life Sci. 61 (10), 1191–1204. doi:10.1007/s11427-018-9342-2.

Zhou, W., Wang, Y., Tang, H., Wang, X., Yan, Y., 2020. Deep learning in drug discovery: Challenges and opportunities. Curr. Top. Med. Chem. 20 (21), 1922–1934.

Zitnik, M., Agrawal, M., Leskovec, J., 2018. Modeling polypharmacy side effects with graph convolutional networks. Bioinformatics 34 (13), i457–i466.

10

Artificial intelligence-enabled tools used in drug designing

Deepak Verma[a] and Shruti Kapoor[b]
[a]*Department of Oncology, Johns Hopkins Medicine, Baltimore, MD, United States*
[b]*University of California Santa Cruz, Santa Cruz, CA, United States*

1 Introduction

Over the last decade, advancements in algorithms, data access, and computing power have driven the development of an ecosystem of artificial intelligence (AI)-enabled tools that influence nearly every phase of the discovery process: target identification and validation, hit finding, de novo molecule design, docking and binding pose prediction, property and ADMET prediction, retrosynthesis planning, lead optimization, and drug repurposing. These tools vary from open-source libraries and benchmarks that make cutting-edge techniques accessible to the public to industrial platforms that combine AI with automation and high-content screening. This chapter explores the landscape, core tasks, and data fundamental to AI in drug design, along with key methods and tools, their successes and limitations, and their integration into model-informed and data-driven discovery strategies (Kim et al., 2020; Vamathevan et al., 2019). A workflow for drug design, along with other essential components, is illustrated in Fig. 10.1.

If you work in drug discovery, you've likely noticed the change. A few years ago, AI in pharma was mainly promises and pitch decks. Today, it's a collection of specific tools that teams actively use to make practical decisions: which targets to pursue, what molecules to generate, what to test first, and how to synthesize them. This chapter focuses on that real-world application. It's a guided overview of named AI tools you can apply across the small-molecule and biological pipeline, what they do, where they fit, and what to be aware of when using them.

Why focus on tools rather than theory? Because in discovery, speed and context matter. The difference between a model on paper

The AI Frontier in Molecular Modelling and Drug Designing. https://doi.org/10.1016/B978-0-443-40338-5.00002-0

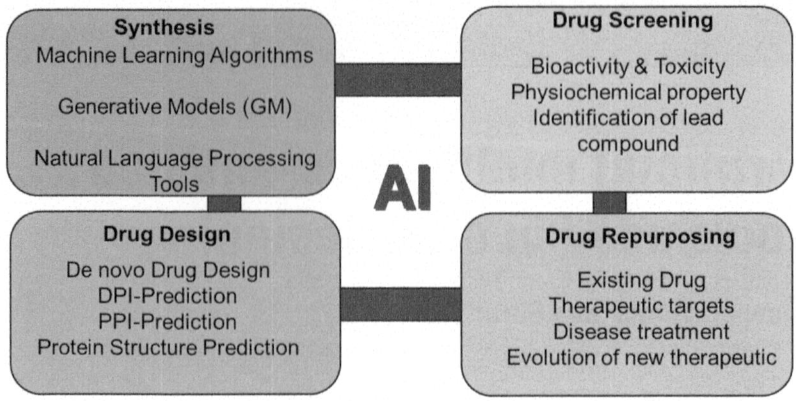

Fig. 10.1 Workflow of drug designing. All the components are listed for AI-based drug designing.

and a tool in your hands is whether it's connected to the data you have, the decisions you need to make this week, and the constraints of your lab and budget. When a medicinal chemist sits down to plan the next cycle, they don't want to build a model from scratch; they want a trustworthy way to generate candidate compounds that satisfy potency, selectivity, ADMET, and synthetic feasibility constraints. When a biology lead is exploring new disease biology, they want to identify which targets are most promising based on genetic and clinical evidence. The "what, where, and how" of tools is the shortest path from AI to impact (Kim et al., 2020).

1.1 Three things made artificial intelligence tools in drug design usable

Firstly, data has become more accessible and easier to process. Public resources, such as the Open Targets Platform, combine genetics, omics, and clinical evidence with machine learning assistance, enabling you to evaluate targets in minutes rather than weeks. The AlphaFold database offers high-quality structural predictions for most proteins you will encounter, enabling pocket prediction, epitope mapping, and structure-guided design even when crystals are unavailable (Ren et al., 2023; Visan and Negut, 2024).

Secondly, models have transitioned into ready-to-use products. Instead of needing a GitHub repository to train, you now have web apps and application programming interface (APIs) such as ADMETlab (Fu et al., 2024), IBM RXN (Cardinale et al., 2023) for chemistry, and BioNeMo-hosted generative models with safeguards for synthesizability. Commercial platforms, such as Chemistry42 (Ivanenkov et al., 2023) or Iktos (Parrot et al., 2023), integrate multiparameter optimization (MPO), retrosynthesis scoring, and portfolio-aware constraints to better align proposals with actual production.

Third, organizations learned how to integrate. It's now common to see pipelines where ideation tools feed into ADMET filters and synthesizability gates, which then pass to retrosynthesis planners linked to vendor catalogs. Real-world discovery relies on repeatable loops: design, triage, plan, make, test, learn, and repeat—ideally in a weekly sprint cycle (Kim et al., 2020).

1.2 What this looks like in practice

Imagine you're beginning an oncology project. You shortlist targets with strong human evidence using Open Targets, then obtain structures from AlphaFold2 and evaluate ligandability with pocket predictors. You outline a target product profile (including potency goals, central nervous system (CNS) exposure limits, and off-targets to avoid) and set up a design tool like REINVENT (Loeffler et al., 2024) or Chemistry42 to generate compounds that meet your property criteria. Before anyone becomes attached to a scaffold, proposals are screened with ADMETlab and pharmacokinetics using graph-based signatures (pkCSM) (Pires et al., 2015) to identify solubility, cytochrome P450 (CYP), and human Ether-à-go-go–Related Gene (hERG) risks. Next, you run the top candidates through AIZynthFinder (Saigiridharan et al., 2024) or IBM RXN to confirm that routes exist and precursors are accessible. Only the designs that pass this "feasible and safe enough to try" filter proceed to synthesis and testing. Each lab result feeds back into retraining your scoring functions, tightening constraints, and refining structure-activity hypotheses. No docking is required.

This workflow isn't imaginary. It's how many teams already operate, whether with open-source components, commercial platforms, or a combination of both. The specifics differ across therapeutic areas and modalities, but the pattern repeats: AI tools serve as specialized instruments in a lab, each with a clear purpose, calibrated to your context.

2 Role of AI in drug discovery

Target identification and prioritization. Tools here help you move from broad disease biology to specific, testable targets with context. Open Targets combines genetics, clinical trials, and literature evidence into ranked lists. Commercial platforms, such as PandaOmics (Kamya et al., 2024) and BenevolentAI (Niazi, 2025), generate hypotheses from knowledge graphs and omics data. The key is transparency: understanding why a target is recommended and what evidence supports it, so that you can coordinate with your biology and safety teams.

Protein structure and pocket predictions. AlphaFold2 and ESMFold (Zalewski et al., 2025) provide structures when no crystal data are available, along with confidence metrics. Pocket predictors, such as DeepSite or P2Rank (Krivák and Hoksza, 2018), help assess ligandability and guide rational design or binding-surface analysis of biologics. These tools don't account for dynamics but offer a strong starting point for developing mechanistic hypotheses and designing molecules or binders.

De novo small molecule design and multiparameter optimization. This is where generative models begin to resemble copilot tools for medicinal chemists. Open-source frameworks like REINVENT allow you to encode your project's scoring function, balancing potency proxies with physicochemical properties and liabilities. Commercial platforms such as Chemistry42 or NVIDIA's BioNeMo MegaMolBART (BioNeMo's, n.d.) offer more ready-to-use capabilities and are easier to operate at scale. The aim is not just novelty, but novelty that you can create, test, and tailor to your profile.

ADMET and safety prediction. Tools such as ADMETlab 3.0, pkCSM, and industrial suites (e.g., ADMET Predictor) forecast early risks of absorption, distribution, metabolism, excretion, and toxicity. They're imperfect—every model is—but when calibrated to your assays, they help you avoid costly dead ends and prioritize synthesis. Think of them as triage and guidance, not verdicts.

Synthesis planning and chemical accessibility. Great ideas are only helpful if you can execute them. RXN for Chemistry, ASKCOS (Tu et al., 2025), AiZynthFinder, and Synthia offer forward predictions, retrosynthesis, and route scoring. Platforms that link routes to actual supplier catalogs (e.g., PostEra Manifold) help you base your designs on real purchasing options and enable on-demand chemistry. Including these in the design process improves the quality of candidates you send to the lab and shortens cycle times.

Quantitative structure-activity relationship (QSAR) and custom property modeling. Sometimes the best model is the one you train on your data. Tools like Chemprop, AutoML frameworks, and konstanz information miner (KNIME) -based pipelines enable you to create project-specific predictors for potency, selectivity, or ADME endpoints when public models are insufficient. The key is disciplined data curation, proper splits (scaffold or temporal), and tracking uncertainty (Tomorowicz et al., 2020; Romero et al., 2022; Heid et al., 2024; Hammami et al., 2025).

Biologics and modality-specific design. Protein design has progressed quickly. RFdiffusion can generate backbones for binders or new proteins; ProteinMPNN creates sequences suited to those backbones. Antibody-focused tools (ABodyBuilder3, IgFold) help with structure modeling and complementarity-determining region (CDR) loop predictions. These tools complement small-molecule design by targeting protein-protein interfaces and biologic modalities using AI-driven methods (Dauparas et al., 2022; Watson et al., 2023; Kenlay et al., 2024).

3 AI-enabled tools in drug design

In this section, we will discuss various AI-driven tools for drug design. A list of currently available tools is provided in Table 10.1.

3.1 DeepChem (toolkit and model zoo)

DeepChem is an open-source Python library that standardizes featurization, modeling, training, and evaluation for cheminformatics, materials science, and computational biology. It provides unified featurization (e.g., extended-connectivity fingerprint (ECFP fingerprints), atom/bond graph features, 3D conformer-based features, and protein/ simplified molecular input line entry system (SMILES) sequence featurizers) and a broad set of models, including graph convolutional networks (GraphConv, Weave), message-passing neural networks (MPNNs), attention-based graph models, classical ML (random forests, XGBoost), multitask neural nets, and 3D grid/CNN models for protein–ligand tasks. DeepChem's data pipeline includes MoleculeNet dataset loaders, scaffold-aware splits, metric utilities, and hyperparameter search, enabling fair and reproducible benchmarking and rapid experimentation. It is designed to be extensible, serving as scaffolding to integrate new state-of-the-art architectures as they emerge. Example: build a blood–brain barrier permeability (BBBP) classifier by loading the BBBP dataset from MoleculeNet in DeepChem, using scaffold split for validation, featurizing with RDKit-based atom/bond features, training an MPNN, and calibrating predictions for deployment in early CNS screening. Web link: https://deepchem.io/ (code: https://github.com/deepchem/deepchem). The portal homepage is shown in Fig. 10.2.

Table 10.1 Description of machine learning models for drug design and discovery.

Tool	Application	Framework	Method	Input Types	Availability	URL	References
ADMETlab 3.0	ML-based ADMET property prediction suite	–	–	–	–	https://admetmesh.scbdd.com/service/admetlab2/	Fu et al. (2024)
AIZynthFinder	ML-guided retrosynthesis planning	–	–	–	Open source	https://github.com/MolecularAI/aizynthfinder	Saigiridharan et al. (2024)
AlphaFold	Protein structure prediction	Python, JAX	Transformer-based MSA	Amino acid sequence	Open source	https://github.com/deepmind/alphafold/	Varadi et al. (2022)
ASKCOS	Template/template-free retrosynthesis and planning	–	–	–	–	https://askcos.mit.edu/	Tu et al. (2025)
Atomwise AtomNet	CNN-based structure-based virtual screening	Caffe	DCNN	3D molecular structures	Open source	https://www.atomwise.com/	Eyster et al. (1932)
CDDD	Continuous data-driven molecular descriptors	–	–	–	Open source	https://github.com/jrwnter/cddd	Winter et al. (2019)
Chemical VAE	Molecular property learning	TensorFlow	DNN	SMILES	Open source	https://github.com/aspuru-guzik-group/chemical_vae/	Gómez-Bombarelli et al. (2018)
Chemistry42 (Insilico)	Generative design platform (multiobjective)	–	–	–	–	https://insilico.com/platform/chemistry42	Ivanenkov et al. (2023)
DeepAffinity	Drug–target binding affinity prediction	Python, TensorFlow	CNN + RNN	SMILES, protein sequences	Open source	https://github.com/Shen-Lab/DeepAffinity	Karimi et al. (2019)
DeepBar	Binding affinity estimation	Python	Deep Generative Models	Molecular descriptors	Documentation available	https://fastmbar.readthedocs.io/en/latest/	Perini et al. (2021)

DeepBind Model	Binding specificity prediction	PyTorch	Reinforcement Learning	DNA/RNA sequences	Open source	https://github.com/MedChaabane/DeepBind-withPyTorch	Alipanahi et al. (2015)
DeepChem	Cheminformatics, drug discovery	TensorFlow, PyTorch	Scikit-learn, TensorFlow, XGBoost	SMILES, graphs	Open source	https://github.com/deepchem/deepchem	Bharath Ramsundar et al. (2019)
DeepConv-DTI	Drug–target interaction prediction	TensorFlow	CNN	SMILES, sequences	Open source	https://github.com/GIST-CSBL/DeepConv-DTI	Lee et al. (2019)
DeepCPI	Compound–protein interaction prediction	TensorFlow	Multimodal DNN	SMILES, protein sequences	Open source	https://github.com/FangpingWan/DeepCPI	Wan et al. (2019)
DeepDrug	DTI & DDI prediction	PyTorch	Deep GNN	SMILES, protein sequences, graphs	Open source	https://github.com/wanwenzeng/deepdrug	Yin et al. (2023)
DeepDTA	Drug–target interaction prediction	TensorFlow	CNN	SMILES, protein sequences	Open source	https://github.com/hkmztrk/DeepDTA	Öztürk et al. (2018)
DeepGraphMol	Molecular generation	TensorFlow, RL frameworks	Graph CNN + RL	Graphs	Open source	https://github.com/dbkgroup/prop_gen	Khemchandani et al. (2020)
DeepPocket	Protein–ligand binding site prediction	Python, PyTorch	3D CNN	3D protein structures	Open source	https://github.com/DeepRank/DeepPocket	Renaud et al. (2021)
DeepPurpose	Drug–target interaction prediction	PyTorch	CNN + RNN	SMILES, sequences	Open source	https://github.com/kexinhuang12345/DeepPurpose	Huang et al. (2020)
DeepScreen	Drug–target interaction prediction	Python	DCNN	Molecular graphs, sequences	Web-based	http://deepscreening.xielab.net/	Rifaioglu et al. (2020)

Continued

Table 10.1 Description of machine learning models for drug design and discovery—cont'd

Tool	Application	Framework	Method	Input Types	Availability	URL	References
DeepSite	DNA–protein binding prediction	TensorFlow	BLSTM + CNN	DNA sequences	Open source	https://github.com/greenelab/deep-review/issues/677	Zhang et al. (2020)
DeepTox	Toxicity prediction	Python	SVM + Random Forest	SMILES	Web-based	http://www.bioinf.jku.at/research/DeepTox/	Mayr et al. (2016)
DGL-LifeSci	GNN toolkit for molecular/protein tasks (built on DGL)	Python	GNN	–	Open source	https://lifesci.dgl.ai/	Zhu et al. (2022)
DiffDock	Diffusion model for protein–ligand pose prediction	Python	–	pdb	Open source	https://github.com/gcorso/diffdock	Herron et al. (2025)
EquiBind	SE(Ren et al., 2023)-equivariant ligand docking	–	–	–	Open source	https://github.com/HannesStark/EquiBind	EquiBind: Geometric Deep Learning for Drug Binding Structure Prediction (2022)
ESMFold	Fast single-sequence protein folding (transformers)	–	–	–	Open source	https://github.com/facebookresearch/esm	Zalewski et al. (2025)
GNINA	CNN-based docking and rescoring	–	–	–	Open source	https://github.com/gnina/gnina	McNutt et al. (2025)
Graph-Level Learning	Drug discovery via graph learning	TensorFlow	NN	Molecular graphs	Open source	https://github.com/ZJULearning/graph-level-drugdiscovery	Ma et al. (2018)

Link-INVENT	Generative linker design (e.g., PROTAC linkers)	–	–	–	Open source	https://github.com/MolecularAI/Link-INVENT	Guo et al. (2023)
MoleculeNet	Molecular property benchmarks	TensorFlow, scikit-learn	Scikit-learn, TensorFlow, XGBoost	SMILES, descriptors	Open source	https://moleculenet.org/	Wu et al. (2018)
MolTrans	Drug–target interaction prediction	Python	Transformer	SMILES, protein sequences	Open source	https://github.com/kexinhuang12345/MolTrans	Huang et al. (2021)
NVIDIA BioNeMo	Foundation models for molecules/proteins (e.g., MegaMolBART, ESMFold)	–	–	–	–	https://developer.nvidia.com/bionemo	BioNeMo's (n.d.)
OpenFold	Open-source reimplementation of AlphaFold	–	–	–	Open source	https://github.com/aqlaboratory/openfold	Ahdritz et al. (2024)
PADME	Drug–target interaction prediction	Python, TensorFlow	Graph Convolutional Network	Molecular graphs, protein sequences	Open source	https://github.com/chaninn/PADME	Feng et al. (2018)
PathDSP	Cancer drug sensitivity	Keras	FNN	Pathways, gene expression	Open source	https://github.com/TangYiChing/PathDSP	Tang and Gottlieb (2021)
pkCSM	Graph-based signatures for ADMET predictions	–	–	–	–	http://biosig.unimelb.edu.au/pkcsm/	Pires et al. (2015)
RDKit	Cheminformatics and feature generation	–	–	–	Open source	https://www.rdkit.org/	RDKit It. Introduction to RDKit (n.d.)
REINVENT	RL-based de novo molecular generation	–	–	–	Open source	https://github.com/MolecularAI/Reinvent	Loeffler et al. (2024)

Continued

Table 10.1 Description of machine learning models for drug design and discovery—cont'd

Tool	Application	Framework	Method	Input Types	Availability	URL	References
RoseTTAFold	Protein structure prediction (tri-track network)	–	–	–	Open source	https://github.com/RosettaCommons/RoseTTAFold	Baek et al. (2021)
RXNMapper	Attention-based atom mapping for reactions	–	–	–	Open source	https://github.com/rxn4chemistry/rxnmapper	Chen et al. (2024)
SELFIES	Robust molecular string representation for generative models	–	–	–	Open source	https://github.com/aspuru-guzik-group/selfies	Krenn et al. (2020)
TorchDrug	Drug discovery platform	PyTorch	Graph Isomorphism Network	Graphs, SMILES	Open source	https://torchdrug.ai/	Zhu et al. (2022)
WideDTA	Drug–target binding affinity prediction	Python, Keras	CNN	SMILES, protein sequences	Open source	https://github.com/hkmztrk/WideDTA	Öztürk et al. (2019), Öztürk et al. (2019)

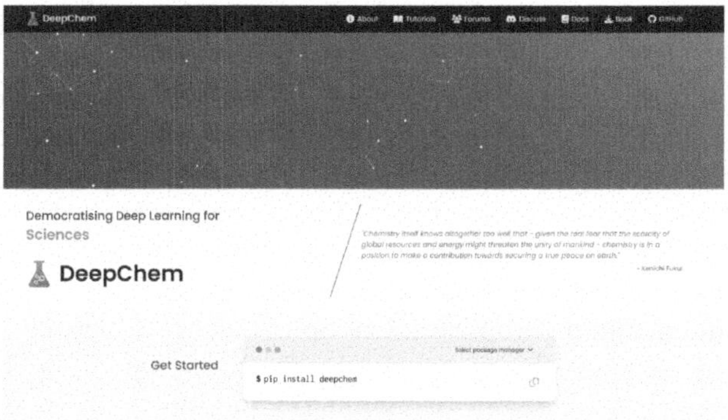

Fig. 10.2 Homepage of DeepChem. DeepCam is an open-source tool and can be accessed through https://deepchem.io/.

3.2 Chemprop (directed message passing for property prediction)

Chemprop is a state-of-the-art framework for molecular property prediction built on the directed MPNN (D-MPNN). It passes messages along directed bonds rather than nodes, improving information flow and reducing message "tottering," and learns from RDKit-derived atomic and bond features while optionally concatenating global molecular descriptors to boost data efficiency. The global graph embedding is pooled and fed through feed-forward layers, with support for multitask learning, class imbalance handling, and model calibration. Robust generalization is encouraged via ensembling, scaffold splits, and uncertainty estimation (e.g., MC dropout or ensemble variance), which are vital in low-data regimes typical of drug discovery. Chemprop also supports extensions for 3D/conformer-aware inputs and domain-specific heads for ADMET, potency, and selectivity. Example: train a D-MPNN ensemble on the MoleculeNet "β-site APP-cleaving enzyme (BACE)" classification task to predict beta-secretase inhibitors, use a scaffold split to mimic real-world novelty, and add calculated descriptors (e.g., logP, topological polar surface area (TPSA)) for improved performance under limited data. Web link: https://chemprop.readthedocs.io/ (code: https://github.com/chemprop/chemprop).

3.3 AlphaFold (protein structure prediction)

AlphaFold is a transformer-based model that predicts protein 3D structures from sequences, enabling downstream tasks such as binding-site mapping and structure-based design. It uses multiple sequence alignments (MSAs) and template hits to build sequence and pairwise representations that capture coevolutionary signals. The Evoformer block employs triangular updates and attention to propagate constraints across the MSA and pair tracks, while the structure module uses invariant point attention to assemble 3D coordinates; iterative "recycling" refines predictions. Confidence outputs (per-residue predicted local distance difference test score (pLDDT) and predicted aligned error (PAE)) inform which regions of the model are reliable for docking or design, and AlphaFold-Multimer extends the approach to protein complexes. Example: retrieve a high-confidence AlphaFold structure for a novel enzyme from the AlphaFold DB, mask low-confidence loops using pLDDT, identify pockets, and dock fragment libraries into the confident regions to seed a structure-based campaign. Web link: https://alphafold.com/ (code: https://github.com/google-deepmind/alphafold; database: https://alphafold.ebi.ac.uk/). The AlphaFold homepage is shown in Fig. 10.3.

3.4 MoleculeNet (benchmarking suite and datasets)

MoleculeNet is a curated collection of molecular datasets with standardized splits and metrics, designed to systematically benchmark AI models in drug discovery. It covers physicochemical, biophysics, quantum chemistry, and ADMET tasks with careful label curation and quality control. Standard splits include random, stratified, and scaffold splits to assess both in-distribution performance and scaffold-level generalization—critical for realistic evaluation in medicinal chemistry. MoleculeNet provides baselines ranging from fingerprint-based methods with random forests/gradient boosting to several graph neural

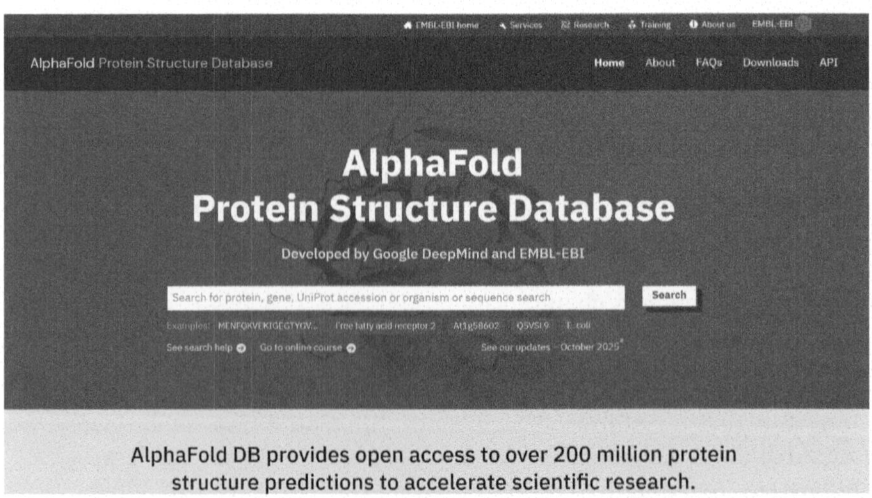

Fig. 10.3 Homepage of AlphaFold. This is the homepage of widely used AlphaFold.

networks, using consistent metrics (ROC-receiver operating characteristic - area under the curve (AUC), precision-recall - area under the curve (PR-AUC), root mean squared error (RMSE), mean absolute error (MAE)) and workflows to ensure reproducibility. For example, compare Chemprop versus a GraphConv baseline on estimated solubility (ESOL), hydration free energy (FreeSolv), and Tox21 (toxicity) across scaffold splits, then select the best-calibrated model for prospective screening. Web link: https://moleculenet.org/ (also available via DeepChem: https://deepchem.io/molecule-net). The homepage of the MoleculeNet machine learning project is shown in Fig. 10.4.

3.5 Generative tensorial reinforcement learning (for de novo design)

Generative tensorial reinforcement learning (GENTRL) is a generative RL framework for de novo molecular design targeting multiple objectives, including potency, novelty, ADMET, and synthesizability. It starts with a variational autoencoder (VAE) trained on molecular strings (e.g., SMILES) to learn a continuous latent space of chemical structures, then applies policy-gradient reinforcement learning to bias sampling toward molecules with high composite rewards computed by predictive models (QSAR, docking) and synthetic feasibility assessments. Its "tensorial" aspect comes from tensor-train (low-rank tensor) parameterizations that help scale modeling of distributions over high-dimensional latent variables. Careful reward shaping balances potency, selectivity, diversity/novelty, and synthetic accessibility to avoid mode collapse and impractical designs, and the workflow alternates generative updates with external scoring for fast iteration. Example: optimize a kinase inhibitor series by rewarding predicted DDR1 potency (QSAR), docking score to the target, SA score, and

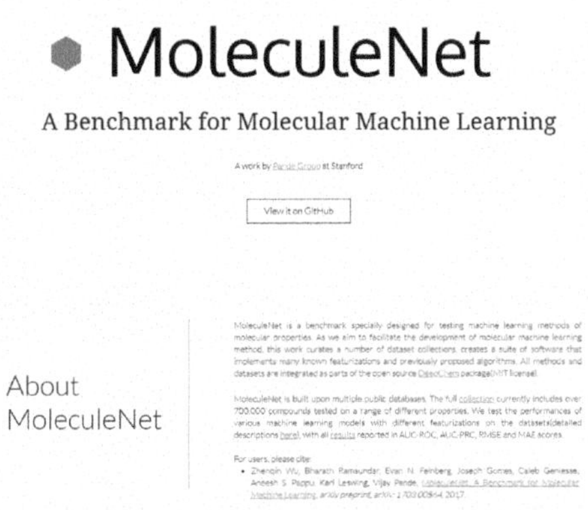

Fig. 10.4 Homepage of MoleculeNet, A benchmark tool for machine learning.

novelty vs. the existing chemotype, then filter generated candidates with retrosynthetic analysis and ADMET screens before synthesis. Web link: https://github.com/insilicomedicine/GENTRL.

3.6 IBM RXN for chemistry (transformer-based reaction prediction and retrosynthesis)

IBM RXN is a cloud platform that uses sequence-to-sequence transformers for forward reaction prediction, single-step retrosynthesis, and multistep synthesis planning, treating reactions as tokenized sequences (e.g., SMILES) trained on large corpora such as united states patent and trademark office (USPTO) patents. It supports both forward prediction (products from reactants/reagents) and retrosynthesis (precursor suggestions), uses beam search with chemical validity checks and constraints (e.g., reagent availability, protection/deprotection logic), and leverages attention for atom mapping (via RXNMapper) to improve interpretability and data augmentation. Planning stitches single steps using guided search and cost considerations. Example: propose a three-step route to a fragment-like amide by starting with retrosynthesis in IBM RXN, constraining building blocks to a vendor catalog, validating atom mappings with RXNMapper, and exporting a route for lab execution. Web link: https://rxn.res.ibm.com/ (docs and tools: RXNMapper: https://github.com/rxn4chemistry/rxnmapper). The homepage for the IBM-RXN portal is shown in Fig. 10.5.

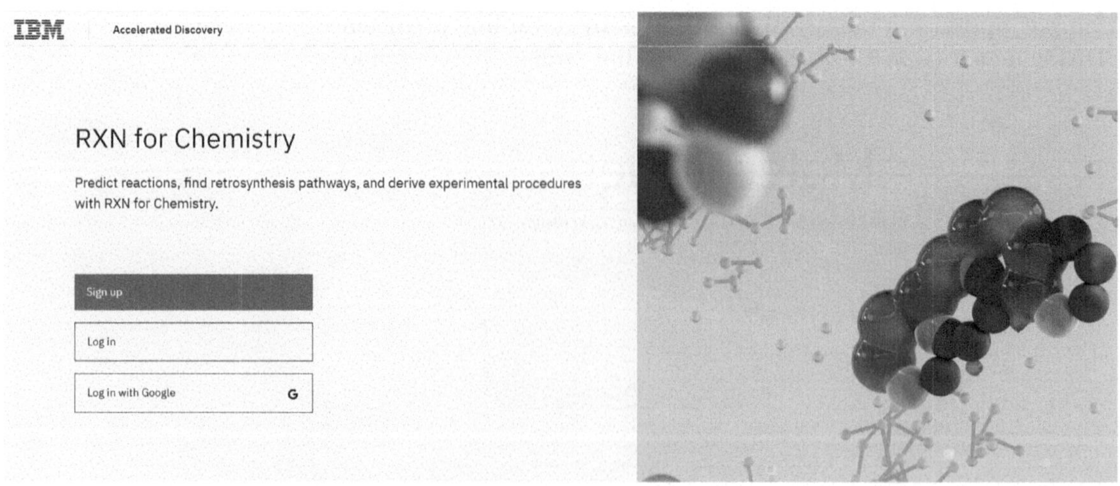

Fig. 10.5 Home page of IBM-RXNMapper. This is the IBM-RXNMapper homepage and can be accessed through: https://rxn.res.ibm.com/.

3.7 AutoDock-GPU + AI scorers (physics-based docking enhanced by ML rescoring)

AutoDock-GPU is a GPU-accelerated docking engine that speeds up the Lamarckian genetic algorithm and local search to explore ligand poses and conformations efficiently. Traditional scoring functions estimate intermolecular energies (van der Waals, electrostatics, hydrogen bonding, desolvation) to rank poses; AI-based scorers—commonly 3D convolutional neural network (CNNs) or graph neural network (GNNs) trained on datasets like PDBbind—can rescore the docked poses to improve early enrichment and pose selection. In practice, consensus strategies combine physics-based and ML scores or ensemble multiple models to reduce bias across chemotypes, and active learning can iteratively update ML scorers using new experimental SAR or higher-fidelity calculations (e.g., free energy perturbation (FEP)). Example: run a virtual screen of 100k compounds against a GPCR using AutoDock-GPU, rescore the top 10% poses with GNINA's 3D CNN (trained on cross-docked sets), select consensus hits, and follow up with short MD and rescoring to prioritize synthesis. Web link: AutoDock accelerated on graphics processing units (AutoDock-GPU) https://github.com/ccsb-scripps/AutoDock-GPU; GNINA (AI rescoring) https://github.com/gnina/gnina.

4 Workflow example: AI-powered drug design

Target selection using AI-first discovery integrates multiomics (transcriptomics, proteomics), genetic evidence genome-wide association study (GWAS)/ expression quantitative trait locus (eQTL), and perturbation screens to identify disease-relevant proteins with actionable biology and tractability. For instance, use Open Targets to score target–disease associations from genetics and literature, then verify essentiality and dependency in disease-relevant cell lines via DepMap clustered regularly interspaced short palindromic repeats (CRISPR) screens. If DNA damage response1 (DDR1), a receptor tyrosine kinase, shows strong genetic support in fibrosis and oncology, shortlist DDR1 based on disease connection, pathway importance, druggability (kinase pocket), and safety signals from human genetics. Links: Open Targets https://platform.opentargets.org/; DepMap https://depmap.org/portal/.

Protein structure prediction involves predicting or retrieving the 3D structure to enable structure-guided design. For targets with only sequence data or novel isoforms, run AlphaFold locally or obtain a model from the AlphaFold DB, and inspect per-residue pLDDT and PAE to identify reliable regions for binding-site work. Map potential ligandable pockets using standard tools (e.g.,

Fpocket) and deprioritize low-confidence loops for initial docking. For DDR1, AlphaFold generally provides high-confidence kinase-domain cores suitable for adenosine triphosphate (ATP) -pocket exploration and the design of type II inhibitors. Links: AlphaFold DB https://alphafold.ebi.ac.uk/; AlphaFold code https://github.com/google-deepmind/alphafold.

Virtual screening (briefly) involves training or applying Chemprop (D-MPNN) and DeepChem baselines to quickly score very large vendor libraries (e.g., ZINC/Enamine REAL) for target activity or proxy endpoints (e.g., kinase-likeness). Use scaffold splits, model ensembling, and calibration for robust prioritization; forward top-scored, diverse scaffolds to docking. Links: Chemprop https://chemprop.readthedocs.io/; DeepChem https://deepchem.io/; Enamine REAL https://enamine.net/hit-finding/real-compounds/real-database; ZINC https://zinc20.docking.org/.

Hit selection and optimization: Move from initial hits to leads using generative design with explicit multiobjective control. GENTRL learns a latent chemical space via a VAE and applies reinforcement learning to maximize a composite reward (e.g., predicted DDR1 potency from a Chemprop model, docking score to the ATP pocket, synthetic accessibility, novelty/diversity, quantitative estimate of Drug-likeness (QED)). Alternatively, REINVENT fine-tunes a SMILES generator with policy gradients against similar rewards and can incorporate reaction filters for synthesizability. In practice, you seed the model with known kinase-like chemotypes, constrain ring systems and PAINS filters, and iterate generation–scoring–selection in short cycles. Example: optimize a quinazoline core toward DDR1 by rewarding lower docking scores, higher ensemble potency predictions, SA score ≤5, and Tanimoto distance ≥0.3 from known DDR1 scaffolds to maintain novelty. Links: GENTRL https://github.com/insilicomedicine/GENTRL; REINVENT https://github.com/MolecularAI/Reinvent; RDKit (descriptors/filters) https://www.rdkit.org/.

ADMET evaluation triage designs involve quick in silico safety and pharmacokinetic screens before synthesis. pkCSM predicts key properties such as hERG liability, CYP inhibition, clearance, and permeability from graph-based signatures, while DeepTox-style deep models assess multiendpoint toxicity (e.g., Tox21). For DDR1 candidates, exclude molecules with predicted hERG risk, strong CYP3A4 inhibition, or poor HLM stability; retain those with acceptable solubility and Caco-2 permeability. Supplement with internal QSARs or public tools (e.g., ADMETlab) as needed, and employ conformal prediction or calibrated probabilities to manage risk when models are extrapolating. Links: pkCSM http://biosig.unimelb.edu.au/pkcsm/; DeepTox (reference implementation) https://github.com/bioinf-jku/DeepTox; ADMETlab 2.0 https://admetmesh.scbdd.com/.

Validation (docking, MD, experiments) involves validating top-ranked designs both computationally and experimentally. First, dock into the AlphaFold or experimental structure using AutoDock-GPU, then rescore the poses with a trained 3D CNN (e.g., GPU-accelerated neural network-enhanced AutoDock (GNINA)) to enhance pose ranking, focusing on hinge H-bonds and gatekeeper interactions typical for kinase inhibitors. Next, run short MD simulations in explicit solvent (e.g., OpenMM or GROningen MAchine for chemical simulations (GROMACS)) to evaluate pose stability and protein–ligand interactions; optionally, compute end-point energies molecular mechanics/generalized born surface area (MM/GBSA) for prioritization. Advance a diverse subset to the bench: confirm binding via biochemical assays (enzyme inhibition), then characterize binding kinetics/affinity surface plasmon resonance (SPR)/isothermal titration calorimetry (ITC) and evaluate cell potency and selectivity across kinome panels. Incorporate experimental SAR data back into the Chemprop predictors and the generative reward to complete the active-learning loop. Links: AutoDock-GPU https://github.com/ccsb-scripps/AutoDock-GPU; GNINA https://github.com/gnina/gnina; OpenMM https://openmm.org/; GROMACS https://www.gromacs.org/.

5 Benefits and challenges

5.1 What makes a tool "good" for a project?

What makes a tool "good" for your project isn't its citation count but its suitability to your team's needs and constraints. The best tools align inputs and outputs with what you actually have and require: do you possess the right data types (sequences, structures, labeled activities, property targets), and does the tool return results your team can act on (such as SMILES, ranked targets, or routes with precursors)? They provide evidence and explainability, so you can understand why a target was ranked or why a property prediction is high or low. Even basic confidence scores or applicability-domain metrics aid in triage. They integrate seamlessly with your stack, supporting RDKit, CSV, and REST, and offer KNIME nodes, Python SDKs, and web APIs—making workflows reproducible and auditable. They suit your cost and licensing posture: open source offers flexibility, whereas commercial options provide robustness and support. Many teams sensibly combine both, using open-source for prototyping and specific tasks, and commercial tools for enterprise-critical processes. They support governance and compliance requirements through versioning, traceability, and documented validation, ensuring model versions, data lineage, and logs are preserved for audits and technical transfer. Finally, they are backed by an active community, responsive support, and regular updates that reduce operational risk.

5.2 Common pitfalls

Common pitfalls are predictable and avoidable. Teams often overtrust generic models: a public ADMET model that performs well on benchmarks may struggle with your chemotypes, so calibrate or retrain it with internal data and monitor correlations with new assays over time. Another trap is deferring synthesizability until the end; if you generate thousands of molecules only to learn they're impractical to make, you've wasted effort—put retrosynthesis or make-on-demand filters up front. Single-structure blindness is also common: AlphaFold models are valuable, but proteins move and pockets reshape, so consider multiple conformers or homologs and triangulate pocket predictions to reduce false negatives. In de novo design, scoring-function sprawl can derail progress; start simple with one or two potency proxies and a few property targets, expand as you learn, and track diversity to avoid mode collapse. Data leakage and unrealistic splits can inflate model performance; prefer scaffold or temporal splits and keep an eye on applicability domain and uncertainty. Above all, don't neglect human-in-the-loop; experienced chemists and biologists should steer AI tools, with reviews and checkpoints built into your loops.

5.3 Validation: Turning predictions into decisions

Validation turns predictions into decisions by being right enough, often enough, to change what you do next. Prioritize prospective tests: run small, real experiments based on tool outputs to gauge utility—did the ADMET filter reduce hERG hits, or did the retrosynthesis tool shorten cycle time? Complement this with backtesting under guardrails: re-run past projects using only data available at the time to see whether outcomes would have changed, while guarding against hindsight bias. Set calibrated expectations up front and decide the role of each prediction—hard gate, soft ranker, or gentle nudge—document thresholds and revisit them as evidence accumulates. Maintain continuous learning by incorporating new assay results into QSAR models and scoring functions, retiring models that drift or underperform, and versioning all updates so that you can roll back when needed.

5.4 Data quality

Data quality influences how far AI tools can go, and you don't need a huge data lake to begin; you need the basics. Standardize clean chemical representations by deduplicating molecules, handling salts and tautomers consistently, and applying clear neutralization rules. Unambiguously define assays by harmonizing protocols and units and tracking changes over time; if two assays both claim to measure solubility under different conditions, they are not the same. Keep data secure yet accessible by protecting sensitive IP while enabling the tools and people who need it—use APIs, governed workspaces, and role-based access. Create feedback loops that record outcomes, such as noting when a route fails due to reagent unavailability so that planning tools can improve with experience.

5.5 Organizational adoption

Organizational adoption is most successful when you treat AI tools like new laboratory equipment. Begin with motivated teams facing clear challenges and a champion willing to iterate, since early successes generate momentum. Offer training sessions and practical guides that teach users how to set scoring functions, interpret uncertainty, and know when to seek a second opinion. Clarify roles so it's obvious who manages data, maintains configurations, and approves moving a design into synthesis; transparency speeds up processes. Track impact using metrics that matter to you—such as the time from concept to synthesis, the proportion of designs passing ADMET filters, and the number of cycles to reach a lead—and share these results broadly. Keep humans involved and celebrate both chemist-generated ideas that AI overlooked and AI-suggested ideas that surprised the team; the aim is augmentation, not replacement.

5.6 Ethics, intellectual property (IP), and risk management

Ethics, intellectual property, and risk management require careful attention as AI tools become more prevalent. Understand the source of training data for generative tools and the applicable license terms, while clarifying IP ownership of AI-generated designs in contracts and internal policies. Monitor bias and fairness: if your training data underrepresents certain chemotypes or protein families, your models will reflect those gaps, so aim for diversity and assess performance across relevant segments. Ensure reproducibility and audit trails by versioning models, data, and configurations, especially in regulated environments where explanations of decisions may be needed years later. Protect proprietary structures, sequences, and assays through secure, compliant deployment options, preferring on-premises or fortified cloud solutions as appropriate.

5.7 Vignettes: Applying principles

A few vignettes illustrate how to apply these principles. In small-molecule ideation for CNS, a team targets a G-protein–coupled receptor (GPCR) implicated by human genetics, confirms evidence with Open Targets, and uses AlphaFold to model extracellular domains. Working within tight CNS constraints, such as low polar surface area and P-gp avoidance, they configure a generative tool to propose candidates. Early triage with ADMETlab flags P-gp liabilities; a quick return from the scoring function reduces them, and AiZynthFinder filters out 40% of proposals that lack feasible routes. The remaining designs proceed to synthesis, and within two cycles, the team achieves a three-fold improvement in brain exposure, validating the value of including ADMET and synthesis planning early in the process.

In a kinase project aimed at redesigning the route to unlock SAR, the team's preferred scaffold stalls because the only feasible route requires a scarce chiral building block. By inputting the scaffold and constraints into IBM RXN and Synthia, they discover an alternative disconnection that utilizes a different, readily available chiral pool. Make-on-demand catalogs confirm availability, enabling the team to resume SAR exploration and identify a subseries with improved selectivity. This advancement wouldn't have been possible if synthesis planning had remained outside the design process.

For protein binder design against an extracellular target without a crystal structure, the team relies on AlphaFold-Multimer to model a dimer interface. It uses RFdiffusion to suggest binders for a conserved pocket. ProteinMPNN generates sequence variants, while an antibody modeling tool assesses CDR loop liabilities. After expression and a small binding panel, they feed back results and iterate, converging within a few rounds on a stable binder with nanomolar affinity, cutting months off the traditional cycle.

6 Future directions

The advent of AI in drug design and discovery has been successful in achieving the goal of producing high-quality data, reducing costs and time, and impacting the entire process. Even so, it poses many unresolved challenges. First, it is worth mentioning that AI, and AI methods in particular, are often seen as "black boxes" or "dark secrets," meaning there is uncertainty about the conclusions AI models provide. The black-box nature of AI models limits their interpretability in decision-making, posing challenges for applying their pharmaceutical or biological implications. The second challenge lies in overfitting and the requirement for large datasets. The size and condition of the datasets used to train the model influence the model's success and, in turn, limit its performance and authenticity. Additionally, the data used to generate these models or databases are not publicly accessible and are often restricted. The third challenge involves selecting models and adjusting the framework. With newer models frequently being proposed, multiple frameworks are available, making it vital to choose the right model for the required tasks.

One major challenge of using AI is managing the various types of bias, including algorithmic, data-driven, and human biases. Data-driven bias can emerge when the training data lacks sufficient variability. Inaccurately or inadequately constructed algorithms struggle to detect patterns in training datasets, resulting in inconclusive outcomes in the screening of lead compounds or drugs. To address this challenge, it is essential to enhance experiment reproducibility, run multiple experiments, utilize a combination of permutation algorithms, employ diverse training groups from various cohorts, and develop methods to detect data biases early. Incorporating these strategies can reduce biases and promote a robust drug discovery process. Last but not least, well-trained AI professionals who can effectively implement AI methods are the need of the hour, and regulatory frameworks must evolve to address AI-driven drug discovery, ensuring safe, transparent, and ethical use.

7 Conclusions

AI has revolutionized the field of drug design, discovery, and development. Once hesitant to deploy AI, companies and laboratories are now promoting and actively utilizing it to advance potential drugs into clinical trials. AI has proven to be a potent tool for discovering new therapeutic chemical moieties, predicting potential drug targets, and assessing chemical and molecular properties with high accuracy and efficiency, accelerating processes and being cost-effective. As technology continues to evolve, there will be an upsurge in advanced, sophisticated algorithms, paving the way for innovative therapeutic solutions. By addressing current gaps and embracing combinatorial approaches, AI will undoubtedly transform medicine, ensuring faster, more effective treatments to address global healthcare needs.

Incorporating AI tools in drug discovery entails both innovation and practicality, exemplified by specific methodologies and frameworks. For instance, target identification and validation are greatly enhanced by AI algorithms like DeepBind, which use sequence data to predict protein-DNA binding. A notable example is its application in identifying critical transcription factors involved in oncogenesis, aiding in early cancer drug development. Similarly, molecular design benefits from tools such as AutoDock, where machine learning aids docking simulations, as shown in research identifying novel Alzheimer's disease inhibitors by analyzing beta-amyloid interactions. Generative models, such as MolGAN, extend these capabilities by creating new molecular entities tailored to specific requirements, demonstrated in drug discovery for antimicrobial resistance, where traditional methods have faltered. Structure-based drug design tools, exemplified by AlphaFold, provide unprecedented insights into protein folding, with applications such as elucidating the structure of SARS-CoV-2 spike proteins, which have led to vaccine and therapeutic developments. Additionally, IBM Watson for Drug Discovery's NLP capabilities have been pivotal in extracting actionable knowledge from vast literature, such as repurposing thalidomide for cancer treatment by identifying its angiogenesis-inhibitory properties. Together, these tools not only accelerate discovery processes but also open avenues for addressing complex biomedical challenges.

AI disclosure

During the preparation of this work, the author(s) used Grammarly Pro in order to tailor the sentences and improve the overall clarity and readability of the chapter. After using this tool/service, the author(s) reviewed and edited the content as needed and take full responsibility for the content of the publication.

References

Ahdritz, G., Bouatta, N., Floristean, C., Kadyan, S., Xia, Q., Gerecke, W., O'Donnell, T.J., Berenberg, D., Fisk, I., Zanichelli, N., Zhang, B., Nowaczynski, A., Wang, B., Stepniewska-Dziubinska, M.M., Zhang, S., Ojewole, A., Guney, M.E., Biderman, S., Watkins, A.M., Ra, S., Lorenzo, P.R., Nivon, L., Weitzner, B., Ban, Y.-E.A., Chen, S., Zhang, M., Li, C., Song, S.L., He, Y., Sorger, P.K., Mostaque, E., Zhang, Z., Bonneau, R., AlQuraishi, M., 2024. OpenFold: retraining AlphaFold2 yields new insights into its learning mechanisms and capacity for generalization. Nat. Methods 21, 1514–1524. doi:10.1038/s41592-024-02272-z.

Alipanahi, B., Delong, A., Weirauch, M.T., Frey, B.J., 2015. Predicting the sequence specificities of DNA- and RNA-binding proteins by deep learning. Nat. Biotechnol. 1546-1696. 33 (8), 831–838. Available from: http://www.nature.com/nbt/index.html. doi:10.1038/nbt.3300.

Baek, M., DiMaio, F., Anishchenko, I., Dauparas, J., Ovchinnikov, S., Lee, G.R., Wang, J., Cong, Q., Kinch, L.N., Schaeffer, R.D., Millán, C., Park, H., Adams, C., Glassman, C.R., DeGiovanni, A., Pereira, J.H., Rodrigues, A.V., Van Dijk, A.A., Ebrecht, A.C., Opperman, D.J., Sagmeister, T., Buhlheller, C., Pavkov-Keller, T., Rathinaswamy, M.K., Dalwadi, U., Yip, C.K., Burke, J.E., Garcia, K.C., Grishin, N.V., Adams, P.D., Read, R.J., Baker, D., 2021. Accurate prediction of protein structures and interactions using a three-track neural network. Science. 1095-9203. 373 (6557), 871–876. Available from: https://science.sciencemag.org/content/373/6557/871.full. doi:10.1126/science.abj8754.

Bharath Ramsundar, P.E., Walters, P., Pande, V., Leswing, K., Zhenqin, W., 2019. Deep Learning for the Life Sciences: Applying Deep Learning to Genomics, Microscopy, Drug Discovery, and more O'Reilly Media, Inc.

BioNeMo's, n.d. N. NVIDIA BioNeMo's. https://github.com/NVIDIA/bionemo-framework.

Cardinale, A., Castrogiovanni, A., Gaudin, T., Geluykens, J., Laino, T., Manica, M., Probst, D., Schwaller, P., Sobczyk, A., Toniato, A., Vaucher, A.C., Wolf, H., Zipoli, F.,

2023. Fueling the digital chemistry revolution with language models. Chimia 77, 484–488. doi:10.2533/chimia.2023.484.

Chen, S., Sunggi, A., Babazade, R., Jung, Y., 2024. Precise atom-to-atom mapping for organic reactions via human-in-the-loop machine learning. Nat. Commun. 2041-1723. 15 (1). doi:10.1038/s41467-024-46364-y.

Dauparas, Anishchenko, Bennett, Bai, Ragotte, Milles, Wicky, Courbet, de Haas, Bethel, Leung, Huddy, Pellock, Tischer, Chan, Koepnick, Nguyen, Kang, Sankaran, Bera, King, Baker, 2022. Robust deep learning–based protein sequence design using ProteinMPNN. Science 378 (6615), 49–56. doi:10.1126/science.add2187.

EquiBind: Geometric Deep Learning for Drug Binding Structure Prediction, 2022.

Eyster, Matsuzaki, S., Pranay, A., Giorgione, J.R., Faakye, A., Ahmed, M., et al., 1932. Mechanistic studies of PFKFB2 reveal a novel inhibitor of its kinase activity.

Feng, Q., Dueva, E., Cherkasov, A., Ester, M., 2018. PADME: a deep learning-based framework for drug-target interaction prediction. arXiv. 2331-8422. Available from: https://arxiv.org. doi:10.48550/arxiv.1807.09741.

Fu, L., Shi, S., Yi, J., Wang, N., He, Y., Wu, Z., Peng, J., Deng, Y., Wang, W., Wu, C., Lyu, A., Zeng, X., Zhao, W., Hou, T., Cao, D., 2024. ADMETlab 3.0: an updated comprehensive online ADMET prediction platform enhanced with broader coverage, improved performance, API functionality and decision support. Nucleic Acids Res. 52. doi:10.1093/nar/gkae236

Gómez-Bombarelli, R., Wei, J.N., Duvenaud, D., Hernández-Lobato, J.M., Sánchez-Lengeling, B., Sheberla, D., Aguilera-Iparraguirre, J., Hirzel, T.D., Adams, R.P., Aspuru-Guzik, A., 2018. Automatic chemical design using a data-driven continuous representation of molecules. ACS Cent. Sci. 2374-7951. 4 (2), 268–276. Available from: http://pubs.acs.org/journal/acscii. doi:10.1021/acscentsci.7b00572.

Guo, J., Knuth, F., Margreitter, C., Janet, J.P., Papadopoulos, K., Engkvist, O., Patronov, A., 2023. Link-INVENT: generative linker design with reinforcement learning. Digit. Discov. 2635-098X. 2 (2), 392–408. Available from: https://www.rsc.org/journals-books-databases/about-journals/digital-discovery/. doi:10.1039/d2dd00115b.

Hammami, M., Yeddes, W., Gadhoumi, H., Yazidi, R., Tounsi, M.S., Msaada, K., 2025. Machine learning-driven bioavailability prediction in early-stage drug development: a KNIME-based computational workflow for digital health applications. Xenobiotica 55 (5), 339–348. doi:10.1080/00498254.2025.2508804.

Heid, E., Greenman, K.P., Chung, Y., Li, S.-C., Graff, D.E., Vermeire, F.H., Wu, H., Green, W.H., McGill, C.J., 2024. Chemprop: a machine learning package for chemical property prediction. J. Chem. Inf. Model. 64, 9–17. doi:10.1021/acs.jcim.3c01250.

Herron, L., Dakka, J., Yao, K., Shi, D., Zhang, Y., Jerome, S.V., 2025. DiffDock-Glide: a hybrid physics-based and data-driven approach to molecular docking. bioRxiv. doi:10.1101/2025.06.02.657461.

Huang, K., Fu, T., Glass, L.M., Zitnik, M., Xiao, C., Sun, J., 2020. DeepPurpose: a deep learning library for drug-target interaction prediction. Bioinformatics. 1460-2059. 36 (22-23), 5545–5547. Available from: http://bioinformatics.oxfordjournals.org/. doi:10.1093/bioinformatics/btaa1005.

Huang, K., Xiao, C., Glass, L.M., Sun, J., 2021. MolTrans: molecular interaction transformer for drug-target interaction prediction. Bioinformatics. 1460-2059. 37 (6), 830–836. Available from: http://bioinformatics.oxfordjournals.org/. doi:10.1093/bioinformatics/btaa880.

Ivanenkov, Y.A., Polykovskiy, D., Bezrukov, D., Zagribelnyy, B., Aladinskiy, V., Kamya, P., Aliper, A., Ren, F., Zhavoronkov, A., 2023. Chemistry42: an AI-driven platform for molecular design and optimization. J. Chem. Inf. Model. 63, 695–701. doi:10.1021/acs.jcim.2c01191.

Kamya, P., Ozerov, I.V., Pun, F.W., Tretina, K., Fokina, T., Chen, S., Naumov, V., Long, X., Lin, S., Korzinkin, M., Polykovskiy, D., Aliper, A., Ren, F., Zhavoronkov, A., 2024.

PandaOmics: an AI-driven platform for therapeutic target and biomarker discovery. J. Chem. Inf. Model. 64, 3961–3969. doi:10.1021/acs.jcim.3c01619.

Karimi, M., Wu, D., Wang, Z., Shen, Y., 2019. DeepAffinity: interpretable deep learning of compound-protein affinity through unified recurrent and convolutional neural networks. Bioinformatics 35 (18), 3329–3338. doi:10.1093/bioinformatics/btz111.

Kenlay, H., Dreyer, F.A., Cutting, D., Nissley, D., Deane, C.M., 2024. ABodyBuilder3: improved and scalable antibody structure predictions. Bioinformatics. 1367-4811. 40 (10). Available from: http://bioinformatics.oxfordjournals.org/. doi:10.1093/bioinformatics/btae576.

Khemchandani, Y., O'Hagan, S., Samanta, S., Swainston, N., Roberts, T.J., Bollegala, D., Kell, D.B., 2020. DeepGraphMol, a multi-objective, computational strategy for generating molecules with desirable properties: a graph convolution and reinforcement learning approach. bioRxiv. 2692-8205. Available from: https://www.biorxiv.org. doi:10.1101/2020.05.25.114165.

Kim, H., Kim, E., Lee, I., Bae, B., Park, M., Nam, H., 2020. Artificial intelligence in drug discovery: a comprehensive review of data-driven and machine learning approaches. Biotechnol. Bioprocess Eng. 25 (6), 895–930. doi:10.1007/s12257-020-0049-y.

Krenn, M., Häse, F., Nigam, A., Friederich, P., Aspuru-Guzik, A., 2020. Self-referencing embedded strings (SELFIES): a 100% robust molecular string representation. Mach. Learn. Sci. Technol. 2632-2153. 1 (4), 045024. doi:10.1088/2632-2153/aba947.

Krivák, R., Hoksza, D., 2018. P2Rank: machine learning based tool for rapid and accurate prediction of ligand binding sites from protein structure. J. Cheminform. 1758-2946. 10 (1). Available from: http://www.springer.com/chemistry/theoretical+and+computational+chemistry/journal/13321. doi:10.1186/s13321-018-0285-8.

Lee, I., Keum, J., Nam, H., Briggs, J.M., 2019. DeepConv-DTI: prediction of drug-target interactions via deep learning with convolution on protein sequences. PLoS Comput. Biol. 1553-7358. 15 (6), e1007129. doi:10.1371/journal.pcbi.1007129.

Loeffler, H.H., He, J., Tibo, A., Janet, J.P., Voronov, A., Mervin, L.H., Engkvist, O., 2024. Reinvent 4: modern AI–driven generative molecule design. J. Cheminform. 16. doi:10.1186/s13321-024-00812-5

Ma, T., Xiao, C., Zhou, J., Wang, F. 2018 Drug similarity integration through attentive multi-view graph auto-encoders. In: IJCAI International Joint Conference on Artificial Intelligence. 9780999241127. International Joint Conferences on Artificial Intelligence, United Kingdom, pp. 3477–3483. http://www.ijcai.org/. doi:10.24963/ijcai.2018/483.

Mayr, A., Klambauer, G., Unterthiner, T., Hochreiter, S., 2016. DeepTox: toxicity prediction using deep learning. Front. Environ. Sci. 2296-665X. 3. doi:10.3389/fenvs.2015.00080.

McNutt, A.T., Li, Y., Meli, R., Aggarwal, R., Koes, D.R., 2025. GNINA 1.3: the next increment in molecular docking with deep learning. J. Cheminform. 1758-2946. 17 (1). Available from: https://jcheminf.biomedcentral.com/. doi:10.1186/s13321-025-00973-x.

Niazi, S.K., 2025. Artificial intelligence in small-molecule drug discovery: a critical review of methods, applications, and real-world outcomes. Pharmaceuticals. 1424-8247. 18 (9), 1271. doi:10.3390/ph18091271.

Öztürk, H., Özgür, A., Ozkirimli, E., 2018. DeepDTA: deep drug–target binding affinity prediction. Bioinformatics. 1367-4803. 34 (17), i821. doi:10.1093/bioinformatics/bty593.

Öztürk, H., Ozkirimli, E., Özgür, A., 2019. WideDTA: prediction of drug-target binding affinity. arXiv. 2331-8422. Available from: https://arxiv.org. doi:10.48550/arxiv.1902.04166.

Parrot, M., Tajmouati, H., da Silva, V.B.R., Atwood, B.R., Fourcade, R., Gaston-Mathé, Y., Huu, N.D., Perron, Q., 2023. Integrating synthetic accessibility with AI-based generative drug design. J. Cheminform. 15. doi:10.1186/s13321-023-00742-8

Perini, M., Piazza, A., Panelli, S., Papaleo, S., Alvaro, A., Vailati, F., Corbella, M., Saluzzo, F., Gona, F., Castelli, D., Farina, C., Marone, P., Cirillo, D.M., Cavallero, A., Zuccotti, G.V., Comandatore, F., 2021. Hypervariable-locus melting typing (HLMT): a novel, fast and inexpensive sequencing-free approach to pathogen typing based on high resolution melting (HRM) analysis. bioRxiv. 2692-8205. Available from: https://www.biorxiv.org. doi:10.1101/2021.07.01.450706.

Pires, D.E.V., Blundell, T.L., Ascher, D.B., 2015. pkCSM: predicting small-molecule pharmacokinetic and toxicity properties using graph-based signatures. J. Med. Chem. 58, 4066–4072. doi:10.1021/acs.jmedchem.5b00104.

RDKit It. Introduction to RDKit, n.d. https://education.molssi.org/python-data-science-chemistry/rdkit_descriptors/rdkit.html.

Ren, F., Ding, X., Zheng, M., Korzinkin, M., Cai, X., Zhu, W., Mantsyzov, A., Aliper, A., Aladinskiy, V., Cao, Z., Kong, S., Long, X., Liu, B.H.M., Liu, Y., Naumov, V., Shneyderman, A., Ozerov, I.V., Wang, J., Pun, F.W., Polykovskiy, D.A., Sun, C., Levitt, M., Aspuru-Guzik, A., Zhavoronkov, A., 2023. AlphaFold accelerates artificial intelligence powered drug discovery: efficient discovery of a novel CDK20 small molecule inhibitor. Chem. Sci. 2041-6520. 14 (6), 1443–1452. doi:10.1039/d2sc05709c.

Renaud, N., Geng, C., Georgievska, S., Ambrosetti, F., Ridder, L., Marzella, D.F., Réau, M.F., Bonvin, A.M.J.J., Xue, L.C., 2021. DeepRank: a deep learning framework for data mining 3D protein-protein interfaces. Nat. Commun. 2041-1723. 12 (1). doi:10.1038/s41467-021-27396-0.

Rifaioglu, A.S., Nalbat, E., Atalay, V., Martin, M.J., Cetin-Atalay, R., Doğan, T., 2020. DEEPScreen: high performance drug-target interaction prediction with convolutional neural networks using 2-D structural compound representations. Chem. Sci. 11, 2531–2557. doi:10.1039/c9sc03414e.

Romero, R.A.A., Deypalan, M.N.Y., Mehrotra, S., Jungao, J.T., Sheils, N.E., Manduchi, E., Moore, J.H., 2022. Benchmarking AutoML frameworks for disease prediction using medical claims. BioData Min. 15. doi:10.1186/s13040-022-00300-2

Saigiridharan, L., Hassen, A.K., Lai, H., Torren-Peraire, P., Engkvist, O., Genheden, S., 2024. AiZynthFinder 4.0: developments based on learnings from 3 years of industrial application. J. Cheminform. 16. doi:10.1186/s13321-024-00860-x

Tang, Y.C., Gottlieb, A., 2021. Explainable drug sensitivity prediction through cancer pathway enrichment. Sci. Rep. 2045-2322. 11 (1). Available from: https://www.nature.com/srep/index.html. doi:10.1038/s41598-021-82612-7.

Tomorowicz, Ł., Sławiński, J., Żołnowska, B., Szafrański, K., Kawiak, A., 2020. Synthesis, antitumor evaluation, molecular modeling and quantitative structure–activity relationship (Qsar) of novel 2-[(4-amino-6-n-substituted-1,3,5-triazin-2-yl) methylthio]-4-chloro-5-methyl-n-(1h-benzo[d]imidazol-2(3h)-ylidene)benzenesulfonamides. Int. J. Mol. Sci. 1422-0067. 21 (8). Available from: https://www.mdpi.com/1422-0067/21/8/2924/pdf. doi:10.3390/ijms21082924.

Tu, Z., Choure, S.J., Fong, M.H., Roh, J., Levin, I., Yu, K., Joung, J.F., Morgan, N., Li, S.-C., Sun, X., Lin, H., Murnin, M., Liles, J.P., Struble, T.J., Fortunato, M.E., Liu, M., Green, W.H., Jensen, K.F., Coley, C.W., 2025. ASKCOS: open-source, data-driven synthesis planning. Acc. Chem. Res. 58 (11), 1764–1775. doi:10.1021/acs.accounts.5c00155.

Vamathevan, J., Clark, D., Czodrowski, P., Dunham, I., Ferran, E., Lee, G., Li, B., Madabhushi, A., Shah, P., Spitzer, M., Zhao, S., 2019. Applications of machine learning in drug discovery and development. Nat. Rev. Drug Discov. 1474-1776. 18 (6), 463–477. doi:10.1038/s41573-019-0024-5.

Varadi, M., Anyango, S., Deshpande, M., Nair, S., Natassia, C., Yordanova, G., Yuan, D., Stroe, O., Wood, G., Laydon, A., Žídek, A., Green, T., Tunyasuvunakool, K.,

Petersen, S., Jumper, J., Clancy, E., Green, R., Vora, A., Lutfi, M., Figurnov, M., Cowie, A., Hobbs, N., Kohli, P., Kleywegt, G., Birney, E., Hassabis, D., Velankar, S., 2022. AlphaFold protein structure database: massively expanding the structural coverage of protein-sequence space with high-accuracy models. Nucleic Acids Res. 0305-1048. 50 (D1), D439. doi:10.1093/nar/gkab1061.

Visan, A.I., Negut, I., 2024. Integrating artificial intelligence for drug discovery in the context of revolutionizing drug delivery. Life. 2075-1729. 14 (2), 233. doi:10.3390/life14020233.

Wan, F., Zhu, Y., Hu, H., Dai, A., Cai, X., Chen, L., Gong, H., Xia, T., Yang, D., Wang, M.-W., Zeng, J., 2019. DeepCPI: a deep learning-based framework for large-scale in silico drug screening. Genomics, Proteomics & Bioinformatics. 1672-0229. 17 (5), 478–495. doi:10.1016/j.gpb.2019.04.003.

Watson, J.L., Juergens, D., Bennett, N.R., Trippe, B.L., Yim, J., Eisenach, H.E., Ahern, W., Borst, A.J., Ragotte, R.J., Milles, L.F., Wicky, B.I.M., Hanikel, N., Pellock, S.J., Courbet, A., Sheffler, W., Wang, J., Venkatesh, P., Sappington, I., Vázquez Torres, S., Lauko, A., De Bortoli, V., Mathieu, E., Ovchinnikov, S., Barzilay, R., Jaakkola, T.S., DiMaio, F., Baek, M., Baker, D., 2023. De novo design of protein structure and function with RFdiffusion. Nature 620, 1089–1100. doi:10.1038/s41586-023-06415-8.

Winter, R., Montanari, F., Noé, F., Clevert, D.A., 2019. Learning continuous and data-driven molecular descriptors by translating equivalent chemical representations. Chem. Sci. 2041-6539. 10 (6), 1692–1701. Available from: http://pubs.rsc.org/en/journals/journal/sc. doi:10.1039/c8sc04175j.

Wu, Z., Ramsundar, B., Feinberg, E.N., Gomes, J., Geniesse, C., Pappu, A.S., Leswing, K., Pande, V., 2018. MoleculeNet: a benchmark for molecular machine learning. Chem. Sci. 9, 513–530. doi:10.1039/c7sc02664a.

Yin, Q., Fan, R., Cao, X., Liu, Q., Jiang, R., Zeng, W., 2023. DeepDrug: a general graph-based deep learning framework for drug-drug interactions and drug-target interactions prediction. Quant. Biol. 2095-4689. 11 (3), 260–274. doi:10.15302/j-qb-022-0320.

Zalewski, M., Wallner, B., Kmiecik, S., 2025. Protein–peptide docking with ESMFold language model. J. Chem. Theory Comput. 1549-9618. 21 (6), 2817–2821. doi:10.1021/acs.jctc.4c01585.

Zhang, Y., Qiao, S., Ji, S., Li, Y., 2020. DeepSite: bidirectional LSTM and CNN models for predicting DNA–protein binding. Int. J. Mach. Learn. Cybern. 1868-8071. 11 (4), 841–851. doi:10.1007/s13042-019-00990-x.

Zhu, Z., Shi, C., Zhang, Z., Liu, S., Xu, M., Yuan, X., Zhang, Y., Chen, J., Cai, H., Lu, J., Ma, C., Liu, R., Xhonneux, L.P., Qu, M., Tang, J., 2022. TorchDrug: a powerful and flexible machine learning platform for drug discovery. arXiv. 2331-8422. Available from: https://arxiv.org. doi:10.48550/arxiv.2202.08320.

11

AI driven clinical trials

Shruti Kapoor[a] **and Deepak Verma**[b]
[a]*University of California Santa Cruz, Santa Cruz, CA, United States*
[b]*Department of Oncology, Johns Hopkins Medicine, Baltimore, MD, United States*

1 Introduction

Clinical development is one of the most capital-intensive and uncertain ventures in science. Years of research and billions of pounds can depend on a handful of trials, most of which fail to achieve their primary endpoints. Simultaneously, the volume of relevant data from electronic health records, medical images, multiomics, previous trial archives, and continuous signals from wearables has surged. Artificial intelligence(AI) and machine learning (ML) sit at the crossroads of these pressures and opportunities. Fig. 11.1 depicts the AI workflow to utilize the data for patients. When utilized effectively, they can assist sponsors in asking more precise questions, designing more intelligent studies, and predicting outcomes before enrolling a single patient (Olawade et al., 2026; Sergi and Sesso, 2025).

This chapter explores how AI/ML methods are transforming clinical trials by predicting outcomes and optimizing decisions throughout the development process. Instead of viewing a trial as a one-off experiment, AI enables a learning system: historical and real-world data (RWD) are distilled into models that estimate the likelihood of success for a program, forecast effect sizes under different endpoints, highlight safety or operational risks, and suggest sites and eligibility criteria that might speed up participant recruitment. These tools can also identify subpopulations more likely to respond, justify smaller or external control arms where suitable, and facilitate adaptive designs that reassign patients to more promising arms in real time (Olawade et al., 2026; Sergi and Sesso, 2025).

The core methods of this transformation are robust and diverse. For tabular program features—such as target class, modality, genetic evidence, and early readouts—regularized regression, gradient boosting, and Bayesian hierarchical models provide calibrated estimates of technical and regulatory success. In complex biomedical contexts, graph neural networks (GNNs) utilize knowledge graphs linking genes,

The AI Frontier in Molecular Modelling and Drug Designing. https://doi.org/10.1016/B978-0-443-40338-5.00001-9

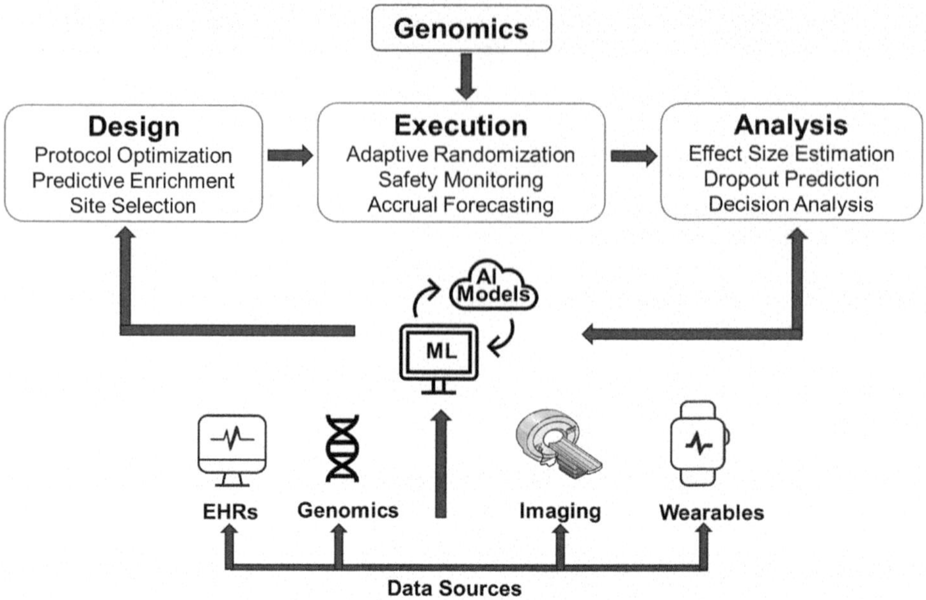

Fig. 11.1 AI integration across clinical trial phases. Data sources such as EHRs, genomics, imaging, and wearables feed into AI models that support trial design, execution, and analysis—enabling more innovative protocols, adaptive operations, and predictive insights.

pathways, diseases, and past outcomes to reveal patterns that are invisible to simple models, as shown in Fig. 11.2 (Serra et al., 2025; Walters and Barzilay, 2021).

Longitudinal biomarkers and time-to-event outcomes benefit from mixed-effects and joint models. At the same time, transformers extract information from unstructured protocols, publications, and clinical notes to identify design pitfalls and feasibility constraints. Causal inference methods such as propensity-based estimators, targeted learning, and causal forests enable credible comparisons to external or synthetic controls when randomized data are limited. Across these techniques runs a common theme: uncertainty is quantified and presented to decision-makers, facilitating transparent go/no-go decisions and risk-aware portfolio management (Walters and Barzilay, 2021; Zhavoronkov et al., 2019; Niazi, 2025).

The promise of AI-driven trials is clear and tangible. Over recent years, partnerships between academic institutions, AI-focused biotech firms, and major pharmaceutical companies have produced real results: AI-selected targets advancing into preclinical stages, AI-designed small molecules entering first-in-human trials, and, in some cases, progressing to mid-stage trials. These case studies demonstrate how computational discovery can shorten the design, synthesis, and testing cycles, explore vast chemical and biological spaces, and create candidates that meet clinical requirements. They also highlight key lessons on when AI provides the most significant benefit, which validations are necessary to build confidence, and how computational insights can be integrated with medicinal chemistry, translational biology, and clinical expertise (Walters and Barzilay, 2021; Zhavoronkov et al., 2019; Niazi, 2025).

Recognizing the benefits of AI in clinical development requires more than clever algorithms. Data must be curated, harmonized, and governed with the same rigor as any GxP process. Models should be trained and evaluated on cohorts separated by time and location to test generalization, then piloted in "shadow mode" before they influence irreversible decisions. Performance must be monitored for drift, and subgroup audits are essential to identify and reduce bias. Regulators are increasingly receptive to RWD, external controls, and AI-enabled tools when they are fit-for-purpose and well-documented; aligning model development and validation with evolving guidance is therefore vital (FDA, 2023a, 2018a, 2025f). AI should support, not substitute for, clinical expertise. Predictions are most valuable when accompanied by explanations that clinicians, statisticians, and operations teams can scrutinize. Clear statements on intended use, decision thresholds linked to business and ethical considerations, and well-designed workflows ensure that models influence behavior in the clinic and the boardroom, not just as benchmarks.

1.1 Why clinical trials need AI now

Clinical development faces a widening efficiency gap, underscoring the urgent need for AI: bringing a new medicine to market typically takes close to a decade and costs hundreds of millions to billions of dollars, with recent estimates ranging from roughly $1 billion to over $2.8 billion per approved therapy. The timelines generally span 7–12+

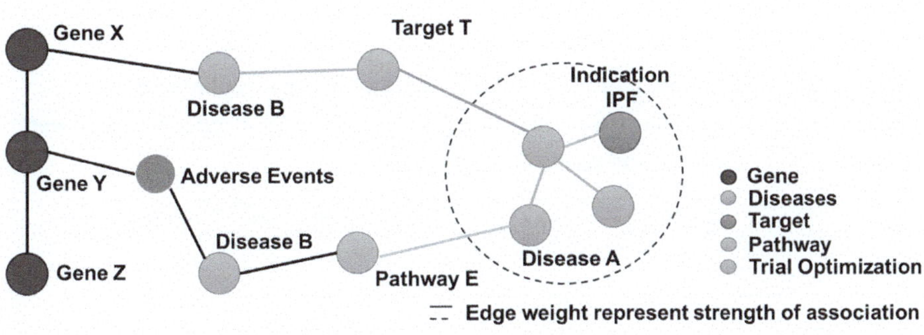

Fig. 11.2 Biomedical knowledge graph linking genes, pathways, diseases, and trial outcomes. Graph neural networks use these relationships to propagate evidence and improve prediction accuracy in underpowered settings.

years from discovery to approval (Wouters et al., 2020; DiMasi et al., 2016; Paul et al., 2010). Despite these substantial investments, most programs fail in the clinic; overall success rates from first-in-human trials to approval hover around 7%–14%. Table 11.1 depicts the time reduction for multiple important events in clinical trials. Late-stage failures, though less frequent, are disproportionately costly because they occur after the most significant expenditures on patients, manufacturing scale-up, and pivotal infrastructure (Hay et al., 2014; Kola and Landis, 2004). Meanwhile, the volume and diversity of biomedical data have soared: widespread adoption of electronic health records, high-throughput genomics and other "omics," large-scale imaging, wearable and digital health streams, and extensive registries/biobanks create unprecedented opportunities for faster learning. However, these also introduce heterogeneity, missing data, bias, and privacy risks that cannot be managed with traditional methods alone (Krumholz, 2014; EMA, 2025a).

AI-driven clinical trials address these challenges by integrating three capabilities throughout design and execution. First, predictive modeling enables enrichment—identifying patients, sites, and windows of responsiveness most likely to benefit—enhancing statistical power while reducing sample sizes and exposure to ineffective treatments when properly prespecified and validated (FDA, 2019b; Thall, 2022). Second, modern causal inference and the robust use of RWD help estimate treatment effects more reliably outside or alongside randomized settings—for instance, in external control arms or endpoint ascertainment—provided that the trial design emulates target trials, confounding is addressed, and diagnostics are transparent (Hern´an and Robins, 2024; Schuemie et al., 2020). Third, adaptive experimentation employs Bayesian and other adaptive designs, including response-adaptive randomization and platform trials, which learn as the trial progresses. This approach reallocates resources to promising regimens, stops futile arms earlier, and

Table 11.1 Comparative efficiency metrics between traditional and AI-enhanced trials. AI-driven approaches significantly reduce time to first patient, total duration, cost per approved therapy, and required sample size.

Metric	Traditional value	AI-enhanced value	Reduction (%)
Time to first patient	100	21	79
Total trial duration	100	57	43
Cost per approved therapy	100	75	25
Sample size required	100	87	13

speeds up decision-making while maintaining statistical rigor under prespecified and regulatory guidelines. When implemented with appropriate governance such as data standards and provenance, bias and performance monitoring, external validation, privacy-preserving analytics like federated learning, and alignment with evolving regulators' expectations—AI does not replace clinical judgment; it enhances it, increasing the chances of success, reducing waste, and turning the data avalanche into more ethical, quicker, and more informative trials (EMA, 2025a; Berry, 2011; Rieke et al., 2020). Recent advancements in AI have significantly reduced the time, as described in Table 11.1.

2 Data foundations for AI in trials

Robust AI for clinical trials relies on a layered data foundation that combines historical trial evidence, RWD, multimodal omics and imaging, digital health streams, and structured biological knowledge, each curated, standardized, and linked with clear provenance to support regulatory-grade decisions. Historical trials offer the priors: registries such as ClinicalTrials.gov and European Union Clinical Trials Regulation (EU CTR)/Clinical Trials Information System (CTIS), published reports aligned with Consolidated Standards of Reporting Trials (CONSORT), and protocols aligned with Standard Protocol Items: Recommendations for Interventional Trials (SPIRIT), along with internal archives of feasibility and operational metrics, all containing patterns that predict eligibility bottlenecks, screen-failure rates, site productivity, event rates, and likely effect sizes. When text and tabular data from these sources are normalized to standards like Clinical Data Interchange Standards Consortium (CDISC) study data tabulation model (SDTM)/analysis data model (ADaM) and systematically mined, they inform enrolment forecasting, endpoint selection, and risk mitigation before first patient in (Zarin et al., 2011; Schulz et al., 2010). Real-world data (RWD) identified EHRs, claims, registries, and patient-reported outcomes harmonized through networks such as Sentinel, Patient-Centered Outcomes Research Network (PCORnet), and Observational Health Data Sciences and Informatics (OHDSI)'s Observational Medical Outcomes Partnership (OMOP) standard data model add external context to test the feasibility of inclusion/exclusion criteria, calibrate background event rates, and, when fit-for-purpose, support external comparators or endpoint verification. These uses demand careful causal design (target-trial emulation), rigorous confounding control, data quality checks, and transparent diagnostics consistent with evolving FDA/EMA guidance on RWD/real-world evidence (RWE) (FDA, 2018a; EMA, 2025a; Hern´an and Robins, 2024; Fleurence et al., 2014; Hripcsak et al., 2015). Omics and imaging deepen biological resolution: genomic, transcriptomic, and proteomic features can stratify patients and define sensitive, mechanism-linked endpoints (Verma et al., 2024); radiomics extracts quantitative signatures from routine scans that correlate with prognosis and treatment response, enabling enrichment and early decision rules when analytically validated and locked down prospectively (Aerts et al., 2014a; Lambin et al., 2012; MacLean, 2021). Digital health technologies wearables, smartphones, and home sensors enable continuous, real-time measurement of function, physiology, and behaviour, turning sporadic visits into dense time series that are more responsive to change; properly validated, these streams can generate novel endpoints, reduce site burden, and broaden access, under device-appropriate consent, cybersecurity, and reliability controls (FDA, 2023b; Raja et al., 2019; Turakhia et al., 2019; CTTI, 2019). Finally, knowledge graphs integrate curated relationships among genes, targets, diseases, pathways, drugs, and past trial outcomes, allowing AI models to embed biological context, propagate evidence across related entities, and generate mechanistically plausible hypotheses for enrichment, combination selection, or endpoint refinement (Himmelstein et al., 2017; Ochoa et al., 2021). Across all levels, success depends on data governance and interoperability—linking modalities via privacy-preserving record linkage, using interoperable standards (e.g., Health Level Seven - Fast Healthcare Interoperability Resources (HL7 FHIR) for electronic health records (EHR), digital imaging and communications in medicine (DICOM) for imaging), monitoring bias and drift, and applying techniques such as federated learning to respect confidentiality while enabling multisite model training. Without these foundations—fit-for-purpose data, harmonization, provenance, and safeguards against re-identification and spurious correlations AI models risk being fragile or biased; with them, they can reliably inform design, prediction, and adaptive execution to make trials faster, more ethical, and more likely to succeed (Rieke et al., 2020; Sweeney, 2002).

3 Predicting clinical trial outcomes: Methods and use cases

3.1 Program- and trial-level success prediction

Decisions to start, continue, or redesign a program benefit from explicit, data-driven estimates of the probability of technical and regulatory success (PoS). Baseline empirical rates differ by indication, modality, biomarker use, and phase transition, and can serve as priors; large-scale analyses report aggregate PoS from first-in-human to approval in the 7%–14% range overall, with substantial variation by therapeutic area and higher success when mechanistic biomarkers are used (Wong et al., 2019; BIO, 2021). Predictors of success at the program/trial level typically include target class and mechanism, indication and line of therapy, modality, genetic support for the target–disease link, preclinical and early clinical readouts, competitive landscape (including standard-of-care dynamics), endpoint selection, and sponsor/site track record (BIO, 2021; Nelson et al., 2015; King et al., 2019). Supervised learning methods, such as gradient boosting machines and random forests, provide strong baselines with variable importance diagnostics that help teams understand drivers of predicted risk and opportunity (Breiman, 2001; Friedman, 2001). Regularized logistic regression and Bayesian hierarchical models produce well-calibrated probabilities and credible intervals, while enabling partial pooling across related indications, modalities, or endpoints to prevent overfitting where data are sparse (Gelman et al., 2013; Hastie and Friedman, 2009). To capture biological context beyond flat covariate lists, GNNs trained over curated biomedical knowledge graphs can propagate evidence along gene–target–pathway–disease edges and incorporate historical trial outcomes to improve prediction in underpowered settings (Himmelstein et al., 2017; Thomas and Welling, 2017; Hamilton, 2020; Zitnik et al., 2018). Multitask learning further shares statistical strength across related indications or modalities, improving generalization when many features are partially observed (Caruana, 1997; Ruder, 2017). Outputs include phase-specific PoS with uncertainty, scenario analyses that quantify the impact of endpoint choices or biomarker-enriched eligibility on PoS, and portfolio optimization that prioritizes programs by expected value adjusted for risk and resource constraints, borrowing ideas from decision analysis and modern portfolio theory to balance upside and downside within budget and time constraints (BIO, 2021; Markowitz, 1952; Claxton and Posnett, 1996).

3.2 Endpoint and effect-size forecasting

A key question in design is whether a planned study can detect a clinically meaningful effect under plausible outcome trajectories. Mixed-effects models use historical and pilot data to estimate between- and within-patient variability for continuous or ordinal endpoints, guiding effect-size assumptions and covariance structures in power calculations (Laird and Ware, 1982; Fitzmaurice et al., 2011). For longitudinal biomarkers, modern sequence models (e.g., recurrent networks, temporal convolutional networks, or transformers) can capture nonlinearity, seasonality, and irregular sampling to forecast change over time at the patient and site levels; coupled with uncertainty quantification, these forecasts translate to distributions of treatment differences at planned analyses (Lipton et al., 2016; Bai et al., 2018; Lim et al., 2021). When endpoints are linked (e.g., a biomarker trajectory influencing time-to-event outcomes), joint models coherently connect longitudinal change to hazard, enhancing efficiency and reducing bias from informative dropout (Sudell et al., 2016; Tsiatis and Davidian, 2004). These predictive distributions inform power and sample-size calculations that extend beyond single point effect assumptions, such as computing predictive power under multiple effect/variance scenarios, along with subgroup- and site-level sensitivity analyses and adaptive sample-size re-estimation if early data diverge from priors (Schoenfeld, 1983; Chow et al., 2017; Hampson and Jennison, 2012).

3.3 Safety, dropout, and operational risk prediction

Proactively anticipating safety and operational risks prevents costly delays and early terminations. For adverse events (AEs), Bayesian hierarchical models share information across sites, subgroups, and related events to stabilize rate estimates and enable early detection of emerging safety signals, while controlling for multiplicity and small-sample noise (Gelman et al., 2013; Berry, 2006). Unsupervised and semisupervised anomaly detection on AE incidence, labs, and vitals can flag outlier patterns suggestive of risk or data quality issues, especially when combined with clinical curation (Chandola et al., 2009). Free-text narratives and MedDRA-coded reports can be mined with domain-adapted transformers (e.g., BioBERT, ClinicalBERT) to improve case classification, seriousness prediction, and clustering of safety phenotypes, complementing traditional disproportionality analyses (Devlin et al., 2019a; Lee et al., 2019; Alsentzer et al., 2019). Patient attrition is naturally modeled with time-to-dropout survival models that incorporate demographics, comorbidities, site burden, and visit schedules; in settings where dropout depends on unobserved outcomes, joint modeling helps correct informative censoring (Sudell et al., 2016; Collett, 2014). Outputs feed risk mitigation plans—preemptive monitoring or dose adjustments, targeted patient support to reduce burden, and endpoint choices that balance sensitivity with tolerability aligned with risk-based quality management frameworks (FDA, 2018b, 2013; Teodoro et al., 2025).

3.4 Accrual and site performance forecasting

Enrollment shortfalls are a major cause of delays and weak results; therefore, predicting site performance and accrual patterns is vital for execution. Historical enrollment data, investigator networks, proximity to eligible patient populations, and operational capacity (e.g., start-up times, screen failure rates) can be combined in supervised models to identify high- and low-yield sites and to customize feasibility packages. Gradient boosting and related methods offer strong discrimination while maintaining interpretability for feasibility teams (Friedman, 2001; Hastie and Friedman, 2009). At the program level, accrual dynamics are effectively captured by survival- and Poisson-process-based recruitment models that include center heterogeneity and calendar-time effects, enabling proactive redistribution of sites or budgets to meet milestones (Anisimov and Fedorov, 2007; Anisimov, 2011). Public registries can provide priors for screen failure rates and competition within a specific indication and geography, while internal archives calibrate model expectations to sponsor-specific processes (Anisimov and Fedorov, 2007). Forecast outputs include site rankings, region-level enrollment potential, and scenario-based accrual curves under different outreach or inclusion/exclusion strategies.

3.5 Dose-finding and early-phase design

Early-phase studies aim to identify doses with acceptable safety and promising activity swiftly and ethically. Model-based dose-escalation designs, such as the continual reassessment method and the Bayesian optimal interval approach, outperform rule-based designs in finding the maximum tolerated dose (or the optimal biologic dose), reducing the number of patients exposed to subtherapeutic or excessively toxic levels (O'Quigley et al., 1990; Yuan et al., 2016). For combinations and dual endpoints (toxicity/efficacy), Bayesian frameworks naturally extend to model trade-offs and guide smooth escalation and de-escalation (Wang and Tatsuoka, 2025; Yan et al., 2018). Model-informed drug development (MIDD) links preclinical PK/PD, first-in-human exposures, and mechanism-based quantitative systems pharmacology (QSP) models to predict human therapeutic windows and guide dose selection and scheduling—an approach endorsed and piloted by regulators (Zhu et al., 2019; Bradshaw et al., 2019; FDA, 2025b). Adaptive expansion cohorts can then dynamically reallocate patients to promising doses or biomarker-defined subgroups, using Bayesian posterior probabilities or group-sequential rules to enrich where benefit is most likely, as demonstrated by platform trials in oncology (Trippa and Xu, 2023; Wang and Yee, 2019; Collignon, 2022).

3.6 Predictive enrichment and precision enrollment

Enrolling patients who are most likely to benefit or to show measurable change increases statistical power and reduces exposure. Enrichment strategies, prognostic, predictive, or both, are supported by regulatory guidance when prespecified and justified by biology (FDA, 2019b). Genomic and transcriptomic signatures (e.g., polygenic risk scores or expression panels) can identify subpopulations with higher event rates or treatment sensitivity; radiomics and other image-derived phenotypes offer orthogonal signals for stratification; and composite digital endpoints capture functional change at higher resolution than episodic clinical measures when analytically and clinically validated (Torkamani et al., 2018; Ou et al., 2019; Aerts et al., 2014a; FDA, 2023b). To optimize inclusion criteria, uplift modeling estimates individual treatment effects to prioritize features that maximize treatment–control separation rather than overall response, using causal forests, metalearners, or Bayesian individualized treatment effect models with careful attention to positivity and confounding (Athey and Imbens, 2016; Wager and Athey, 2018; Künzel et al., 2019). These tools translate into eligibility criteria and stratification plans that improve the chance of detecting benefit while maintaining generalizability through parallel cohorts or preplanned validation.

3.7 Protocol optimization and feasibility

Protocol complexity causes screen failures, deviations, and amendments; AI can identify risky design elements before the first patient is enrolled. Natural language processing of previous protocols and publications extracts structured eligibility criteria, visit schedules, and operational outcomes; mapped to standards such as OMOP and CDISC, these data reveal overly restrictive, conflicting, or difficult-to-operationalize clauses and recommend safer relaxations based on historical evidence (Shivade et al., 2016; Kim et al., 2023). Beyond heuristic edits, reinforcement learning and simulation can explore "what-if" eligibility scenarios tightening or relaxing criteria, adding a biomarker, or adjusting visit burdens to evaluate trade-offs among screen failure rates, event occurrence, and generalizability while maintaining clinical and ethical constraints; policy-search techniques from the dynamic treatment regime literature guide these analyses (Murphy, 2003; Sutton and Barto, 2018; Zhao et al., 2012). During implementation, predictive monitoring models identify sites at high risk of deviations or data quality issues based on early patterns in query rates, timeliness, and protocol-specific procedures, facilitating targeted training and risk-based quality management aligned with ICH E6(R2) and current regulatory standards (FDA, 2018b, 2013; Bhagat et al., 2020).

3.8 External and synthetic controls

When appropriate, external and synthetic controls can reduce or replace internal control arms, particularly in rare diseases and oncology, provided rigorous design and diagnostics are employed.

The causal inference toolkit, propensity scores, inverse probability weighting, matching, doubly robust estimators, targeted maximum likelihood estimation (TMLE), and machine-learning-based learners such as Bayesian additive regression trees and causal forests assist in controlling for measured confounding and estimating counterfactual outcomes from RWD aligned with a target trial protocol (Wager and Athey, 2018; Austin, 2011; Williamson and Ravani, 2017; van der Laan and Rose, 2011; Hill, 2011). Key practices include explicit eligibility alignment, prespecification, covariate balance diagnostics, negative/positive controls, and sensitivity analyses for unmeasured confounding—consistent with FDA/EMA guidance on RWD/RWE (FDA, 2023c; Schuemie et al., 2018; EMA, 2024). Synthetic or "digital twin" approaches generate patient-level counterfactual trajectories using generative and prognostic models trained on longitudinal data; when validated on held-out controls and subjected to strict calibration and balance checks, they can enhance small-sample trials and support decision-making during interim analyses (van der Laan and Rose, 2011; Schulam and Saria, 2017; Bica et al., 2020; Brophy et al., 2023). Transparency about assumptions, uncertainty assessment, and compliance with regulatory expectations are crucial for establishing credibility.

3.9 Uncertainty and decision analysis

Good predictions are well-calibrated, transparent about uncertainty, and linked to decisions. Calibration can be evaluated and improved with reliability curves, Brier scores, and posthoc calibration methods such as Platt scaling and isotonic regression; conformal prediction provides distribution-free prediction intervals that preserve nominal coverage under minimal assumptions, enabling teams to understand the range of plausible outcomes at the trial or program level (Murphy and Winkler, 1992; Menon et al., 2012; Lin et al., 2007; Angelopoulos and Bates, 2021). Value-of-information (VOI) analysis converts uncertainty into expected economic or clinical value, helping to determine whether additional data—such as adaptive interim looks, biomarker assays, or an extra arm—are worthwhile before resources are committed (Morton et al., 2022; Heath et al., 2021; Vervaart et al., 2021). For go/no-go decisions, decision-curve analysis assesses net benefit across threshold preferences, explicitly weighing the costs of false positives (advancing a futile program) versus false negatives (terminating a viable one), thus supporting transparent governance among clinical, statistical, and commercial stakeholders (Vickers and Holland, 2021; Vickers et al., 2019).

4 Making development more efficient and cost-effective

Making development more efficient and cost-effective requires a coordinated mix of quantitative decision-making, innovative trial designs, operational excellence, and portfolio discipline. First, fewer futile trials can be achieved by instituting early stop/go decisions based on calibrated success probabilities. Interim monitoring using conditional power or Bayesian predictive probabilities allows sponsors to halt futility or success before complete enrolment when data suggest a very low or high likelihood of ultimate success, conserving resources and patient exposure while maintaining statistical integrity (FDA, 2019a; Jennison and Turnbull, 2000; Freidlin and Korn, 2009). Second, smarter designs, adaptive, platform, and basket trials enable evaluation of more hypotheses with fewer patients and shorter timelines. Adaptive designs can modify randomization ratios, sample sizes, or enrolment criteria based on interim data without compromising validity, while master protocols (including platform, umbrella, and basket trials) share infrastructure and control arms to test multiple interventions or biomarkers efficiently in parallel (FDA, 2019a, 2022a; Woodcock and LaVange, 2017). Real-world examples such as I-SPY 2, REMAP-CAP, and RECOVERY have demonstrated how response-adaptive randomization, Bayesian decision rules, and perpetual platform designs can accelerate learning and deliver conclusive answers on multiple therapies within a single, continuously operating trial structure (Angus et al., 2020; Horby et al., 2021). Third, improved enrolment enhances speed and reduces costs by decreasing screen failure and attrition and increasing recruitment rate. Data-driven site selection and prescreening with electronic health records, patient-centric decentralization, and remote monitoring can broaden reach, match patients more precisely to studies, and lower burdens that cause drop-out, thereby compressing timelines and avoiding cost overruns (FDA, 2025c; Kho et al., 2011; Getz and Campo, 2018). Fourth, smaller sample sizes are achievable with predictive enrichment and sensitive endpoints. Enrichment strategies focus on enrolling patients more likely to respond, such as biomarker-positive subgroups or those with disease features predictive of benefit, increasing power per participant and reducing the total number needed for a given effect size; similarly, validated surrogate or more sensitive endpoints can detect treatment effects earlier or with less variability, enabling smaller, faster trials without compromising evidentiary standards (FDA, 2019b; Woodcock and LaVange, 2017). Fifth, reducing the control burden through scientifically and regulatorily justified external controls and synthetic comparators can lower the number of patients assigned to placebo or standard care and decrease costs, especially in rare diseases or settings where traditional randomized controls are impractical; emerging guidance on the use of RWD and rigorous methods for constructing external comparators helps ensure validity and minimize bias (Corrigan-Curay et al., 2018; FDA, 2023d). Lastly, portfolio return on investment improves when capital is allocated to programs with the highest risk-adjusted value. Using empirically based phase-transition probabilities and VOI frameworks to prioritize assets and exclude underpowered or low-probability concepts early enhances the expected productivity of R&D investment, a vital factor when development costs are high and success rates remain modest (Wong et al., 2019; Schuhmacher et al., 2025; Sertkaya et al., 2024).

5 Methodological toolbox at a glance

A pragmatic methodological toolbox for clinical development and portfolio analytics utilizes complementary strengths across traditional machine learning, deep learning, causal inference, adaptive algorithms, federated learning, and explainability, each selected and adapted to the clinical question, data limitations, and regulatory requirements. Traditional machine learning remains a valuable baseline for risk prediction, trial feasibility, and survival analysis. Penalized logistic and Cox regression using shrinkage via L1 (lasso), L2 (ridge), or elastic net penalties provide interpretable coefficients, manage collinearity, and offer robustness in high-dimensional contexts common to EHR and omics, supported by well-established software and performance guarantees (Tibshirani, 2011; Zhang and Muller, 2024; Miao et al., 2024). Gradient boosting machines are a reliable default for tabular data, employing additive trees to model nonlinearities and interactions, and can incorporate monotone constraints and missing-data handling to reflect clinical domain knowledge better while enhancing calibration (Friedman, 2001; Chen and Guestrin, 2016; Ke et al., 2017).

Deep learning broadens the scope and enhances performance for unstructured data and cross-modal signals. Transformers enable cutting-edge text mining for protocols, literature, and clinical notes, supporting tasks such as named entity recognition, relation extraction, evidence retrieval, and summarization; domain-specific models pretrained on scientific and biomedical corpora, including bidirectional encoder representations from transformers (BERT), SciBERT, PubMedBERT, and ClinicalBERT, generally outperform general language models in these contexts (Alsentzer et al., 2019; Vaswani et al., 2023; Devlin et al., 2019b; Beltagy et al., 2019; Gu et al., 2021). GNNs are well-suited to knowledge graphs linking biology, mechanisms, targets, drugs, diseases, and past trial outcomes; by learning over heterogeneous nodes and edges, GNNs can capture relational structures for tasks such as target-indication mapping, safety signal propagation, and drug repurposing (Himmelstein et al., 2017; Hamilton, 2020; Zitnik et al., 2018; Kipf and Welling, 2017). Multimodal fusion methods combine tabular clinical features, imaging, omics, and longitudinal time series to produce more complete phenotypes and improve predictive and prognostic performance. Fusion can be early (feature-level), late (decision-level), or joint via attention and shared latent spaces, demonstrating empirical success in oncology, critical care, and precision medicine (Ngiam et al., 2011; Baltrušaitis et al., 2019; Cheerla and Gevaert, 2019; Shickel et al., 2017).

Causal inference methods are vital for effect estimation and decision-making when randomization is impractical or complemented by real-world evidence. TMLE offers a flexible semiparametric framework with double robustness and asymptotic efficiency, provided that the outcome or treatment mechanism is correctly specified. It also accommodates modern machine learning techniques within causal estimation while ensuring valid inference (Hern´an and Robins, 2024; van der Laan and Rose, 2011). Doubly robust estimators, including augmented inverse probability weighting, help reduce bias from model misspecification and can be combined with cross-fitting to minimize overfitting (Wei et al., 2022; Chernozhukov et al., 2018). Instrumental variables can identify causal effects when a valid instrument influences treatment but not the outcome except through treatment; nevertheless, the relevance, independence, and exclusion criteria of instruments must be carefully evaluated, as weak instruments can introduce bias (Hern´an and Robins, 2024; Dukes et al., 2024; Baiocchi et al., 2020). Sensitivity analyses assess the robustness to unmeasured confounding, with frameworks like the E-value and Rosenbaum bounds providing transparent measures of how strong unobserved biases need to be to negate the estimated effects (VanderWeele and Ding, 2017).

Adaptive algorithms enable more efficient experimentation and trial operations. Multiarmed bandits formalize the exploration-exploitation trade-off to allocate patients to arms that are performing better while maintaining opportunities to learn. This approach potentially reduces patient exposure to inferior treatments and promotes ethical efficiencies; Thompson sampling is a Bayesian heuristic with strong empirical and theoretical support and has been studied for response-adaptive randomization. However, operating characteristics (such as type I error and bias) need careful validation through simulations under realistic accrual and drift (Thompson, 1933; Scott, 2010). These algorithms can be integrated within adaptive designs governed by prespecified rules and independent data monitoring, complementing established methods like sample-size re-estimation and response-adaptive randomization.

Federated learning facilitates model training across institutions without sharing patient-level data, thereby reducing privacy risks and legal or friction costs, while also increasing sample diversity and external validity. Practical implementations depend on communication-efficient aggregation (FedAvg), secure aggregation to prevent server-side reconstruction, and differential privacy to limit information leakage; in healthcare, federated learning has been demonstrated to match or surpass centralized performance in multihospital imaging and EHR prediction tasks while preserving data locality. It is also compatible with audit trails and data minimization principles under general data protection regulation (GDPR) (McMahan et al., 2017; Bonawitz et al., 2017; Dayan et al., 2021; Kairouz et al., 2021). Governance should include documentation of participating data controllers, contribution logs, model-card reporting, and bias monitoring to ensure compliance and scientific rigor across non-independent and identically distributed (non-IID) sites.

Explainability methods assist reviewers, clinicians, and scientists in understanding and trusting model behavior. SHapley Additive exPlanations (SHAP) values offer locally precise, additive explanations that align with Shapley axioms, allowing case-by-case attribution and overall feature importance with theoretical guarantees; they have been effectively used in clinical risk prediction and monitoring to identify actionable factors influencing predictions (Lundberg and Lee, 2017; Lundberg et al., 2020). Partial dependence and individual conditional expectation plots clarify marginal relationships and heterogeneity across patients, supporting model critique and hypothesis development, though they require caution with correlated features (Goldstein et al., 2015). Counterfactual explanations outline minimal input modifications that would change a prediction, aiding decision support and fairness assessments; these should be based on feasible clinical interventions and, where possible, aligned with causal structures rather than purely associative perturbations (Wachter et al., 2018; Pearl, 2009). Collectively, these tools provide a comprehensive framework for constructing, validating, deploying, and overseeing models that enhance development efficiency while upholding scientific rigor and transparency.

6 Validation, governance, and regulation

6.1 Validation strategy

6.1.1 Design for out-of-sample generalization

Use temporal splits that respect clinical timelines and prevent data leakage (e.g., train on earlier accrual or calendar periods; validate on later periods). Standard k-fold cross-validation is often overly optimistic when temporal autocorrelation exists; utilize blocked or rolling-origin validation with suitable gap intervals to reduce lookahead bias (Roberts et al., 2020; Hyndman and Athanasopoulos, 2020).

Geographic and site-level holdouts evaluate transportability across institutions and regions, reflecting variations in practice patterns, coding, case mix, and data pipelines. When data are federated or involve multiple centers, reserve entire centers for external validation and report performance stratified by region and center (Varoquaux and Cheplygina, 2022).

External validation on genuinely independent datasets is required for high-stakes clinical applications: include calibration metrics (Brier score, expected calibration error), discrimination measures (ROC-AUC/PR-AUC for imbalanced outcomes), and net-benefit decision-curve analysis to assess clinical utility.

6.1.2 Prospective shadow or silent mode

Before influencing patient allocation or operational decisions, run the model passively alongside ongoing studies, logging prespecified key performance indicators, alert volumes, calibration drift, and operational impact. This phase reveals integration issues, label/lag problems, and workflow frictions without risk to participants (Li et al., 2020; Wiens et al., 2019).

6.1.3 Continuous monitoring and change management

Monitor distributional changes in input data using statistical shift tests and distance measures, such as the population stability index, the Kolmogorov–Smirnov test, and the Jensen–Shannon divergence. Also, track concept drift changes in outcomes or mappings through performance monitoring over time and drift detectors (Gama et al., 2014; Varoquaux and Cheplygina, 2022).

Establish trigger thresholds and runbooks: when drift triggers activate, options include recalibration, constrained retraining, or reverting to a validated champion model. All changes must follow the documented change control, risk assessment, and revalidation processes (Sklavenitis and Kalles, 2025; Sculley et al., 2015).

6.2 Quality and compliance

6.2.1 GxP-compliant MLOps

Establish complete traceability for data, code, models, and environments: use immutable versioning (data snapshots and hashes), dependency pinning, containerization, and reproducible pipelines.

Keep audit logs for data ingestion, feature generation, training runs, hyperparameters, and deployment events; adhere to ALCOA+ principles for data integrity (MHRA, 2018).

Validate computerized systems with a risk-based approach, including planning, specifying, testing, and acceptance. Apply established Computer System Validation principles (installation qualification (IQ)/operational qualification (OQ)/performance qualification (PQ)) and provide evidence proportional to the risk; utilize current best practices such as International Society for Pharmaceutical Engineering (ISPE) Good Automated Manufacturing Practice, Version 5 (GAMP) 5, second edition, and FDA's draft Computer Software Assurance framework. Focus testing on intended use and critical functions (FDA, 2025d).

Maintain a validation plan that covers intended use, risk analysis International Council for Harmonisation - Quality Risk Management, Revision 1 (ICH Q9(R1)), requirements, verification and acceptance criteria, and a lifecycle standard operating procedure (SOP) suitc (including data management, model development, validation, deployment, monitoring, and decommissioning). Use model cards and datasheets to standardize documentation (Mitchell et al., 2019; Gebru et al., 2021).

6.2.2 21 CFR part 11 and EU Good Manufacturing Practice annex 11

Ensure compliance with electronic records and signatures: implement secure, computer-generated, time-stamped audit trails; establish user access controls; validate systems; maintain record retention; and develop procedures for electronic signature management (FDA, 2023e; European Commission, 2023).

Change control and configuration management must be formalized with impact assessment and approvals; all production models and supporting tools are treated as GxP computerized systems when they influence regulated data, decision-making, or submissions.

6.2.3 Data and model governance

Establish data-provenance catalogs and quality controls aligned with the European Medicines Agency (EMA) / Heads of Medicines Agencies (HMA) Data Quality Framework for regulatory-grade RWD (EMA, 2023a). Implement risk management in accordance with National Institute of Standards and Technology - Artificial Intelligence Risk Management Framework (NIST AI RMF) 1.0 and ISO/IEC 23894:2023, including mapping, measurement, and handling of AI risks such as security, robustness, and human factors (NIST, 2023; ISO, 2023).

6.3 Bias and fairness

6.3.1 Subgroup performance auditing

Assess discrimination, calibration, and error rates across important clinical subgroups (e.g., sex, age brackets, race/ethnicity, site, socioeconomic status, comorbidities). Review threshold-dependent metrics (false positives/negatives, positive predictive value (PPV)/negative predictive value (NPV)) and calibration curves by subgroup; evaluate intersectional subgroups where possible (Pleiss et al., 2017; Mehrabi et al., 2021). Utilize suitable fairness metrics appropriate to the context, such as equalized odds or equal opportunity for risk triage, and balance them against clinical utility and safety. Report trade-offs transparently (Hardt et al., 2016; Caton and Haas, 2024).

6.3.2 Mitigations

Preprocessing: reweighting or stratified sampling to improve representation; robust labeling and adjudication.

In-processing: constrained optimization (reductions approach), adversarial debiasing, group-aware calibration (Celis et al., 2019).

Postprocessing: adjusting thresholds by subgroup when justified and documented; human-in-the-loop review for edge cases.

6.3.3 Transparency and human oversight

Provide clear documentation of intended use, limitations, failure modes, data dependencies, and required human judgment. Align with Good Machine Learning Practice guiding principles, emphasizing data quality, model transparency, and monitoring (FDA, 2025e).

Establish escalation routes for discrepancies, with oversight from a governance committee, and ensure corrective actions are managed under change control.

6.4 Regulatory outlook

6.4.1 RWD and external controls

Regulators increasingly accept fit-for-purpose RWD and, in specific contexts (e.g., rare diseases, gene therapies, oncology), external controls or natural history comparators when randomized controlled trials are infeasible or unethical. Acceptance depends on the relevance, reliability, and rigorous design and analysis of the data to mitigate biases (FDA, 2018a; EMA, 2021).

Sponsors should initiate early scientific discussions with regulators to agree on data sources, curation, endpoints, and analytical methods. They should follow emerging best practices from the HMA-EMA Big Data Steering Group on RWE in decision-making (EMA, 2024).

6.4.2 AI/ML in drug development

Agencies have published positions and draft guidance outlining expectations. FDA's discussion paper and draft guidance on AI/ML in drug development emphasize data integrity, risk-proportionate validation, model monitoring, and transparency of algorithms used in discovery, trial optimization, and manufacturing (FDA, 2023a, 2025f).

EMA's reflection paper on AI in the medicinal product lifecycle underscores governance, documentation, model risk classification, robustness, explainability proportional to impact, and human-in-the-loop oversight in clinical trials and pharmacovigilance (EMA, 2023b).

For adaptive and algorithm-informed trials, adhere to FDA guidance on adaptive designs and the Complex Innovative Trial Designs program; demonstrate operating characteristics through simulation with independent data monitoring (FDA, 2022b).

6.4.3 Cross-cutting compliance

Under 21 CFR Part 11 and EU Good Manufacturing Practice Annex 11, ensure that computerized systems used to generate, transform, or analyze regulated data are validated, traceable, and controlled.

In the EU, the AI Act establishes obligations for high-risk AI systems regarding risk management, data governance, technical documentation, transparency, and postmarket monitoring. While internal AI used for drug development may not always be classified as high-risk, sponsors should prepare for alignment with AI governance requirements and implement proportionate controls (EAA, 2024).

ICH E6(R3) and E8(R1) promote risk-based quality management and data collection that are fit for purpose; sponsors should integrate these principles into ML-enabled trial operations and evidence generation (ICH, 2022, 2025).

7 From discovery to clinic: Recent AI-driven outcomes from collaborations

7.1 Insilico medicine and partners (idiopathic pulmonary fibrosis, INS018_055)

INS018_055, a small molecule discovered entirely through Insilico's Pharma.AI platform (target discovery + generative chemistry + preclinical optimization), has progressed past first-in-human trials into Phase II clinical studies starting in 2023. Insilico describes the target as novel and not publicly disclosed, and has announced the initiation of Phase II studies in China with plans for global expansion.

It is one of the earliest publicly documented instances of an AI-discovered target with an AI-designed molecule advancing into mid-stage clinical trials for a complex, high-need condition (IPF) (Insilico Medicine, 2023-2024).

7.2 Benevolent AI and AstraZeneca (target discovery in CKD and IPF)

AstraZeneca started a multiyear partnership with BenevolentAI in 2019 to use AI for target identification in chronic kidney disease (CKD) and idiopathic pulmonary fibrosis (IPF). In 2022, AstraZeneca extended and broadened the collaboration, citing strong productivity, including the nomination and internal validation of new targets that feed into AstraZeneca's discovery pipeline.

It is one of the most prominent examples of AI-guided target discovery adopted by a major biopharma, resulting in tangible target nominations across complex biological areas (BenevolentAI, 2022). BenevolentAI investor communications have reiterated ongoing progress and expansion (BenevolentAI, 2022).

Exscientia, in collaboration with Sumitomo Pharma and other partners, is advancing AI-first medicinal chemistry into Phase I.

Several AI-designed small molecules have entered early clinical testing through Exscientia's collaborations. With Sumitomo Pharma, DSP-1181 (for OCD) was widely reported as the first AI-designed molecule to enter a Phase I trial (Japan) in 2020; the program was subsequently discontinued after early clinical assessment.

Exscientia's selective A2A receptor antagonist EXS21546 entered Phase I trials to assess safety, PK/PD, and immunomodulatory effects; later, Exscientia shifted its focus away from immuno-oncology, discontinuing EXS21546 but continuing other clinical and preclinical programs. These efforts established rapid design–make–test cycles and demonstrated that AI-led medicinal chemistry can deliver clinical candidates quickly, while also highlighting the realities of attrition in early development (Exscientia plc, 2022–2024).

Recursion with Roche/Genentech and Bayer (industrial-scale phenomics advancing programs into discovery and preclinical stages)

Recursion's mapping of cellular phenotypes at scale (machine learning on high-content microscopy) supports large, multitarget collaborations. Collaborations with Roche/Genentech (initiated in 2021) and Bayer (commenced in 2020) have publicly reported progress across multiple joint programs into discovery and preclinical stages, with Recursion disclosing milestone achievements and ongoing advancement across neuroscience, oncology, and fibrosis.

These are among the most extensive AI-enabled discovery partnerships in biopharma and highlight phenomics as a systematic route to generating target hypotheses and preclinical candidates across therapeutic areas (Recursion Pharmaceuticals, 2021).

7.3 XtalPi with leading pharmas (physics- and structure-informed AI for development optimization)

XtalPi's platform combines quantum mechanics, molecular simulation, and machine learning to guide crystal form selection, property prediction, ADMET optimization, and lead design. Global pharmaceutical collaborators have announced the use of XtalPi's tools to enhance developability and, in several collaborations, to nominate preclinical candidates.

Physics-informed AI is increasingly used to tackle downstream risks (solid-state form, PK, safety) that often derail otherwise promising chemistry, enhancing translational readiness.

Healx collaborates with patient organizations and academics on AI-prioritized repurposing and combination therapies for rare diseases.

Healx's Healnet platform and Rare Treatment Accelerator have been used to identify repurposed and combination regimens for rare diseases. In Fragile X syndrome, collaborations with FRAXA Research Foundation and academic partners have prioritized combinations for clinical evaluation; Healx has announced progress of AI-selected regimens toward trials and study launches in small patient populations.

AI-supported repurposing can facilitate quicker, more cost-effective evidence gathering in rare diseases where conventional processes face difficulties, particularly when supported by patient group collaborations (Healx, 2020-2023).

Isomorphic Labs collaborates with Novartis and Eli Lilly (deep AI integration for Big Pharma discovery).

In late 2023, Isomorphic Labs announced multitarget discovery collaborations with Novartis and Eli Lilly to apply AI-enabled structure-based design across various disease areas, with sizable, milestone-based deal structures. By 2024, these alliances were in early discovery stages, aiming to translate AI insights into development candidates.

These deals demonstrate growing confidence in AI-first, structure-guided design at a leading pharmaceutical scale and foster deeper co-discovery operating models.

8 AI-driven clinical trials—into practice

Implementing AI in clinical trial practice begins with defining the scope and making error trade-offs early, such as deciding on phase go/no-go, endpoint choice, site or country allocation, and forecasting enrollment—based on clear estimands and study quality by design. Use ICH E9(R1) to specify what is being estimated during relevant intercurrent events, and ICH E8(R1) to incorporate quality-by-design principles (ICH, 2022). Develop reliable data and feature pipelines by harmonizing trial data to CDISC (SDTM/ADaM) and RWD to OMOP, documenting data lineage and quality checks, and applying FAIR principles to ensure findability, accessibility, interoperability, and reuse. Privacy and auditability should be built in from the outset, with role-based access and traceable transformations, especially when integrating digital health technologies for remote data collection under FDA DHT guidance (FDA, 2023b).

Model choices should be fit-for-purpose: start with simple, well-calibrated baselines and add complexity only when it materially improves decision utility; quantify uncertainty (e.g., intervals, prediction coverage) and stress-test for domain shift. Validate prospectively in shadow mode and preregister evaluation plans using SPIRIT-AI and report outcomes with CONSORT-AI; align operational governance with GCP (ICH E6) and adopt an AI risk management framework (e.g., NIST AI RMF) to tier models by impact, define change control, and monitor calibration, discrimination, drift, and subgroup performance (NIST, 2023; Liu et al., 2020). Embed human-in-the-loop workflows for clinicians, statisticians, and trial operations, pairing predictions with explanations and clear actions, and measure ROI through cycle-time reductions, fewer amendments, improved enrollment metrics, and portfolio-level VOI gains.

9 Future directions

9.1 Multimodal digital endpoints: Continuous passive monitoring combined with clinical and imaging data for earlier efficacy readouts

This enables a new class of endpoints that combine passively collected signals from wearables and smartphones (e.g., mobility, sleep, heart rhythm), structured clinical measures (e.g., labs, patient-reported outcomes (PROs)), and quantitative imaging or radiomics to detect treatment effects earlier and more sensitively than traditional episodic measures. Continuous data enhance signal-to-noise ratio, while imaging quantification can detect subtle structural or functional changes.

9.1.1 Evidence and precedents

Regulators are already accepting specific digital measures. The EMA issued a qualification opinion for Stride Velocity 95th centile (SV95C) derived from wearable accelerometry as a secondary endpoint in Duchenne muscular dystrophy, setting a precedent for activity-based digital endpoints in pivotal trials (Servais et al., 2024).

The FDA's final guidance on Digital Health Technologies for Remote Data Acquisition in Clinical Investigations offers practical expectations for endpoint validation, data integrity, and participant safety when utilizing digital sensors in trials (FDA, 2023b).

Radiomics and quantitative imaging can transform standard scans into high-dimensional biomarkers that are prognostic for outcomes, potentially acting as sensitive efficacy indicators in oncology and other diseases (Lambin et al., 2012; Gillies et al., 2016).

Unsupervised multimodal representations from EHRs have demonstrated strong predictive performance, highlighting the potential to integrate clinical, sensor, and imaging data into unified endpoints (Miotto et al., 2016).

Practical playbooks and evidence standards have been developed to guide endpoint selection, validation, and operations for digital measures (Digital Medicine Society Digital Measures Playbook: https://www.dimesociety.org/toolkits/digital-measures-playbook/).

9.1.2 Implementation considerations

Harmonize devices and data streams, define clinically meaningful change thresholds, manage missing data and drift, and prespecify analysis plans consistent with ICH E9(R1) estimand principles (ICH, 2019).

9.2 Generative design of trials: AI that drafts protocols and simulates outcomes under multiple scenarios to recommend adaptive decision rules

This enables generative AI to accelerate protocol development (objectives, endpoints, procedures) by leveraging templates and prior work. At the same time, simulation engines test various randomization, stopping, and enrichment strategies to enhance power, ethics, and timelines. The integrated workflow can also propose adaptive decision rules that are prespecified in the protocol and Statistical Analysis Plan.

9.2.1 Evidence and precedents

Adaptive design has a well-established regulatory framework that highlights extensive simulations to justify operating features, making it a natural integration point for AI-driven trial design (FDA, 2019a; EMA, 2025b).

Complex innovative trial designs (e.g., Bayesian platform trials) show how simulation-driven decision rules can accelerate development and enhance learning—demonstrated by I-SPY 2's Bayesian adaptive randomization and graduation criteria in breast cancer (Wang and Yee, 2019).

9.2.2 Implementation considerations

Utilize LLMs to draft protocol sections and alternatives, then subject them to expert and statistical review; channel options into simulation to assess Type I error, power, and expected sample size under plausible scenarios.

9.3 Guardrails are essential: Follow estimand frameworks (ICH E9[R1]), keep traceability of design choices, and ensure transparency of priors and adaptation rules

For any AI-generated content, implement governance in line with emerging guidance on the safe and responsible use of AI in health (WHO, 2025). Connect AI-guided discovery, translational science, and clinical development with shared representations to preserve biological signals across stages.

This enables Shared, semantically consistent representations of biology (targets, pathways, biomarkers, mechanisms) from in silico discovery, preclinical models, and translational assays through to clinical phenotypes to reduce "signal loss" at stage transitions. This helps ensure that the mechanistic rationale underlying a candidate persists in patient selection, endpoint choice, and dose/exposure-response decisions.

9.3.1 Evidence and precedents

MIDD is an established regulatory pathway that links PK/PD, exposure–response, and systems models across different phases, facilitating more efficient dose selection and decision-making (FDA MIDD Pilot Program) (FDA, 2025b).

QSP integrates mechanistic knowledge with data-driven components to bridge preclinical and clinical biology, supporting biomarker strategy and trial design (Ermakov et al., 2019).

FAIR data principles and cross-study standards minimize friction and maintain context when linking datasets throughout the pipeline (Wilkinson et al., 2016).

9.3.2 Implementation considerations

Build a "semantic layer" that maps omics, imaging, and clinical features to mechanisms and outcomes, and aligns with controlled vocabularies and standards (CDISC, SNOMED CT).

Co-develop translational biomarkers with endpoints; predefine decision criteria based on biologically anchored models; maintain provenance and versioning for models and data across stages.

9.4 Privacy-preserving collaboration: Federated analytics and differential privacy facilitate cross-institutional learning without sharing raw data

This enables multiinstitutional learning on sensitive clinical and imaging data without centralizing records. Algorithms train where data reside; only model updates or statistics move, with privacy guards to prevent re-identification. This expands diversity and scale while respecting governance and local regulations.

9.4.1 Evidence and precedents

Federated learning has demonstrated feasibility and performance across hospitals and modalities, such as multisite medical imaging and EHR prediction tasks (Rieke et al., 2020).

A large international consortium employed federated learning to predict COVID-19 outcomes without sharing patient-level data, demonstrating strong generalization across sites (Dayan et al., 2021).

Differential privacy provides formal guarantees for protecting individuals when sharing model updates or statistics (Dwork and Roth, 2014; Abadi et al., 2016).

Genomics and health-data communities have established practical standards for secure data exchange and computation (GA4GH Crypt4GH secure file format: https://www.ga4gh.org/news/crypt4gh/).

9.4.2 Implementation considerations

Assess privacy budgets, membership inference risks, and potential gradient leakage; combine federated learning with secure aggregation and differential privacy.

Establish common data models and harmonization procedures to ensure federated updates are comparable; maintain audit trails and governance in accordance with site policies and regulations.

9.5 Transparent regulation and standards: Ongoing development of guidance, benchmarks, and best practices to ensure the safe, effective, and fair use of AI in trials

This enables clear expectations for the validation, monitoring, and updating of AI models and digital endpoints; common data standards to ensure interoperability; reporting guidelines to enhance reproducibility; and ethics frameworks to foster equity and accountability.

9.5.1 Evidence and precedents

Digital endpoints and remote data capture are addressed in the FDA's Digital Health Technologies (DHT) guidance (FDA, 2023b).

For AI/ML-enabled devices, the FDA's final guidance on Predetermined Change Control Plans (PCCP) outlines how sponsors can proactively describe and validate future model updates. This approach is relevant to trial-support tools when they interface with regulated functions (FDA, 2025g).

The EMA's *Reflection Paper* describes how AI can be utilized throughout the medicinal product lifecycle, covering data quality, model governance, and clinical evaluation aspects (EMA, 2023b).

The United Kingdom - Medicines and Healthcare products Regulatory Agency (UK MHRA)'s "*Software and AI as a Medical Device Change Program*" offers a roadmap for risk assessment, evidence requirements, and postmarket monitoring of AI systems (MHRA, 2021).

The ICH E6(R3) update to *Good Clinical Practice* modernizes quality management and supports digital technologies in trials; it should be cross-referenced when deploying AI-enabled endpoints and operations (ICH, 2025).

Community standards and guidelines help ensure robustness and transparency for ML models in healthcare, including reporting frameworks for AI prediction models (Collins et al., 2024).

Practical industry standards encourage interoperable data exchange and automation of trial processes (TransCelerate Digital Data Flow: https://www.transceleratebiopharmainc.com/digital-data-flow/; CDISC: https://www.cdisc.org/standards).

9.5.2 Implementation considerations

Build compliance by design: establish verification and validation plans, real-time monitoring, and update controls (e.g., PCCP) for AI components.

Participate in consortia to co-develop benchmarks for digital endpoints and AI models; publish protocols and performance following established reporting standards; evaluate bias and fairness through stratified analyses and stakeholder input.

Overall, these directions focus on a data- and model-centric clinical development ecosystem where continuous, multimodal measurement, rigorous simulation, end-to-end biological continuity, privacy-preserving collaboration, and transparent governance collectively enhance trial sensitivity, efficiency, and trust. As guidance and standards evolve, the emphasis should be on reproducible validation, equitable performance across populations, and operational robustness from discovery to postmarket learning.

10 Conclusion

AI is revolutionizing clinical trials, transforming them from static, one-off experiments into data-driven, adaptive learning systems. Throughout the development process, models can now integrate multimodal clinical, imaging, and digital sensor data to forecast outcomes, improve patient selection, and detect early signals of efficacy and safety. Coupled with established regulatory frameworks for adaptive designs and digital health technologies, this evolution enables trials that learn continuously, adjusting randomization or enrichment strategies based on ongoing evidence, and remotely monitoring patient trajectories with validated digital measures.

By predicting outcomes, improving design, and optimizing operations, AI can reduce timelines and costs while increasing the likelihood of success. In design, AI-assisted protocol drafting and extensive simulation help select decision rules that maintain type I error while maximizing power and ethical efficiency, especially for adaptive or platform trials. In operations, models aid in site and country selection, eligibility screening from EHRs, and proactive risk-based monitoring, each area demonstrating improved speed and data quality under appropriate governance. In measurement, validated digital endpoints and quantitative imaging can provide earlier, more sensitive readouts to speed up "go/no-go" decisions and, where suitable, serve as secondary or exploratory endpoints in pivotal studies.

The past few years have produced concrete examples of AI-generated targets and molecules entering the clinic through collaborations across academia and industry. Exscientia reported multiple AI-designed small molecules advancing into first-in-human studies with partners, including DSP-1181 and EXS-21546. Insilico Medicine announced an AI-discovered fibrosis candidate (INS018_055) progressing to Phase 2 for idiopathic pulmonary fibrosis. Beyond de novo design, AI has contributed to rapid repurposing: BenevolentAI prioritized baricitinib for COVID-19, subsequently supported in randomized trials and authorized treatment regimens. These cases, while early-stage and subject to attrition, illustrate a credible path from in silico hypotheses to clinical testing when embedded in rigorous translational workflows and partnered with experienced sponsors.

Realizing the potential of AI-driven clinical development goes beyond algorithms. Organizations that integrate high-quality, representative data, strong causal and predictive methods, and responsible governance will be best positioned to make an impact. Methodologically, alignment with the estimand framework, external validation, sensitivity analyses, and biologically grounded priors are essential to prevent false results and ensure transportability across populations and settings. Operationally, privacy-preserving collaboration through federated learning with secure aggregation and differential privacy can unlock diverse, multiinstitutional datasets without sharing raw records, enhancing generalization while maintaining patient trust. Governance should be compliance-by-design: including verification and validation plans, monitoring for drift, and transparent update procedures; these are now reflected in device-focused AI guidance that can inform trial-support tools where applicable.

Multidisciplinary collaboration is the essential enabler. Biostatisticians, clinicians, data scientists, trial operations specialists, ethicists, and regulators must collaborate to develop meaningful endpoints, protocols, and analytical plans that are clinically relevant, statistically robust, and operationally workable. Shared data models and standards, such as CDISC, along with initiatives like TransCelerate's Digital Data Flow, reduce obstacles, enhance interoperability, and help maintain biological signals from discovery to clinical evidence generation. MIDD and QSP frameworks further underpin decisions with mechanistic understanding, supporting rational dose choice, biomarker strategies, and efficient early proof-of-concept.

The trajectory is clear: as evidence standards, guidance, and tooling develop, AI will increasingly enhance every aspect of clinical development, boosting measurement sensitivity, streamlining design, and improving operational reliability while upholding safety, fairness, and transparency. Success will be measured not only by faster processes and reduced costs but also by delivering robust, reproducible benefits to patients across diverse populations. Through disciplined methods, privacy-protecting collaboration, and cohesive end-to-end integration, AI can help transform the clinical trial enterprise from episodic data collection to a continuous learning system that speeds up the translation of science into medicines.

References

Abadi, M., Chu, A., Goodfellow, I., McMahan, H.B., Mironov, I., Talwar, K., et al., 2016. Deep learning with differential privacy. In: Proceedings of the 2016 ACM SIGSAC conference on computer and communications security, Association for Computing Machinery, Vienna, Austria. pp. 308–318.

Aerts, H.J., Velazquez, E.R., Leijenaar, R.T., Parmar, C., Grossmann, P., Carvalho, S., Bussink, J., et al., 2014a. Decoding tumour phenotype by noninvasive imaging using a quantitative radiomics approach. Nat. Commun. 2041-1723. 5, 4006. doi:10.1038/ncomms5006.

Alsentzer, E., Murphy, J., Boag, W., Weng, W.-H., Jindi, D., Naumann, T., et al., editors, 2019. Publicly Available Clinical BERT Embeddings. Association for Computational Linguistics, Minneapolis, Minnesota, USA.

Angelopoulos, A.N., Bates, S., 2021. A gentle introduction to conformal prediction and distribution-free uncertainty quantification. arXiv. doi:10.48550/arXiv.2107.07511.

Angus, D.A.-O., Berry, S., Lewis, R.A.-O., Al-Beidh, F.A.-O.X., Arabi, Y., van Bentum-puijk, W., et al., 2020. The REMAP-CAP (randomized embedded multifactorial adaptive platform for community-acquired pneumonia) study. Rationale and design. Ann. Am. Thorac. Soc. 2325-6621. 17 (7), 879–891. doi:10.1513/AnnalsATS.202003-192SD.

Anisimov, V.V., 2011. Statistical modeling of clinical trials (recruitment and randomization). Commun. Stat. Theory Methods 40 (19-20), 3684–3699.

Anisimov, V.V., Fedorov, V.V., 2007. Modelling, prediction and adaptive adjustment of recruitment in multicentre trials. 0277-6715.

Athey, S., Imbens, G., 2016. Recursive partitioning for heterogeneous causal effects. Proc. Natl. Acad. Sci. U. S. A. 113 (27), 7353–7360.

Austin, P.C., 2011. An introduction to propensity score methods for reducing the effects of confounding in observational studies. 1532-7906.

Bai, S., Kolter, J.Z., Koltun, V., 2018. An empirical evaluation of generic convolutional and recurrent networks for sequence modeling. ArXiv https://arxiv.org/abs/1803.01271.

Baiocchi, M., Cheng, J., Small, D.S. 2020. Instrumental variable methods for causal inference. 1097-0258.

Baltrušaitis, T., Ahuja, C., Morency, L.P., 2019. Multimodal machine learning: a survey and taxonomy. IEEE Trans. Pattern Anal. Mach. Intell. 41 (2), 423–443.

Beltagy, I., Lo, K., Cohan, A. 2019. SciBERT: a pretrained language model for scientific text. pp. 3613–3618.

BenevolentAI. 2022. AstraZeneca-BenevolentAI collaboration productivity update. BenevolentAI FY2022/FY2023 Annual Reports. BenevolentAI RNS/press,14 Apr 2022.

Berry, D.A. 2006. Bayesian clinical trials. 1474-1776.

Berry, D.A., 2011. Adaptive clinical trials: the promise and the caution. J. Clin. Oncol. 29 (6), 606–609.

Bhagat, R.A.-O., Bojarski, L., Chevalier, S., Görtz, D.R., Le Meignen, S., Makowski, M., et al., 2020. Quality tolerance limits: framework for successful implementation in clinical development. 2168-4804

Bica, I., Alaa, A.M., Schaar, M.V.D., 2020. Time series deconfounder: estimating treatment effects over time in the presence of hidden confounders. In: Proceedings of the 37th International Conference on Machine Learning: JMLR.org. p. 83.

BIO, 2021. Clinical development success rates and contributing factors 2011-2020: informa pharma intelligence & QLS advisors. Available from: https://www.bio.org/clinical-development-success-rates-and-contributing-factors-2011-2020.

Bonawitz, K., Ivanov, V., Kreuter, B., Marcedone, A., McMahan, H.B., Patel, S., et al., 2017. Practical secure aggregation for privacy-preserving machine learning. In: Proceedings of the 2017 ACM SIGSAC Conference on Computer and Communications Security. Association for Computing Machinery, Dallas, Texas, USA. pp. 1175–1191.

Bradshaw, E.L., Spilker, M.E., Zang, R., Bansal, L., He, H., Jones, R.D.O., Le, K, Penney, M, Schuck, E, Topp, B, Tsai, A, Xu, C, Nijsen, M.J.M.A., Chan, J.R., 2019. Applications of quantitative systems pharmacology in model-informed drug discovery: perspective on impact and opportunities. CPT Pharmacomet. Syst. Pharmacol. 2163-8306. 8 (11), 777–791. doi:10.1002/psp4.12463.

Breiman, L., 2001. Random forests. Mach. Learn. 45 (1), 5–32.

Brophy, E., Wang, Z., She, Q., Ward, T., 2023. Generative adversarial networks in time series: a systematic literature review. ACM Comput. Surv. 55 (10), 199.

Caruana, R., 1997. Multitask learning. Mach. Learn. 28 (1), 41–75.

Caton, S., Haas, C., 2024. Fairness in machine learning: a survey. ACM Comput. Surv. 56 (7), 166.

Celis, L.E., Huang, L., Keswani, V., Vishnoi, N.K., 2019. Classification with fairness constraints: a meta-algorithm with provable guarantees. In: Proceedings of the Conference on Fairness, Accountability, and Transparency, Association for Computing Machinery, Atlanta, GA, USA. pp. 319–328.

Chandola, V., Banerjee, A., Kumar, V., 2009. Anomaly detection: a survey. ACM Comput. Surv. 41 (3), 15.

Cheerla, A., Gevaert, O., 2019. Deep learning with multimodal representation for pan-cancer prognosis prediction. Bioinformatics 35 (14), i446–i54.

Chen, T., Guestrin, C., 2016. XGBoost: a scalable tree boosting system. In: Proceedings of the 22nd ACM SIGKDD International Conference on Knowledge Discovery and Data Mining, Association for Computing Machinery, San Francisco, California, USA. pp. 785–794.

Chernozhukov, V., Chetverikov, D., Demirer, M., Duflo, E., Hansen, C., Newey, W., et al., 2018. Double/debiased machine learning for treatment and structural parameters. Econom. J. 21 (1), C1–C68.

Chow, S.-C., Shao, J., Wang, H., Lokhnygina, Y., 2017. Sample Size Calculations in Clinical Research, third ed. Chapman and Hall/CRC.

Claxton, K., Posnett, J., 1996. An economic approach to clinical trial design and research priority-setting. Health Econ. 1057-9230. 5 (6), 513–524. doi:10.1002/(SICI)1099-1050(199611)5:6<513::AID-HEC237>3.0.CO;2-9.

Collett, D., 2014, Modelling Survival Data in Medical Research, third ed. Chapman and Hall/CRC, New York.

Collignon, O., 2022. An economic perspective on platform trials—the gift and the curse. JAMA Netw. Open 5 (7), e2221149.

Collins, G.S., Moons, K.G.M., Dhiman, P., Riley, R.D., Beam, A.L., Van Calster, B., et al., 2024. TRIPOD+AI statement: updated guidance for reporting clinical prediction models that use regression or machine learning methods. BMJ 385, e078378.

Corrigan-Curay, J., Sacks, L., Woodcock, J. 2018. Real-world evidence and real-world data for evaluating drug safety and effectiveness. JAMA. 1538-3598. 320 (9), 867–868. doi:10.1001/jama.2018.10136.

CTTI, 2019. Original digital health trials projects Available from: https://ctti-clinicaltrials.org/about/ctti-projects/original-digital-health-trials-projects/.

Dayan, I., Roth, H.R., Zhong, A., Harouni, A., Gentili, A., Abidin, A.Z., et al., 2021. Federated learning for predicting clinical outcomes in patients with COVID-19. Nat. Med. 27 (10), 1735–1743.

Devlin, J., Chang, M.-W., Lee, K., Toutanova, K. (editors.), 2019a. BERT: Pre-training of Deep Bidirectional Transformers for Language Understanding. Association for Computational Linguistics, Minneapolis, Minnesota.

Devlin, J., Chang, M.-W., Lee, K., Toutanova, K.B.E.R.T., 2019b.Pre-training of deep bidirectional transformers for language understanding. pp. 4171–4186.

DiMasi, J.A., Grabowski, H.G., Hansen, R.W., 2016. Innovation in the pharmaceutical industry: new estimates of R&D costs. J. Health Econ. 1879-1646. 47, 20–33.

Dukes, O., Richardson, D.B., Shahn, Z., Robins, J.M., Tchetgen Tchetgen, E.J., 2024. Using negative controls to identify causal effects with invalid instrumental variables. Biometrika 112 (1), asae064. doi:10.1093/biomet/asae064.

Dwork, C., Roth, A., 2014. The algorithmic foundations of differential privacy. Found. Trends Theor. Comput. Sci. 9 (3–4), 211–407. doi:10.1561/0400000042.
EAA, 2024. Regulation of the European Parliament and of the Council laying down harmonised rules on artificial intelligence (AI Act) Available from: https://artificialintelligenceact.eu/the-act/.
EMA, 2021 Guideline on registry-based studies - Scientific guideline 2021 Available from: https://www.ema.europa.eu/en/guideline-registry-based-studies-scientific-guideline.
EMA, 2023a. Data quality framework for medicines regulation.
EMA, 2023b Reflection paper on the use of artificial intelligence in the lifecycle of medicines Available from: https://www.ema.europa.eu/en/news/reflection-paper-use-artificial-intelligence-lifecycle-medicines.
EMA, 2024. Guidance on regulatory use of Real-World Evidence (RWE). EMA/152628/2024.
EMA, 2025a. EBD. Data in regulation: big data and other sources Available from: https://www.ema.europa.eu/en/about-us/how-we-work/data-regulation-big-data-other-sources.
EMA, 2025b. ICHE20adaptive designs for clinical trials—Scientific guideline Available from: https://www.ema.europa.eu/en/ich-e20-adaptive-designs-clinical-trials-scientific-guideline.
Ermakov, S., Schmidt, B.J., Musante, C.J., Thalhauser, C.J., 2019. A survey of software tool utilization and capabilities for quantitative systems pharmacology: what we have and what we need. CPT Pharmacometrics Syst. Pharmacol. 8 (2), 62–76.
European Commission, 2023. EudraLex—Volume 4—Good Manufacturing Practice (GMP) guidelines. Available from: https://health.ec.europa.eu/medicinal-products/eudralex/eudralex-volume-4_en.
Exscientia plc, 2022–2024. Annual report and investor updates on AI-designed clinical candidates.
FDA, 2013. Oversight of clinical investigations—a risk-based approach to monitoring. FDA-2011-D-597.
FDA, 2018a. Real-world evidence Available from: https://www.fda.gov/science-research/science-and-research-special-topics/real-world-evidence.
FDA, 2018b. E6(R1) I.E6(R2) good clinical practice: integrated addendum to ICHE6(R1). Enter for biologics evaluation and research center for drug evaluation and research.
FDA, 2019a. Adaptive design clinical trials for drugs and biologics guidance for industry.
FDA, 2019b. Enrichment strategies for clinical trials to support approval of human drugs and biological products Available from: https://www.fda.gov/regulatory-information/search-fda-guidance-documents/enrichment-strategies-clinical-trials-support-approval-human-drugs-and-biological-products.
FDA, 2022a. Master protocols: efficient clinical trial design strategies to expedite development of oncology drugs and biologics guidance for industry Available from: https://www.fda.gov/regulatory-information/search-fda-guidance-documents/master-protocols-efficient-clinical-trial-design-strategies-expedite-development-oncology-drugs-and.
FDA, 2022b. Submitting documents using real-world data and real-world evidence to FDA for drug and biological products.
FDA, 2023a. Artificial intelligence in software as a medical device Available from: https://www.fda.gov/medical-devices/software-medical-device-samd/artificial-intelligence-software-medical-device.
FDA, 2023b. Digital Health Technologies for Remote Data Acquisition in Clinical Investigations.

FDA, 2023c. F. Considerations for the Design and Conduct of Externally Controlled Trials for Drug and Biological Products Available from: https://www.fda.gov/regulatory-information/search-fda-guidance-documents/considerations-design-and-conduct-externally-controlled-trials-drug-and-biological-products.

FDA, 2023d. Considerations for the use of real-world data and real-world evidence to support regulatory decision-making for drug and biological products.FDA-2021-D-1214.

FDA, 2023e. Part 11, Electronic Records; Electronic Signatures—Scope and Application.FDA-2003-D-143.

FDA, 2025b. Model-informed drug development paired meeting program updated 2023-2027. Available from: https://www.fda.gov/drugs/development-resources/model-informed-drug-development-paired-meeting-program.

FDA, 2025c. FDA use of real-world evidence in regulatory decision making.

FDA, 2025d. Computer software assurance for production and quality system software. FDA-2022-D-795.

FDA, 2025e. Good machine learning practice for medical device development: guiding principles Available from: https://www.fda.gov/medical-devices/software-medical-device-samd/good-machine-learning-practice-medical-device-development-guiding-principles.

FDA, 2025f. Artificial intelligence for drug development.

FDA, 2025g Marketing submission recommendations for a predetermined change control plan for artificial intelligence-enabled device software functions 2025 [FDA-2022-D-628]. Available from: https://www.fda.gov/regulatory-information/search-fda-guidance-documents/marketing-submission-recommendations-predetermined-change-control-plan-artificial-intelligence.

Fitzmaurice, G.M., Laird, N.M., Ware, J.H., 2011. Applied Longitudinal Analysis, Wiley.

Fleurence, R.L., Curtis, L.H., Califf, R.M., Platt, R., Selby, J.V., Brown, J.S., 2014. Launching PCORnet, a national patient-centered clinical research network. J. Am. Med. Inform. Assoc. 21 (4), 578–582.

Freidlin, B., Korn, E.L. 2009. Stopping clinical trials early for benefit: impact on estimation. 1740-7745.

Friedman, J.H., 2001. Greedy function approximation: a gradient boosting machine. Ann. Stat. 29 (4), 1189–1232.

Gama, J., Žliobaitė, I., Bifet, A., Pechenizkiy, M., Bouchachia, A., 2014. A survey on concept drift adaptation. ACM Comput. Surv. 46 (4), 44.

Gebru, T., Morgenstern, J., Vecchione, B., Vaughan, J.W., Wallach III, H., et al., 2021. Datasheets for datasets. Commun. ACM 64 (12), 86–92.

Gelman, A., Carlin, J.B., Stern, H.S., Dunson, D.B., Vehtari, A., Rubin, D.B., 2013. Bayesian Data Analysis, third ed. Chapman and Hall/CRC.

Getz, K.A., Campo, R.A. New benchmarks characterizing growth in protocol design complexity. 20182168-4804.

Gillies, R.J., Kinahan, P.E., Hricak, H., 2016. Radiomics: images are more than pictures, they are data. Radiology. 1527-1315. 278 (2), 63–77. doi:10.1148/radiol.2015151169.

Goldstein, A., Kapelner, A., Bleich, J., Pitkin, E., 2015. Peeking inside the black box: visualizing statistical learning with plots of individual conditional expectation. J. Comput. Graph. Stat. 24 (1), 44–65.

Gu, Y., Tinn, R., Cheng, H., Lucas, M., Usuyama, N., Liu, X., et al, 2021. Domain-specific language model pretraining for biomedical natural language processing. ACM Trans. Comput. Healthc. 3 (1), 2.

Hamilton, W.L., 2020. Graph representation learning. Synthesis Lectures on Artificial Intelligence and Machine Learning. Springer.

Hampson, L.V., Jennison, C., 2012. Group sequential tests for delayed responses (with discussion). J. R. Stat. Soc. Ser. B Stat. Methodol. 75 (1), 3–54.

Hardt, M., Price, E., Srebro, N., 2016. Equality of opportunity in supervised learning. In: Proceedings of the 30th International Conference on Neural Information Processing Systems, Curran Associates Inc., Barcelona, Spain. pp. 3323–3331.
Hastie, T., Friedman, J., 2009. The Elements of Statistical Learning, Springer, New York, NY.
Hay, M., Thomas, D.W., Craighead, J.L., Economides, C., Rosenthal, J., 2014. Clinical development success rates for investigational drugs. Nat. Biotechnol. 32 (1), 40–51.
Healx, 2020-2023.Healx newsroom and blog updates on AI-prioritized repurposing for rare diseases.
Heath, A.A.-O., Strong, M.A.-O., Glynn, D.A.-O., Kunst, N., Welton, N.J., Goldhaber-Fiebert, J.D. , 2021. Simulating study data to support expected value of sample information calculations: a tutorial. Med. Decis. Mak. 1552-681X. doi:10.1177/0272989X211026292.
Hern´an, M.A., Robins, J.M., 2024. Causal inference: what if.
Hill, J.L., 2011. Bayesian nonparametric modeling for causal inference. J. Comput. Graph. Stat. 20 (1), 217–240.
Himmelstein, D.A.-O., Lizee, A., Hessler, C., Brueggeman, L., Chen, S.L., Hadley, D., et al., 2017. Systematic integration of biomedical knowledge prioritizes drugs for repurposing. eLife. 2050-084X. 6, e26726. doi:10.7554/eLife.26726.
Horby, P., Lim, W.S., Emberson, J.R., Mafham, M., Bell, J.L., Linsell, L.A.-O., et al., 2021. Dexamethasone in hospitalized patients with Covid-19. N. Engl. J. Med. 1533-4406. doi:10.1056/NEJMoa2021436.
Hripcsak, G., Duke, J.D., Shah, N.H., Reich, C.G., Huser, V., Schuemie, M.J., et al., 2015. Observational health data sciences and informatics (OHDSI): opportunities for observational researchers. Stud. Health Technol. Inform. 1879-8365. 216, 574–578.
Hyndman, R.J., Athanasopoulos, G., 2020. Forecasting: Principles and Practice, third ed. OTexts, Melbourne, Australia. Available from: https://otexts.com/fpp3/.
ICH, 2019. ICHE9(R1). Statistical principles for clinical trials Available from: https://www.ich.org/page/efficacy-guidelines.
ICH, 2022. ICHE8General considerations for clinical studies—Scientific guideline Available from: https://www.ema.europa.eu/en/ich-e8-general-considerations-clinical-studies-scientific-guideline.
ICH, 2025. ICHE6Good clinical practice—Scientific guideline Available from: https://www.ema.europa.eu/en/ich-e6-good-clinical-practice-scientific-guideline.
Insilico Medicine, 2023-2024. INS018_055 advances into Phase II clinical studies for idiopathic pulmonary fibrosis. Insilico Medicine newsroom.
ISO, 2023. 23894:2023 II. Information technology—Artificial intelligence—Guidance on risk management Available from: https://www.iso.org/standard/77304.html.
Jennison, C., Turnbull, B.W., 2000. Group Sequential Methods with Applications to Clinical Trials, Chapman & Hall/CRC, Boca Raton.
Kairouz, P., McMahan, H.B., Avent, B., Bellet, A., Bennis, M., Bhagoji, A.N., et al., 2021. Advances and open problems in federated learning. Found. Trends Mach. Learn. 14 (1–2), 1–210.
Ke, G., Meng, Q., Finley, T., Wang, T., Chen, W., Ma, W., et al. 2017. LightGBM: a highly efficient gradient boosting decision tree. In: Proceedings of the 31st International Conference on Neural Information Processing Systems, Curran Associates Inc., Long Beach, California, USA. pp. 3149–3157.
Kho, A.N., Pacheco, J.A., Peissig, P.L., Rasmussen, L., Newton, K.M., Weston, N., Crane, P.K., et al., 2011. Electronic medical records for genetic research: results of the eMERGE consortium. 1946-6242. doi:10.1126/scitranslmed.3001807.
Kim, J., Izower, M., Quintana, Y., 2023. Parsable clinical trial eligibility criteria representation using natural language processing. AMIA Annu. Symp. Proc. 1942-597X. 2022, 616–624. Available from: https://pmc.ncbi.nlm.nih.gov/articles/PMC10148319/.

King, E.A.-O., Davis, J.W., Degner, J.F., 2019. Are drug targets with genetic support twice as likely to be approved? Revised estimates of the impact of genetic support for drug mechanisms on the probability of drug approval. 1553-7404.
Kipf, T.N., Welling, M., 2017. Semi-supervised classification with graph convolutional networks. .
Kola, I., Landis, J., 2004. Can the pharmaceutical industry reduce attrition rates? Nat. Rev. Drug Discov. 3 (8), 711–716.
Krumholz, H.M., 2014. Big data and new knowledge in medicine: the thinking, training, and tools needed for a learning health system. Health Aff. (Millwood). 2694-233X. 33 (7), 1163–1170. doi:10.1377/hlthaff.2014.0053. PMID: 25006142.
Künzel, S.R., Sekhon, J.S., Bickel, P.J., Yu, B. Metalearners for estimating heterogeneous treatment effects using machine learning. 2019(1091-6490.
Laird, N.M., Ware, J.H., 1982. Random-effects models for longitudinal data. Biometrics. 0006-341X. 38 (4), 963–974.
Lambin, P., Rios-Velazquez, E., Leijenaar, R., Leijenaar, R., Carvalho, S., Carvalho, S., van Stiphout, R.G.P.M., van Stiphout, R.G., Granton, P., Granton, P., Zegers, C.M.L., et al., 2012. Radiomics: extracting more information from medical images using advanced feature analysis. Eur. J. Cancer. 1879-0852. 48 (4), 441–446. doi:10.1016/j.ejca.2011.11.036. PMID: 22257792.
Lee, J., Yoon, W., Kim, S., Kim, D., Kim, S., So, C.H., et al., 2019. BioBERT: a pre-trained biomedical language representation model for biomedical text mining. Bioinformatics 36 (4), 1234–1240.
Li, R.C., Asch, S.M., Shah, N.H., 2020. Developing a delivery science for artificial intelligence in healthcare. Npj Digit. Med. 3 (1), 107.
Lim, B., Arık, S.Ö., Loeff, N., Pfister, T., 2021. Temporal fusion transformers for interpretable multi-horizon time series forecasting. Int. J. Forecast. 37 (4), 1748–1764.
Lin, H.-T., Lin, C.-J., Weng, R.C., 2007. A note on Platt's probabilistic outputs for support vector machines. Mach. Learn. 68 (3), 267–276.
Lipton, Z.C. Kale, D.C. Wetzell, R., 2016. Modeling missing data in clinical time series with RNNs. In: Proceedings of Machine Learning for Healthcare, vol. 56. pp. 253–270. doi:10.48550/arXiv.1606.04130.
Liu, X., Cruz Rivera, S., Moher, D., Calvert, M.J., Denniston, A.K., Chan, A.-W., et al., 2020. Reporting guidelines for clinical trial reports for interventions involving artificial intelligence: the CONSORT-AI extension. Nat. Med. 26 (9), 1364–1374.
Lundberg, S.M., Erion, G., Chen, H., DeGrave, A., Prutkin, J.M., Nair, B., et al., 2020. From local explanations to global understanding with explainable AI for trees. 2522-5839.
Lundberg, S.M., Lee, S.-I., 2017. A unified approach to interpreting model predictions. In: Proceedings of the 31st International Conference on Neural Information Processing Systems, Curran Associates Inc., Long Beach, California, USA. pp. 4768–4777.
MacLean, F., 2021. Knowledge graphs and their applications in drug discovery. Expert Opin. Drug Discov. 1746-045X. 16 (9), 1057–1069. doi:10.1080/17460441.2021.1910673.
Markowitz, H., 1952. Portfolio selection. J. Finance 7 (1), 77–91.
McMahan, B., Moore, E., Ramage, D., Hampson, S., Arcas, B. 2017. Communication-efficient learning of deep networks from decentralized data. pp. 1273–1282.
Mehrabi, N., Morstatter, F., Saxena, N., Lerman, K., Galstyan, A., 2021. A survey on bias and fairness in machine learning. ACM Comput. Surv. 54 (6), 115.
Menon, A.K., Jiang, X.J., Vembu, S., Elkan, C., Ohno-Machado, L., 2012. Predicting accurate probabilities with a ranking loss.
MHRA, 2018.MHRA GxP data integrity definitions and guidance for industry. Available from: https://www.gov.uk/government/news/mhra-gxp-data-integrity-definitions-and-guidance-for-industry.
MHRA, 2021. Software and AI as a medical device change programme.

Miao, G., Yu, L., Yang, J., Bennett, D.A., Zhao, J., Wu, S.S., 2024. Learning from vertically distributed data across multiple sites: an efficient privacy-preserving algorithm for Cox proportional hazards model with variable selection. J. Biomed. Inform. 149, 104581.

Miotto, R., Li, L., Kidd, B.A., Dudley, J.T., 2016. Deep patient: an unsupervised representation to predict the future of patients from the electronic health records. Sci. Rep. 6(1), 26094.

Mitchell, M., Wu, S., Zaldivar, A., Barnes, P., Vasserman, L., Hutchinson, B., et al., 2019. Model cards for model reporting. In: Proceedings of the Conference on Fairness, Accountability, and Transparency, Association for Computing Machinery, Atlanta, GA, USA. pp. 220–229.

Morton, R.L., Tuffaha, H., Blaya-Novakova, V., Spencer, J., Hawley, C.M., Peyton, P., et al., 2022. Approaches to prioritising research for clinical trial networks: a scoping review. Trials 23 (1), 1000.

Murphy, A.H., Winkler, R.L., 1992. Diagnostic verification of probability forecasts. Int. J. Forecast. 7 (4), 435–455.

Murphy, S.A., 2003. Optimal dynamic treatment regimes. J. R. Stat. Soc. Ser. B Stat. Methodol. 65 (2), 331–355.

Nelson, M.R., Tipney, H., Painter, J.L., Shen, J., Nicoletti, P., Shen, Y., et al., 2015. The support of human genetic evidence for approved drug indications. Nat. Genet. 47 (8), 856–860.

Ngiam, J., Khosla, A., Kim, M., Nam, J., Lee, H., Ng, A.Y. 2011. Multimodal deep learning. In: Proceedings of the 28th International Conference on International Conference on Machine Learning, Omnipress, Bellevue, Washington, USA. pp. 689–696.

Niazi, S., 2025. Artificial intelligence in small-molecule drug discovery: a critical review of methods, applications, and real-world outcomes. Pharmaceuticals 18 (9), 1271. doi:10.3390/ph18091271. PMID 41011141.

NIST, 2023. AI risk management framework. Available from: https://www.nist.gov/itl/ai-risk-management-framework.

O'Quigley, J., Pepe, M., Fisher, L., 1990. Continual reassessment method: a practical design for phase 1 clinical trials in cancer. Biometrics 46 (1), 33–48. doi:10.2307/2531628. PMID: 2350571.

Ochoa, D., Hercules, A., Carmona, M., Suveges, D., Gonzalez-Uriarte, A., Malangone, C., et al., 2021. Open targets platform: supporting systematic drug-target identification and prioritisation. Nucleic Acids Res. 49 (D1), D1302–D1310.

Olawade, D.B., Fidelis, S.C., Marinze, S., Egbon, E., Osunmakinde, A., Osborne, A., 2026. Artificial intelligence in clinical trials: a comprehensive review of opportunities, challenges, and future directions. Int. J. Med. Inform. 206, 106141.

Ou, F.S., An, M.W., Ruppert, A.S., Mandrekar, S.J., 2019. Discussion of trial designs for biomarker identification and validation through the use of case studies. JCO Precis. Oncol. 2473-4284. PO.19.00051. doi:10.1200/po.19.00051.

Paul, S.M., Mytelka, D.S., Dunwiddie, C.T., Persinger, C.C., Munos, B.H., Lindborg, S.R., et al, 2010. How to improve R&D productivity: the pharmaceutical industry's grand challenge. Nat. Rev. Drug Discov. 9 (3), 203–214.

Pearl, J., 2009, Causality, Second ed. Cambridge University Press, Cambridge.

Pleiss, G., Raghavan, M., Wu, F., Kleinberg, J., Weinberger, K.Q., 2017. On fairness and calibration. In: Proceedings of the 31st International Conference on Neural Information Processing Systems, Curran Associates Inc., Long Beach, California, USA. pp. 5684–5693.

Raja, J.M., Elsakr, C., Roman, S., Cave, B., Pour-Ghaz, I., Nanda, A., et al., 2019. Apple watch, wearables, and heart rhythm: where do we stand? Ann. Transl. Med. 7 (17), 417. doi:10.21037/atm.2019.06.79.

Recursion Pharmaceuticals, 2021. Recursion and Roche/Genentech strategic collaboration announcement.

Rieke, N.A.-O., Hancox, J., Li, W.A.-O., Milletarì, F., Roth, H.A.-O., Albarqouni, S.A.-O., et al., 2020. The future of digital health with federated learning. Npj Digit. Med. 2398-6352. 3, 119. doi:10.1038/s41746-020-00323-1. PMID: 33015372.
Roberts, M.E., Stewart, B.M., Nielsen, R.A., 2020. Replication Data for: Adjusting for Confounding with Text Matching. In: Roberts ME, editor. V1 ed: Harvard Dataverse.
Ruder, S., 2017. An overview of multi-task learning in deep neural networks. ArXiv https://arxiv.org/abs/1706.05098.
Schoenfeld, D.A. , 1983. Sample-size formula for the proportional-hazards regression model. Biometrics 39 (2), 499–503. doi:10.2307/2531021. PMID: 6354290.
Schuemie, M.A.-O., Ryan, P.B., Hripcsak, G., Madigan, D., Suchard, M.A., 2018. Improving reproducibility by using high-throughput observational studies with empirical calibration. Philos. Trans. R. Soc. A: Math., Phys. Eng. Sci. 1471-2962. 20170356. doi:10.1098/rsta.2017.0356.
Schuemie, M.J., Ryan, P.B., Pratt, N., Chen, R., You, S.C., Krumholz, H.M., et al., 2020. Principles of large-scale evidence generation and evaluation across a network of databases (LEGEND). J. Am. Med. Inform. Assoc. 27 (8), 1331–1337. doi:10.1093/jamia/ocaa103. PMID: 32909033.
Schuhmacher, A., Hinder, M., Brief, E., Gassmann, O., Hartl, D., 2025. Benchmarking R&D success rates of leading pharmaceutical companies: an empirical analysis of FDA approvals (2006–2022). Drug Discov. Today 30(2), 104291.
Schulam, P.F., Saria, S., eds. 2017. Reliable Decision Support Using Counterfactual Models. Neural Information Processing Systems.
Schulz, K.F., Altman, D.G., Moher, D., 2010. CONSORT 2010 statement: updated guidelines for reporting parallel group randomised trials. BMJ. 1756-1833. 1 (2), 100–107. doi:10.4103/0976-500X.72352. PMID: 21350618.
Scott, S.L., 2010. A modern Bayesian look at the multi-armed bandit. Appl. Stoch. Models Bus. Ind. 26 (6), 639–658.
Sculley, D., Holt, G., Golovin, D., Davydov, E., Phillips, T., Ebner, D., et al., 2015. Hidden technical debt in machine learning systems. In: Proceedings of the 29th International Conference on Neural Information Processing Systems - Volume 2, MIT Press, Montreal, Canada. pp. 2503–2511.
Sergi, C.M., Sesso, H.D., 2025. Artificial Intelligence and the future of clinical trials. Contemp. Clin. Trials Commun. 2451-8654. 47, 101545. doi:10.1016/j.conctc.2025.101545. PMID: 41050844.
Serra, A., Fratello, M., Federico, A., Greco, D., 2025. An update on knowledge graphs and their current and potential applications in drug discovery. Expert Opin. Drug Discov. 20 (5), 599–619.
Sertkaya, A., Beleche, T., Jessup, A., Sommers, B.D., 2024. Costs of drug development and research and development intensity in the US, 2000-2018. JAMA Netw. Open 7(6), e2415445-e.
Servais, L., Strijbos, P., Poleur, M., Mirea, A., Butoianu, N., Sansone, V.A., et al., 2024. Evidentiary basis of the first regulatory qualification of a digital primary efficacy endpoint. Sci. Rep. 14 (1), 29681.
Shickel, B., Tighe, P.J., Bihorac, A., Rashidi, P., 2017. Deep EHR: a survey of recent advances in deep learning techniques for electronic health record (EHR) analysis. IEEE J. Biomed. Health Inform. 22 (5), 1589–1604. doi:10.1109/JBHI.2017.2767063. PMID: 29989977.
Shivade, C., Hebert, C., Regan, K., Fosler-Lussier, E., Lai, A.M., 2016. Automatic data source identification for clinical trial eligibility criteria resolution. 1942-597X
Sklavenitis, D., Kalles, D., 2025. A scoping review and assessment framework for technical debt in the development and operation of AI/ML competition platforms. Appl. Sci. 15 (13), 7165.

Sudell, M.A.-O., Kolamunnage-Dona, R., Tudur-Smith, C. Joint models for longitudinal and time-to-event data: a review of reporting quality with a view to meta-analysis. 2016, 1471-2288.

Sutton, R.S., Barto, A.G., 2018. Reinforcement Learning an Introduction Second Edition, The MIT Press.

Sweeney, L., 2002. k-anonymity: a model for protecting privacy. Int. J. Uncertain. Fuzziness Knowl.-Based Syst. 10 (5), 557–570.

Teodoro, D., Naderi, N., Yazdani, A., Zhang, B., Bornet, A., 2025. A scoping review of artificial intelligence applications in clinical trial risk assessment. Npj Digit. Med. 8 (1), 486.

Thall, P.F., 2022. Adaptive enrichment designs in clinical trials. Annu. Rev. Stat. Appl. 2326-8298. 8 (1), 393–411. doi:10.1146/annurev-statistics-040720-032818. PMID: 36212769.

Thomas, N.K., Welling, M., 2017. Semi-supervised classification with graph convolutional networks. In: ICLR 2017.

Thompson, W.R., 1933. On the likelihood that one unknown probability exceeds another in view of the evidence of two samples. Biometrika 25 (3-4), 285–294.

Tibshirani, R., 2011. Regression shrinkage and selection via the Lasso: a retrospective. J. R. Stat. Soc. Ser. B Stat. Methodol. 73 (3), 273–282.

Torkamani, A., Wineinger, N.E., Topol, E.J., 2018. The personal and clinical utility of polygenic risk scores. Nat. Rev. Genet. 19 (9), 581–590.

Trippa, L., Xu, Y., 2023. Comment: advancing clinical trials with novel designs and implementations. Stat. Sci. 38 (2), 216–218. doi:10.1214/23-sts865c. PMID: 37654478.

Tsiatis, A.A., Davidian, M., 2004. Joint modeling of longitudinal and time-to-event data: an overview. Statistica Sinica 14 (3), 809–834.

Turakhia, M.P., Desai, M., Hedlin, H., Rajmane, A., Talati, N., Ferris, T., et al., 2019. Rationale and design of a large-scale, app-based study to identify cardiac arrhythmias using a smartwatch: the Apple Heart Study. Am. Heart J. 1097-6744. 207, 66–75.

van der Laan, M.J., Rose, S., 2011. Targeted Learning: Causal Inference for Observational and Experimental Data, Springer.

VanderWeele, T.J., Ding, P. Sensitivity analysis in observational research: introducing the E-Value. 2017(1539-3704).

Varoquaux, G., Cheplygina, V., 2022. Machine learning for medical imaging: methodological failures and recommendations for the future. Npj Digit. Med. 5 (1), 48.

Varoquaux, G., Cheplygina, V., 2022. Machine learning for medical imaging: methodological failures and recommendations for the future. Npj Digit. Med. 5 (1), 48. doi:10.1038/s41746-022-00592-y.

Vaswani, A., Shazeer, N., Parmar, N., Uszkoreit, J., Jones, L., Gomez, A.N., et al., 2023. Attention Is All You Need. doi:10.65215/r5bs2d54.

Verma, D., Kapoor, S., Kumari, S., Sharma, D., Singh, J., Benjamin, M., et al., 2024. Decoding the genetic symphony: profiling protein-coding and long noncoding RNA expression in T-acute lymphoblastic leukemia for clinical insights. PNAS Nexus 3 (2), pgae011. doi:10.1093/pnasnexus/pgae011. PMID: 38328782.

Vervaart, M.A.-O., Strong, M.A.-O., Claxton, K.P., Welton, N.J., Wisløff, T.A.-O.X., Aas, E., 2021. An efficient method for computing expected value of sample information for survival data from an ongoing trial. 1552-681X.

Vickers, A.A.-O., van Calster, B., Steyerberg, E.W., 2019. A simple, step-by-step guide to interpreting decision curve analysis. 2397-7523.

Vickers, A.J., Holland, F., 2021. Decision curve analysis to evaluate the clinical benefit of prediction models. Spine J. 21 (10), 1643–1648.

Wachter, S., Mittelstadt, B., Russell, C., 2018. Counterfactual explanations without opening the black box: automated decisions and the GDPR. Harv. J. Law Technol. 31, 841–887. doi:10.2139/ssrn.3063289.

Wager, S., Athey, S., 2018. Estimation and inference of heterogeneous treatment effects using random forests. J. Am. Stat. Assoc. 113 (523), 1228–1242.
Walters, W.A.-O., Barzilay, R., 2021. Applications of deep learning in molecule generation and molecular property prediction. Acc. Chem. Res. 54 (2), 263–270.
Wang, G.-M., Tatsuoka, C., 2025. Bayesian ordered lattice design for phase I clinical trials. Stat. Med. 45 (6–7), e70456. doi:10.1002/sim.70456. PMID: 41781808.
Wang, H., Yee, D., 2019. I-SPY 2: a neoadjuvant adaptive clinical trial designed to improve outcomes in high-risk breast cancer. Curr. Breast Cancer Rep. 11 (4), 303–310. doi:10.1007/s12609-019-00334-2.
Wei, K., Qin, G., Zhang, J., Sui, X., 2022. Doubly robust estimation in causal inference with missing outcomes: with an application to the Aerobics Center Longitudinal Study. Comput. Stat. Data Anal. 168, 107399.
WHO, 2025. Ethics and governance of artificial intelligence for health: guidance on large multi-modal models 2025 Available from: https://www.who.int/publications/i/item/9789240084759.
Wiens, J., Saria, S., Sendak, M., Ghassemi, M., Liu, V.X., Doshi-Velez, F., et al., 2019. Do no harm: a roadmap for responsible machine learning for health care. Nat. Med. 25 (9), 1337–1340.
Wilkinson, M.D., Dumontier, M., Aalbersberg, I.J., Appleton, G., Axton, M., Baak, A., et al., 2016. The FAIR guiding principles for scientific data management and stewardship. Sci. Data 3 (1), 160018.
Williamson, T., Ravani, P., 2017. Marginal structural models in clinical research: when and how to use them? Nephrol. Dial. Transplant. 32 (suppl_2), ii84–ii90. doi:10.1093/ndt/gfw341.
Wong, C.H., Siah, K.W., Lo, A.W., 2019. Estimation of clinical trial success rates and related parameters. Biostatistics 20 (2), 366. doi:10.1093/biostatistics/kxy072.
Woodcock, J., LaVange, L.M., 2017. Master protocols to study multiple therapies, multiple diseases, or both. N. Engl. J. Med. 377 (1), 62–70. doi:10.1056/NEJMra1510062.
Wouters, O.J., McKee, M., Luyten, J., 2020. Estimated research and development investment needed to bring a new medicine to market, 2009-2018. JAMA 323 (9), 844–853.
Yan, F., Thall, P.F., Lu, K.H., Gilbert, M.R., Yuan, Y., 2018. Phase I-II clinical trial design: a state-of-the-art paradigm for dose finding. Ann. Oncol. 29 (3), 694–699. doi:10.1093/annonc/mdx795.
Yuan, Y., Hess, K.R., Hilsenbeck, S.G., Gilbert, M.R., 2016. Bayesian optimal interval design: a simple and well-performing design for phase I oncology trials. 1557-3265.
Zarin, D.A., Tse, T., Williams, R.J., Califf, R.M., Ide, N.C., 2011. The clinicaltrials.gov results database–update and key issues. 1533-4406.
Zhang, Y., Muller, S., 2024. Robust variable selection methods with Cox model—a selective practical benchmark study. Brief. Bioinform. 25 (6), bbae508. doi:10.1093/bib/bbae508.
Zhao, Y., Zeng, D., Rush, A.J., Kosorok, M.R., Kosorok, M.R., 2012. Estimating individualized treatment rules using outcome weighted learning. 0162-1459
Zhavoronkov, A.A.-O., Ivanenkov, Y.A., Aliper, A., Veselov, M.S., Aladinskiy, V.A., Aladinskaya, A.V., et al, 2019. Deep learning enables rapid identification of potent DDR1 kinase inhibitors. Nat. Biotechnol. 1546-1696. 37, 1038–1040.
Zhu, H., Huang, S.M., Madabushi, R., Strauss, D.G., Wang, Y., Zineh, I. 2019. Model-informed drug development: a regulatory perspective on progress. 1532-6535.
Zitnik, M., Agrawal, M., Leskovec, J., 2018. Modeling polypharmacy side effects with graph convolutional networks. Bioinformatics 34 (13), i457–i66.

12

Artificial intelligence, network biology and multiomics data in drug discovery

Manjusa Singh[a], Atifa Hafeez[a], Shiv Kumar Yadav[b], Upasna Srivastava[c], Pankaj Singh[d], and Manish Kumar Gupta[a]

[a]*Department of Biotechnology, Faculty of Science, Veer Bahadur Singh Purvanchal University, Jaunpur, Uttar Pradesh, India*

[b]*Department of Mathematics, Faculty of Engineering and Technology, Veer Bahadur Singh Purvanchal University, Jaunpur, Uttar Pradesh, India*

[c]*Department of Neurology, Yale University, New Haven, CT, United States*

[d]*Department of Biotechnology, Dr. Rammanohar Lohia Avadh University, Ayodhya, Uttar Pradesh, India*

1 Introduction

Traditional statistical modeling has long been used to analyze and interpret complex datasets. However, artificial intelligence (AI) has recently become a revolutionary influence across several domains, including biomedicine and drug discovery (Reel et al., 2021). The formal definition of AI was established during the Dartmouth Conference in 1956 (McCarthy et al., 2006). The rapidly developing field of AI has incorporated machine learning (ML) and deep learning (DL) techniques, which allow computers to learn from data and make educated decisions (Soori et al., 2023). In biomedical research, the analysis of single-omics data frequently fails to elucidate the complex nature of biological systems. Integrating multiomics datasets, such as proteomics, metabolomics, and genomics, offers a more comprehensive understanding of health and disease. AI techniques are essential for navigating this complexity, identifying hidden biological patterns, and forecasting results, thereby accelerating progress in precision medicine and personalized therapy (Osipov et al., 2024).

AI has become increasingly essential in clinical applications, particularly in personalizing drug dosages and predicting adverse reactions. By analyzing patient-specific data, AI optimizes drug administration and enhances treatment safety (Alowais et al.,

The AI Frontier in Molecular Modelling and Drug Designing. https://doi.org/10.1016/B978-0-443-40338-5.00016-0

2023). Moreover, it enables accurate in silico simulations for evaluating properties like toxicity and bioactivity, reducing reliance on traditional large-scale screening methods (Paul et al., 2021). Significant milestones have demonstrated AI's potential in real-world drug discovery. In 2020, Exscientia introduced the first AI-designed drug into clinical trials. AlphaFold predicted over 330,000 protein structures in 2021, including those linked to the human genome. DeepMind resolved 102 crystal structures in a single run, while Insilico Medicine launched a Phase I trial for an AI-identified molecule in 2022. In 2023, AbSci used AI to generate antibodies submitted for Food and Drug Administration (FDA) review, and Insilico achieved FDA Orphan Drug Designation for an AI-developed compound now in Phase II trials. These advancements illustrate AI's critical role in target identification and protein structure prediction (Maleki Varnosfaderani and Forouzanfar, 2024; Senior et al., 2020).

Drug discovery is currently being revolutionized by the combination of AI with multiomics data and network biology. While AI deciphers large-scale, complex datasets, network biology maps cellular interactions, offering a holistic view of disease mechanisms. When combined with multiomics, this interdisciplinary approach enhances target identification, predicts drug efficacy, and supports the development of safer, more effective therapies (Maleki Varnosfaderani and Forouzanfar, 2024; Paul et al., 2021; Senior et al., 2020). The ongoing integration of AI with systems biology and multiomics technology presents significant potential for revolutionizing drug development processes. Future advancements may provide real-time modeling of disease progression and AI-guided clinical trial designs. Personalized therapies, customized to an individual's genetic and molecular profile, are becoming more feasible, driven by advancements in integrated omics and AI. The increasing abundance of biological data, along with the advancement of computer models, is anticipated to enhance precision medicine, shorten drug development timeframes, and address complex, multifactorial diseases with greater accuracy (Esteva et al., 2019; Hasin et al., 2017; Jiang et al., 2017).

2 Multiomics data and application in understanding disease

2.1 Overview of multiomics data

The fundamental principle of molecular biology is that genetic information is transferred in biological systems via the transcription of DNA into messenger RNA (mRNA), which is then translated into proteins. This directional flow of information provides a framework for understanding cellular functions and gene regulation. This biological route allows the decoding of complex molecular interactions necessary for sustaining life, comparable to how a computer system analyzes and provides data (Reel et al., 2021). Understanding complex biological systems often requires combining information from various "omics" approaches. Researchers now integrate data from genomics, proteomics, transcriptomics, and metabolomics to better understand how biomolecules interact. This approach has proven useful in improving disease diagnosis, predicting patient outcomes, and developing more targeted therapies (Subramanian et al., 2020). Researchers apply various high-throughput techniques across different omics domains to unravel biological complexity. In genomics, tools such as whole-genome and whole-exome sequencing are commonly used to identify genetic variations. Transcriptomic studies often rely on RNA sequencing (RNA-seq) to assess gene expression levels. Epigenomic landscapes can be characterized using bisulfite sequencing for DNA methylation, Chromatin Immunoprecipitation-Sequencing (ChIP-seq) for mapping histone modifications, and Assay for Transposase Accessible Chromatin-Sequencing (ATAC-seq) for assessing chromatin accessibility. Chromatin interaction analysis by paired-end tag sequencing and Hi–C are two techniques used to investigate the spatial organization of the genome. In addition, proteomic and metabolomic analyses, largely driven by mass spectrometry (MS) technologies, provide insight into protein expression and metabolic pathways (Mukherjee et al., 2024).

In the context of precision medicine, strategies for drug discovery have evolved to target specific molecular mechanisms that drive disease progression. This approach emphasizes accurate target identification and lead compound development, with a strong focus on molecular perturbations. The success of such targeted therapies increasingly depends on the effective use of big data to convert vast biological datasets into actionable insights that enhance clinical outcomes. The exponential growth and complexity of omics data indicate that biomedical research has entered the big data era. As a result, there is a growing consensus among researchers on the critical need to integrate diverse layers of omics information, collectively termed multiomics, to achieve a thorough understanding of disease biology and therapeutic responses (Ewans et al., 2022; Katsila et al., 2016; Yu and Zeng, 2018; Mukherjee et al., 2024).

2.1.1 Genomics

Genomic research has been essential in elucidating the genetic foundations of complex disorders and pinpointing prospective treatment targets. These investigations frequently entail extensive statistical analyses that must address significant obstacles, including multiple hypothesis testing, tiny effect sizes, and complex interactions among genetic variations. Addressing these problems requires robust analytical frameworks that can handle high-dimensional data and derive significant connections from complex genomic environments (Mukherjee et al., 2024). An effective method for identifying hundreds of genetic variations linked to complex disorders in several human populations is genome-wide association studies (GWAS) (Hasin et al., 2017). Using genome-scale methods like whole-genome sequencing, genomics aims to describe the roles of every genetic component in an organism. It may be used to map biochemically active genomic areas such as transcriptional enhancers, predict gene functions, find biomarkers for patient stratification, and establish genotype-phenotype associations. The interpretability of molecular datasets in comparative genomics has been significantly improved by advances in network-based biological analytic techniques, such as gene family networks, genome networks, and sequence similarity networks. To identify disease subtypes and find new therapeutic targets, these network-based approaches first integrate gene expression and interaction data, which are subsequently converted into biologically significant processes, ultimately facilitating the identification of disease subtypes and the discovery of novel drug targets (You et al., 2022).

2.1.2 Transcriptomics

The study of transcriptomics examines an organism's transcriptome, which is the complete set of RNA transcripts synthesized within certain cell types or under particular conditions (Lowe et al., 2017). By using high-throughput sequencing (HTS) technology to examine the dynamics of gene expression, it highlights the diversity of the cellular transcriptome across space and time. RNA-seq, massively parallel signature sequencing, serial analysis of gene expression, and gene expression microarrays are just a few of the transcriptomic techniques that have been developed as a result of the advent of HTS. Third-generation methods like Drop-Seq and inDrop, as well as single-cell RNA-seq , represent further advancements. These techniques assist in several applications in the biomedical and life sciences by making it easier to investigate transcriptional regulation, disease processes, and pathway responses to therapeutic treatments (Yang et al., 2020).

2.1.3 Proteomics

Proteins are vital biomolecules that efficiently connect biological processes, disease phenotypes, and genetic information. When it comes to evaluating different drug categories, MS is superior to immunoassays due to its excellent sensitivity and specificity. Because of its applications in diagnostics, finding new drug targets, directing treatments, offering prognostic insights, and investigating possible biomarker candidates, MS-based clinical proteomics has significantly improved medical procedures (Birhanu, 2023). Proteomic techniques are becoming increasingly popular for analyzing disease mechanisms and identifying disease-specific biomarkers in both model systems and human samples. These methods provide high-throughput, quantitative, and unbiased analyses relevant to a diverse range of proteins (Hedl et al., 2019). Recent advancements have facilitated the development of single-cell proteomics technologies, enabling the quantification of thousands of proteins in individual mammalian cells (Ma et al., 2024). In addition, the integration of proteomic techniques with computational tools has enhanced target identification, thereby improving the efficiency of drug discovery. Computational modeling utilizes chemical and biological data regarding ligands and targets to design and enhance prospective therapeutics. This approach facilitates the *in silico* filtering of compounds exhibiting suboptimal ADMET profiles, thereby optimizing the selection of viable candidates. The rapid growth of this field is driven by advancements in software capabilities and computational power, as well as the increasing accessibility of publicly available protein structure databases that aid in molecular target identification (Jhanker et al., 2012).

2.1.4 Metabolomics

Metabolomics, which involves analyzing metabolites within biofluids, tissues, and cells, has become a standard approach for identifying potential biomarkers. Advances in analytical methods, informatics, and the integration of complementary biological techniques have broadened its scope, enabling system-wide assessments of metabolite functions. Due to its high sensitivity, metabolomics can detect even minor changes in biological pathways, shedding light on the mechanisms underlying both normal physiology and disease states (Johnson et al., 2016). This field is fundamentally supported by technologies initially developed for analytical chemistry to identify and characterize a broad range of chemical compounds. High-field nuclear magnetic resonance spectroscopy, in conjunction with liquid chromatography and high-resolution MS, represents the two primary platforms utilized. The primary aim of metabolomics is to thoroughly characterize metabolomes in various organisms, facilitating the identification of new drug candidates. Plants and humans represent valuable sources for drug scaffolds, emphasizing the role of metabolomics in identifying novel leads from plant, microbial, or mammalian sources (Wishart, 2008).

2.1.5 Epigenomics

Recent advances in epigenomics have enabled the analysis of chromatin states and regulatory modifications at the resolution of individual cells, representing a significant step forward in decoding cellular heterogeneity (Wang and Chang, 2018). In parallel, the identification of novel cytosine modifications, such as 5-hydroxymethylcytosine, along with a growing catalog of noncoding RNAs, has broadened the understanding of how epigenetic mechanisms contribute to pharmacokinetics (PKs) and pharmacodynamics (PDs). These molecular modifications influence gene expression networks that govern drug metabolism, distribution, and action, thereby contributing to patient-specific variability in therapeutic outcomes (Ivanov et al., 2012). Moreover, circulating epigenetic signatures, particularly those derived from cell-free nucleic acids, are emerging as informative biomarkers, offering promising avenues for stratified or personalized treatment strategies. Complementing these discoveries, recent innovations in epigenetic therapies have yielded compounds capable of modulating gene activity at the pretranscriptional level. These agents exhibit high target specificity and enable temporal control of gene regulation, potentially reducing dosing frequency while enhancing safety. Such features may significantly broaden the clinical applicability of epigenome-targeted therapeutics across various disease settings (Feehley et al., 2023).

2.1.6 Lipidomics

Since its inception in 2003, lipidomics has made significant strides, mostly as a result of the advancement of MS (Yang and Han, 2016). Lipidomics refers to the comprehensive study of the lipidome, which consists of a compilation of all the lipids in a biological system. The exploration of lipids and their metabolic pathways offers significant opportunities for the discovery of novel biomarkers and the development of innovative therapeutic strategies, as lipids serve an assortment of physiological purposes and are affected by a wide range of diseases (Hafeez et al., 2024). Lipidomics can be crucial to mechanistic research, risk assessment, and treatment monitoring associated with metabolic syndromes (cardiovascular diseases, diabetes, and obesity) (Meikle et al., 2014), neurological syndromes (Alzheimer's disease) (Han, 2005), and eye disorders (inflammation and neuroprotection) (Pieragostino et al., 2015). Cancer cells naturally experience significant alterations in lipid homeostasis and metabolism, which presents novel possibilities for diagnosis and treatment that lipidomics may help to uncover (Yang and Han, 2016). For high-risk individuals with breast cancer, lipidomics, a promising detection technique, may offer a unique prognostic strategy (Chen et al., 2016). It has made it possible to find new signaling molecules, uncover the fundamental mechanisms behind patho(physio)logical conditions, identify promising biomarkers for early disease diagnosis and prognosis, screen drug targets and/or test drug efficacy, direct nutritional intervention, and achieve personalized medicine, thanks to lipidomics (Yang and Han, 2016).

2.1.7 Glycomics

Comprehensive glycome analysis, called glycomics, is a promising field of study for finding new and more precise cancer biomarkers. Deciphering the glycome and its dynamic regulation is crucial to identifying the molecular causes of diseases and converting glycomic discoveries into novel diagnostic and treatment approaches (Onigbinde et al., 2025). AI approaches are increasingly embedded into predictive bioinformatics frameworks, driving advances in glycoscience through the emerging field of glycoinformatics (Bojar and Lisacek, 2022). In addition, glycans play a significant role in two different but related fields of drug development: either alone as saccharide-based therapies or as a component of glycoprotein treatments, which modulate protein activity and stability (Shriver et al., 2004).

2.1.8 Immunomics

The investigation of immunology involves combining data from transcriptomics, proteomics, and genomics with the goal of bringing molecular immunology into clinical practice. The collection of antigens or epitopes that interact with the host immune system is known as the immunome (Dai and Shen, 2022). To comprehend immune responses in cancer, immunomics integrates immunology with multiomics data (Jin and Kim, 2024). Immunomics is an integrative interdisciplinary approach that has tremendous potential to promote 21st-century antigen identification and effective vaccine design against complex pathogens (De Sousa and Doolan, 2016). Immunomics has improved disease detection, diagnosis, and prevention. It can also transform our understanding of vaccine formulation and antigen identification (Hafeez et al., 2024). During the COVID-19 pandemic, immunomics has been a key factor in advancing vaccine technology. The ability to analyze intricate immune responses at the molecular level is made possible by immunomics, providing insights that are crucial for creating efficient therapies and preventative strategies. By precisely aligning vaccine development with global immunological landscapes, immunomics integration ensures dynamic vaccine personalization. Immunomics establishes personalized therapeutic strategies by deciphering complex pathogen-host immune system interactions, greatly improving patient outcomes (Gao et al., 2024).

3 Artificial intelligence in therapeutic discovery

Traditional wet laboratory testing, validation procedures, and synthesis steps in drug discovery are often time-consuming and expensive. By enabling more efficient data processing, predictions, and decision-making, AI, with a focus on DL and ML, has completely changed the drug discovery process. These technologies are presently crucial for a number of stages of the drug development process, including target structure modeling, drug-target binding affinity studies, de novo drug design, and drug–target interaction (DTI) prediction (Chen et al., 2023; Farnoud et al., 2022).

AI approaches have significantly enhanced the efficacy of virtual screening initiatives. By analyzing large datasets such as molecular structures, ligand-target interactions, and binding affinities, AI algorithms can quickly identify promising therapeutic candidates (Abbas et al., 2024). This capability enables researchers to select compounds for experimental validation, conserving both time and resources.

Furthermore, AI has demonstrated considerable potential in identifying successful therapy combinations, especially for complex disorders that involve numerous biological pathways. Through the integration of genetic data, patient information, and synthetic lethality research, AI can identify synergistic target combinations that may improve therapeutic outcomes (Pun et al., 2023). Moreover, AI is enhancing drug repurposing and predicting novel therapeutic applications, further broadening its utility in modern pharmacology (Abbas et al., 2024).

3.1 Machine learning in drug discovery

ML plays a vital role in advancing drug discovery by utilizing extensive pharmacological datasets and improving prediction accuracy. ML, in contrast to conventional hypothesis-driven methods, uses adaptable and reusable analytical techniques to turn complicated biological data into actionable insights. Drug development employs a range of ML algorithms, such as support vector machine (SVM), multiple linear regression, naive Bayes classification, logistic regression (LR), random forest (RF), linear discriminant analysis, probabilistic neural networks, and multilayer perceptron (MLP). Unsupervised learning, which finds hidden patterns or clusters in unlabeled data, and supervised learning, which concentrates on classification and regression tasks using labeled data to predict outcomes, are the two basic learning paradigms into which these approaches are usually divided, as shown in Table 12.1 and Fig. 12.1 (Dara et al., 2022).

3.1.1 Supervised learning in drug discovery

Supervised learning is the development of prediction models generated by the relationships between input and output data, predominantly utilizing classification and regression approaches. In drug discovery, classified models are used for disease diagnosis by grouping samples into distinct subtypes, while regression models predict drug efficacy

Table 12.1 Comprehensive list of supervised and unsupervised machine learning tools used in drug discovery.

S. No.	Machine learning type	Tools	Application	Description	Citations
1.	Supervised	XGBoost	Bioactive molecule prediction using extreme gradient boosting	Ensemble of classification and regression tree (CART) and a variant of the gradient boosting machine, was investigated for the prediction of biological activity based on quantitative description of the compound's molecular structure.	Mustapha and Saeed (2016)
2.	Supervised	Random Forest (RF)	QSAR modeling, ADMET prediction, virtual screening.	Built-in performance assessment, a measure of the relative importance of descriptors, a measure of compound similarity weighted by the relative importance of descriptors, high prediction accuracy, and its collection of desired features make Random Forest uniquely suited for modeling in cheminformatics.	Svetnik et al. (2003)
3.	Supervised	Support vector machine (SVM)	Predicting active compounds and molecular properties.	SVM approach is applicable to compound classification and ranking, multiclass predictions, and, in algorithmically modified form, regression modeling.	Rodríguez-Pérez and Bajorath (2022)
4.	Supervised	k-Nearest Neighbors (k-NN)	Proposed for rapid biopharmaceutical process diagnosis and process performance monitoring.	A kNN-based similarity method for supporting drug manufacturing has been developed; it measures the spatial distance between batches, identifies the most similar historical batches, and ranks them in order of similarity.	Ren et al. (2020)
5.	Supervised	Naive Bayesian	Target protein of a drug was involved in side effects of drugs, metabolic enzymes of the drugs, and drug transporters.	An algorithm for the prediction of effective drug combinations. The new method is suitable for small data sets and is able to construct more stable and accurate predictive models compared to other machine learning models.	Bai et al. (2018)

(*Continued*)

Table 12.1 Comprehensive list of supervised and unsupervised machine learning tools used in drug discovery—cont'd

S. No.	Machine learning type	Tools	Application	Description	Citations
6.	Unsupervised	LigandScout	3-D Pharmacophores Derived from Protein-Bound Ligands and Their Use as Virtual Screening Filters	Pharmacophore to identify the compound, which was part of the pharmacophore creation process. Ligand conformations are conserved from the PDB in this database, which provides direct access to the underlying PDB complex through the compound name for each hit.	Wolber and Langer (2005)
7.	Unsupervised	alvaDesc	Calculate and analyze molecular descriptors and fingerprints	Proposed molecular descriptors and fingerprints, and generally the attention paid by the scientific community to the development of novel methodologies to represent chemical structures, are evidence of the relevance of these representations in the prediction of chemical properties.	Mauri (2020)
8.	Unsupervised	Self-organizing maps (SOMs)	Druglike property space by self-organizing maps	Analysis and comparison of various supplier catalogs, and thereby for the exploration and exploitation of currently unpopulated parts of the purchasable and druglike chemical space, using physicochemical properties as descriptors.	Takács et al. (2022)
9.	Hybrid (Supervised + Unsupervised)	KNIME	Data preprocessing, QSAR, classification.	The potential of KNIME in drug discovery and data mining has been demonstrated through the development of workflows for detecting drug scaffolds, retrieving PDB files, molecular filtering, virtual drug screening, chemical library design, and improving the accuracy of machine learning models based on pharmacophoric features and molecular shape.	Joshi et al. (2024)
10.	Hybrid (Supervised + Unsupervised) =	Orange	Simplify image analysis by integrating deep learning embeddings, machine learning procedures, and data visualization.	Orange supports the construction of data analysis workflows by assembling components for data preprocessing, visualization, and modeling. The Orange framework, with its extension for image analytics, provides a user-friendly interface for unsupervised and supervised mining of images from various domains of biomedicine.	Godec et al. (2019)

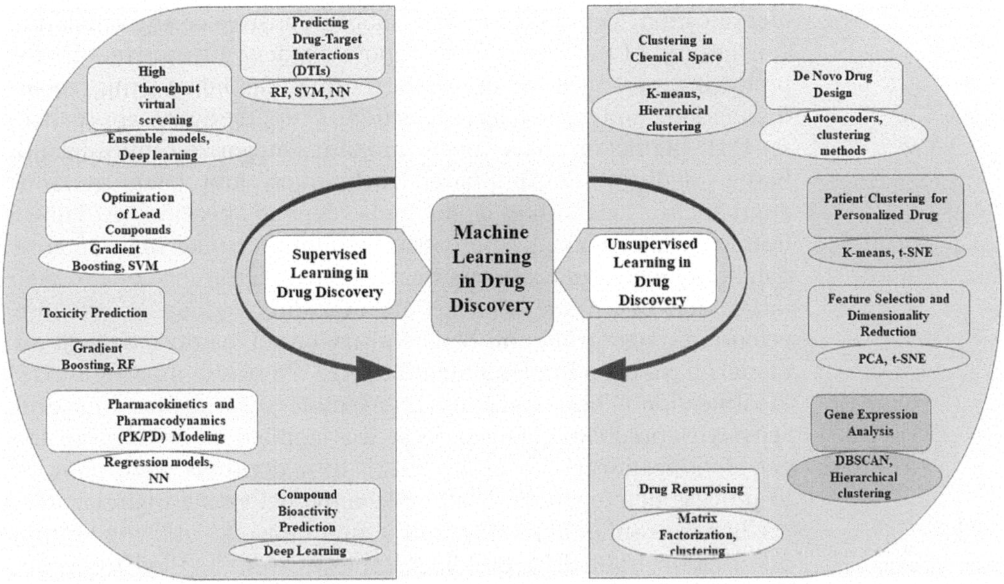

Fig. 12.1 An overview of machine learning-based methods in drug discovery. It highlighting both supervised and unsupervised learning approaches. Supervised learning techniques, such as random forests (RF), support vector machines (SVM), gradient boosting, and deep neural networks, are applied to tasks including drug–target interaction prediction, toxicity prediction, lead compound optimization, and PK/PD modeling. In contrast, unsupervised learning methods, including K-means, hierarchical clustering, PCA, t-SNE, and autoencoders, are utilized in areas such as chemical space clustering, gene expression analysis, dimensionality reduction, and drug repurposing.

and Absorption, Distribution, Metabolism, Excretion, and Toxicity (ADMET) properties (Mak and Pichika, 2019). After training, these models can be utilized on multiomics datasets to determine critical data aspects linked to specific biomarkers. In classification tasks, the output variable is categorical, facilitating the discovery of biomarker groupings with molecular characteristics distinguishing healthy and diseased states. In contrast, regression tasks involve continuous output variables, exemplified by estimating survival risk throughout disease development. The adaptability of supervised learning makes it an effective technique for tackling classification and regression problems in biological research (Picard et al., 2021; Sun et al., 2023).

Drug–target interactions

The study of DTIs has contributed significantly to drug repositioning, adverse drug reaction prediction, and pharmacological insights. Developments in molecular biology have enabled a broader understanding of the biological and chemical processes involved in DTIs, supported by public databases such as SuperTarget, Kyoto Encyclopedia of Genes and Genomes (KEGG), DrugBank, and Therapeutic Target Database (TTD). However, conventional DTI identification techniques remain labor-intensive, costly, and time-consuming. AI has emerged as a more efficient alternative, offering promising strategies for drug repurposing, candidate drug recommendation, and side effect detection. Computational approaches to DTI prediction have been broadly categorized into ligand-based methods, docking-based techniques, and chemogenomic approaches. Ligand-based methods depend heavily on known ligands, while docking approaches require accurate 3D structural data. Chemogenomic strategies have gained importance due to their integration of diverse information, including sequence, structure, evolution, fingerprint, and biochemistry-based features. Several ML models have been implemented: Biased SVM was employed for DTI identification (Chen et al., 2021). Ensemble SVM was used for drug sensitivity prediction; Linear SVM was applied to novel drug target identification (Dara et al., 2022); RF algorithms were reported to process heterogeneous data efficiently, delivering high-accuracy predictions (Shi et al., 2019); and neural networks utilizing entropy information from drug-protein complexes were applied to predict drug-target binding affinities (Xu et al., 2021).

High throughput virtual screening

In the pharmaceutical industry, ML techniques have been widely used for virtual screening, reducing the necessity for comprehensive high-throughput screening (HTS) by selecting specific substances (Ekins et al., 2019). Virtual screening facilitates the fast examination of huge chemical libraries to identify potential hit molecules against biological targets. This method is divided into two categories: ligand-based virtual screening and structure-based virtual screening. The integration of AI in virtual screening promotes hit rates, predicts ADMET characteristics, enhances drug analysis, and accurately evaluates compound-target interactions (Abbas et al., 2024). Ensemble modeling has been utilized to predict mutagenicity, docking scores, solubility, drug-likeness, and other in-vitro biological activities (Simmons et al., 2008). DL improves virtual screening by enhancing ligand docking accuracy and accelerating computational processes (Schneider, 2018).

Optimization of lead compounds

Lead optimization is an essential stage in drug development, during which structurally promising molecules are modified to improve efficacy and safety. This step aims to minimize adverse effects by implementing specific structural modifications of active analogues. GLPG1690, an optimized autotaxin inhibitor, has advanced to clinical trials for the treatment of pulmonary fibrosis (Dara et al., 2022). AI techniques, including multitask neural networks, are progressively utilized to evaluate critical ADME/T properties—absorption, distribution, metabolism, excretion, and toxicity—during the optimization process. SVM, first developed for classification tasks, are increasingly utilized for regression issues, thereby improving predictive modeling. Boosting techniques improve model accuracy and reduce overfitting (Wang et al., 2016).

Toxicity prediction

One of the most important steps in the drug discovery process is assessing the toxicological profile of potential drugs. In vivo toxicity assessment has always relied mostly on animal models, which makes it an expensive and morally difficult procedure. AI has become a useful substitute for this, providing quicker and more economical methods for toxicity prediction. Several AI-powered algorithms have been created to more accurately and scalably assess harmful chemical effects. Computational toxicity models have been developed and benchmarked by the "Toxicology in the 21st Century (Tox21)" program. A prominent illustration is DeepTox, which uses a three-layer deep neural network (DNN) to precisely forecast a chemical compound's toxicity (Chen et al., 2023). Using a variety of data sets, including gene expression profiles and high-content cell imaging, AI models are now often used to evaluate off-target effects, genotoxicity, organ-specific toxicity, and mitochondrial toxicity (Abbas et al., 2024). Strong prediction skills have been demonstrated by ML techniques, particularly quantitative structure-activity relationship (QSAR) models. Ensemble methods such as RF and SVMs frequently outperform conventional toxicological evaluations, enhancing model robustness and predictive accuracy. To further improve prediction precision, support vector classifiers and gradient boosting approaches have also shown efficiency in identifying structural components associated with toxicity (Malothu, 2024).

Pharmacokinetics and pharmacodynamics modeling

Nowadays, PK and PD modeling is essential to drug development, providing mathematical tools to measure the pharmacological effects, distribution, metabolism, excretion, and absorption of medicinal substances. At several phases of drug development, mechanism-based PK/PD models have been effectively incorporated to improve therapeutic effectiveness and optimize dose strategies. While PD models describe the time-dependent biological response to drugs, including mechanisms of action and important rate-limiting biological processes, PK models focus on characterizing drug transport through the body. These models aid in the quantitative establishment of connections between treatment response and drug exposure. They also take into consideration how different parameters, such as formulation-specific factors (like release and internalization rates), drug-specific factors (like clearance and receptor affinity), and system-specific factors (like blood flow, enzyme expression, and transporter activity), affect this exposure-response relationship. In addition, PK/PD modeling has been used to optimize a variety of drug delivery systems, including antibody-drug conjugates, liposomes, protein modifications, and extended-release formulations (Zou et al., 2020). Recent developments in DL have led to a rise in the use of neural networks in pharmacological modeling. Research has demonstrated that when modeling exposure-response interactions, artificial neural networks (ANNs) can perform better than conventional regression techniques, producing predictions that are less biased and more accurate (Tang, 2023). Although the temporal dynamics of PK/PD data are challenging for traditional ANN models to handle, their incorporation into hybrid modeling frameworks is becoming increasingly popular to enhance drug development prediction performance.

Compound bioactivity prediction

Predicting drug bioactivity has changed dramatically as a result of the integration of AI into drug screening procedures, which is a crucial factor in evaluating therapeutic potential. AI-based models are increasingly used to identify novel targets and predict the binding affinity of compounds to specific proteins or receptors, enhancing both drug efficacy assessment and mechanistic understanding. One of the major hurdles in early-stage drug development is determining whether a compound, especially one derived from natural products, exhibits sufficient bioactivity for therapeutic use. Conventional methods, relying on in vitro and in vivo testing, are often time-consuming and resource-intensive. AI approaches offer a cost-effective and scalable alternative for bioactivity prediction, enabling the identification of pharmacological properties such as anticancer, antiviral, and antibacterial activities. For example, a directed message-passing neural network has been employed to predict antimicrobial properties by converting SMILES notations into molecular graphs and extracting comprehensive feature vectors. This method demonstrates high accuracy in evaluating antibacterial potential, streamlining the discovery of new therapeutic agents (Abbas et al., 2024). QSAR modeling also makes extensive use of ML architectures, including convolutional neural networks (CNNs), recurrent neural networks (RNNs), and fully connected feed-forward neural networks. Although single-layer neural networks have been used for a long time in QSAR research, deeper, multilayer architectures have become increasingly popular for more reliable and accurate bioactivity predictions due to improvements in computing power and data availability (Chen et al., 2018).

3.1.2 Unsupervised learning in drug discovery

Unsupervised learning approaches aim to identify hidden patterns and vital structures within unlabeled datasets, allowing for the classification of data into significant clusters (Vamathevan et al., 2019). These techniques are especially useful in situations where labeled data is not available, as they enable models to identify latent similarities across samples by utilizing common characteristics. The efficacy of unsupervised ML depends on the characteristics of the input data and is susceptible to outliers. Consequently, the choice of method usually requires a compromise between computational efficiency and the capacity of the model to detect intricate, physiologically relevant patterns. Primarily with large-scale biological datasets, unsupervised learning often aims to find natural groupings or correlations among data points. In multiomics, unsupervised approaches are commonly utilized for disease categorization, subtype identification, and the identification of biomarkers or disease-associated modules. Many contemporary methodologies examine multiple outcome variables in isolation rather than within an integrated multivariate framework (Mukherjee et al., 2024). Techniques like Mode of Action by NeTwoRk Analysis (MANTRA) and Prediction of Drug-Target Interactions and Indications (PREDICT) illustrate the utilization of unsupervised learning in drug development, specifically in predicting the therapeutic effectiveness of medicines and their target proteins, even those with unidentified mechanisms. These tools have demonstrated efficacy in drug repurposing efforts and in clarifying the molecular basis of therapeutic actions (Paul et al., 2021).

Clustering in chemical space

Clustering has been an essential aspect of unsupervised learning, with broad applications in many scientific fields (Gul and Rehman, 2023). In drug discovery, especially within computer-aided frameworks, grouping small molecules has played a key role in improving both virtual and laboratory screening efforts. Organizing chemical compounds into defined regions of the chemical space allows researchers to select datasets either randomly or with a specific goal in mind. This approach has proven helpful in multiple ways. One major use involves dividing datasets into training and validation sets while building QSAR and cheminformatics models. Doing so ensures broader chemical space coverage, improving the model's reliability and reducing biases by keeping very similar compounds out of both sets. In addition, clustering helps identify new regions in chemical space for novel compounds or to focus on known areas for designing targeted libraries. Another benefit involves selecting in silico hits for lab testing. Because only a limited number of candidates can be tested due to financial or resource constraints, clustering is employed to select a chemically diverse subset of in silico hits for experimental validation, ensuring broader coverage of the chemical space within the available testing capacity (Talevi and Bellera, 2024).

K-means clustering, a common method, divides data into *k* groups, assigning each point to the group with the nearest average value. This helps identify central patterns in the data, though its results can vary depending on how the initial group centers are chosen (Mukherjee et al., 2024). Hierarchical clustering provides an alternative: either starting with the full dataset and breaking it into smaller groups (divisive) or starting with individual elements and combining the most similar ones (agglomerative) to form clusters (Lupolova et al., 2019).

De novo drug design

By allowing the synthesis of totally novel chemical compounds with desired characteristics, AI has significantly enabled advancements in de novo drug discovery. Unlike traditional AI applications that predict molecular behavior, these approaches focus on generating novel molecular structures to explore uncharted regions of chemical space. Two main strategies are commonly applied: Holistic Generation builds complete molecules from scratch, supporting early-phase discovery, while Iterative Generation assembles molecules step by step, allowing refinement of promising leads (Crucitti et al., 2024). Molecular patterns and novel molecules with desired properties have been learned using generative models such as variational autoencoders (VAEs) and generative adversarial networks (GANs). For example, a VAE-based method enables molecular generation by optimizing points in a learned latent space. Deep reinforcement learning has also been integrated into de novo design, where a generative model proposes structures and a predictive model evaluates them (Abbas et al., 2024). Another approach, DeepGRMF, combines graph models, neural networks, and matrix factorization to predict drug responses by integrating chemical structure and cellular response data (Ren et al., 2021). These AI-driven innovations offer powerful tools to design novel compounds beyond existing chemical libraries.

Patient clustering for personalized drug

An unsupervised method called integrative multiomics clustering uses various types of omics data to find biologically significant groups of samples or characteristics. This approach plays a critical role in disease subtyping, particularly in cancer research, where it has been employed to classify tumors into meaningful subtypes and uncover potential therapeutic targets. Applications in breast, lung, and stomach cancers have demonstrated its value in precision medicine and translational research (Zhang et al., 2022). Numerous techniques, such as iCluster, iClusterPlus, iClusterBayes, intNMF, Integrative Sparse K-means, Cancer Integration by Multikernel Learning, and Patient-specific Data Fusion, help achieve these integrative objectives. Furthermore, traditional clustering algorithms like K-means use distance-based separation to group data points into predetermined clusters based on similarity (Suyal and Sharma, 2024). For visualizing high-dimensional omics or assay data, t-Distributed Stochastic Neighbor Embedding (t-SNE) is commonly applied. It reduces dimensionality and helps uncover distinct clusters when paired with algorithms like K-means, particularly in large-scale exploratory datasets (Balamurali and Melkumyan, 2016).

Feature selection and dimensionality reduction

Dimensionality reduction techniques are essential for simplifying complex biomedical datasets, such as those used to assess antidepressant medication utilization. These methods reduce data complexity while preserving essential patterns, allowing for easier visualization of patient characteristics without intensive mathematical processing. Although some detail is inevitably lost through feature selection and discretization, the core structure of the data is maintained, and noise is effectively filtered out. In fact, such reduced data representations have performed comparably to traditional models like LR and decision trees in predictive accuracy (Huang et al., 2009). Dimensionality reduction and visualization methods have become crucial tools for hit detection and hit-to-lead optimization in the framework of early-stage drug development. Principal Component Analysis (PCA), self-organizing maps (SOM), stochastic proximity embedding (SPE), and stochastic neighbor embedding (SNE), among other techniques, facilitate this process. Retaining much of the original variance, PCA, a linear method, transforms linked features into a smaller collection of uncorrelated variables. SOM, a type of neural network, maps high-dimensional chemical data onto a two-dimensional space, revealing patterns and clusters. SPE focuses on maintaining pairwise data proximities in lower dimensions, whereas SNE and its optimized version, t-SNE, provide clearer separation of natural clusters by using a more efficient cost function and a Student-t distribution. These methods enhance the interpretability of complex datasets, supporting informed decision-making during drug development (Reutlinger and Schneider, 2012).

Gene expression analysis

Analyzing gene *expression* plays a crucial role in understanding gene functions and identifying genes involved in similar biological processes. Genes with correlated expression profiles often participate in related functional pathways. Clustering techniques are widely used to detect coexpressed gene groups and identify unique expression patterns across datasets. These methods help derive meaningful insights from large-scale gene expression data, contributing to advances in disease prevention, prognosis, and therapeutic development. Among clustering approaches, hierarchical clustering is known for its ability to reveal nested relationships among gene clusters. Despite its interpretability and scalability, the method can be computationally intensive. It operates in two primary modes: agglomerative (bottom-up) and divisive (top-down). In comparative analyses, clustering algorithms such as k-means (partition-based), Agglomerative nesting (AGNES) a hierarchical technique, Clustering in Quest (CLIQUE)-a grid-based technique, and A Density-Based Spatial Clustering of Applications with Noise (DBSCAN) have been explored. Notably, density-based methods like DBSCAN excel in identifying clusters of varying shapes and densities, offering improved performance and speed in complex datasets (Nies et al., 2019).

Drug repurposing

AI has emerged as a transformative tool in drug repurposing, leveraging its analytical strength to uncover hidden associations between existing drugs and novel disease targets. By analyzing large-scale datasets, including drug repositories, clinical outcomes, and genomic profiles, AI facilitates the identification of potential therapeutic applications beyond a drug's original use. In this field, methods including matrix factorization, feature-based techniques, and network-based techniques have proven crucial. One of the key advantages of AI-supported drug repurposing lies in bypassing early-stage trials, owing to the preestablished safety of approved drugs. This significantly reduces development timelines and costs, enabling direct progression to Phase II trials. Particularly promising are DNNs and GANs, which can categorize medications according to their toxicity and effectiveness and create new molecules that closely resemble genuine molecular structures. Furthermore, graph neural networks (GNNs), such as GraphSAGE, have been applied to predict drug-disease interactions. These models integrate drug and disease features, along with network clustering outputs derived from matrix factorization, to estimate the likelihood of therapeutic relevance (Abbas et al., 2024; Zhang et al., 2022).

3.2 Deep learning in drug discovery

DL has emerged as an effective tool in several scientific and technical domains, including drug discovery. Traditional approaches to drug development often involve long timelines and high costs, making them less effective in responding to newly emerging or rapidly evolving diseases. Consequently, more sophisticated techniques, such as Naive Bayes, SVMs, and neural networks, have been developed to enhance the reliability of predictions utilizing extensive datasets generated by HTS. Among these, DL stands out for its adaptable neural network structures that can handle complex data more efficiently. Its ability to reduce both time and cost offers a promising way to accelerate drug development processes (Zhang et al., 2021). Unlike traditional ML, DL models the human brain by processing data through several layers, with each layer enhancing the input from its predecessor. This stratified methodology facilitates the production of more precise and reliable results, as shown in Table 12.2 and Fig. 12.2 (Mintz and Brodie, 2019).

3.2.1 Convolutional neural networks

One popular DL technique for evaluating structured and visual input is the use of CNNs. In a conventional CNN model, the final prediction or classification tasks are handled by fully connected layers, pooling layers simplify the input by lowering its dimensions, and convolutional layers collect significant features. CNNs have several advantages, one of which is their ability to automatically identify patterns in unprocessed input data without the requirement for explicitly chosen characteristics (Chen et al., 2023). In the field of drug discovery, CNNs have been applied effectively to predict the bioactivity of drug-like compounds (Abbas et al., 2024). For instance, a 2D CNN-based regression model has been developed to estimate protein-ligand binding affinity (ΔG) by capturing specific interactions between protein residues and ligand atoms (Wang et al., 2021). In addition, CNNs have been employed to predict drug toxicity using image-based data, such as nuclei staining, offering a cost-effective and scalable approach for early toxicity screening (Jimenez-Carretero et al., 2018).

3.2.2 Recurrent neural networks

RNNs are a form of DL model specifically built to process data in sequences. Unlike conventional neural networks, RNNs are structured with feedback connections, enabling them to carry information from one step to the next within a sequence. This feature makes them suitable for analyzing patterns over time, such as in language processing, genomic sequences, or drug-related molecular data. Traditional RNNs, although effective in many areas, face difficulties in learning long-term dependencies due to problems like vanishing gradients, which hinder their ability to recognize distant data relationships. To resolve this, more advanced models, including Long Short-Term Memory and Gated Recurrent Units, have been

Table 12.2 Overview of deep learning-based techniques and tools utilized in drug discovery.

S. No.	Techniques	Tools	Applications	Description	Citations
1.	Convolutional neural networks (CNNs)	AtomNet	Structure-based drug design.	The use of deep learning for structure-based drug design is a core technology of Atomwise's best-in-class AI discovery engine, which is differentiated by its ability to find and optimize novel chemical matter.	Wallach et al. (2015)
2.		DEEPScreen	Predicting novel drug–target interactions	DEEPScreen inherently learns complex features from the 2-D representation of compounds to predict drug–target interactions, thus producing highly accurate predictions.	Rifaioglu et al. (2020)
3.		Tox_(R)CNN	*In vitro* screening of drug-induced toxicity	Deep convolutional neural networks (CNNs) were trained to predict toxicity from images of DAPI-stained cells pretreated with a set of drugs exhibiting differing toxicity mechanisms.	Jimenez-Carretero et al. (2018)
4.		CNN-DDI	Predict drug–drug interactions.	Novel semisupervised algorithm using a CNN architecture, named CNN-DDI, to predict drug–drug interactions.	Zhang et al. (2022)
5.		OnionNet	Protein – Ligand Binding Affinity Prediction	Based on rotation-free, element-pair-specific contacts between ligands and protein atoms, the contacts are further grouped into different distance ranges to cover both the local and nonlocal interaction information between the ligand and the protein.	Wang et al. (2021)
6.		Chemi-Net	Predict ADME properties of molecular compounds.	Chemi-Net implements a novel dynamic batching algorithm and a fine-tuning process to further improve the stability and performance of trained models.	Liu et al. (2019)
7.		DeepConv-DTI	Identification of drug–target interactions	Novel DTI prediction model to extract local residue patterns of target protein sequences using a CNN-based deep learning approach.	Lee et al. (2019)
8.		DeepPurpose	Prediction of drug–target interactions (DTI)	Accurate prediction of drug–target interactions (DTI) is crucial for drug discovery. Recently, deep learning (DL) models have shown promising performance for DTI prediction.	Huang et al. (2020)

9.	Recurrent neural networks (RNN)	REINVENT	Generation of novel drug-like molecules with desired properties.	AI–driven molecular design facilitates de novo design, R-group replacement, library design, linker design, scaffold hopping, and molecule optimization.	Loeffler et al. (2024)
10.		MolecularRNN	Generating realistic molecular graphs with optimized properties.	Model generates diverse, realistic molecular graphs after likelihood pretraining on a large database of molecules.	Popova et al. (2019)
11.		GraphRNN	Generating Realistic Graphs with Deep Auto-Regressive Models	GraphRNN learns to generate graphs by training on a representative set of graphs and decomposes the graph generation process into a sequence of node and edge formations, conditioned on the graph structure generated so far.	You et al. (2018)
12.		Pocket2Drug	Select promising drug candidates for pharmacologically relevant target proteins	A novel deep learning model employing an encoder-decoder architecture predicts binding molecules for a ligand-binding site. Pocket2Drug was trained in an end-to-end supervised manner using a large collection of ligand-pocket pairs.	Shi et al., (2022))
13.		GCRNN	Graph convolutional recurrent neural network for compound–protein interaction prediction	Based on the classification according to a binary class of interactions between proteins and compounds, the architectural design of the GCRNN model comes with the integration of the Bi-Recurrent layer on top of the CNN to learn dependencies of motifs on protein sequences and improve the accuracy of the predictions.	Elbasani et al. (2021)
14.		SMILES2vec	Predicting chemical properties, including toxicity, activity, solubility, and solvation energy, while also outperforming contemporary MLP neural networks.	A deep RNN that automatically learns features from SMILES to predict chemical properties, without the need for additional explicit feature engineering, using Bayesian optimization methods to tune the network architecture.	Goh et al. (2017)

(*Continued*)

Table 12.2 Overview of deep learning-based techniques and tools utilized in drug discovery—cont'd

15.	Generative adversarial network (GAN)	MedGAN	De novo molecular generation with improved structural validity and diversity.	A deep learning model based on Wasserstein Generative Adversarial Networks and Graph Convolutional Networks, developed to generate new quinoline-scaffold molecules from complex molecular graphs, including hyperparameter adjustments and evaluations of drug-likeness attributes such as pharmacokinetics, toxicity, and synthetic accessibility.	Macedo et al. (2024)
16.		Feedback GAN	DNA optimizes protein functions	Novel approach to generate realistic data, such as genes, proteins, or drugs, in synthetic biology. Generating synthetic genes coding for antimicrobial peptides and optimizing synthetic genes for the secondary structure of their resulting peptides.	Gupta and Zou (2019)
17.		ADSeqGAN	A novel approach to molecular generation in small-sample datasets.	ADSeqGAN, on a dataset comprising nucleic acid-targeting and protein-targeting small molecules, demonstrates its superior ability to generate nucleic acid binders compared to baseline models. Generated molecules exhibit strong binding affinities, enhanced chemical diversity, and improved synthetic feasibility.	Tang et al. (2025)
18.		InstGAN	Efficient generation of molecules with optimized pharmacological properties.	Employs actor-critic reinforcement learning with instant and global rewards for multiproperty optimization.	Tang et al. (2024)
19.		MolGAN	An implicit generative model for small molecular graphs	An implicit generative model for molecular graphs of small size, through joint training with a GAN and an RL objective, is capable of generating molecular graphs with both higher validity and novelty than previous comparable VAE-based generative models, while not requiring a permutation-dependent likelihood function.	De Cao and Kipf (2018)
20.		ORGAN	Generation of molecules with desired properties by optimizing specific objectives.	Improve certainly desired metrics, achieving better results than recurrent neural networks trained via either MLE or SeqGAN. Even more importantly, data generation can be made subject to a domainspecific reward function while still using the adversarial setting to guarantee the production of nonrepetitious samples.	Guimaraes et al. (2017)
21.		Mol-CycleGAN	A generative model for molecular optimization	A CycleGAN-based model that generates optimized compounds with high structural similarity to the original ones. Namely, given a molecule, our model generates a structurally similar one with an optimized value for the considered property.	(Maziarka et al., 2020)

22.	Autoencoders (AEs)	NP-VAE	Construction of chemical latent spaces for natural product libraries and the generation of novel compounds.	Natural product-oriented variational autoencoder, based on a variational autoencoder for managing hard-to-analyze datasets from DrugBank and large molecular structures such as natural compounds with chirality, an essential factor in the 3D complexity of compounds.	Ochiai et al. (2023)
23.		ScafoldGVAE	A VAE based on multiview graph neural networks for scaffold generation and hopping.	Auto encoder based on multiview graph neural networks for scaffold generation and scaffold hopping of drug molecules.	Hu et al. (2023)
24.		DrVAE	Improve the accuracy of drug response prediction.	Its semisupervised extension is a latent representation of the underlying gene states before and after drug application that depends on: (i) drug-induced biological changes of each gene and (ii) the overall treatment response outcome.	Rampasek et al. (2017)
25.		AEFS	Potential drug–target interactions (DTIs) in drug discovery and repurposing.	A heterogeneous network is established to integrate the information of drugs, proteins, and diseases. The original drug features are projected into an embedding (protein) space by a multilayer encoder and further projected into a label (disease) space by a decoder.	Sun et al. (2021)
26.	Graph neural networks (GNNs)	DeepDDS	Synergistic drug combinations for further wet-lab experiment validation.	Based on graph neural networks and the attention mechanism to identify drug combinations that can effectively inhibit the viability of specific cancer cells, the feature embeddings of drug molecule structures and gene expression profiles were taken as input to a multilayer feedforward neural network to identify the synergistic drug combinations.	Wang et al. (2022)
27.		PepGB	Facilitating peptide early drug discovery via graph neural networks	a deep learning framework to facilitate peptide early drug discovery by predicting peptide-protein interactions (PepPIs). Employing graph neural networks, PepGB incorporates a fine-grained perturbation module and a dual-view objective with a contrastive learning-based peptide pretrained representation to predict PepPIs.	Lei et al. (2024)
28.		MLGANN	Drug–target interaction mapping	Exhibited significant performance, surpassing existing approaches in comparative experiments, underscoring its immense potential in elevating the efficiency and accuracy of DTI predictions.	Lu et al. (2024)
29.		HOGCN	Prediction of complex biomedical interactions, including drug-drug and drug–target interactions.	Higher-Order Graph Convolutional Network that aggregates information from various neighborhood distances for biomedical interaction prediction.	Kishan et al. (2022)

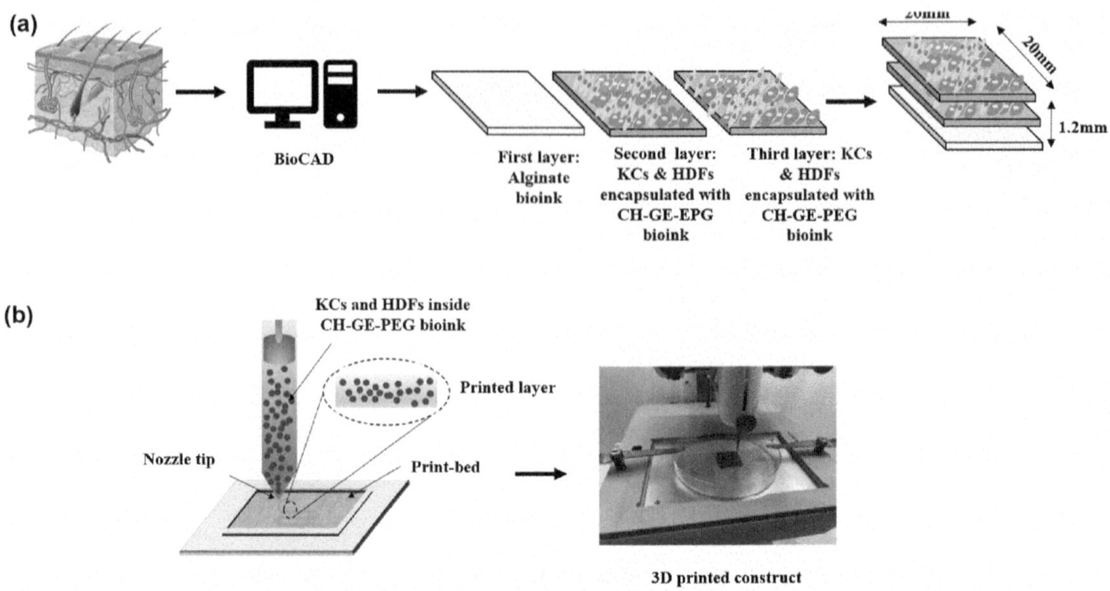

Fig. 12.2 Deep learning-based methods. Methods including convolutional neural networks (CNN), Recurrent Neural Networks (RNN), Generative Adversarial Networks (GAN), Autoencoders (AE), and Graph Neural Networks (GNN) are extensively used in drug discovery. These models enable a broad range of applications, including protein-ligand interaction prediction, toxicity and ADMET prediction, structure-based drug design, sequence-based drug discovery, molecular dynamics simulations, protein-protein interaction predictions, de novo drug design, adversarial property optimization, chemical space exploration, dimensionality reduction, feature extraction, drug repurposing, molecular property prediction, DTI prediction, and synthetic pathway optimization.

developed. These models are designed to store and manage information more effectively across longer sequences, making them more reliable for tasks that require memory of earlier inputs, such as predicting molecular behavior or analyzing protein interactions in drug discovery (Abbas et al., 2024; Jha et al., 2022; Kadupitiya et al., 2022).

3.2.3 Generative adversarial networks

In drug development, GANs have proven to be an effective tool, particularly in investigating novel compounds. Traditional drug discovery methods face challenges in exploring the entire chemical space—the vast range of possible chemical compounds that meet specific conditions. GANs, as DL models, can address this by generating compounds with desired properties. These models can be trained with biological data, encompassing evolutionary knowledge, diversity algorithms, and population patterns. Upon training, GANs can produce several drug variants, which can subsequently be evaluated for efficacy and refined to reduce adverse effects. This iterative method enables the

GAN to perpetually enhance and adjust according to the intended chemical effects. GANs have potential in de novo peptide and protein creation, wherein novel chemical entities are generated without a pre-existing template. Moreover, GANs can predict drug binding affinity to disease proteins, facilitating the identification of potential drug candidates in the discovery process (Tripathi et al., 2022).

3.2.4 Autoencoders

An autoencoder (AE) is a neural network architecture tailored for unsupervised learning, often employed to reduce high-dimensional data and uncover essential features. It operates through three key components: the encoder, the decoder, and a loss function. The encoder condenses the input data into a lower-dimensional latent space, capturing its core structure. The decoder subsequently rebuilds the initial input using this compressed representation, while the loss function evaluates the reconstruction accuracy by comparing the input with its output. The loss function assesses how much information is lost during this process by measuring the difference between the input and its reconstruction, with the goal of minimizing this error during training. Because the model learns to recreate its input without the need for labeled data, it is considered a self-supervised learning approach. The compression step, or "bottleneck," forces the network to focus on capturing only the most essential and informative features of the data. Although PCA is a traditional linear technique used for dimensionality reduction, a basic autoencoder is often regarded as its nonlinear counterpart. The effectiveness of the autoencoder in reducing dimensionality and extracting useful features largely depends on the design of the encoder-decoder structure and the type of input data. Notably, when built using convolutional or recurrent layers, autoencoders (AEs) have shown great potential in processing textual and molecular data, highlighting their value in drug discovery. In particular, the latent representations generated by AEs are being actively explored for drug repurposing, as they can reveal functional similarities among structurally diverse compounds (Bansal et al., 2024; Blaschke et al., 2018).

3.2.5 Graph neural networks

Designed to analyze and learn from graph-structured data, GNNs are a unique kind of neural network in which nodes represent items and edges record the intricate interactions among them. Their adaptability has led to successful applications across domains such as visual recognition, language understanding, network analytics, biological data science, and, increasingly, drug discovery. GNNs are especially suited to modeling molecular graphs and biological networks, allowing them to excel in tasks like molecular property prediction, DTI prediction, and synthetic pathway optimization. These models have delivered promising outcomes in virtual screening, binding affinity estimation, and drug repurposing efforts. Although GNNs have demonstrated strong capabilities across various predictive tasks, their full potential in drug synergy prediction is still being actively investigated. Nonetheless, their comparative effectiveness, especially against established high-performing frameworks like MatchMaker, DeepSynergy, and DTF, continues to underscore their growing role in combination therapy research and pharmaceutical innovation (Besharatifard and Vafaee, 2024).

4 Identifying putative drug targets using AI and multiomics integration

AI has become a pivotal tool in discovering putative therapeutic targets by facilitating accurate modeling of molecular interactions, elucidating disease processes, and synthesizing intricate omics datasets. AI employs DL, ML, and network-based methodologies to enhance systems-level comprehension of disease biology, thereby substantially refining the search for therapeutic targets (Gupta et al., 2021; Ocana et al., 2025; Zhang et al., 2024).

4.1 AI-driven modeling of molecular interactions

AI-driven molecular docking signifies a substantial progression in computer-aided drug discovery, providing considerable benefits compared to conventional virtual screening methods. These include the capacity to analyze intricate, high-dimensional information, predict binding affinities with precision, and accelerate the complete drug discovery process. Advanced ML methods, especially DNNs, are utilized to predict ligand–protein binding poses and affinities by analyzing extensive chemical datasets. These models capture intricate structural, biochemical, and pharmacological relationships that may be overlooked by classical methods (Abramson et al., 2024; Durojaye et al., 2023; Idris et al., 2020).

Unlike traditional approaches, AI models can integrate diverse data types into a unified predictive framework, resulting in a more holistic and accurate virtual screening process. To describe the dynamics of molecular interactions with enhanced accuracy and efficiency, for example, tools like uMol use DL algorithms such as GNNs, CNNs, RNNs, and attention mechanisms. Furthermore, AI-based platforms significantly reduce the need for manual intervention, conserving both time and computational resources. Traditional methods often face limitations in accounting for the flexibility of ligands and protein targets, whereas AI algorithms offer improved flexibility modeling. Virtual screening generally includes both ligand-based and structure-based approaches. Ligand-based techniques, like pharmacophore modeling and QSAR, are applied when structural information on the target is limited, whereas structure-based methods, especially molecular docking, are predominant when target structures are known. Commonly used software tools such as AutoDock, AutoDock Vina, Glide, GOLD, HADDOCK, and ClusPro employ various algorithms for docking simulations and have played a significant role in pharmaceutical research since the 1980s. These platforms laid the groundwork for the integration of AI technologies, which now push the boundaries of accuracy, flexibility, and computational efficiency in drug design (Fadahunsi et al., 2024; Stewart and Buehler, 2025).

4.2 Deciphering disease pathways with network biology

Network-based approaches to understanding human diseases have shown great promise in both biological research and clinical applications. By leveraging the interconnected nature of cellular systems, these methods help uncover disease genes and pathways, potentially leading to more precise drug targets and biomarkers for disease monitoring. For example, metabolic networks can be analyzed in silico through flux balance analysis to predict the impact of enzyme-inhibiting drugs, facilitating the identification of novel antibacterial agents and compensatory therapeutic strategies (Barabási et al., 2011). Protein-protein interaction (PPI) networks are also used to construct dynamic models that identify disease-associated modules or dynamical network biomarkers, providing insights into disease mechanisms at the systems level. Network-based drug-target prediction methods, which do not require structural or sequence information, offer advantages such as simplicity, speed, and robustness. These methods use principles like resource diffusion, collaborative filtering, and random walk algorithms to infer interactions. However, to obtain an accurate understanding of disease responses, it is necessary to integrate several networks, such as PPIs with gene expression data, because no single network type can fully represent the biological complexity (Cho et al., 2012; Jayachandran et al., 2021; Yan et al., 2017; Zhang et al., 2022).

4.3 Drug-target prediction through multiomics data integration

Drug target identification has been established as a fundamental component of modern drug discovery. Although single-omics technologies have been widely employed, they often fail to elucidate the causal relationships between drugs and complex phenotypic outcomes. With advances in large-scale sequencing and high-throughput platforms, the trend has shifted toward the use of integrated multiomics approaches, replacing traditional single-layer analyses. Target screening and identification have been improved with the incorporation of multiomics data. Genomics and transcriptomics integration has revealed the link between gene mutations and expression levels, aiding in the understanding of transcriptional regulation and the discovery of novel targets. Transcriptomics combined with proteomics has helped clarify the relationship between gene expression and protein abundance, providing insights at both RNA and protein levels. Furthermore, integrating proteomics or transcriptomics with metabolomics has enabled the exploration of protein-metabolite associations and the genotype–phenotype relationship, revealing upstream regulatory mechanisms of metabolic traits through a reverse-inference approach. Despite existing challenges, these multiomics strategies have shown remarkable potential in uncovering disease mechanisms and identifying therapeutic targets, marking a major advancement in molecular-level drug development (Du et al., 2024; Wang et al., 2021).

4.4 Network biology in drug discovery

The human body operates as a dynamic system in which millions of biochemical signals are transmitted every second, involving complex interactions among cells, tissues, organs, and environmental stimuli. These interactions underlie vital physiological processes and are driven by molecular mechanisms that remain largely elusive due to their complexity and scale. The emergence of HTS technologies, MS, advanced imaging, and real-time biosensing tools has significantly expanded our capacity to generate, analyze, and interpret biological data at a systems level (Jiang et al., 2025). At the cellular level, most biomolecules (proteins, RNAs, and metabolites) do not function in isolation but exert their roles through networks of interactions. These molecular interactions form the basis of the human interactome, a vast and intricate network comprising over 100,000 nodes, including approximately 25,000 protein-coding genes, functional RNAs, and small molecules. The links between these components represent regulatory, metabolic, signaling, and physical interactions that define the cellular state (Barabási et al., 2011). Network biology provides a comprehensive framework to represent and analyze this molecular connectivity. It captures both direct and indirect relationships among biomolecules, offering insights into the global organization of cellular systems. In the context of drug discovery, network-based approaches enable the identification of disease modules, subnetworks of interacting molecules associated with pathological states, and facilitate the prioritization of candidate drug targets based on their topological and functional importance within these modules.

Moreover, the integration of diverse information, including chemical-protein binding data, gene-disease connections, gene expression profiles, PPIs, and adverse drug response patterns, becomes possible through network representations. This multilayered integration reflects the complexity of biological decision-making and supports the rational selection of targets with better therapeutic potential and minimized off-target effects (Martínez-Jiménez and Marti-Renom, 2016). By embracing the interconnected nature of biological systems, network biology not only improves our understanding of disease mechanisms but also accelerates the development of multitarget drugs and precision medicine strategies.

5 Principles and methodologies of network biology in drug discovery

Network biology leverages various types of biological networks to model and analyze complex biological systems relevant to drug discovery:

5.1 Protein–protein interaction networks

PPI networks illustrate the physical interactions between proteins, which are crucial for biological functions like gene expression, metabolism, and signaling (Yadav et al., 2024). The goal of PPI networks is to represent the interactome, offering an effective framework for comprehending the intricate connections that underpin biological functions. Identifying pharmacological targets, finding cancer driver genes, and functional enrichment are just a few of the many uses for these networks (Ramos et al., 2024). Many cellular functions, such as signaling cascades, metabolic regulation, and structural organization, depend on PPIs. These interactions, while often constrained by the crowded intracellular environment and limited to short-range effects, form intricate networks known as *interactomes*. Such networks facilitate coordinated protein activity across the cell, supporting the complex biological functions necessary for survival (Nada et al., 2024). PPIs occur at specific domain interfaces on protein surfaces and can be either transient or stable. Identifying protein-binding partners is essential for understanding their functional roles within the cell. In this context, PPI networks are modeled with *nodes* representing proteins and *edges* denoting their interactions. From a graph theory perspective, the topological characteristics of these networks, such as degree, centrality, and modularity, are highly informative and often correlate with specific biological functions (Chen et al., 2019).

In drug discovery, targeting PPIs presents unique opportunities but also notable challenges. HTS has been widely used to identify PPI modulators by screening large chemical libraries, particularly those enriched with compounds designed to target protein interfaces. However, some PPIs lack well-defined binding hot spots, limiting the effectiveness of HTS. A similar approach to this problem is fragment-based drug discovery (FBDD). FBDD utilizes low molecular weight fragments that are well-suited to binding the often discontinuous and shallow pockets on PPI interfaces, making it a powerful approach for developing novel modulators (Nada et al., 2024). Integrating the structural comprehension of PPI networks with computational and experimental methodologies provides a comprehensive framework for clarifying illness causes and discovering potential treatment targets.

5.2 Gene regulatory networks

The differentiation of cells and the transitions between cell types are regulated by gene regulatory networks (GRNs). In these networks, each edge connects a transcription factor (TF) to a gene it regulates, ideally representing a direct, directional relationship indicating activation or inhibition (Pratapa et al., 2020). GRNs capture the complexity of gene–gene interactions and predict systems-level responses to perturbations. Different types of GRNs reflect various molecular mechanisms. Signal transduction networks consist of physical interactions, primarily between proteins, transmitting signals through modifications such as phosphorylation, represented by kinase cascades. TF networks define direct gene targets controlled by specific TFs. In addition, expression-derived networks infer regulatory dependencies from gene coexpression patterns, assuming that functionally related genes often exhibit correlated expression (Unger Avila et al., 2024).

Despite their value, existing computational algorithms for GRN construction occasionally introduce ambiguity in regulatory relationships and directionality (Li et al., 2024). GRNs consist of several components, including TFs, cis-regulatory modules, and noncoding RNAs, and facilitate essential activities such as differentiation, homeostasis, and environmental adaptation. **Abnormal regulation** of GRNs has been implicated in various diseases, particularly cancer, where aberrant regulation contributes to proliferation and metastasis. Decoding GRNs in malignant contexts provides insights into molecular mechanisms and aids in identifying potential therapeutic targets, forming the basis for precision medicine (Jiang et al., 2025).

5.3 Metabolic networks

Metabolic networks represent the biochemical reactions within a cell and emphasize metabolic pathways that may serve as therapeutic targets. Metabolomics, as the “omics” layer closest to phenotype, has emerged as a pivotal tool in drug target identification, offering a direct route to understanding drug mechanisms and effects.

High-throughput metabolomics has been utilized to predict DTIs at the whole-genome level, potentially enabling the development of a universal approach for drug-target mapping. Although metabolic pathways are broadly conserved between yeast and mammalian systems, critical differences in nutrient-sensing mechanisms underscore the need to validate these approaches in mammalian cells. Despite substantial advancements, key challenges remain before high-throughput metabolomics can be routinely applied to predict DTIs in complex organisms (Garana and Graham, 2022). Metabolomics enables the detection of phenotypic changes induced by external compounds, overcoming the limitations posed by the disconnect between protein targets and complex cellular phenotypes. This approach has been particularly valuable for elucidating metabolic vulnerabilities and identifying key enzymes and pathways associated with disease states. Metabolomics can be divided into lipidomics and hydrophilic metabolomics based on the nature of metabolites, and into targeted or untargeted methodologies depending on the research objective. Targeted metabolomics enables detailed quantification of specific pathways, while untargeted metabolomics provides a broad-spectrum view for discovering novel metabolic disruptions. Pseudo-targeted metabolomics, which integrates both strategies, has facilitated high-throughput, large-scale studies with improved accuracy and coverage. Before statistical analysis, essential preprocessing steps such as normalization, error correction, and data filtering are performed to mitigate technical variations and enhance reliability. Techniques such as internal-standard normalization and the use of quality control samples ensure robust data adjustment across large datasets. Functional metabolomics further establishes the role of bioactive metabolites in biological processes by linking metabolite functions to metabolic pathways, thereby enabling the identification of therapeutic targets that influence disease phenotypes. Recent studies emphasize phenotype-oriented analysis, revealing significant metabolic shifts associated with pathological conditions. By comparing metabolic profiles between healthy and diseased states, metabolomics has facilitated biomarker discovery, uncovered genetic and phenotypic correlations, and enabled the identification of potential protein targets through pathway association analyses (Pan et al., 2024).

5.4 Signaling pathway networks

Signaling pathways function as essential channels, transmitting extracellular signals to the nucleus and cytoplasm to regulate diverse cellular responses. Mutations or dysregulation in signaling components are frequently associated with cancer and can result in uncontrolled cell growth and division (Kochen et al., 2022). Because of their crucial role in disease progression, these pathways and the proteins they involve are often targeted in therapeutic development.

Traditional drug discovery strategies that focus on inhibiting single targets within a pathway have had limited success in treating complex diseases such as cancer. This is largely due to limited specificity, adverse side effects, and the emergence of resistance, which are often linked to an incomplete understanding of how drugs interact with entire signaling cascades (Kochen et al., 2022). Quantitative modeling of these pathways offers an opportunity to analyze how drugs impact interconnected cellular systems, including cross-talk between pathways and the overall sensitivity of outputs to perturbations.

A large quantity of data has been produced to investigate pharmacogenomic interactions as a result of the development of high-throughput technologies, such as next-generation sequencing, mRNA/microRNA expression analysis, and GWAS. For example, the Connectivity Map has enabled systematic profiling of gene expression in response to over 1300 small molecules in human cell lines, facilitating both drug repositioning and target discovery.

In addition, drug-related databases such as DrugBank, KEGG-DRUG, PharmGKB, and STITCH have provided comprehensive information on drug targets, PK/PD, gene expression changes, and disease-gene associations (Sun et al., 2015). These resources support the construction of detailed signaling pathway networks that link upstream regulators to downstream effectors, aiding in the identification of pivotal genes and interactions influencing drug action. Network-assisted approaches have proven powerful in mapping gene-disease, gene-gene, and drug-target relationships. These systems-based strategies not only uncover novel targets but also enable the repositioning of existing drugs and the design of multitarget regimens to combat resistance and enhance therapeutic efficacy. This approach is particularly valuable for diseases involving complex intersystem interactions, where single-target therapies are often insufficient (Harrold et al., 2013).

5.5 DTI networks

Given the vast number of unknown interactions between chemicals and genomic components, computational methods are being widely employed to predict potential DTIs. These methods enhance the efficiency of drug discovery and help minimize research and development expenses. Furthermore, discovering new DTIs facilitates drug repurposing by uncovering additional targets for drugs that are already on the market. Traditional computational strategies for DTI prediction are mainly divided into molecular docking and ligand-based methods. However, docking simulations are restricted by the absence of 3D crystal structures, particularly for membrane proteins such as G-protein-coupled receptors (GPCRs). Ligand-based approaches also struggle with poor prediction performance when few binding ligands are known. To overcome these limitations, ML-based models have emerged, leveraging large-scale chemogenomics data to extract latent patterns from chemical and genomic features. Among various computational techniques, similarity-based approaches are particularly prominent. They operate under the premise that drugs with similar properties are likely to bind to similar targets. These methods take advantage of established similarity metrics derived from both molecular structures and protein sequences, enabling effective integration of chemical and genomic information. By integrating various similarity metrics into a heterogeneous network, DTI prediction can be reframed as a graph-based link prediction task. Graph embedding techniques have become prominent for encoding topological properties of nodes into low-dimensional vectors suitable for ML models. These approaches have performed better than a number of traditional methods for determining a variety of biological interactions, such as interactions between drugs, proteins, and targets (Amiri Souri et al., 2022).

The development of DTINet exemplifies this direction, integrating diverse drug-related data into a heterogeneous network and learning informative low-dimensional feature representations. This approach significantly improved DTI prediction performance and demonstrated potential for drug repurposing (Luo et al., 2017). In addition, network-based methods rooted in resource diffusion, collaborative filtering, and random walks offer advantages such as independence from 3D structure data and the ability to handle sparse datasets. Their simplicity, speed, and scalability make them practical for large-scale applications (Wu et al., 2018).

Recent advances have focused on enriching model inputs with multimodal biological information, such as side effects, disease associations, molecular graphs, and 3D structural data. These approaches construct more robust heterogeneous networks by capturing both direct and indirect relationships among drugs, targets, diseases, and phenotypes. Instead of relying solely on character-level sequences like Simiplified Molecular Input Line Entry System (SMILES), modern frameworks increasingly utilize molecular graphs, as they preserve atomic-level features critical for accurate interaction prediction (Liao et al., 2025).

6 Integration of AI, multiomics, and network biology in drug discovery

Network-based approaches are commonly employed to capture the complex interactions and regulatory mechanisms in biological systems by modeling molecules such as genes, proteins, and metabolites as nodes, with edges denoting their pairwise interactions. These molecular networks, including PPIs, transcriptional regulation, and metabolic pathways, reveal important topological features such as degree distribution, shortest paths, and modularity. Modules within networks often represent functionally related entities, supporting the “guilt by association” principle. Typically, such inference methods are applied within single omics layers, offering limited insights into cross-layer interactions. To bridge this gap, two main strategies are used: one leverages prior knowledge from curated databases, and the other uses data-driven multivariate statistical methods. Combining both has been proposed to enhance the construction of multiomics networks. Patient Similarity Networks (PSNs) and molecular networks like gene/protein networks are key examples. In PSNs, individual patients or samples are connected based on omics-derived similarities. Two main integration strategies exist: **feature-level fusion** and **network-level fusion**. In feature-level fusion, multiple features are extracted separately from different PSNs and then fused. In contrast, network-level fusion applies methods like Similarity Network Fusion to merge omics-specific networks into a unified structure before feature extraction. In both cases, the resulting low-dimensional network features are used as input for classifiers in ML, such as DNNs or models trained with recursive feature elimination (Bodein et al., 2022; Wang et al., 2022). Large-scale networks such as **HetioNet**, which include 18 types of nodes and 19 types of edges, offer a hierarchical view of human biology for predicting gene-disease associations. Similarly, **MetPriCNet** prioritizes candidate metabolites for specific diseases using a three-level network of genes, metabolites, and disease associations. **OmicsNet** and **MiBioMics** provide web-based tools for constructing and visualizing multiomics networks, integrating data from resources like STRING, KEGG, and ENCODE. While OmicsNet focuses on user-defined molecular inputs, MiBioMics allows direct data upload and offers coinertia analysis and module detection via WGCNA. Time-series data integration has also advanced, with methods like MinardoModel identifying significant temporal shifts and constructing causal graphs across omics layers (Bodein et al., 2022). In drug discovery, heterogeneous networks integrating disease-specific omics profiles with drug-related data such as FDA-approved drugs, experimental compounds, and DTIs have shown strong potential. These networks incorporate both omics and nonomics features (drugs, diseases, targets), with edges representing functional associations such as pharmacological or phenotypic effects. Network diffusion and ML techniques are increasingly used in these integrative frameworks to predict therapeutic outcomes and identify novel drug targets (Agamah et al., 2022).

Drug development has entered a new era of precision and effectiveness due to the combination of AI, network biology, and multiomics technologies, as shown in Fig. 12.3. By providing a thorough understanding of cellular processes, multiomics approaches such as transcriptomics, proteomics, metabolomics, and genomics offer

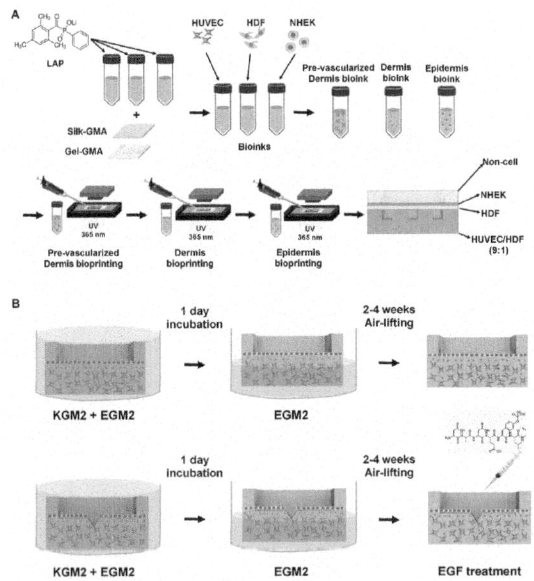

Fig. 12.3 Integration of AI, multiomics, and network biology to enable next-generation drug discovery. Synergizing artificial intelligence with multiomics and network biology to decode disease diagnosis, identify drug targets, and drive next-generation drug discovery.

a comprehensive understanding of disease pathophysiology (Hasin et al., 2017). When integrated, these diverse datasets create a complex but information-rich landscape that can be mined using AI algorithms.

ML and DL models process large-scale omics data to predict disease-associated genes, DTIs, and response variability (Dara et al., 2022; Vamathevan et al., 2019). Network biology enhances this integration by structuring biological data into networks, including PPI networks, GRNs, and metabolic networks. These networks facilitate the identification of core hubs, bottlenecks, and modules that represent potential therapeutic targets (Barabási et al., 2011). To implement this integration, several advanced computational platforms and tools have been developed. AI-driven instruments like PandaOmics (Kamya et al., 2024), NOODAI (Totu et al., 2024), HiOmics (Li et al., 2024), and POINT (He et al., 2025) facilitate the discovery of therapeutic targets and the repurposing of drugs. Multiomics and network-based tools such as OmicsNet 2.0 (Zhou et al., 2022), Mergeomics 2.0 (Ding et al., 2021), COMO (Bessell et al., 2023), KnetMiner (Hassani-Pak et al., 2021), Metascape (Zhou et al., 2019), Cytoscape (Otasek et al., 2019), Galaxy (Hiltemann et al., 2023), AlzGPS (Zhou et al., 2021), and GenoCraft (Lu et al., 2023) facilitate the integration, visualization, and analysis of complex biological data. A comprehensive categorization of these tools, including their roles and utilization in drug discovery, is provided in Table 12.3. Collectively, this integrated approach signifies a paradigm

Table 12.3 AI-enabled network biology tools integrating multiomics data for drug discovery.

S. No.	Tool name	Omics layers supported	Network biology-based	AI-based	Used for drug discovery purpose	URL	Citations
1.	OmicsNet 2.0	Genomics, transcriptomics, proteomics, metabolomics	Yes	No	Identify potential disease-associated genes or proteins	https://www.omicsnet.ca/	Zhou et al. (2022)
2.	Mergeomics 2.0	Genomics, epigenomics, transcriptomics, proteomics, and metabolomics	yes	No	Model a diverse set of diseases, including cardiometabolic disorders such as nonalcoholic fatty liver disease (23), cardiovascular disease (24–26), and type 2 diabetes (27); autoimmunity, including psoriasis (28) and rheumatoid arthritis (29); alcohol dependence (30); brain injury (31); Sjogren's syndrome (32); and environmental contributions to disease (33–35). Importantly, multiple validations of molecular predictions from Mergeomics with in silico, in vitro, and in vivo studies highlight the validity and causal nature of the disease network predictions	https://bioconductor.org/packages/release/bioc/html/Mergeomics.html	Ding et al. (2021)
3.	NOODAI	Genomics, transcriptomics, proteomics, metabolomics	Yes	Yes	Network-oriented multiomics data analysis and integration	https://omicsoracle.com	Totu et al. (2024)

4.	HiOmics	Transcriptomics, metagenomics, and whole-genome sequencing. In addition, it has integrated fundamental data, such as reference genomes and indexes for commonly studied species	Yes	Yes	A cloud-based, one-stop platform for the comprehensive analysis of large-scale omics data	https://henbio.com/en/tools	Li et al. (2024)
5.	POINT	Genomics, transcriptomics, proteomics, metabolomics	Yes	Yes	Including network integration, therapeutic target prediction, functional enrichment of potential targets, and inferring novel drug-disease relationships (i.e., repurposing and screening)	http://point.gene.ac/	He et al. (2025)
6.	GenoCraft	Genomics, transcriptomics, proteomics, and metabolomics	Yes	Yes	Including data normalization, quality control, differential expression analysis, and data visualization	https://genocraft.stanford.edu/	Lu et al. (2023)
7.	COMO	Genomics, transcriptomics, proteomics	Yes	No	Integrates multiomics data processing, context-specific metabolic model development, simulations, drug databases, and disease data to aid drug discovery	https://github.com/HelikarLab/COMO/pkgs/container/como	Bessell et al. (2023)

(*Continued*)

Table 12.3 AI-enabled network biology tools integrating multiomics data for drug discovery—cont'd

S. No.	Tool name	Omics layers supported	Network biology-based	AI-based	Used for drug discovery purpose	URL	Citations
8.	Metascape	Genomics, transcriptomics, proteomics, and metabolomics	Yes	No	Analyzing biological data, specifically for gene set enrichment analysis and functional annotation of gene lists	http://metascape.org	Zhou et al. (2019)
9.	Cytoscape	All (via plugins)	Yes	No	Visualizing interaction networks in drug-target prediction	https://cytoscape.org/	Otasek et al. (2019)
10.	Galaxy	Genomics, transcriptomics, proteomics, metabolomics	Yes	Yes	Workflow integration for omics-based drug discovery	https://galaxyproject.org	Hiltemann et al. (2023)
11.	KnetMiner	Genomics, transcriptomics	Yes	Yes	Network-based gene-trait-drug associations	https://knetminer.com/	Hassani-Pak et al. (2021)
12.	PandaOmics	Genomics, transcriptomics, proteomics	Yes	Yes	Generates novel and repurposed therapeutic targets and biomarker hypotheses with the desired properties	https://pharma.ai/pandaomics	Kamya et al. (2024)
13.	AlzGPS	Genomics, transcriptomics, proteomics, metabolomics	Yes	Yes	A genome-wide positioning systems platform to catalyze multiomics for Alzheimer's drug discovery	https://alzgps.lerner.ccf.org/	Zhou et al. (2021)

change toward data-driven, AI-enhanced, and network-informed drug discovery, improving the precision, speed, and success rate of drug development processes.

7 Conclusion

AI, multiomics technologies, and network biology mark a significant paradigm shift in modern drug discovery. This data-driven and computationally guided framework accelerates target identification, optimizes therapeutic development, and supports precision medicine. By leveraging the complementary strengths of these approaches, researchers can navigate biological complexity more effectively and generate high-confidence predictions for novel drug targets. This integrated strategy has already demonstrated success in addressing complex diseases such as cancer, neurodegenerative disorders, and infectious diseases, offering improved accuracy, scalability, and personalization in therapeutic development. The continuous improvement and synergy among these technologies are driving more effective outcomes, and they are expected to further bridge the gap between biological complexity, therapeutic innovation, and precise drug development strategies.

References

Abbas, M.K.G., Rassam, A., Karamshahi, F., Abunora, R., Abouseada, M., 2024. The role of AI in drug discovery. ChemBioChem. 1439-7633. 25 (14). Available from: http://onlinelibrary.wiley.com/journal/10.1002/(ISSN)1439-7633. doi:10.1002/cbic.202300816.

Abramson, J., Adler, J., Dunger, J., Evans, R., Green, T., Pritzel, A., Ronneberger, O., Willmore, L., Ballard, A.J., Bambrick, J., Bodenstein, S.W., Evans, D.A., Hung, C.C., O'Neill, M., Reiman, D., Tunyasuvunakool, K., Wu, Z., Žemgulytė, A., Arvaniti, E., Beattie, C., Bertolli, O., Bridgland, A., Cherepanov, A., Congreve, M., Cowen-Rivers, A.I., Cowie, A., Figurnov, M., Fuchs, F.B., Gladman, H., Jain, R., Khan, Y.A., Low, C.M.R., Perlin, K., Potapenko, A., Savy, P., Singh, S., Stecula, A., Thillaisundaram, A., Tong, C., Yakneen, S., Zhong, E.D., Zielinski, M., Žídek, A., Bapst, V., Kohli, P., Jaderberg, M., Hassabis, D., Jumper, J.M., 2024. Accurate structure prediction of biomolecular interactions with AlphaFold 3. Nature. 1476-4687. 630 (8016), 493–500. Available from: https://www.nature.com/nature/. doi:10.1038/s41586-024-07487-w.

Agamah, F.E., Bayjanov, J.R., Niehues, A., Njoku, K.F., Skelton, M., Mazandu, G.K., Ederveen, T.H.A., Mulder, N., Chimusa, E.R., 't Hoen, P.A.C., 2022. Computational approaches for network-based integrative multi-omics analysis. Front. Mol. Biosci. 2296-889X. 9. Available from: https://journal.frontiersin.org/journal/molecular-biosciences. doi:10.3389/fmolb.2022.967205.

Alowais, S.A., Alghamdi, S.S., Alsuhebany, N., Alqahtani, T., Alshaya, A.I., Almohareb, S.N., Aldairem, A., Alrashed, M., Bin Saleh, K., Badreldin, H.A., Al Yami, M.S., Harbi, S.A., Albekairy, A.M., 2023. Revolutionizing healthcare: the role of artificial intelligence in clinical practice. BMC Med. Educ. 1472-6920. 23 (1). Available from: https://bmcmededuc.biomedcentral.com/. doi:10.1186/s12909-023-04698-z.

Amiri Souri, E., Laddach, R., Karagiannis, S.N., Papageorgiou, L.G., Tsoka, S., 2022. Novel drug-target interactions via link prediction and network embedding. BMC Bioinformatics. 1471-2105. 23 (1). doi:10.1186/s12859-022-04650-w.

Bai, L.Y., Dai, H., Xu, Q., Junaid, M., Peng, S.L., Zhu, X., Xiong, Y., Wei, D.Q., 2018. Prediction of effective drug combinations by an improved naïve Bayesian algorithm. Int. J. Mol. Sci. 1422-0067. 19 (2). Available from: http://www.mdpi.com/1422-0067/19/2/467/pdf. doi:10.3390/ijms19020467.

Balamurali, M., Melkumyan, A., 2016. t-SNE based visualisation and clustering of geological domain. In: Lecture Notes in Computer Science (Including Subseries Lecture Notes in Artificial Intelligence and Lecture Notes in Bioinformatics), Vol. 9950. Springer Verlag, Australia, pp. 565–572. 16113349. http://springerlink.com/content/0302-9743/copyright/2005/. doi:10.1007/978-3-319-46681-1_67.

Bansal, C., Deepa, P.R., Agarwal, V., Chandra, R., 2024. A clustering and graph deep learning-based framework for COVID-19 drug repurposing. Expert Syst. Appl. 0957-4174. 249, 123560. doi:10.1016/j.eswa.2024.123560.

Barabási, A.L., Gulbahce, N., Loscalzo, J., 2011. Network medicine: a network-based approach to human disease. Nat. Rev. Genet. 1471-0064. 12 (1), 56–68. doi:10.1038/nrg2918.

Besharatifard, M., Vafaee, F., 2024. A review on graph neural networks for predicting synergistic drug combinations. Artif. Intell. Rev. 1573-7462. 57 (3). doi:10.1007/s10462-023-10669-z.

Bessell, B., Loecker, J., Zhao, Z., Aghamiri, S.S., Mohanty, S., Amin, R., Helikar, T., Puniya, B.L., 2023. COMO: a pipeline for multi-omics data integration in metabolic modeling and drug discovery. Brief. Bioinform. 1477-4054. 24 (6). Available from: http://bib.oxfordjournals.org. doi:10.1093/bib/bbad387.

Birhanu, A.G., 2023. Mass spectrometry-based proteomics as an emerging tool in clinical laboratories. Clin. Proteomics. 1559-0275. 20 (1). Available from: https://clinicalproteomicsjournal.biomedcentral.com/. doi:10.1186/s12014-023-09424-x.

Blaschke, T., Olivecrona, M., Engkvist, O., Bajorath, J., Chen, H., 2018. Application of generative autoencoder in de novo molecular design. Mol. Inform. 1868-1751. 37 (1). Available from: http://onlinelibrary.wiley.com/journal/10.1002/(ISSN)1868-1751. doi:10.1002/minf.201700123.

Bodein, A., Scott-Boyer, M.P., Perin, O., Lê Cao, K.A., Droit, A., 2022. Interpretation of network-based integration from multi-omics longitudinal data. Nucleic Acids Res. 1362-4962. 50 (5), E27. Available from: https://academic.oup.com/nar/issue. doi:10.1093/nar/gkab1200.

Bojar, D., Lisacek, F., 2022. Glycoinformatics in the artificial intelligence era. Chem. Rev. 0009-2665. 122 (20), 15971–15988. doi:10.1021/acs.chemrev.2c00110.

Chen, C., Shi, H., Jiang, Z., Salhi, A., Chen, R., Cui, X., Yu, B., 2021. DNN-DTIs: improved drug-target interactions prediction using XGBoost feature selection and deep neural network. Comput. Biol. Med. 0010-4825. 136, 104676. doi:10.1016/j.compbiomed.2021.104676.

Chen, H., Engkvist, O., Wang, Y., Olivecrona, M., Blaschke, T., 2018. The rise of deep learning in drug discovery. Drug Discov. Today. 1878-5832. 23 (6), 1241–1250. Available from: https://www.elsevier.com/locate/drugdiscov. doi:10.1016/j.drudis.2018.01.039.

Chen, S.J., Liao, D.L., Chen, C.H., Wang, T.Y., Chen, K.C., 2019. Construction and analysis of protein-protein interaction network of heroin use disorder. Sci. Rep. 2045-2322. 9 (1). Available from: https://www.nature.com/srep/index.html. doi:10.1038/s41598-019-41552-z.

Chen, W., Liu, X., Zhang, S., Chen, S., 2023. Artificial intelligence for drug discovery: resources, methods, and applications. Mol. Ther. Nucleic Acids. 2162-2531. 31, 691–702. Available from: https://www.journals.elsevier.com/molecular-therapy-nucleic-acids. doi:10.1016/j.omtn.2023.02.019.

Chen, X., Chen, H., Dai, M., Ai, J., Li, Y., Mahon, B., Dai, S., Deng, Y., 2016. Plasma lipidomics profiling identified lipid biomarkers in distinguishing early-stage breast cancer from benign lesions. Oncotarget. 1949-2553. 7 (24), 36622–36631. doi:10.18632/oncotarget.9124.

Cho, D.Y., Kim, Y.A., Przytycka, T.M., 2012. Chapter 5: network biology approach to complex diseases. PLoS Comput. Biol. 1553-7358. 8 (12). Available from: http://www.ploscompbiol.org/article/fetchObjectAttachment.action?uri=info%3Adoi%2F10.1371%2Fjournal.pcbi.1002820&representation=PDF. doi:10.1371/journal.pcbi.1002820.

Crucitti, D., Pérez Míguez, C., Díaz Arias, J.Á., Prada, D.B.F., Orgueira, A.M., 2024. De novo drug design through artificial intelligence: an introduction. Front. Hematol. 2813-3935. 3. Available from: https://www.frontiersin.org/journals/hematology. doi:10.3389/frhem.2024.1305741.

Dai, X., Shen, L., 2022. Advances and trends in omics technology development. Front. Med. 2296-858X. 9. doi:10.3389/fmed.2022.911861.

Dara, S., Dhamercherla, S., Jadav, S.S., Babu, C.M., Ahsan, M.J., 2022. Machine learning in drug discovery: a review. Artif. Intell. Rev. 15737462. 55 (3), 1947–1999. Available from: www.springer.com/journal/10462. doi:10.1007/s10462-021-10058-4.

De Cao, N., Kipf, T., 2018. MolGAN: an implicit generative model for small molecular graphs. arXiv. 2331-8422. Available from: https://arxiv.org. doi:10.48550/arxiv.1805.11973.

De Sousa, K.P., Doolan, D.L., 2016. Immunomics: a 21st century approach to vaccine development for complex pathogens. Parasitology. 1469-8161. 143 (2), 236–244. Available from: http://journals.cambridge.org/action/displayJournal?jid=PAR. doi:10.1017/S0031182015001079.

Ding, J., Blencowe, M., Nghiem, T., Ha, S.M., Chen, Y.W., Li, G., Yang, X., 2021. Mergeomics 2.0: a web server for multi-omics data integration to elucidate disease networks and predict therapeutics. Nucleic Acids Res. 1362-4962. 49 (1), W375. Available from: https://academic.oup.com/nar/issue. doi:10.1093/nar/gkab405.

Du, P., Fan, R., Zhang, N., Wu, C., Zhang, Y., 2024. Advances in integrated multi-omics analysis for drug-target identification. Biomolecules. 2218-273X. 14 (6). Available from: http://www.mdpi.com/journal/biomolecules. doi:10.3390/biom14060692.

Durojaye, O.A., Okoro, N.O., Odiba, A.S., Nwanguma, B.C., 2023. MasitinibL shows promise as a drug-like analog of masitinib that elicits comparable SARS-Cov-2 3CLpro inhibition with low kinase preference. Sci. Rep. 2045-2322. 13 (1). Available from: https://www.nature.com/srep/. doi:10.1038/s41598-023-33024-2.

Ekins, S., Puhl, A.C., Zorn, K.M., Lane, T.R., Russo, D.P., Klein, J.J., Hickey, A.J., Clark, A.M., 2019. Exploiting machine learning for end-to-end drug discovery and development. Nat. Mater. 1476-4660. 18 (5), 435–441. Available from: http://www.nature.com/nmat/. doi:10.1038/s41563-019-0338-z.

Elbasani, E., Njimbouom, S.N., Oh, T.J., Kim, E.H., Lee, H., Kim, J.D., 2021. GCRNN: graph convolutional recurrent neural network for compound–protein interaction prediction. BMC Bioinformatics. 1471-2105. 22. Available from: http://www.biomedcentral.com/bmcbioinformatics/. doi:10.1186/s12859-022-04560-x.

Esteva, A., Robicquet, A., Ramsundar, B., Kuleshov, V., DePristo, M., Chou, K., Cui, C., Corrado, G., Thrun, S., Dean, J., 2019. A guide to deep learning in healthcare. Nat. Med. 1546-170X. 25 (1), 24–29. Available from: http://www.nature.com/nm/index.html. doi:10.1038/s41591-018-0316-z.

Ewans, L.J., Minoche, A.E., Schofield, D., Shrestha, R., Puttick, C., Zhu, Y., Drew, A., Gayevskiy, V., Elakis, G., Walsh, C., Adès, L.C., Colley, A., Ellaway, C., Evans, C.A., Freckmann, M.L., Goodwin, L., Hackett, A., Kamien, B., Kirk, E.P., Lipke, M., Mowat, D., Palmer, E., Rajagopalan, S., Ronan, A., Sachdev, R., Stevenson, W., Turner, A., Wilson, M., Worgan, L., Morel-Kopp, M.C., Field, M., Buckley, M.F., Cowley, M.J., Dinger, M.E., Roscioli, T., 2022. Whole exome and genome sequencing in mendelian disorders: a diagnostic and health economic analysis. Eur. J. Hum. Genet. 1476-5438. 30 (10), 1121–1131. Available from: https://www.nature.com/ejhg/. doi:10.1038/s41431-022-01162-2.

Fadahunsi, A.A., Uzoeto, H.O., Okoro, N.O., Cosmas, S., Durojaye, O.A., Odiba, A.S., 2024. Revolutionizing drug discovery: an AI-powered transformation of molecular docking. Med. Chem. Res. 1554-8120. 33 (12), 2187–2203. Available from: https://www.springer.com/journal/44. doi:10.1007/s00044-024-03253-9.

Farnoud, A., Ohnmacht, A.J., Meinel, M., Menden, M.P., 2022. Can artificial intelligence accelerate preclinical drug discovery and precision medicine?. Expert Opin. Drug Discov. 1746-045X. 17 (7), 661–665. Available from: https://www.tandfonline.com/loi/iedc20. doi:10.1080/17460441.2022.2090540.

Feehley, T., O'Donnell, C.W., Mendlein, J., Karande, M., McCauley, T., 2023. Drugging the epigenome in the age of precision medicine. Clin. Epigenetics. 1868-7083. 15 (1). Available from: https://clinicalepigeneticsjournal.biomedcentral.com/. doi:10.1186/s13148-022-01419-z.

Gao, J., Zhang, C., Wheelock, Å.M., Xin, S., Cai, H., Xu, L., Wang, X.J., 2024. Immunomics in one health: understanding the human, animal, and environmental aspects of COVID-19. Front. Immunol. 1664-3224. 15. Available from: https://www.frontiersin.org/journals/immunology#. doi:10.3389/fimmu.2024.1450380.

Garana, B.B., Graham, N.A., 2022. Metabolomics paves the way for improved drug target identification. Mol. Syst. Biol. 1744-4292. 18 (2). Available from: https://onlinelibrary.wiley.com/journal/17444292. doi:10.15252/msb.202210914.

Godec, P., Pančur, M., Ilenič, N., Čopar, A., Stražar, M., Erjavec, A., Pretnar, A., Demšar, J., Starič, A., Toplak, M., Žagar, L., Hartman, J., Wang, H., Bellazzi, R., Petrovič, U., Garagna, S., Zuccotti, M., Park, D., Shaulsky, G., Zupan, B., 2019. Democratized image analytics by visual programming through integration of deep models and small-scale machine learning. Nat. Commun. 2041-1723. 10 (1). doi:10.1038/s41467-019-12397-x.

Goh, G.B., Siegel, C., Hodas, N., Vishnu, A., 2017. SMILES2vec: an interpretable general-purpose deep neural network for predicting chemical properties. arXiv. 2331-8422. Available from: https://arxiv.org. doi:10.48550/arxiv.1712.02034.

Guimaraes, G., Sanchez-Lengeling, B., Outeiral, C., Farias, P.L.C., Aspuru-Guzik, A., 2017. Objective-reinforced generative adversarial networks (ORGAN) for sequence generation models. arXiv. 2331-8422. Available from: https://arxiv.org. doi:10.48550/arxiv.1705.10843.

Gul, M., Rehman, M.A., 2023. Big data: an optimized approach for cluster initialization. J. Big Data. 2196-1115. 10 (1). Available from: https://journalofbigdata.springeropen.com. doi:10.1186/s40537-023-00798-1.

Gupta, A., Zou, J., 2019. Feedback GAN for DNA optimizes protein functions. Nat. Mach. Intell. 2522-5839. 1 (2), 105–111. doi:10.1038/s42256-019-0017-4.

Gupta, R., Srivastava, D., Sahu, M., Tiwari, S., Ambasta, R.K., Kumar, P., 2021. Artificial intelligence to deep learning: machine intelligence approach for drug discovery. Mol. Divers. 1573-501X. 25 (3), 1315–1360. Available from: https://www.wkap.nl/journalhome.htm/1381-1991. doi:10.1007/s11030-021-10217-3.

Hafeez, A., Gupta, A., Gupta, M.K., 2024. Biological omics databases and tools. In: Integrative Omics: Concept, Methodology, and Application. Elsevier, India, pp. 35–53. Available from: https://www.sciencedirect.com/book/9780443160929. doi:10.1016/B978-0-443-16092-9.00003-5.

Han, X., 2005. Lipid alterations in the earliest clinically recognizable stage of Alzheimers disease: implication of the role of lipids in the pathogenesis of Alzheimers disease. Curr. Alzheimer Res. 1567-2050. 2 (1), 65–77. doi:10.2174/1567205052772786.

Harrold, J.M., Ramanathan, M., Mager, D.E., 2013. Network-based approaches in drug discovery and early development. Clin. Pharmacol. Ther. 1532-6535. 94 (6), 651–658. doi:10.1038/clpt.2013.176.

Hasin, Y., Seldin, M., Lusis, A., 2017. Multi-omics approaches to disease. Genome Biol. 1474-760X. 18 (1). Available from: http://genomebiology.com/. doi:10.1186/s13059-017-1215-1.

Hassani-Pak, K., Singh, A., Brandizi, M., Hearnshaw, J., Parsons, J.D., Amberkar, S., Phillips, A.L., Doonan, J.H., Rawlings, C., 2021. KnetMiner: a comprehensive approach for supporting evidence-based gene discovery and complex trait analysis across species. Plant Biotechnol. J. 1467-7652. 19 (8), 1670–1678. Available from: http://onlinelibrary.wiley.com/journal/10.1111/(ISSN)1467-7652. doi:10.1111/pbi.13583.

He, Z., Liu, L., Han, D., Gao, K., Dong, L., Bu, D., Huo, P., Wang, Z., Deng, W., Liu, J., Guo, J., Zhao, Y., Wu, Y., 2025. Title page POINT: a web-based platform for pharmacological investigation enhanced by multi-omics networks and knowledge graphs Author contributions POINT: a web-based platform for pharmacological investigation enhanced by multi-omics networks and knowledg.

Hedl, T.J., Gil, R.S., Cheng, F., Rayner, S.L., Davidson, J.M., Luca, A.D., Villalva, M.D., Ecroyd, H., Walker, A.K., Lee, A., 2019. Proteomics approaches for biomarker and drug target discovery in als and ftd. Front. Neurosci. 1662-453X. 13. Available from: https://www.frontiersin.org/journals/neuroscience#. doi:10.3389/fnins.2019.00548.

Hiltemann, S., Rasche, H., Gladman, S., Hotz, H.R., Larivière, D., Blankenberg, D., Jagtap, P.D., Wollmann, T., Bretaudeau, A., Goué, N., Griffin, T.J., Royaux, C., Bras, Y.L., Mehta, S., Syme, A., Coppens, F., Droesbeke, B., Soranzo, N., Bacon, W., Psomopoulos, F., Gallardo-Alba, C., Davis, J., Föll, M.C., Fahrner, M., Doyle, M.A., Serrano-Solano, B., Fouilloux, A.C., van Heusden, P., Maier, W., Clements, D., Heyl, F., Grüning, B., Batut, B., 2023. Galaxy training: a powerful framework for teaching!. PLoS Comput. Biol. 1553-7358. 19 (1). Available from: https://journals.plos.org/ploscompbiol/article?id=10.1371/journal.pcbi.1010752. doi:10.1371/journal.pcbi.1010752.

Hu, C., Li, S., Yang, C., Chen, J., Xiong, Y., Fan, G., Liu, H., Hong, L., 2023. ScaffoldGVAE: scaffold generation and hopping of drug molecules via a variational autoencoder based on multi-view graph neural networks. J. Cheminform. 1758-2946. 15 (1). doi:10.1186/s13321-023-00766-0.

Huang, K., Fu, T., Glass, L.M., Zitnik, M., Xiao, C., Sun, J., 2020. DeepPurpose: a deep learning library for drug-target interaction prediction. Bioinformatics. 1460-2059. 36 (22-23), 5545–5547. Available from: http://bioinformatics.oxfordjournals.org/. doi:10.1093/bioinformatics/btaa1005.

Huang, S.H., Wulsin, L.R., Li, H., Guo, J., 2009. Dimensionality reduction for knowledge discovery in medical claims database: application to antidepressant medication utilization study. Comput. Methods Programs Biomed. 0169-2607. 93 (2), 115–123. doi:10.1016/j.cmpb.2008.08.002.

Idris, M.O., Yekeen, A.A., Alakanse, O.S., Durojaye, O.A., 2020. Computer-aided screening for potential TMPRSS2 inhibitors: a combination of pharmacophore modeling, molecular docking and molecular dynamics simulation approaches. J. Biomol. Struct. Dyn. 1538-0254. 1–19. Available from: http://www.tandfonline.com/loi/tbsd20. doi:10.1080/07391102.2020.1792346.

Ivanov, M., Kacevska, M., Ingelman-Sundberg, M., 2012. Epigenomics and Interindividual differences in drug response. Clin. Pharmacol. Ther. 0009-9236. 92 (6), 727–736. doi:10.1038/clpt.2012.152.

Jayachandran, P., Ilango, S., Paital, B., Bhanja, S., Nirmaladevi, R., 2021. Approaches for network based drug discovery. Front. Biosci.—Sch. 1945-0524. 13 (1), 30–433. Available from: https://www.fbscience.com/Scholar/articles/pdf/Scholar551.pdf. doi:10.52586/S551.

Jha, K., Saha, S., Singh, H., 2022. Prediction of protein–protein interaction using graph neural networks. Sci. Rep. 2045-2322. 12 (1). doi:10.1038/s41598-022-12201-9.

Jhanker, Y.M., Kadir, M.F., Khan, R.I., Hasan, R., 2012. Proteomics in drug discovery. J. Appl. Pharm. Sci. 2231-3354. 2 (8), 1–12. Available from: http://www.japsonline.com/admin/php/uploads/583_pdf.pdf. doi:10.7324/JAPS.2012.2801Bangladesh.

Jiang, F., Jiang, Y., Zhi, H., Dong, Y., Li, H., Ma, S., Wang, Y., Dong, Q., Shen, H., Wang, Y., 2017. Artificial intelligence in healthcare: past, present and future. Stroke Vasc. Neurol. 2059-8696. 2 (4), 230–243. Available from: https://svn.bmj.com. doi:10.1136/svn-2017-000101.

Jiang, W., Ye, W., Tan, X., Bao, Y.J., 2025. Network-based multi-omics integrative analysis methods in drug discovery: a systematic review. BioData Min. 1756-0381. 18 (1). Available from: https://biodatamining.biomedcentral.com/. doi:10.1186/s13040-025-00442-z.

Jimenez-Carretero, D., Abrishami, V., Fernández-de-Manuel, L., Palacios, I., Quílez-Álvarez, A., Díez-Sánchez, A., Del Pozo, M.A., Montoya, M.C., 2018. Tox_(R)CNN: deep learning-based nuclei profiling tool for drug toxicity screening. PLoS Comput. Biol. 1553-7358. 14 (11). Available from: http://www.ploscompbiol.org/article/browseVolume.action?field=volume. doi:10.1371/journal.pcbi.1006238.

Jin, J., Kim, J., 2024. Multi-omics and artificial intelligence technology for elucidating disease pathophysiology. Preprints. doi:10.20944/preprints202408.0350.v1.

Johnson, C.H., Ivanisevic, J., Siuzdak, G., 2016. Metabolomics: beyond biomarkers and towards mechanisms. Nat. Rev. Mol. Cell Biol. 1471-0080. 17 (7), 451–459. Available from: http://www.nature.com/molcellbio. doi:10.1038/nrm.2016.25.

Joshi, R., Zheng, Z., Agarwal, P., Hatmal, M.M., Chang, X., Seidler, P., Haworth, I.S., 2024. KNIME workflows for applications in medicinal and computational chemistry. Artif. Intell. Chem. 2949-7477. 2 (1), 100063. doi:10.1016/j.aichem.2024.100063.

Kadupitiya, J.C.S., Fox, G.C., Jadhao, V., 2022. Solving Newton's equations of motion with large timesteps using recurrent neural networks based operators. Mach. Learn. Sci. Technol. 2632-2153. 3 (2). Available from: https://iopscience.iop.org/journal/2632-2153. doi:10.1088/2632-2153/ac5f60.

Kamya, P., Ozerov, I.V., Pun, F.W., Tretina, K., Fokina, T., Chen, S., Naumov, V., Long, X., Lin, S., Korzinkin, M., Polykovskiy, D., Aliper, A., Ren, F., Zhavoronkov, A., 2024. PandaOmics: an AI-driven platform for therapeutic target and biomarker discovery. J. Chem. Inf. Model. 1549-960X. 64 (10), 3961–3969. Available from: http://pubs.acs.org/journal/jcisd8. doi:10.1021/acs.jcim.3c01619.

Katsila, T., Spyroulias, G.A., Patrinos, G.P., Matsoukas, M.T., 2016. Computational approaches in target identification and drug discovery. Comput. Struct. Biotechnol. J. 2001-0370. 14, 177–184. Available from: https://www.csbj.org. doi:10.1016/j.csbj.2016.04.004.

Kishan, K.C., Li, R., Cui, F., Haake, A.R., 2022. Predicting biomedical interactions with higher-order graph convolutional networks. IEEE/ACM Trans. Comput. Biol. Bioinform. 1557-9964. 19 (2), 676–687. Available from: http://ieeexplore.ieee.org/xpl/RecentIssue.jsp?punumber=8857. doi:10.1109/TCBB.2021.3059415.

Kochen, M.A., Andrews, S.S., Wiley, H.S., Feng, S., Sauro, H.M., 2022. Dynamics and sensitivity of signaling pathways. Curr. Pathobiol. Rep. 2167-485X. 10 (2), 11–22. Available from: https://springer.com/medicine/pathology/journal/40139. doi:10.1007/s40139-022-00230-y.

Lee, I., Keum, J., Nam, H., Briggs, J.M., 2019. DeepConv-DTI: prediction of drug-target interactions via deep learning with convolution on protein sequences. PLoS Comput. Biol. 1553-7358. 15 (6), e1007129. doi:10.1371/journal.pcbi.1007129.

Lei, Y., Wang, X., Fang, M., Li, H., Li, X., Zeng, J., 2024. PepGB: facilitating peptide drug discovery via graph neural networks. arXiv. 2331-8422. Available from: https://arxiv.org. doi:10.48550/arXiv.2401.14665.

Li, Y., Du, Y., Wang, M., Ai, D., 2024. CSER: a gene regulatory network construction method based on causal strength and ensemble regression. Frontiers in Genetics, 15. doi:10.3389/fgene.2024.1481787.

Liao, Q., Zhang, Y., Chu, Y., Ding, Y., Liu, Z., Zhao, X., Wang, Y., Wan, J., Ding, Y., Tiwari, P., Zou, Q., Han, K., 2025. Application of artificial intelligence in drug-target interactions prediction: a review. Npj Biomed. Innov. 3005-1444. 2 (1). doi:10.1038/s44385-024-00003-9.

Liu, K., Sun, X., Jia, L., Jun, M., Xing, H., Junqiu, W., Gao, H., Sun, Y., Boulnois, F., Fan, J., 2019. Chemi-Net: a molecular graph convolutional network for accurate drug property prediction. Int. J. Mol. Sci. 1422-0067. 20 (14), 3389. doi:10.3390/ijms20143389.

Loeffler, H.H., He, J., Tibo, A., Janet, J.P., Voronov, A., Mervin, L.H., Engkvist, O., 2024. Reinvent 4: modern AI–driven generative molecule design. J. Cheminform. 1758-2946. 16 (1). Available from: https://jcheminf.biomedcentral.com/. doi:10.1186/s13321-024-00812-5.

Lowe, R., Shirley, N., Bleackley, M., Dolan, S., Shafee, T., 2017. Transcriptomics technologies. PLoS Comput. Biol. 1553-7358. 13 (5), e1005457. doi:10.1371/journal.pcbi.1005457.

Lu, Q., Zhou, Z., Wang, Q., 2024. Multi-layer graph attention neural networks for accurate drug-target interaction mapping. Sci. Rep. 2045-2322. 14 (1). doi:10.1038/s41598-024-75742-1.

Lu, Y., Shen, M., Yue, L., Li, C., Chen, L., Meng, F., Wang, X., Herrington, D., Wang, Y., Zhao, Y., Fu, T., Rechem, C.V., 2023. GenoCraft: a comprehensive, user-friendly web-based platform for high-throughput omics data analysis and visualization. arXiv. 2331-8422. Available from: https://arxiv.org. doi:10.48550/arXiv.2312.14249.

Luo, Y., Zhao, X., Zhou, J., Yang, J., Zhang, Y., Kuang, W., Peng, J., Chen, L., Zeng, J., 2017. A network integration approach for drug-target interaction prediction and computational drug repositioning from heterogeneous information. Nat. Commun. 2041-1723. 8 (1). doi:10.1038/s41467-017-00680-8.

Lupolova, N., Lycett, S.J., Gally, D.L., 2019. A guide to machine learning for bacterial host attribution using genome sequence data. Microb. Genom. 2057-5858. 5 (12). Available from: https://www.microbiologyresearch.org/content/journal/mgen/10.1099/mgen.0.000317. doi:10.1099/mgen.0.000317.

Ma, J., Dong, C., Aibin, H., Xiong, H., 2024. Single-cell multiomics: a new frontier in drug research and development. Front. Drug Discov. 2674-0338. 4. doi:10.3389/fddsv.2024.1474331.

Macedo, B., Ribeiro Vaz, I., Gomes, T.T., 2024. MedGAN: optimized generative adversarial network with graph convolutional networks for novel molecule design. Sci. Rep. 2045-2322. 14 (1). doi:10.1038/s41598-023-50834-6.

Mak, K.K., Pichika, M.R., 2019. Artificial intelligence in drug development: present status and future prospects. Drug Discov. Today. 1878-5832. 24 (3), 773–780. Available from: https://www.elsevier.com/locate/drugdiscov. doi:10.1016/j.drudis.2018.11.014.

Maleki Varnosfaderani, S., Forouzanfar, M., 2024. The role of AI in hospitals and clinics: transforming healthcare in the 21st century. Bioengineering. 2306-5354. 11 (4). Available from: https://www.mdpi.com/journal/bioengineering. doi:10.3390/bioengineering11040337.

Malothu, L.J., 2024. Evaluation of featurizer-model combinations and their interpretability in toxicity prediction. Int. J. Sci., Eng. Technol. 2395-4752. 12 (6), 1–9. doi:10.61463/ijset.vol.12.issue6.359.

Martínez-Jiménez, F., Marti-Renom, M.A., 2016. Should network biology be used for drug discovery?. Expert Opin. Drug Discov. 1746-045X. 11 (12), 1135–1137. Available from: https://www.tandfonline.com/loi/iedc20. doi:10.1080/17460441.2016.1236786.

Mauri, A., 2020. alvaDesc: a tool to calculate and analyze molecular descriptors and fingerprints. In: Methods in Pharmacology and Toxicology. Humana Press Inc., Italy, pp. 801–820. Available from: http://www.springer.com/series/7653 http://www.springer.com/humana+press/book/978-1-934115-23-7?cm_mmc=AD-_-enews-_-HUM1627-_-0&. doi:10.1007/978-1-0716-0150-1_32.

Maziarka, Ł., Pocha, A., Kaczmarczyk, J., Rataj, K., Danel, T., Warchoł, M., 2020. Mol-CycleGAN: a generative model for molecular optimization. J. Cheminform. 1758-2946. 12 (1). doi:10.1186/s13321-019-0404-1.

McCarthy, J., Minsky, M.L., Rochester, N., Shannon, C.E., 2006. A proposal for the Dartmouth summer research project on artificial intelligence. AI Mag. 0738-4602. 27 (4), 12–14.

Meikle, P.J., Wong, G., Barlow, C.K., Kingwell, B.A., 2014. Lipidomics: potential role in risk prediction and therapeutic monitoring for diabetes and cardiovascular disease. Pharmacol. Ther. 0163-7258. 143 (1), 12–23. doi:10.1016/j.pharmthera.2014.02.001.

Mintz, Y., Brodie, R., 2019. Introduction to artificial intelligence in medicine. Minim. Invasive Ther. Allied Technol. 1364-5706. 28 (2), 73–81. doi:10.1080/13645706.2019.1575882.

Mukherjee, A., Abraham, S., Singh, A., Balaji, S., Mukunthan, K.S., 2024. From Data to Cure: A Comprehensive Exploration of Multi-omics Data Analysis for Targeted Therapies. Mol. Biotechnol. 67 (4), 1269–1289. doi:10.1007/s12033-024-01133-6.

Mustapha, I.B., Saeed, F., 2016. Bioactive molecule prediction using extreme gradient boosting. Molecules. 1420-3049. 21 (8), 983. doi:10.3390/molecules21080983.

Nada, H., Choi, Y., Kim, S., Jeong, K.S., Meanwell, N.A., Lee, K., 2024. New insights into protein-protein interaction modulators in drug discovery and therapeutic advance. Signal Transduct. Target. Ther. 2059-3635. 9 (1). Available from: https://www.nature.com/sigtrans. doi:10.1038/s41392-024-02036-3.

Nies, H.W., Zakaria, Z., Mohamad, M.S., Chan, W.H., Zaki, N., Sinnott, R.O., Napis, S., Chamoso, P., Omatu, S., Corchado, J.M., 2019. A review of computational methods for clustering genes with similar biological functions. Processes. 2227-9717. 7 (9). Available from: https://res.mdpi.com/d_attachment/processes/processes-07-00550/article_deploy/processes-07-00550-v2.pdf. doi:10.3390/pr7090550.

Ocana, A., Pandiella, A., Privat, C., Bravo, I., Luengo-Oroz, M., Amir, E., Gyorffy, B., 2025. Integrating artificial intelligence in drug discovery and early drug development: a transformative approach. Biomark. Res. 2050-7771. 13 (1). Available from: https://biomarkerres.biomedcentral.com. doi:10.1186/s40364-025-00758-2.

Ochiai, T., Inukai, T., Akiyama, M., Furui, K., Ohue, M., Matsumori, N., Inuki, S., Uesugi, M., Sunazuka, T., Kikuchi, K., Kakeya, H., Sakakibara, Y., 2023. Variational autoencoder-based chemical latent space for large molecular structures with 3D complexity. Commun. Chem. 2399-3669. 6 (1). doi:10.1038/s42004-023-01054-6.

Onigbinde, S., Adeniyi, M., Daramola, O., Chukwubueze, F., Bhuiyan, M.M.A.A., Nwaiwu, J., Bhattacharjee, T., Mechref, Y., 2025. Glycomics in human diseases and its emerging role in biomarker discovery. Biomedicines. 2227-9059. 13 (8). Available from: https://www.mdpi.com/journal/biomedicines. doi:10.3390/biomedicines13082034.

Osipov, A., Nikolic, O., Gertych, A., Parker, S., Hendifar, A., Singh, P., Filippova, D., Dagliyan, G., Ferrone, C.R., Zheng, L., Moore, J.H., Tourtellotte, W., Van Eyk, J.E., Theodorescu, D., 2024. The molecular twin artificial-intelligence platform integrates multi-omic data to predict outcomes for pancreatic adenocarcinoma patients. Nat. Cancer. 2662-1347. 5 (2), 299–314. Available from: https://www.nature.com/natcancer/. doi:10.1038/s43018-023-00697-7.

Otasek, D., Morris, J.H., Bouças, J., Pico, A.R., Demchak, B., 2019. Cytoscape automation: empowering workflow-based network analysis. Genome Biol. 1474-760X. 20 (1). Available from: http://genomebiology.com/. doi:10.1186/s13059-019-1758-4.

Pan, S., Yin, L., Liu, J., Tong, J., Wang, Z., Zhao, J., Liu, X., Chen, Y., Miao, J., Zhou, Y., Zeng, S., Xu, T., 2024. Metabolomics-driven approaches for identifying therapeutic targets in drug discovery. MedComm. 2688-2663. 5 (11). Available from: https://onlinelibrary.wiley.com/journal/26882663. doi:10.1002/mco2.792.

Paul, D., Sanap, G., Shenoy, S., Kalyane, D., Kalia, K., Tekade, R.K., 2021. Artificial intelligence in drug discovery and development. Drug Discov. Today. 1878-5832. 26 (1), 80–93. Available from: https://www.elsevier.com/locate/drugdiscov. doi:10.1016/j.drudis.2020.10.010.

Picard, M., Scott-Boyer, M.P., Bodein, A., Périn, O., Droit, A., 2021. Integration strategies of multi-omics data for machine learning analysis. Comput. Struct. Biotechnol. J. 2001-0370. 19, 3735–3746. Available from: https://www.csbj.org. doi:10.1016/j.csbj.2021.06.030.

Pieragostino, D., D'Alessandro, M., Di Ioia, M., Di Ilio, C., Sacchetta, P., Boccio, P.D., 2015. Unraveling the molecular repertoire of tears as a source of biomarkers: beyond ocular diseases. Proteomics Clin. Appl. 1862-8346. 9 (1-2), 169–186. doi:10.1002/prca.201400084.

Popova, M., Shvets, M., Oliva, J., Isayev, O., 2019. MolecularRNN: generating realistic molecular graphs with optimized properties. arXiv. 2331-8422. Available from: https://arxiv.org. doi:10.48550/arxiv.1905.13372.

Pratapa, A., Jalihal, A.P., Law, J.N., Bharadwaj, A., Murali, T.M., 2020. Benchmarking algorithms for gene regulatory network inference from single-cell transcriptomic data. Nat. Methods. 1548-7105. 17 (2), 147–154. Available from: http://www.nature.com/nmeth/. doi:10.1038/s41592-019-0690-6.

Pun, F.W., Ozerov, I.V., Zhavoronkov, A., 2023. AI-powered therapeutic target discovery. Trends Pharmacol. Sci. 1873-3735. 44 (9), 561–572. Available from: www.elsevier.com/locate/tips. doi:10.1016/j.tips.2023.06.010.

Ramos, R.H., de Oliveira Lage Ferreira, C., Simao, A., 2024. Human protein–protein interaction networks: a topological comparison review. Heliyon. 2405-8440. 10 (5), e27278. doi:10.1016/j.heliyon.2024.e27278.

Rampasek, L., Hidru, D., Smirnov, P., Haibe-Kains, B., Goldenberg, A., 2017. Dr.VAE: drug response variational autoencoder.

Reel, P.S., Reel, S., Pearson, E., Trucco, E., Jefferson, E., 2021. Using machine learning approaches for multi-omics data analysis: a review. Biotechnol. Adv. 0734-9750. 49. Available from: https://www.elsevier.com/inca/publications/store/5/2/5/4/5/5/index.htt. doi:10.1016/j.biotechadv.2021.107739.

Ren, J., Zhou, R., Farrow, M., Peiris, R., Alosi, T., Guenard, R., Romero-Torres, S., 2020. Application of a kNN -based similarity method to biopharmaceutical manufacturing. Biotechnol. Prog. 8756-7938. 36 (2). doi:10.1002/btpr.2945.

Ren, S., Tao, Y., Yu, K., Xue, Y., Schwartz, R., Lu, X., 2021. De novo prediction of cell-drug sensitivities using deep learning-based graph regularized matrix factorization. bioRxiv. 2692-8205. Available from: https://www.biorxiv.org. doi:10.1101/2021.10.11.462450.

Reutlinger, M., Schneider, G., 2012. Nonlinear dimensionality reduction and mapping of compound libraries for drug discovery. J. Mol. Graph. Model. 1093-3263. 34, 108–117. doi:10.1016/j.jmgm.2011.12.006.

Rifaioglu, A.S., Nalbat, E., Atalay, V., Martin, M.J., Cetin-Atalay, R., Doğan, T., 2020. DEEPScreen: high performance drug-target interaction prediction with convolutional neural networks using 2-D structural compound representations. Chem. Sci. 2041-6539. 11 (9), 2531–2557. Available from: http://pubs.rsc.org/en/journals/journal/sc. doi:10.1039/c9sc03414e.

Rodríguez-Pérez, R., Bajorath, J., 2022. Evolution of support vector machine and regression modeling in chemoinformatics and drug discovery. J. Comput. Aided Mol. Des. 0920-654X. 36 (5), 355–362. doi:10.1007/s10822-022-00442-9.

Schneider, G., 2018. Automating drug discovery. Nat. Rev. Drug Discov. 1474-1784. 17 (2), 97–113. Available from: http://www.nature.com/nrd/index.html. doi:10.1038/nrd.2017.232.

Senior, A.W., Evans, R., Jumper, J., Kirkpatrick, J., Sifre, L., Green, T., Qin, C., Žídek, A., Nelson, A.W.R., Bridgland, A., Penedones, H., Petersen, S., Simonyan, K., Crossan, S.,

Kohli, P., Jones, D.T., Silver, D., Kavukcuoglu, K., Hassabis, D., 2020. Improved protein structure prediction using potentials from deep learning. Nature. 1476-4687. 577 (7792), 706–710. Available from: http://www.nature.com/nature/index.html. doi:10.1038/s41586-019-1923-7.

Shi W. Singha M. Srivastava G. Pu L. Ramanujam J. Brylinski M. 2022 Pocket2Drug: An encoder-decoder deep neural network for the target-based drug design Front. Pharmacol. 13 doi:10.3389/fphar.2022.837715

Shi, H., Liu, S., Chen, J., Li, X., Ma, Q., Yu, B., 2019. Predicting drug-target interactions using Lasso with random forest based on evolutionary information and chemical structure. Genomics, 111 (6), 1839–1852. doi:10.1016/j.ygeno.2018.12.007.

Shriver, Z., Raguram, S., Sasisekharan, R., 2004. Glycomics: a pathway to a class of new and improved therapeutics. Nat. Rev. Drug Discov. 1474-1776. 3 (10), 863–873. doi:10.1038/nrd1521.

Simmons, K., Kinney, J., Owens, A., Kleier, D.A., Bloch, K., Argentar, D., Walsh, A., Vaidyanathan, G., 2008. Practical outcomes of applying ensemble machine learning classifiers to high-throughput screening (HTS) data analysis and screening. J. Chem. Inf. Model. 1549-960X. 48 (11), 2196–2206. Available from: http://pubs.acs.org/journal/jcisd8. doi:10.1021/ci800164u.

Soori, M., Arezoo, B., Dastres, R., 2023. Artificial intelligence, machine learning and deep learning in advanced robotics, a review. Cogn. Robot. 2667-2413. 3, 54–70. doi:10.1016/j.cogr.2023.04.001.

Stewart, I., Buehler, M.J., 2025. Molecular analysis and design using generative artificial intelligence via multi-agent modeling. Mol. Syst. Des. Eng. 2058-9689. 10 (4), 314–337. Available from: https://www.rsc.org/journals-books-databases/about-journals/molecular-systems-design-engineering/. doi:10.1039/d4me00174e.

Subramanian, I., Verma, S., Kumar, S., Jere, A., Anamika, K., 2020. Multi-omics data integration, interpretation, and its application. Bioinform. Biol. Insights. 1177-9322. 14. Available from: http://insights.sagepub.com/journal.php?journal_id=39&tab=volume. doi:10.1177/1177932219899051.

Sun, C., Cao, Y., Wei, J.M., Liu, J., 2021. Autoencoder-based drug-target interaction prediction by preserving the consistency of chemical properties and functions of drugs. Bioinformatics. 1460-2059. 37 (20), 3618–3625. Available from: http://bioinformatics.oxfordjournals.org/. doi:10.1093/bioinformatics/btab384.

Sun, J., Zhao, M., Jia, P., Wang, L., Wu, Y., Iverson, C., Zhou, Y., Bowton, E., Roden, D.M., Denny, J.C., Aldrich, M.C., Xu, H., Zhao, Z., 2015. Deciphering signaling pathway networks to understand the molecular mechanisms of metformin action. PLoS Comput. Biol. 1553-7358. 11 (6). Available from: http://www.ploscompbiol.org/article/browseVolume.action?field=volume. doi:10.1371/journal.pcbi.1004202.

Sun, M., Li, L., Xiao, H., Feng, J., Wang, J., Wan, S., 2023. Editorial: bioinformatics analysis of omics data for biomarker identification in clinical research, Volume II. Front. Genet. 1664-8021. 14. doi:10.3389/fgene.2023.1256468.

Suyal, M., Sharma, S., 2024. A review on analysis of K-means clustering machine learning algorithm based on unsupervised learning. J. Artif. Intell. Syst. 6 (1), 85–95. doi:10.33969/ais.2024060106.

Svetnik, V., Liaw, A., Tong, C., Culberson, J.C., Sheridan, R.P., Feuston, B.P., 2003. Random Forest: a classification and regression tool for compound classification and QSAR modeling. J. Chem. Inf. Comput. Sci. 0095-2338. 43 (6), 1947–1958. doi:10.1021/ci034160g.

Takács, G., Sándor, M., Szalai, Z., Kiss, R., Balogh, G.T., 2022. Analysis of the uncharted, druglike property space by self-organizing maps. Mol. Divers. 1573-501X. 26 (5), 2427–2441. Available from: https://www.wkap.nl/journalhome.htm/1381-1991. doi:10.1007/s11030-021-10343-y.

Talevi, A., Bellera, C.L., 2024. Clustering of small molecules: new perspectives and their impact on natural product lead discovery. Front. Nat. Prod. 2813-2602. 3. doi:10.3389/fntpr.2024.1367537.

Tang, A., 2023. Machine learning for pharmacokinetic/pharmacodynamic modeling. J. Pharm. Sci. 0022-3549. 112 (5), 1460–1475. doi:10.1016/j.xphs.2023.01.010.

Tang, H., Li, C., Kamei, S., Yamanishi, Y., Morimoto, Y., 2024. Molecular generative adversarial network with multi-property optimization. arXiv. 2331-8422. Available from: https://arxiv.org. doi:10.48550/arXiv.2404.00081.

Tang, H., Long, J., Wang, J., 2025. Auxiliary discrminator sequence generative adversarial networks (ADSeqGAN) for few sample molecule generation. arXiv. 2331-8422. Available from: https://arxiv.org. doi:10.48550/arXiv.2502.16446.

Totu, T., Tomasoni, M., Bolck, H.A., Buljan, M., 2024. NOODAI: a webserver for network-oriented multi-omics data analysis and integration pipeline. doi: 10.1101/2024.11.08.622488.

Tripathi, S., Augustin, A.I., Dunlop, A., Sukumaran, R., Dheer, S., Zavalny, A., Haslam, O., Austin, T., Donchez, J., Tripathi, P.K., Kim, E., 2022. Recent advances and application of generative adversarial networks in drug discovery, development, and targeting. Artif. Intell. Life Sci. 2667-3185. 2. Available from: https://www.journals.elsevier.com/artificial-intelligence-in-the-life-sciences. doi:10.1016/j.ailsci.2022.100045.

Unger Avila, P., Padvitski, T., Leote, A.C., Chen, H., Saez-Rodriguez, J., Kann, M., Beyer, A., 2024. Gene regulatory networks in disease and ageing. Nat. Rev. Nephrol. 1759-507X. 20 (9), 616–633. Available from: https://www.nature.com/nrneph/. doi:10.1038/s41581-024-00849-7.

Vamathevan, J., Clark, D., Czodrowski, P., Dunham, I., Ferran, E., Lee, G., Li, B., Madabhushi, A., Shah, P., Spitzer, M., Zhao, S., 2019. Applications of machine learning in drug discovery and development. Nat. Rev. Drug Discov. 1474-1784. 18 (6), 463–477. Available from: http://www.nature.com/nrd/index.html. doi:10.1038/s41573-019-0024-5.

Wallach, I., Dzamba, M., Heifets, A., 2015. AtomNet: a deep convolutional neural network for bioactivity prediction in structure-based drug discovery. arXiv preprint arXiv:1510.02855.

Wang, C., Lue, W., Kaalia, R., Kumar, P., Rajapakse, J.C., 2022. Network-based integration of multi-omics data for clinical outcome prediction in neuroblastoma. Sci. Rep. 2045-2322. 12 (1). Available from: https://www.nature.com/srep/index.html. doi:10.1038/s41598-022-19019-5.

Wang, C., Lye, X., Kaalia, R., Kumar, P., Rajapakse, J.C., 2021. Deep learning and multi-omics approach to predict drug responses in cancer. BMC Bioinformatics. 1471-2105. 22. Available from: https://bmcbioinformatics.biomedcentral.com/. doi:10.1186/s12859-022-04964-9.

Wang, K.C., Chang, H.Y., 2018. Epigenomics technologies and applications. Circ. Res. 1524-4571. 122 (9), 1191–1199. Available from: http://circres.ahajournals.org. doi:10.1161/CIRCRESAHA.118.310998.

Wang, N.N., Dong, J., Deng, Y.H., Zhu, M.F., Wen, M., Yao, Z.J., Lu, A.P., Wang, J.B., Cao, D.S., 2016. ADME properties evaluation in drug discovery: prediction of Caco-2 cell permeability using a combination of NSGA-II and boosting. J. Chem. Inf. Model. 1549-960X. 56 (4), 763–773. Available from: http://pubs.acs.org/journal/jcisd8. doi:10.1021/acs.jcim.5b00642.

Wishart, D.S., 2008. Applications of metabolomics in drug discovery and development. Drugs R D. 1174-5886. 9 (5), 307–322. doi:10.2165/00126839-200809050-00002.

Wolber, G., Langer, T., 2005. LigandScout: 3-D pharmacophores derived from protein-bound ligands and their use as virtual screening filters. J. Chem. Inf. Model. 1549-9596. 45 (1), 160–169. doi:10.1021/ci049885e.

Wu, Z., Li, W., Liu, G., Tang, Y., 2018. Network-based methods for prediction of drug-target interactions. Front. Pharmacol. 1663-9812. 9. doi:10.3389/fphar.2018.01134.

Xu, L., Ru, X., Song, R., 2021. Application of machine learning for drug-target interaction prediction. Front. Genet. 1664-8021. 12. doi:10.3389/fgene.2021.680117.

Yadav, S.K., Hafeez, A., Kumar, R., Gupta, M.K., Gutti, R.K., 2024. Biomolecular networks. In: Integrative Omics: Concept, Methodology, and Application. Elsevier, India, pp. 351–367. Available from: https://www.sciencedirect.com/book/9780443160929. doi:10.1016/B978-0-443-16092-9.00021-7.

Yan, J., Risacher, S.L., Shen, L., Saykin, A.J., 2017. Network approaches to systems biology analysis of complex disease: integrative methods for multi-omics data. Brief. Bioinform. 1477-4054. 19 (6), 1370–1381. Available from: http://bib.oxfordjournals.org. doi:10.1093/bib/bbx066.

Yang, K., Han, X., 2016. Lipidomics: techniques, applications, and outcomes related to biomedical sciences. Trends Biochem. Sci. 0968-0004. 41 (11), 954–969. doi:10.1016/j.tibs.2016.08.010.

Yang, X., Kui, L., Tang, M., Li, D., Wei, K., Chen, W., Miao, J., Dong, Y., 2020. High-throughput transcriptome profiling in drug and biomarker discovery. Front. Genet. 1664-8021. 11. doi:10.3389/fgene.2020.00019.

You, J., Ying, R., Ren, X., Hamilton, W.L., Leskovec, J., 2018. GraphRNN: generating realistic graphs with deep auto-regressive models. In: 35th International Conference on Machine Learning, ICML 2018, Vol. 13. 9781510867963. International Machine Learning Society (IMLS), United States. pp. 9072–9081.

You, Y., Lai, X., Pan, Y., Zheng, H., Vera, J., Liu, S., Deng, S., Zhang, L., 2022. Artificial intelligence in cancer target identification and drug discovery. Signal Transduct. Target. Ther. 2059-3635. 7 (1). Available from: https://www.nature.com/sigtrans. doi:10.1038/s41392-022-00994-0.

Yu, X.T., Zeng, T., 2018. Integrative analysis of omics big data. Methods Mol. Biol. 1754, 109–135. Available from: http://www.springer.com/series/7651. doi:10.1007/978-1-4939-7717-8_7.

Zhang, X., Zhou, Z., Xu, H., Liu, C.T., 2022. Integrative clustering methods for multi-omics data. Wiley Interdiscip. Rev. Comput. Stat. 1939-0068. 14 (3). Available from: http://onlinelibrary.wiley.com/journal/10.1002/(ISSN)1939-0068. doi:10.1002/wics.1553.

Zhang, Y., Wang, Y., Wu, C., Zhan, L., Wang, A., Cheng, C., Zhao, J., Zhang, W., Chen, J., Li, P., 2024. Drug-target interaction prediction by integrating heterogeneous information with mutual attention network. arXiv. 2331-8422. Available from: https://arxiv.org. doi:10.48550/arXiv.2404.03516.

Zhang, Y., Ye, T., Xi, H., Juhas, M., Li, J., 2021. Deep learning driven drug discovery: Tackling severe acute respiratory syndrome coronavirus 2. Front. Microbiol. 12. doi:10.3389/fmicb.2021.739684.

Zhou, G., Pang, Z., Lu, Y., Ewald, J., Xia, J., 2022. OmicsNet 2.0: a web-based platform for multi-omics integration and network visual analytics. Nucleic Acids Res. 0305-1048. 50 (W1), W527. doi:10.1093/nar/gkac376.

Zhou, Y., Fang, J., Bekris, L.M., Kim, Y.H., Pieper, A.A., Leverenz, J.B., Cummings, J., Cheng, F., 2021. AlzGPS: a genome-wide positioning systems platform to catalyze multi-omics for Alzheimer's drug discovery. Alzheimers Res. Ther. 1758-9193. 13 (1). Available from http://alzres.com/. doi:10.1186/s13195-020-00760-w.

Zhou, Y., Zhou, B., Pache, L., Chang, M., Khodabakhshi, A.H., Tanaseichuk, O., Benner, C., Chanda, S.K., 2019. Metascape provides a biologist-oriented resource for the analysis of systems-level datasets. Nat. Commun. 2041-1723. 10 (1). Available from: http://www.nature.com/ncomms/index.html. doi:10.1038/s41467-019-09234-6.

Zou, H., Banerjee, P., Leung, S.S.Y., Yan, X., 2020. Application of pharmacokinetic-pharmacodynamic modeling in drug delivery: development and challenges. Front. Pharmacol. 1663-9812. 11. Available from: http://www.frontiersin.org/Pharmacology. doi:10.3389/fphar.2020.00997.

13

Artificial intelligence-driven personalized medicine and biomarker discovery

Samvedna Singh[a], Aman Chandra Kaushik[b], and Shakti Sahi[a]

[a]*School of Biotechnology, Gautam Buddha University, Greater Noida, Uttar Pradesh, India*

[b]*Technology Dissemination and Computational Biology Division, CSIR-Central Institute of Medicinal and Aromatic Plants, Lucknow, Uttar Pradesh, India*

1 Introduction

Precision medicine relies heavily on biomarkers, which are quantifiable markers of biological states or diseases that help with precise diagnosis, prognosis, and treatment monitoring (Ahmad et al., 2023). The term "precision medicine" is a subset of personalized medicine. Precision medicine refers to the diagnosis and treatment plan that is customized according to patients' genetic information, lifestyle, and clinical data. Although the terms "personalized medicine" and "precision medicine" are sometimes used interchangeably, precision medicine is more specific and data-driven. However, not all personalized treatment strategies are precision medicine. The past few years have seen a rise in publicly available high-dimensional biological information due to developments in high-throughput technologies in biomedicine. These high-dimensional data have opened new avenues for scientific inquiry. Artificial intelligence (AI) can play a pivotal role at all relevant stages of clinical development. Therapeutic techniques can also be optimized for individual patients by utilizing AI algorithms to determine the most effective therapies for certain subpopulations.

A person's unique genetics, phenotype, epigenetics, and lifestyle are taken into account when designing preventive, diagnostic, and therapeutic plans in personalized medicine. In the case of cancer, where biomarker-driven therapy is essential, recent advancements in the methods of biomarker identification have been especially noteworthy (Das et al., 2024). For example, researchers are using biomarkers for the identification of mutations in tumor cells to target subgroups

The AI Frontier in Molecular Modelling and Drug Designing. https://doi.org/10.1016/B978-0-443-40338-5.00007-X

within different forms of cancer types (Parekh et al., 2023). AI and machine learning (ML) algorithms enhance treatment strategies by using phenotypic prediction, risk analysis, medical imaging, and gene expression analysis. Precision medicine allows the identification of a subpopulation within a large population, should its habitat, physiology, and other characteristics differ from those of the larger population. Such differences would affect disease patterns, risk, prognosis, detection, and treatment response (Singh et al., 2024)

Data-intensive assays are essential for identifying the most suitable targets for intervention and strategies for personalizing medicines. Emerging AI approaches are ready to make use of this data and change the scientific method from being hypothesis-driven to being data-driven. Contemporary statistical and ML techniques facilitate knowledge discovery and predictive modeling, providing critical insights into the molecular pathological mechanisms of diseases. They also enable the identification of novel drug targets and the creation of cost-effective assays to improve response prediction for clinical use. With the development of enhanced AI/ML-based diagnostic tools and the identification of more biomarkers, personalized treatment strategies will advance. This will assist physicians in finding more specialized treatments for a wider spectrum of diseases, leading to better patient outcomes.

AI-driven decision-making processes facilitate three essential aspects of big data analysis: integration of scientific knowledge, multimodal analysis, and decision support systems. . Furthermore, they can identify various single-cell parameters, encompassing genomic and signature analysis of genomic and epigenomic data, profiling of immunological markers, and morphological evaluations. This informs the choice of target-based medications, which is made possible by AI/ML-based precision medicine. However, processing multimodal datasets requires advanced computer systems, which is a major limitation of computational precision medicine. The "V's" of big data stand for volume, velocity, variety, veracity, variability, and value (Leff and Yang, 2015). These are the main obstacles to successful and efficient biomedical and health informatics. Volume refers to the enormous amount of data produced by sources such as electronic health records, clinical data, medical imaging, and genomic data from sequencing, which requires models to handle large datasets. Velocity describes how quickly data is processed in the case of real-time patient monitoring, which necessitates quick data management. Variety reflects the various types of data, and AI can enable the detection of patterns from multiple high-dimensional datasets. Veracity pertains to the precision and dependability of data; in cases of missing or inconsistent data, results can lead to inaccurate conclusions. Variability highlights the anomalies and changes in data over time.

Finally, value represents the ability to derive meaningful and useful conclusions from data. The intricacy of processing and utilizing big data in personalized medicine and healthcare innovation is encapsulated by these V's collectively.

This chapter also points out how AI/ML are used in the treatment approaches for different diseases like cancer and diabetes. Although AI holds enormous advantages, it should be used cautiously. AI can handle voluminous data and build individualized treatment plans. Conventional approaches in personalized medicine are constrained by the challenges of processing the large amounts of data needed to create personalized treatment regimens. Using AI-based algorithms to perform omics-level analysis and detect patterns in large datasets can help overcome such challenges. Details on how AI/ML models are enhancing personalized treatment strategies are discussed in this chapter with the help of insightful case studies on multiple diseases.

2 The role of AI in early drug discovery: Enabling precision medicine and biomarker discovery

Discovery and development of a new drug are anticipated to cost more than USD 3 billion, and compounds reaching clinical trials have an approximate approval rate of about 13% (Boniolo et al., 2021). Personalized medicine is possible by tailoring therapies to the distinct features of patients, including their genetic profile, environmental variables, and lifestyle. This has raised high hopes for improving patient outcomes and the success rate of clinical trials. This approach has expanded quickly in many medical and healthcare applications since its introduction, with cancer leading the way in setting its use (Garraway et al., 2013). Fig. 13.1 illustrates the role of AI in personalized medicine. In addition, current research on cardiovascular diseases, cancer, and type 2 diabetes has emphasized how precision medicine is becoming increasingly important for the entire healthcare industry (Sethi et al., 2023).

Identification of biomarkers can accelerate the complete drug discovery and approval process by increasing success rates at lower costs. AI can perform complete molecular characterization of patients, allowing early disease management, and hence it is a valuable tool in precision medicine (Wong et al., 2019). Disease subtyping is one of the crucial steps in the development of treatment strategies. AI improves the chances of disease subtyping by integrating multiple types of data, hence propelling progress in the field of personalized medicine (Guinney et al., 2015). Similarly, ML in pharmacogenomics can predict responses to monotherapy using molecular data from cell cultures, potentially uncovering new predictive

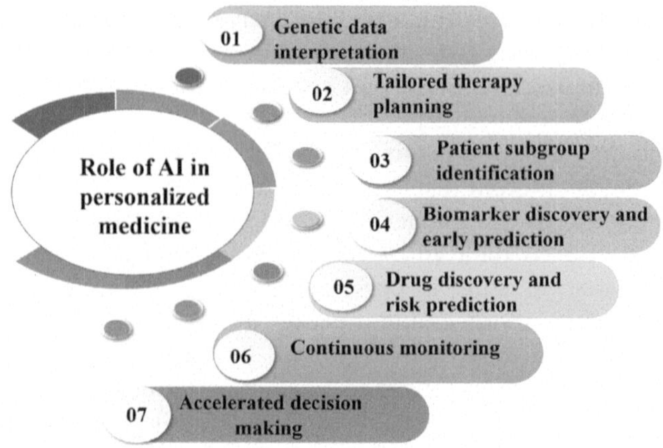

Fig. 13.1 AI in personalized medicine. The figure illustrates the role of AI in different areas of personalized medicine that can be used to enhance treatment strategies and individualized treatment plans.

biomarkers through model interpretation (Menden et al., 2013). In addition, AI has made notable strides in identifying effective drug combinations (Preuer et al., 2018). The ultimate form of precision medicine is represented by personalized medicine, in which individual demands are taken into account while developing therapies that are not just based on biomarkers. One of the well-known examples of how AI has contributed to the development of personalized medicine is the designing of personalized cancer vaccines, targeting antigen peptides specific to an individual's tumor and major histocompatibility complex (MHC) genotype. These vaccines are designed to enhance the patient's immune system (Sahin et al., 2017). AI also enables the prediction of diseases associated with genetic mutations. For instance, the ExPecto algorithm, designed by Zhou et al. (2018), predicts tissue-level gene expression levels from regulatory regions that contain 40-kb promoter-proximal sequences.

2.1 AI-based disease subtyping for biomarker discovery

Disease subtyping is another useful approach for patient stratification. This allows for reducing the dimensionality of the data in cases of complicated diseases, where disease features are broken into more manageable signs. The development of significant and reliable disease subgroups has been made more feasible through the use of AI. One of the prominent examples is cancer, where disease subtyping has proven successful in developing treatment strategies (Zhao et al., 2019).

Colorectal cancer research does not identify a single genetic biomarker for drug sensitivity analysis and, therefore, has been at the forefront of using ML-based gene expression subtyping. Six notable colorectal cancer research groups conducted a significant study utilizing random forest (RF) classification to identify four consensus molecular subtypes. The identified subtypes were established as the optimal number of biologically significant clusters, and their prognostic value was subsequently validated in clinical trials (Mooi et al., 2018). In the case of other cancers lacking clear genetic biomarkers, such as bladder and pancreatic cancer (Orth et al., 2019), gene expression subtyping has been successfully utilized. This approach can generate different molecular subtypes to help predict disease progression and therapeutic response. The primary characteristics of these cancer subtypes often relate to the differentiation stages of the tumor. For instance, well-differentiated or classical subtypes tend to be more responsive toward therapies and less aggressive than undifferentiated basal tumors. The subtyping initiative employed ML techniques, such as unsupervised methods like independent component analysis and nonnegative matrix factorization, to ascertain and validate the optimal number of subtype signatures. The majority of tumor subtyping initiatives usually concentrate on a single data modality, frequently ignoring the complementary data and interdependencies found at many molecular levels. Recently, efforts have focused on creating ML methods for multiomics integration to overcome this constraint. Using multiomics approaches, such as combining data from different omics types—proteomics, transcriptomics, genomics, epigenomics, as well as metabolomics—enables analyses such as gene expression analysis, mutation analysis, and single-cell analysis, which can deepen the understanding of biological pathways and processes involved in the disease. This approach provides a more detailed and enhanced understanding of the disease mechanism and can improve the accuracy of models compared to single-modality approaches. Methods like canonical correlation analysis and component analysis have allowed researchers to discover variations in pathways while modeling data from different molecular sources (Yang and Uhler, 2019).

Recent AI techniques like variational autoencoders can enhance data integration. Autoencoder-like techniques allow analysis of omics layers in the data (Argelaguet et al., 2020). In conclusion, disease subtyping is driven by unsupervised learning methods that explore molecular patterns. When combined with domain expert knowledge, such approaches can generate interpretable and actionable biomarkers. This method augments the existing precision medicine paradigm, which mostly focuses on single-gene correlations. Utilizing AI-based methods to detect disease subtypes can improve treatment strategies. The integration of these subtypes with single-gene biomarkers that have been established will increase patient stratification and make the development of subtype-specific treatments in the short-term possible.

2.2 AI-based methods for personalized vaccine design and drug therapy

Personalized medicine is an integrated approach that combines the information of an individual based on their proteome, metabolome, and transcriptome. The goal of this combination is to achieve an understanding of the molecular mechanism of the patient's disease, which may enable the creation of personalized treatment plans that can reduce side effects and maximize therapeutic results. This can also allow the distribution of drugs based on the genotypes of the patient instead of the symptoms. It covers the stages of disease diagnosis, analysis, prevention, and therapy. The goal of personalized medicine may be achieved using such approaches, which can create direct effectiveness while reducing side effects.

Cancer immunotherapies target and evade cancer by harnessing the immune system of the patients. Neoepitopes are distinctive peptides produced by genetic alterations that occur when cancer progresses, and they are an essential part of this technique (Xu et al., 2021). These neoepitopes are linked to the MHC, which allows them to differentiate between healthy and cancer cells. The immunotherapy design depends upon the accurate selection of neoepitopes. AI has significantly enhanced the ability to identify the neoepitope-MHC binding and immunogenicity. Adoptive T-cell therapies and customized cancer vaccines are more accurate and effective because of the AI-based techniques that improve the selection of potent neoepitopes. AI is also a pivotal component when considering its role in the development of personalized cancer vaccines (Ott et al., 2017). It is the key approach when considered for use in the entire process, from identifying and assembling these neoepitopes into successful vaccinations to predicting which ones will be present in a patient's modified peptide pool.

3 The role of big data analytics in personalized medicine

Big data has enabled substantial transformation in the space of personalized medicine. The cutting-edge technologies and tools used for enhancing the patient treatment plan and care have been efficient due to big data analytics. Large data, when analyzed using sophisticated AI-based methods, may enable tailored and more precise treatment plans. Big data may be useful in therapy optimization based on an individual's needs, which can be predicted using AI/ML models based on a patient's genetic data. These models can be used on multiomics data to customize cancer therapies for specific individuals (Cai et al., 2022). To accurately determine which course of therapy would be most effective for a given individual, ML techniques have been applied to vast amounts of data obtained from genome sequencing. ML models on the vast data, such as genome sequencing data, have been highly beneficial in determining disease mechanisms.

The integration of diversified data of a patient, when analyzed using AI, may lead to robust and updated findings of biomarkers for a range of disease diagnoses. To unlock the full potential of personalized medicine, we need the help of AI and ML-based approaches (Fröhlich et al., 2018; Sahu et al., 2022). Identifying subgroups of patients who belong to a large subset, for instance, in the case of a patient group whose survival rates exceed the mean of the rest, is one of the requirements when it comes to classification challenges. Phenotype prediction is another challenge, where AI, along with big data analytics, can help expedite the process of drug discovery, providing a better understanding of the varying genetic pathways underlying disease development (Cernea et al., 2020). Researchers (Oikonomou et al., 2022) highlighted the use of big data in identifying people at risk for diseases like cardiovascular disease by demonstrating how polygenic risk scores produced from big data may predict disease risk. Colombian healthcare institutions designed a digital health platform that combines sophisticated analytics with clinical and operational data sources, which can enhance decision-making, leading to improved disease management (López-Martínez et al., 2020).

AI algorithms allow the integration of data sources, which can create the best classification. These data can be derived from different sources, for example, genetic, genomic, epigenomic, or even transcriptomic sources. All of them include different datasets, literature, electronic health records, and/or medical images (Table 13.1). These data can be effectively used in classifiers, such as regression models, to predict the values of real and continuous variables. Fig. 13.2 shows an integrative framework of how data from electronic health records (EHRs), wearable devices, and other sources can be used for the prediction of disease progression. Data from such sources can be used to predict blood cholesterol levels, monitor glucose levels, and blood pressure levels based on other biomarkers (Hassan et al., 2022). Furthermore, when aggregating information from multiple data sources to predict events or outcomes, ML methods are a

Table 13.1 Major global consortia dedicated to personalized medicine.

S. No	Big data consortia	Research focus	Link
1	The Encyclopedia of DNA Elements (ENCODE)	Genomic functional elements	https://encodeproject.org
2	Cancer cell line encyclopedia	Cancer target validation and defining drug efficacy	https://sites.broadinstitute.org/ccle/
3	Human genome diversity project (HGDP)	Broad genomic research	https://hgdp.org
4	Genomics of drug sensitivity in cancer (GDSC)	Genomic marker, drug response, and sensitivity data	https://www.cancerrxgene.org/
5	Global network of Personal Genome Projects (PGP)	General genomic studies	https://personalgenomes.org
6	International human epigenome consortium (IHEC)	Human epigenome research	https://ihec-epigenomes.org
7	NIH Roadmap Epigenomics Mapping Consortium (Roadmap)	Epigenomic mapping	https://roadmapepigenomics.org

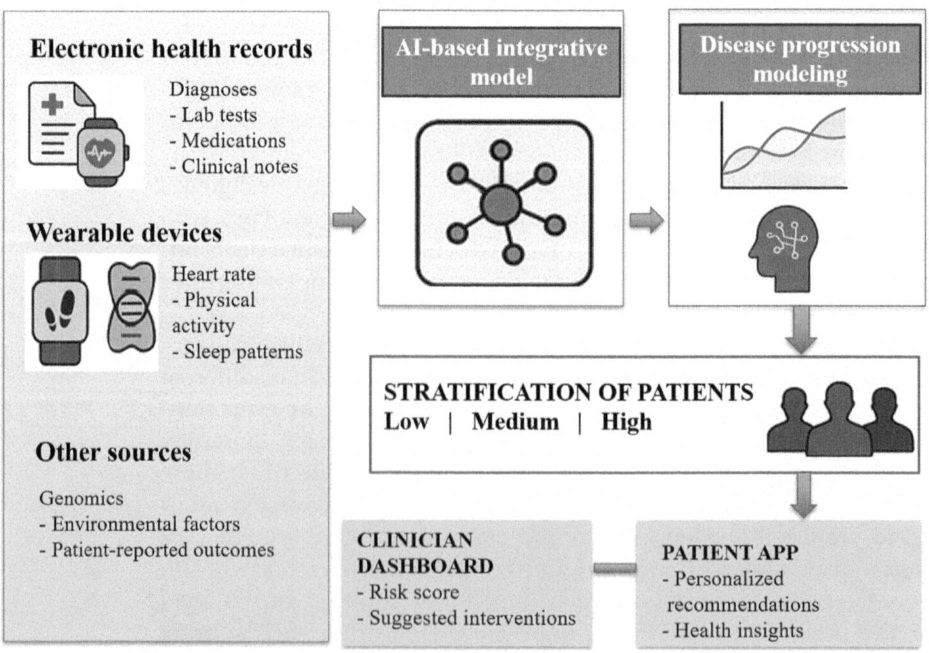

Fig. 13.2 An integrative AI-driven framework for utilizing longitudinal health data to predict disease progression and enable personalized interventions. The figure illustrates AI-based approaches used to process data from different sources to identify patient risks and outcomes, which can facilitate personalized treatment plans.

valuable asset (Cirillo and Valencia, 2019). For instance, Generalized Linear Models have a general form where variables and outcomes are linearly related by a link function. Model parameters can then be estimated, typically by employing models such as Bayesian models and maximum likelihood. Biological data exhibit structured patterns, such as genes clustered with related functions, which might require improved predictive modeling. AI-based supervised multiview feature selection uses structural regularization methods like Bayesian models, such as naïve Bayes, or sparse group Least Absolute Shrinkage and Selection Operator (LASSO). These models can perform probabilistic reasoning to determine clinical outcomes depending on the features. Therefore, they increase decision-making under uncertain scenarios. Similarly, in the case of regularization methods, such as LASSO, it can allow the creation of structured groups, for example, a group of genes within the same pathway, which may improve the ability of the model to observe patterns and groups in the biological data. Methods like these can enable more accurate and biologically relevant predictions, supporting tasks like disease classification, prognosis, and biomarker discovery.

In a study, Banerjee et al. (2019) examined the usage of big data to accomplish the designing of personalized medicine, targeted drug delivery, and higher precision in customized medicine. Population health analytics leverages big data to understand disparities, disease trends, and healthcare utilization patterns at the population level. By analyzing population-level data from different sources like public health databases and health surveys, healthcare organizations can identify high-risk populations, prioritize interventions, and allocate resources effectively. Population health analytics also informs policy decisions, community-based interventions, and quality improvement initiatives aimed at preventing diabetes, reducing health inequalities, and promoting healthy behaviors.

It is expected that big data in healthcare will have a major influence on personalized medicine and pharmacogenetics. Even the same chemotherapy drugs can have different reactions in patients with the same cancer type. For instance, variations in the CYP2D6 gene are known to influence responses to Tamoxifen (Malash et al., 2020). In addition, recent studies have identified multiple gene signatures that correlate with the effectiveness of chemoradiotherapy for rectal cancer (Qian et al., 2022) BRAF mutations, specifically Y472C, are associated with differential responses to Dasatinib in non-small cell lung cancer (Nguyen-Ngoc et al., 2015).

The PanCancer project was started by The Cancer Genome Atlas research network to examine different tumor forms and molecular anomalies, allowing the identification of novel genetic aberrations. Utilizing and integrating data can help unearth discoveries, such as biomarkers and the mutation profiles of various cancer types

(Tomczak et al., 2015). It is believed that a factor in the differences in drug reactions among individuals is genomic instability. Discovering the intricate relationships between genomes and chemotherapeutic sensitivity, resistance, and toxicity has been the focus of a recent study. Large genomic databases are being built as part of efforts like the Genomics of Drug Sensitivity in Cancer (Garnett et al., 2012) and the Cancer Cell Line Encyclopedia to investigate the relationships between drug sensitivity and genomic biomarkers in a variety of cancer cell lines. Recent research suggests that drug-response data and genomic profiles might improve computational methods for drug prediction for particular cell lines, hence supporting the possibility of large pharmacogenetic databases to predict drug responses, improving the outcomes of personalized medicine.

4 AI/ML algorithms in the development of personalized medicine

AI models and algorithms have played a crucial role in advancing drug discovery, biomarker identification, and personalized medicine by integrating various sophisticated approaches (Paul et al., 2021). AI/ML models advance biomarker prediction, leading to optimal personalized therapies. The role of AI algorithms in the stages of biomarker identification in personalized medicine is shown in Fig. 13.3.

AI/ML algorithm approaches are categorized into six key subcategories. Multitask learning improves predictive performance by using shared representation in related tasks. Prediction response can

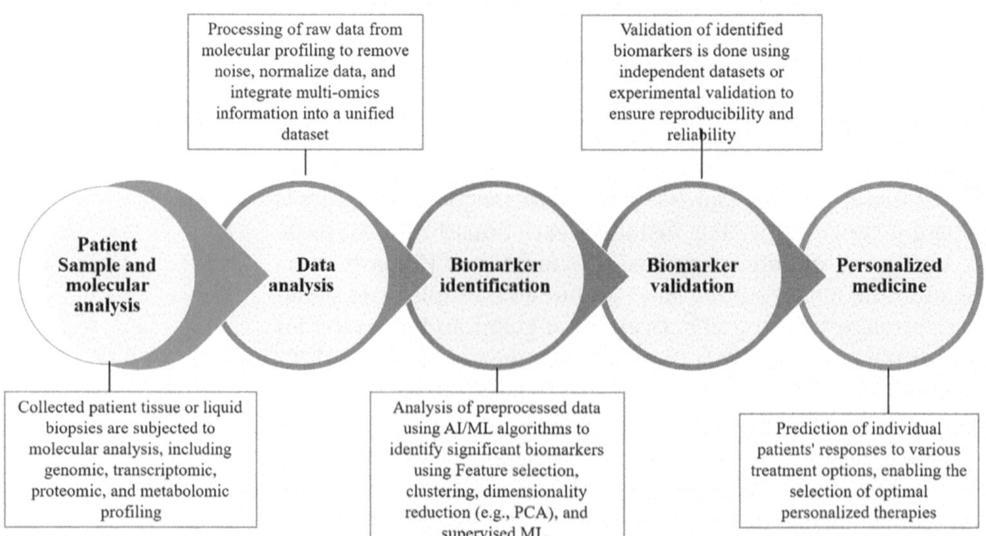

Fig. 13.3 Application of AI in the stages of biomarker identification and personalized medicine. The figure demonstrates the integration of AI in different stages of biomarker identification.

be useful in various drug trials and can also be used while identifying biomarkers related to different conditions. Reinforcement learning is another model where models learn through the trial-and-error method in a dynamic environment. Such models help design treatment strategies in the drug development process. Another model is unsupervised learning, which enables the identification of hidden patterns in larger datasets. This model is particularly helpful in developing personalized treatment plans when it can be trained to identify subgroups of patients based on high-dimensional data. It can be employed to identify novel molecular signatures and molecular subtypes. Semisupervised learning allows for improving the accuracy of the models by combining a small dataset with a large labeled dataset. This methodology is most useful in labeled sets of data, i.e., authorized biomarkers or tagged clinical results, and is usually slow and costly, while extensive quantities of raw omics or imaging data remain unlabeled. Using both sets of data, semisupervised learning allows predictions to become more accurate. It also enables the uncovering of important biological patterns. An overview of these algorithms, along with their applications, is given in Table 13.2. Together, these AI-based strategies enable more efficient and targeted approaches to developing new therapies, identifying biomarkers, and tailoring treatments to individual patient needs.

5 Deep learning in personalized treatment and biomarker discovery

Deep learning (DL) is one of the most innovative techniques that has been developed in biomedical sciences. It allows highly robust biomarker identification along with various analyses that are crucial to personalized medicine. Artificial neural networks (ANN) are one of the assets in DL; it is an ML approach that is used for the analysis. These algorithms allow big data analysis by taking a massive amount of data and analyzing it using neural network (NN) topologies (Papadakis et al., 2019). These algorithms also allow the identification of hidden patterns and insights that can be overlooked by a conventional approach. This section reviews key applications of DL in these areas, emphasizing its role in advancing personalized medicine and identifying new biomarkers.

Personalized medicine aims to replace general therapies and instead generate more dedicated treatment plans that are specifically based on an individual patient's profile. Another goal is to develop plans focusing on disease susceptibility evaluations. Data such as omics data are essential for this aim, derived from various parameters. Omics data can enable gene expression analysis, analysis of DNA sequences, and also assist in medical imaging results, which can help

Table 13.2 Overview of applications of different AI and ML algorithms for improved individualized treatment strategies.

S. No	Algorithm	Description	Research focus	Links and references
1	Neural networks (NN)	Computational models known as neural networks imitate the intricate workings of the human brain. Neural networks are composed of linked neurons or nodes that analyze and learn from input, allowing machine learning tasks like pattern recognition and decision-making.	a) Medical Image Analysis, b) analyzing skin cancer images for personalized treatment	Esteva et al. (2017), Litjens et al. (2017).
2	Random forest	A flexible supervised machine learning technique called Random Forest builds and combines many decision trees to form a "forest."	a) Predicted survival of colorectal patients using ML models, b) development of personalized medicine approaches in immune-mediated chronic inflammatory diseases, c) RF as a predictor for medical data classification using feature ranking, d) prediction of drug activity against cancer cells	Lind et al. (2019), Alam et al. (2019), Cardoso et al. (2023)
3	Support-vector machines	An approach that can be used in cases of both classification and regression.	a) Alzheimer's disease diagnosis using brain volume determined by structural MRI, b) understanding cancer genomics, c) development of personalized treatment plans	Carrillo-Pérez et al. (2022), Vichianin et al. (2021), Huang et al. (2018)
4	k-nearest neighbors (KNN)	A non-parametric classifier that classifies the grouping of a single data point using proximity.	Prediction of various diseases, such as cardiovascular disorders,	Choudhary et al. (2023), Uddin et al. (2022)
5	Gradient boosting machines (GBM)	In machine learning, a set of ensemble approaches known as the GBM algorithm builds models progressively to minimize mistakes.	Predicting the progression of chronic kidney disease	Ji et al. (2022), Hussein and Majumder (2023).
6	Reinforcement learning (RL)	A branch of machine learning, known as reinforcement learning (RL), gives AI-based systems the ability to operate in a dynamic environment to maximize reward.	a) Developing cancer chemotherapy treatment strategies, b) optimizing personalized treatment plans in sepsis	Komorowski et al. (2018), Yang et al. (2023)

7	Deep learning (DL)	DL is built on the design of ANN. ANN uses layers of linked nodes, termed neurons, to analyze and learn from the data.	Stress/Rest Myocardial Perfusion Imaging-Based Prediction of All-Cause Mortality (MPI)	Cheng et al. (2022)
8	Deep convolutional neural network	The type of neural network most commonly used to find patterns in images and videos is the traditional ANN, which has made way for DCNNs that employ a three-dimensional neural pattern.	DCCN for endotracheal tube position classification on plain chest radiography with automatic trachea and tube segmentation	Jung et al. (2022)
9	Deep reinforcement learning	Deep reinforcement learning (DRL) is an artificial intelligence method that blends deep neural networks with reinforcement learning. It gains the ability to respond to inputs in the form of reward or penalty signals.	Improving segmentation of COVID-19 CT Images	Allioui et al. (2022)
10	Recursive feature elimination (RFE)	RFE can be used for removing less significant characteristics while focusing on those that improve predictive accuracy. Until a desirable feature subset is identified, RFE evaluates the relevance of each feature, eliminates the least important, and rebuilds the model.	Gene expression profiles to predict customized medication responses.	Chen et al. (2022), Huang et al. (2017)

identify variations in biological processes. ML technologies are frequently evolving, and it is a rapidly expanding industry. Because of this, as advantageous as these approaches are, they might also possess some significant limitations, which can be resolved by using DL models (Rajkomar et al., 2019). For example, feature extraction is a natural approach inbuilt in a DL model, whereas when analyzing data using ML models, the performance of the model significantly depends on the preprocessing of the data to extract the required features (Eraslan et al., 2019). Personalized medicine has also significantly benefited from the combination of DL models with genetic data. In the case of personalized medicine, genetic sequences of an individual patient can be examined thoroughly to identify mutation signatures and patterns that are linked to the disease. DL can also allow the prediction of genetic polymorphisms, which are important for understanding genetic disease mechanisms (Naito, 2019).

In a research study, the two prediction models were used in combination. One was the ML model that was based on genomic characteristics, and the other was the deep NN that was based on base sequences. The combination of these models was used to predict exonic splicing mutations in the Fifth Critical Assessment of Genome Interpretation Massively Parallel Splicing Assay challenge, with encouraging outcomes. According to the study's inferences, performance was considerably enhanced when multiple predictive models were combined utilizing the stacked generalization approach. Furthermore, feature values produced by a DNN-based splice site prediction tool, named DSSP, improved prediction accuracy, even though the majority of genomic features utilized in ML models had already been published. Predicting splicing disruptions has been made easier by understanding sequence patterns linked to regular splicing and how mutations affect splicing site probability. These findings aid in the generation of more individualized treatment plans. DL has also become essential in cancer research across various domains, including multiomics analysis, biomarker identification, and image analysis. With the decreasing costs of genome sequencing, analyzing genomic data now involves processing between 1000 and 100,000 mutations within a single tumor sample. The AI-based approaches are important for determining meaningful insights from the data. In the case of multi task and single-task learning, DL is particularly beneficial. In addition, it performs well when used for the analysis of different types of combinations of data. As cancer is one of the most heterogeneous and complex diseases, combining diverse data sources becomes crucial. In those scenarios, DL can be used for the most effective outcomes (Zehir et al., 2017; Shimizu and Nakayama, 2020).

DL-based approaches in cancer are beneficial for the identification of drug targets, biomarker identification, drug target interaction prediction, analysis of data to determine patterns from genomic data, and various other applications like drug optimization that are crucial to personalized treatment development. In a study, (Bibault et al., 2018) introduced a DL model based on a radiomics system that can be applied to forecast the outcome of neoadjuvant chemoradiation, especially in the case of localized rectal cancer. This approach was specifically designed to identify individuals who would benefit from the conventional treatment instead of resection.

In other diseases as well, DL has shown numerous applications. For example, in the case of neurodegenerative disorders like Alzheimer's, a convolutional NN (CNN), a DL-based approach, was used in the clinical setting to identify patterns from diverse data and large datasets. CNN-based approaches are being used in multiple diseases, such as Type 2 diabetes mellitus (T2DM). In T2DM, a CNN model can predict treatment strategies, risk prediction, and patient outcomes. This can include analyzing multiple disease-specific variables. In the case of diabetes, variables include gender, age, comorbidities, genetic predisposition, and prior treatment response. Similarly, ANN models can also identify high-risk patients, which can help in providing preventive interventions (Krishnan et al., 2023; Katiyar et al., 2024). CNN has also significantly improved the early diagnosis of AD, as recently introduced by Ding et al. The technique, which makes use of 18f fludeoxyglucose positron emission tomography brain images, obtained an average specificity of 82% at 100% sensitivity, approximately 75.8 months ahead of schedule for the final diagnosis. This development may significantly increase the availability of early treatment therapies (Ding et al., 2019).

One of the crucial key elements for successful personalized treatment is accurately predicting reactions to different drugs. In a study, Ahmed et al. (2022) suggested unifying cell line information to integrate gene expression, mutation profiles, and drug reaction data. Principal component analysis and models such as support vector machine (SVM) and logistic regression (LR) were employed for feature reduction. These models enhanced accuracy and lowered the mean square error by approximately 25% when the AI models were tested with and without it. The proposed DL model also utilizes dimension-reduction encoders, which are trained to equate input and output through unsupervised learning. By employing the Pearson correlation coefficient (PCC), the model was found to be more accurate compared to the newer models. Despite a huge database of genes and drugs, the enhanced deep drug response (Enhanced Deep-DR) model yielded the highest PCC values, which indicated its high capacity and performance. Overall, the integration of AI and DL models in personalized medicine considerably enhances the accuracy of drug response prediction, thereby optimizing cancer treatment protocols and outcomes.

6 AI-based Tools, pipelines and platforms for enhanced personalized medicine and treatment strategies

Different AI-powered tools and websites have also been developed by researchers to facilitate the identification of biomarkers as well as approaches for personalized medicine. For example, the AI pipeline DrugCell, developed by Kuenzi et al. (2020), was created for the purpose of predicting the number of drugs that will impact cell response. It utilizes an ANN with three hidden layers that are linked to each other. Model training was conducted using 509,294 combinations of drugs and cell lines, varying from 684 drugs to 1235 tumor cell lines. The Genomics of Drug Sensitivity in Cancer database (GDSC) and the Cancer Therapeutics Response Portal v2—these two databases—were used for obtaining the training datasets. The model's performance was validated using the Spearman rho method. The PyTorch library was used to execute the DrugCell model. The predictions of DrugCell to boost progression-free survival in cell lines were astounding. In addition, the model demonstrated promising potential in the classification of therapeutic effects for patients with ER-positive breast cancer. A list of such tools, along with their description, is provided below in Table 13.3.

7 Case studies in cancer

The intrinsic variability of cancer necessitates individualized treatment plans. AI may help oncologists create personalized treatment regimens by combining data specific to each patient, such as medical reports, imaging reports, and genetic profiles (Tripathi et al., 2024). AI-based methods are also used to identify prognostic indicators, drug targets, and possible treatments (Huang et al., 2022; Kaushik et al., 2020). Researchers introduced T-cell recognition potential of HLA-I presented peptides (TRAP) (https://github.com/ChloeHJ/TRAP), a sophisticated DL-based platform designed to predict CD8+ T-cell epitopes from MHC-I presented pathogenic and self-peptides. To address the challenge of data that is significantly different, referred to as out-of-distribution generalization, researchers developed separate models for pathogenic and self-derived peptides. This distinction helps improve prediction

Table 13.3 AI-based tools and pipelines for personalized medicine and biomarker discovery.

S. No	Tool/pipeline name	Algorithm	Description	Links and references
1	GenoML	Automated machine learning (AutoML)	A genomic data automated ML package that supports the generation of prediction models	Makarious et al. (2021) https://genoml.com/
2	CancerIDP	Deep learning	An interpretable neural network using individualized transcriptomes and prescription drugs to forecast the survival of cancer patients	Sun and Chen (2023)
3	PandaOmics	Deep learning	AI approaches to biological text data and multimodal omics for the identification of therapeutic targets and biomarkers	Kamya et al. (2024)
4	PADME	Deep learning	Drug target identification	Feng et al. (2018)
5	DeepDTA	Deep learning	Identification of drug-target binding affinity	Öztürk et al. (2018) https://github.com/hkmztrk/DeepDTA.
6	DeepDR	Deep learning	In silico repurposing of drugs using biological networks	Zeng et al. (2019) https://github.com/ChengF-Lab/deepDR
7	DrugnomeAI	Semisupervised ML	Druggability prediction of each gene in the human exome coding for a protein can be determined	Zeng et al. (2019), Raies et al. (2022) http://drugnomeai.public.cgr.astrazeneca.com
8	ORGANIC	Reinforcement learning	De novo designing of polymers and organic compounds can be performed using ORGANIC	Chen et al. (2020) https://github.com/aspuru-guzik-group/ORGANIC
9	PrOctor	Random forest	The potential for toxicity in clinical trials can be anticipated by PrOCTOR	Gayvert et al. (2016) https://github.com/kgayvert/PrOCTOR
10	iDrug-target	Synthetic Minority Oversampling Technique (SMOTE) and Neighborhood Cleaning Rule	Determines how drugs interact with nuclear receptors, ion channels, GPCRs, and enzymes	Xiao et al. (2015) http://www.jci-bioinfo.cn/iDrug-Target/
11	PLINK	Logistic regression and linear regression	A whole-genome association analysis toolbox, intended to carry out several fundamental and extensive studies in a computationally effective way	Purcell et al. (2007) https://zzz.bwh.harvard.edu/plink/

Continued

Table 13.3 AI-based tools and pipelines for personalized medicine and biomarker discovery—cont'd

S. No	Tool/pipeline name	Algorithm	Description	Links and references
12	DeepChem	Deep learning	A deep learning toolset for drug discovery and biomarker identification that is available as an open-source platform	https://github.com/deepchem/deepchem
13	AutoPrognosis	Automated machine learning (AutoML)	An automated machine learning framework for predicting clinical outcomes and discovering biomarkers	Imrie et al. (2023) https://github.com/vanderschaarlab/autoprognosis
14	IntelliGenes	Recursive feature elimination, RF, SVM, XGBoost, k-NN	A unique ML pipeline to find highly accurate biomarkers important for disease prediction using multigenomics exploration	DeGroat et al. (2023) https://github.com/drzeeshanahmed/IntelliGenes
15	DeepHRD	Deep learning	Homologous Recombination Deficiency (HRD) in cancer genomes may be predicted using this method. It makes use of DL techniques to increase the precision of HRD identification, which is essential for directing the use of targeted medicines	Bergstrom et al. (2024) https://github.com/AlexandrovLab/DeepHRD/pulls
16	TRAP	Deep learning	A powerful framework for CD8 + T-cell epitope prediction using MHC-pathogenic and self-peptides was what I showed	Lee et al. (2022)
17	DrugCell	VNN	A "visible" neural network (VNN) that models the hierarchical structure of a human cancer cell to anticipate how an anticancer treatment will operate	Kuenzi et al. (2020)
18	Autosurv	Deep learning	A deep learning framework that integrates clinical and multiomics data for cancer survival analysis	Jiang et al. (2024)
19	AdaMedGraph	Graph neural networks (GNN)	Adaboosting graph neural networks for personalized medicine	Lian et al. (2023)

accuracy by tailoring the learning process to the distinct characteristics of each peptide type. More specific information on the physicochemical, electrostatic, and biophysical characteristics of amino acids was obtained by encoding peptide sequences using protein transformer-based pretrained language models to overcome data limitations. A one-dimensional CNN (1D CNN) was used to obtain T-cell identification motifs. "A 1D CNN was selected for this task because it can efficiently process sequential data, like amino acid chains, making it suitable for identifying position-specific motifs in peptides without requiring spatial (2D) features". The highly accurate NetMHCpan (https://services.healthtech.dtu.dk/services/NetMHCpan-4.1/) algorithm predicted the MHC binding rank score, which was used to include MHC binding information. Peptides with low-confidence prediction rates, those that were different from the training data, were assessed and removed using an out-of-distribution detection module. This brand-new computational platform reliably predicts CD8+ T-cell epitopes, facilitating the creation of efficient personalized treatments and a better understanding of antigen-specific T-cell responses.

Breast cancer is highly heterogeneous, requiring individualized treatment strategies. In a study, Cardoso et al. (2016) examined drug sensitivity data and human breast cancer cell lines for possible medications using cell line data from the Cancer Cell Line Encyclopedia (CCLE) and Genomics of Drug Sensitivity in Cancer (GDSC) databases. LASSO, Elastic Net, and Ridge were the three main ML models used to validate the results. Next, using information from the Cleveland database, the top-ranked biomarkers for radiation resistance were analyzed based on their significance in breast cancer. Palbociclib, Panobinostat, PD-0325901, PLX4720, Selumetinib, and Tanespimycin were the six medications shown to have a substantial effect on breast cancer cell lines by researchers. TNFSF15, DCAF6, KDM6A, PHETA2, and IFNGR1 were the five biomarkers that were also sensitive to all six of the nominated medications.

Accurate diagnosis is one of the main aims of personalized medicine. MammaPrint (https://www.agendia.com/mammaprint/), a breast cancer predictive diagnostic based on 70 gene signatures, was authorized by the FDA. Using fresh tissue or formalin-fixed paraffin-embedded tissue for microarray analysis, MammaPrint is a signature method based on the microarray technique. In addition, the BluePrint (https://www.agendia.com/blueprint/) test has shown expression data, which may help the Microarray In Node-negative and 1 to 3 positive lymph node Disease may Avoid ChemoTherapy (MINDACT) and Measuring the Impact of MammaPrint on Adjuvant and Neoadjuvant Treatment in Breast Cancer Patients (IMPACT) studies with personalized therapy (Viale et al., 2018). Seven deep-learning algorithms were developed in a study to identify tissue sections with metastases from women with breast cancer that were stained with hematoxylin and eosin. The algorithms outperformed a group of eleven pathologists, with the best algorithm achieving an area under the curve (AUC) of 0.994, while the best performance by the pathologists was 0.884 (Bejnordi et al., 2017).

Triple-Negative Breast Cancer Treatment (TNBC) drug therapies driven by ML. Because TNBC lacks HER2 receptors, progesterone, and estrogen, it is difficult to treat. Kaushik et al. (2021) and Kaushik and Zhao (2023) assessed the effects of drugs on TNBC cell lines using ML techniques. Six successful drugs were found by analyzing data from the CCLE and GDSC databases: Panobinostat, PLX4720, lapatinib, nilotinib, selumetinib, and tanespimycin. It has been discovered that biomarkers like SETD7 can predict a drug's reaction, which suggests the possibility of individualized treatment plans.

In another study, the long noncoding RNAs (lncRNA) signature for prognosis in TNBC was investigated. lncRNAs serve important biological roles and are frequently used as cancer prognostic indicators. First, the lncRNA expression data from the TANRIC (https://bioinformatics.mdanderson.org/public-software/tanric/) collection were gathered by filtering out samples with insufficient tumor purity. TNBC patients were then split into two prognostic classifications based on whether they lived for three years or less. Based on the differences in lncRNA expression between the shorter and longer survival groups, researchers employed the RF ML technique to select lncRNA features. The predictive model was built using the stochastic gradient boosting technique. A total of 353 lncRNAs exhibited distinct transcription patterns in the longer and shorter survival groups. Two lncRNAs were further selected using the recursive feature elimination method. Researchers achieved 69.69% accuracy and an AUC of 0.6475 using stochastic gradient boosting as the training method. The results of the study revealed that the two lncRNAs could serve as potential biomarkers for prognostic classification in patients suffering from TNBC. Many lncRNAs were found to be dysregulated in TNBC using an ML-based approach, even though the majority of them were likely involved in the biology of cancer. These lncRNAs may be useful biomarkers because some of them were associated with TNBC prognosis.

These advancements indicate significant developments in the application of AI and ML in the clinical field. Platforms like TRAP must undergo comprehensive validation in prospective clinical trials and be integrated into workflows before they can be utilized in real-world settings. AI-based pipelines, AI transparency, and data privacy are also crucial. The use of EHR, real-time patient data, and evolving AI platforms will dictate the next phase of personalized treatment and precision oncology, where treatment options are continuously optimized and dynamically tailored for each patient.

8 Case studies in type 2 diabetes

The identification of T2DM biomarkers and personalized treatment plans is being developed by AI. It allows the highlighting of intricate data patterns in a limited time, which may assist in the identification of disease-related biomarkers. This process accelerates the identification of disease-related biomarkers, helping in the early diagnosis and development of efficient treatment plans. By leveraging advanced algorithms, ML models, and DL algorithms, AI provides a paradigm shift in efficiency, accuracy, and personalized understanding that ultimately improves outcomes by enabling risk prediction, delivering personalized prognostic models, and eventually leading to early diagnosis and treatment (Khalifa and Albadawy, 2024)

In the Systolic Blood Pressure Intervention Trial (SPRINT), researchers developed an effective tool for people with T2DM and without T2DM to personalize their treatment choice between two groups: one with intensive blood pressure management and the other with usual systolic blood pressure management. They achieved this by developing personalized benefit estimates from phenotypic representations of clinical trials using an ML model. They compared intensive (systolic blood pressure <120 mm Hg) and normal (systolic blood pressure <140 mm Hg) systolic blood pressure control in T2DM-free participants. Using iterative Cox regression analysis based on 59 baseline variables, they estimated personalized treatment effect estimates for MACE to define the phenotypes of the population under study. Thereafter, an extreme gradient boosting algorithm (XGBoost) was modeled to estimate the individual benefit of intensive blood pressure control, and its efficacy was tested in T2DM patients who were randomized in the Action to Control Cardiovascular Risk in Diabetes (ACCORD) BP trial. AI also enables the identification of prognostic and diagnostic biomarkers for precision medicine approaches, playing an important role in discovery by mining omics data to identify molecular signatures associated with diabetes risk, treatment response, and progression (Mohsen et al., 2023).

In a different study, Borzouei and Soltanian (2018) used a NN model to determine the most significant demographic risk variables for a diagnosis of T2DM. A sample of 234 people, whose hemoglobin A1c values were used to diagnose T2DM, was analyzed. A multilayer perceptron in ANN was employed to evaluate the importance of demographic risk factors for type 2 diabetes. Various clinical, lifestyle, and demographic factors were analyzed for their relevance to diabetes risk to identify the most significant predictors of type 2 diabetes.

The model was expanded to include variables that were noted as significant, with a $p < 0.2$, including parameters such as body mass index (BMI), hypertension, age, stress, consumption of vegetables, family history, fruit diet, sex, and walking in a univariate logistic regression analysis. Seven stages of NN modeling revealed BMI (78.2%), smoking (49.3%), waist circumference (100.0%), age (78.5%), hypertension (69.4%), and stress as significant factors. These results indicated how ANN-based models can aid personalized diabetes management according to patient risk profiles.

9 Case studies in neurodegenerative disorders

Neurodegenerative disorders like Alzheimer's disease (AD), Parkinson's disease (PD), and Huntington's disease require an understanding of the underlying disease mechanisms, genomic profiles of the patients, and identification of novel therapeutic targets. Personalized medicine strategies aim to break the 'one size fits all' approach of traditional treatment options. It focuses on generating treatment opportunities with individualized profiling, pathophysiological profiling, or genomic profiling of the patients. This may allow for the identification of disease patterns, prevention, and the development of personalized therapies. On this basis, various studies have focused on utilizing AI to expedite the process of disease management, including strategies like phenotyping to assist in clinical trial design and classification of diseases (Dorsey et al., 2020). To examine disease causes, progression markers, and risk factors, large, well-characterized groups like the Parkinson's Progression Markers Initiative (PPMI) (Marek et al., 2018) and the AD Neuroimaging Initiative (Jones-Davis and Buckholtz, 2015) provide invaluable insights with imaging, biometric, and genetic data.

An ML-based GenoML platform was developed (Makarious et al., 2021) for the analysis of PD patients. The PD Biomarker Program dataset was used to validate this model after it was trained on multimodal data from the PPMI. The AUC values, which determine the quality of a classification model, were 85.03% and 89.72%, respectively. The higher AUC value in relation to 100% reflects the ability of the model to separate between classes. Here, the higher value suggests the accuracy of the GenoML platform. Such a platform demonstrates the benefits of combining different and larger datasets for the prediction of risk among patients and therapeutic targets.

In a study, Huang et al. (2024) identified diagnostic markers for the treatment of PD. In addition to this, they studied the impact of immune cell infiltrations on the pathogenesis of the disease. They analyzed Gene Expression Omnibus datasets to identify differentially expressed genes (DEGs). A training model was used based on the human substantia nigra. DEGs were analyzed using Robust Rank Aggregation analysis. The identification of protein-protein interaction-based hub genes was analyzed using Cytoscape. Potential diagnostic genes were found using a Lasso-Cox regression model. For validation, the GSE20292 dataset was utilized. A CIBERSORT method was employed to screen 62 infiltrating immune cells. DEGs, namely TAC1, PCDH8, KIAA0319, AGTR1, SLC18A2, AXIN1 and PDH6H were identified by combining protein interaction networks and LASSO-Cox regression analysis. These seven significant DEGs demonstrated high sensitivity (true positive rate) and specificity (true negative rate) in diagnosing PD, which highlighted the critical role played by immune cell infiltration in the disease.

In another study, Hampel et al. (2020) used genome-wide analysis for the identification of biomarkers that are linked with AD. The AD Cooperative Study-Activities of Daily Living scale (ADCS-ADL) and the Mini-Mental State Examination (MMSE) were modified in a Phase 2a trial of blarcamesine (ANAVEX2-73), a selective agonist of the sigma-1 receptor (SIGMAR1). The experiment was conducted to assess the clinical characteristics, safety, effectiveness, and pharmacokinetics. They performed whole exome sequencing on a cohort of 21 patients' transcriptomic data. They used the Knowledge Extraction and Management (KEM) framework and unsupervised formal concept analysis (FCA) for the assessment of effective biomarkers. The baseline MMSE score (MMSE slope: $P < .015$), the genomic variants SIGMAR1 p. Gln2Pro (ΔMMSE: $P < .039$; ΔADCS-ADL: $P < .063$), the mean plasma concentration of blarcamesine (MMSE slope: $P < .041$), and COMT p. Leu146fs (ΔMMSE: $P < .039$; ΔADCS-ADL: $P < .063$) were found to be significant biomarkers influencing clinical outcomes at week 57. Using linear mixed-effect models, the impact of these biomarkers on treatment response was validated at week 148. Ongoing Phase 2b/3 studies are further evaluating these patient selection markers. Such studies exemplify how AI-driven personalized medicine and biomarkers can be game changers in the field of science.

10 Success stories of AI-driven personalized medications in the pharmaceutical industry

Evaxion Biotech (https://www.evaxion-biotech.com/) has been using various cutting-edge AI-based methods to enhance the development of vaccines and immunotherapies. AI is utilized in immune system modeling and neoepitope prediction for cancer immunotherapy to find new antigens arising from mutations in cancer cells. The development of customized cancer vaccines that target specific mutations unique to each patient depends on these neoepitopes.

ML algorithms are used to evaluate enormous volumes of biological data, identify complex patterns, and discover novel antigen targets for vaccine development that may be missed by traditional methodologies. DL is applied to improve prediction accuracy. AI-powered biophysical models mimic molecular interactions, such as antigen binding to MHC molecules. This is important because it helps in vaccine design by predicting which peptides T cells would be exposed to. Among their efforts are platforms like EDEN, which has been confirmed preclinically in seven bacterial pathogens and recognizes B-cell antigens that resemble highly protective proteins. This results in strong immune responses against a variety of bacterial diseases. Another platform, named Peptide Innovation for Early Diabetes Treatment (PIONEER), selects tumor-specific epitopes that trigger robust T-cell responses to target and destroy tumor cells with minimal effect on healthy cells and precisely identifies patient-specific neoantigens for personalized cancer immunotherapies. Identifying vaccine candidates against any virus, existing, new, or mutating is the main goal of the Reimagining Available Vaccines and Envisioning Novelty (RAVEN) platform. Targeting both T and B cells, RAVEN-generated vaccines provide a wider, more dependable, and variant-agnostic vaccine solution, even for viruses that have shown resistance to prior vaccination attempts. They also support long-lasting humoral and cellular responses. RAVEN antigens include peptides, proteins, mRNA, and DNA.

In a phase 2 study, EVX-01, a liposomal/peptide immunotherapy, is being used in conjunction with pembrolizumab (Keytruda) (NCT05309421), a PD-1 inhibitor manufactured by Merck & Co., to treat patients with metastatic or unresectable melanoma who have not yet responded to checkpoint inhibitors. Patients demonstrated a higher response rate in phase 1 trials compared to historical controls. For this continuing collaboration, pembrolizumab is supplied by Merck & Co., which is referred to as MSD outside of North America.

Phase 1/2a clinical studies are now ongoing for EVX-02 (NCT04455503), a personalized DNA therapeutic vaccine for adjuvant melanoma that targets resected disease. The vaccine was well-tolerated, and interim results revealed T-cell responses in every patient, supporting the DNA-delivery technology's proof of mechanism. A further discovery is that, in preclinical models, EVX-03, a targeted DNA therapeutic vaccine optimized with an antigen-presenting cell (APC)-targeting unit, has shown tumor shrinkage at low doses and a distinct dose response. APCs are the immune system's main components, which include B cells, dendritic cells, and macrophages. Using MHC molecules, APCs process and present antigens (such as peptides derived from tumors or neoantigens) on their surfaces, activating T cells and leading to adaptive immunity. By adding an APC-targeting component, EVX-03 improves the efficiency of T-cell activation and boosts the overall antitumor immune response by directly delivering tumor-specific antigens to these immune sentinels. Since the tumor microenvironment is typically immunosuppressive, improved immunogenicity is particularly crucial in non-small-cell lung cancer, which is the focus of EVX-03's clinical development.

The findings of a collaborative preclinical research study between Evaxion and Pantherna Therapeutics, which examined the delivery of tumor neoantigens discovered by Evaxion's PIONEER platform utilizing Pantherna's lipid-nanoparticle mRNA technology, were recently reported. The results of this collaboration included complete inhibition of tumor development and a robust immune response. Endogenous retroviruses, often known as ERVs, are patient-specific viral targets. Throughout development, ERVs are remnants of extinct viral infections that have been integrated into the human genome. Certain ERVs are patient-specific viral targets for immunotherapy. Due to their propensity to become aberrantly expressed in cancer cells, they are typically dormant. The company's newest cancer AI platform, ObsERV, will discover these targets and create a new target pool for personalized cancer vaccines. Offering a unique treatment paradigm for malignancies that often do not respond well to immunotherapy is the aim of this approach.

Transgene, which is working with Nippon Electric Company (NEC) Corporation to develop a personalized therapeutic cancer vaccine, is another company that is employing AI. Transgene is using viral vectors instead of mRNA vaccines to teach patients' immune systems to defend against certain cancer targets. Presented at American Association for Cancer Research (AACR) 2024, the encouraging TG4050 Phase I findings demonstrated robust immunogenicity, a sustained cellular immune response, and indications of therapeutic benefit for patients. Only those in the control arm suffered a recurrence; all patients who received TG4050 were disease-free at the time of analysis. Due to these positive findings, Transgene and its partner, NEC, have decided to move forward with a Phase II extension of the randomized study. The Phase II NCT04183166 (Frankart et al., 2022) study aims to further explore the use of single-agent TG4050 in the adjuvant context after surgery and chemoradiotherapy for patients with recently diagnosed, locoregionally progressed, HPV-negative squamous cell carcinoma of the head and neck (SCCHN). A substantial medical need still exists for these patients, even in the adjuvant context, despite modest progress in the treatment of SCCHN. After surgery and adjuvant treatment, 30% to 40% of patients are predicted to relapse within 24 months under the current standard of care. Immune checkpoint drugs have not shown significant benefit for these individuals, despite completing Phase III trials. As an adjuvant therapy for head and neck cancer, TG4050 is the only personalized neoantigen cancer vaccine that is presently being studied in a randomized study.

11 Limitations and challenges of AI in personalized medicine

In the realm of personalized treatment, the integration of AI shows significant promise but is accompanied by numerous limitations and challenges that require careful consideration. Although AI advancements have achieved success in enabling high-quality data production, reducing the time and cost involved, and impacting the drug discovery process, several challenges remain unsolved. One of the main challenges is that AI methods tend to be "black boxes" due to the lack of transparency in how such models arrive at their conclusions (Chan et al., 2019). A basic challenge is the quality and diversity of data used for AI-based analysis. Since the quality and size of these datasets directly affect the performance and reliability of AI models, issues such as overfitting and the need for large datasets are significant. Although EHR and genomic information are useful, their heterogeneity may introduce bias and restrict the generalizability of AI models. Moreover, most database data is not publicly available and must be paid for. The transparency and interpretability of AI algorithms remain a concern, especially in interpreting clinical outcomes and data.

The absence of uniform protocols and regulatory guidelines for AI-powered interventions is a regulatory and ethical concern, particularly in terms of data privacy, patient consent, and security (Selvaraj et al., 2022). The integrity of AI-created data, the need for skilled human resources to deploy AI, financial constraints, and the challenge of choosing a model and framework from multiple AI options are some of the additional challenges (Tripathi et al., 2021). One other challenge experienced is the decision regarding the model and framework, as there are many frameworks, especially DL ones, being created, which require selecting them very cautiously according to the specific task demands. Another issue faced by AI/ML-based platforms in developing end-to-end drug discovery systems is the skewed nature of data toward popular targets, leaving many potential targets unexplored and hindering the overall drug target identification process. These limitations can be addressed through an integrated effort to elevate the quality of the data, ensure regulatory supervision, enhance the transparency of algorithms, and promote fair access to healthcare resources. This will maximize the potential of

AI to improve patient outcomes within personalized medicine as well as in treatment plans.

12 Discussion

AI is transforming healthcare by improving the understanding of diseases that involve various biological pathways and molecular interactions. AI-based algorithms can efficiently analyze vast datasets, including genomic information, patient records, and synthetic lethality data, to uncover synergistic combinations of targets and mechanisms that could lead to more effective therapies (Alowais et al., 2023). In the context of personalized medicine, conventional wet lab experiments, including models like in vitro and in vivo, are costly and also require a lot of time and resources. However, when combined with these conventional methods, AI models can significantly accelerate the discovery process with fewer limitations. These AI-driven approaches, particularly DL, have already shown promising results across various diseases, offering new hope for more personalized and effective treatments.

Precision medicine has significantly impacted healthcare, particularly through genotype-guided treatment. Clinicians now use genetic information to tailor drug therapies, such as determining the correct dose of warfarin based on a patient's genotype. To help clinicians optimize treatment with genetic test results, the Clinical Pharmacogenetics Implementation Consortium has even released genotype-based drug guidelines. Furthermore, developing tailored treatment regimens for patients with diseases like lung cancer, breast cancer, and cardiovascular disorders relies heavily on genomic profiling (Marques et al., 2024; Ingelman-Sundberg and Pirmohamed, 2024)

AI in personalized medicine has the potential to completely transform the way healthcare is delivered. To fully realize this potential, future research should focus on developing AI algorithms that are more precise and effective, improving the quality of data and accessibility, and addressing privacy and ethical concerns. If these challenges are overcome, AI could significantly enhance patient outcomes and the overall quality of healthcare. In this field, IBM Watson (https://developer.ibm.com/articles/introduction-to-watson-natural-language-processing/system) stands out as a pioneer. With its integrated ML and natural language processing modules, Watson has shown remarkable outcomes in oncology, with 99% of its therapy suggestions aligning with medical conclusions. Furthermore, Watson has partnered with Quest Diagnostics to offer AI-driven genetic diagnostic analysis, further demonstrating its potential in personalized medicine. More recent DL-based architectures, such as NNs like recurrent NNs, generative adversarial networks, and techniques like transfer learning, have received more recognition than traditional ML methods. These models have been applied to a variety of healthcare applications, including aging research, de novo small-molecule design, and pharmacological drug prediction based on the transcriptional data of drug-perturbed cell lines (Bajwa et al., 2021).

This chapter delves into the growing influence of DL algorithms at different stages of disease therapy. In the past two years, AI has revolutionized this process by offering benchmark datasets and a combination of innovative algorithms. We believe that the AI and ML integration, specifically DL models, will be instrumental in unraveling complex diseases and their biological pathways and interactions, enabling the identification of novel treatment strategies. An overview of fundamental AI algorithms, concepts, and applications in biomarker identification and personalized medicine is discussed in this chapter. It addresses key techniques and emerging applications for AI-based pipelines, tools, and algorithms. Readers will gain insight into the diverse applications of AI for enhancing personalized treatment through various success stories and case studies. Along with discussing the challenges and limitations of AI, the chapter also explores the challenges and scenarios in clinical research. It shows how employing advanced AI algorithms can help advance clinical research. It compares different algorithms and assesses their results, providing insights into potential future advancements.

References

Ahmad, A., Imran, M., Ahsan, H., 2023. Biomarkers as biomedical bioindicators: approaches and techniques for the detection, analysis, and validation of novel biomarkers of diseases. Pharmaceutics. 1999-4923. 15 (6), 1630. doi:10.3390/pharmaceutics15061630.

Ahmed, H., Hamad, S., Shedeed, H.A., Hussein, A.S., 2022. Enhanced deep learning model for personalized cancer treatment. IEEE Access. 2169-3536. 10, 106050–106058. Available from: http://ieeexplore.ieee.org/xpl/RecentIssue.jsp?punumber=6287639. doi:10.1109/ACCESS.2022.3209285.

Alam, M.Z., Rahman, M.S., Rahman, M.S., 2019. A random forest based predictor for medical data classification using feature ranking. Inform. Med. Unlocked. 2352-9148. 15, 100180. doi:10.1016/j.imu.2019.100180.

Allioui, H., Mohammed, M.A., Benameur, N., Al-Khateeb, B., Abdulkareem, K.H., Garcia-Zapirain, B., Damaševičius, R., Maskeliūnas, R., 2022. A multi-agent deep reinforcement learning approach for enhancement of COVID-19 CT image segmentation. J. Pers. Med. 2075-4426. 12 (2). Available from: https://www.mdpi.com/2075-4426/12/2/309/pdf. doi:10.3390/jpm12020309.

Alowais, S.A., Alghamdi, S.S., Alsuhebany, N., Alqahtani, T., Alshaya, A.I., Almohareb, S.N., Aldairem, A., Alrashed, M., Saleh, K.B., Badreldin, H.A., Yami, M.S.A., Harbi, S.A., Albekairy, A.M., 2023. Revolutionizing healthcare: the role of artificial intelligence in clinical practice. BMC Med. Educ. 1472-6920. 23 (1). Available from: https://bmcmededuc.biomedcentral.com/. doi:10.1186/s12909-023-04698-z.

Argelaguet, R., Arnol, D., Bredikhin, D., Deloro, Y., Velten, B., Marioni, J.C., Stegle, O., 2020. MOFA+: a statistical framework for comprehensive integration of multi-modal single-cell data. Genome Biol 21 (1). doi:10.1186/s13059-020-02015-1.

Bajwa, J., Munir, U., Nori, A., Williams, B., 2021. Artificial intelligence in healthcare: transforming the practice of medicine. Future Healthc. J. 2514-6645. 8 (2), e188. doi:10.7861/fhj.2021-0095.

Banerjee, A., Chakraborty, C., Kumar, A., Biswas, D., 2019. Emerging trends in IoT and big data analytics for biomedical and health care technologies. In: Handbook of Data Science Approaches for Biomedical Engineering. Elsevier, Singapore, pp. 121–152. Available from: http://www.sciencedirect.com/science/book/9780128183182. doi:10.1016/B978-0-12-818318-2.00005-2.

Bejnordi, B.E., Veta, M., van Diest, P.J., van Ginneken, B., Karssemeijer, N., Litjens, G., van der Laak, J.A.W.M., Hermsen, M., Manson, Q.F., Balkenhol, M., Geessink, O., Stathonikos, N., van Dijk, M.C.R.F., Bult, P., Beca, F., Beck, A.H., Wang, D., Khosla, A., Gargeya, R., Irshad, H., Zhong, A., Dou, Q., Quanzheng, L., Chen, H., Lin, H.-J., Heng, P.-A., Haß, C., Bruni, E., Wong, Q., Halici, U., Ümit Öner, M., Cetin-Atalay, R., Berseth, M., Khvatkov, V., Vylegzhanin, A., Kraus, O., Shaban, M., Rajpoot, N., Awan, R., Sirinukunwattana, K., Qaiser, T., Tsang, Y.-W., Tellez, D., Annuscheit, J., Hufnagl, P., Valkonen, M., Kartasalo, K., Latonen, L., Ruusuvuori, P., Liimatainen, K., Albarqouni, S., Mungal, B., George, A., Demirci, S., Navab, N., Watanabe, S., Seno, S., Takenaka, Y., Matsuda, H., Phoulady, H.A., Kovalev, V., Kalinovsky, A., Liauchuk, V., Bueno, G., Milagro Fernandez-Carrobles, M., Serrano, I., Deniz, O., Racoceanu, D., Venâncio, R., 2017. Diagnostic assessment of deep learning algorithms for detection of lymph node metastases in women with breast cancer. JAMA. 0098-7484. 318 (22), 2199. doi:10.1001/jama.2017.14585.

Bergstrom, E.N., Abbasi, A., Díaz-Gay, M., Galland, L., Ladoire, S., Lippman, S.M., Alexandrov, L.B., 2024. Deep learning artificial intelligence predicts homologous recombination deficiency and Platinum response from histologic slides. J. Clin. Oncol. 1527-7755. Available from: https://ascopubs.org/loi/jco. doi:10.1200/JCO.23.02641.

Bibault, J.-E., Giraud, P., Housset, M., Durdux, C., Taieb, J., Berger, A., Coriat, R., Chaussade, S., Dousset, B., Nordlinger, B., Burgun, A., 2018. Deep learning and radiomics predict complete response after neo-adjuvant chemoradiation for locally advanced rectal cancer. Sci. Rep. 2045-2322. 8 (1). doi:10.1038/s41598-018-30657-6.

Boniolo, F., Dorigatti, E., Ohnmacht, A.J., Saur, D., Schubert, B., Menden, M.P., 2021. Artificial intelligence in early drug discovery enabling precision medicine. Expert Opin. Drug Discov. 1746-045X. 16 (9), 991–1007. Available from: https://www.tandfonline.com/loi/iedc20. doi:10.1080/17460441.2021.1918096.

Borzouei, S., Soltanian, A.R., 2018. Application of an artificial neural network model for diagnosing type 2 diabetes mellitus and determining the relative importance of risk factors. Epidemiol. Health. 2092-7193. 40 (40), e2018007. doi:10.4178/epih.e2018007.

Cai, Z., Poulos, R.C., Liu, J., Zhong, Q., 2022. Machine learning for multi-omics data integration in cancer. iScience. 2589-0042. 25 (2), 103798. doi:10.1016/j.isci.2022.103798.

Cardoso, F., Van't Veer, L.J., Bogaerts, J., Slaets, L., Viale, G., Delaloge, S., Pierga, J.Y., Brain, E., Causeret, S., DeLorenzi, M., Glas, A.M., Golfinopoulos, V., Goulioti, T., Knox, S., Matos, E., Meulemans, B., Neijenhuis, P.A., Nitz, U., Passalacqua, R., Ravdin, P., Rubio, I.T., Saghatchian, M., Smilde, T.J., Sotiriou, C., Stork, L., Straehle, C., Thomas, G., Thompson, A.M., Hoeven, J.M.V.D., Vuylsteke, P., Bernards, R., Tryfonidis, K., Rutgers, E., Piccart, M., 2016. 70-gene signature as an aid to treatment decisions in early-stage breast cancer. N. Engl. J. Med. 1533-4406. 375 (8), 717–729. Available from: http://www.nejm.org/doi/pdf/10.1056/NEJMoa1602253.

doi:10.1056/NEJMoa1602253.
Cardoso,, Parro, C., Peres, V., Curado, S., Fernandes, M.P., Filho, G.A.W., et al., 2023. Machine learning for predicting survival of colorectal cancer patients. Sci. Rep. 13, 8874.
Carrillo-Perez, F., Morales, J.C., Castillo-Secilla, D., Gevaert, O., Rojas, I., Herrera, L.J., 2022. Machine-learning-based late fusion on multi-omics and multi-scale data for non-small-cell lung cancer diagnosis. J. Pers. Med. 2075-4426. 12 (4). Available from: https://www.mdpi.com/2075-4426/12/4/601/pdf. doi:10.3390/jpm12040601.
Cernea, A., Fernández-Martínez, J.L., Deandrés-Galiana, E.J., Fernández-Ovies, F.J., Alvarez-Machancoses, O., Fernández-Muñiz, Z., Saligan, L.N., Sonis, S.T., 2020. Robust pathway sampling in phenotype prediction. Application to triple negative breast cancer. BMC Bioinformatics. 1471-2105. 21. Available from: https://bmcbioinformatics.biomedcentral.com/. doi:10.1186/s12859-020-3356-6.
Chan, H.C.S., Shan, H., Dahoun, T., Vogel, H., Yuan, S., 2019. Advancing drug discovery via artificial intelligence. Trends Pharmacol. Sci. 1873-3735. 40 (8), 592–604. Available from: https://www.elsevier.com/locate/tips. doi:10.1016/j.tips.2019.06.004.
Chen, G., Shen, Z., Iyer, A., Ghumman, U.F., Tang, S., Bi, J., Chen, W., Li, Y., 2020. Machine-learning-assisted de novo design of organic molecules and polymers: opportunities and challenges. Polymers. 2073-4360. 12 (1). Available from: https://res.mdpi.com/d_attachment/polymers/polymers-12-00163/article_deploy/polymers-12-00163-v2.pdf. doi:10.3390/polym12010163.
Chen, X., Yang, J., Lu, Z., Ding, Y., 2022. A 70-RNA model based on SVR and RFE for predicting the pancreatic cancer clinical prognosis. Methods. 1095-9130. 204, 278–285. Available from: http://www.elsevier.com/inca/publications/store/6/2/2/9/1/4/index.htt. doi:10.1016/j.ymeth.2022.02.011.
Cheng, D.C., Hsieh, T.C., Hsu, Y.J., Lai, Y.C., Yen, K.Y., Wang, C.C.N., Kao, C.H., 2022. Prediction of all-cause mortality based on stress/rest myocardial perfusion imaging (MPI) using deep learning: a comparison between image and frequency spectra as input. J. Pers. Med. 2075-4426. 12 (7). Available from: https://www.mdpi.com/2075-4426/12/7/1105/pdf?version=1657015913. doi:10.3390/jpm12071105.
Choudhary, R., Tyagi, S., Goyal, H., Prasad, Y., Tyagi, A., Choudhury, T., 2023. Comparative analysis of heart disease prediction using machine learning algorithms. In: Algorithms for Intelligent Systems. Springer Science and Business Media LLC, pp. 297–308. doi:10.1007/978-981-99-1620-7_23.
Cirillo, D., Valencia, A., 2019. Big data analytics for personalized medicine. Curr. Opin. Biotechnol. 0958-1669. 58, 161–167. doi:10.1016/j.copbio.2019.03.004.
Das, S., Dey, M.K., Devireddy, R., Gartia, M.R., 2024. Biomarkers in cancer detection, diagnosis, and prognosis. Sensors. 1424-8220. 24 (1), 37. doi:10.3390/s24010037.
DeGroat, W., Mendhe, D., Bhusari, A., Abdelhalim, H., Zeeshan, S., Ahmed, Z., Martelli, P.L., 2023. IntelliGenes: a novel machine learning pipeline for biomarker discovery and predictive analysis using multi-genomic profiles. Bioinformatics. 1367-4811. 39 (12). doi:10.1093/bioinformatics/btad755.
Ding, Y., Sohn, J.H., Kawczynski, M.G., Trivedi, H., Harnish, R., Jenkins, N.W., Lituiev, D., Copeland, T.P., Aboian, M.S., Aparici, C.M., Behr, S.C., Flavell, R.R., Huang, S.Y., Zalocusky, K.A., Nardo, L., Seo, Y., Hawkins, R.A., Pampaloni, M.H., Hadley, D., Franc, B.L., 2019. A deep learning model to predict a diagnosis of Alzheimer disease by using 18 F-FDG PET of the brain. Radiology. 1527-1315. 290 (3), 456–464. Available from: https://pubs.rsna.org/doi/pdf/10.1148/radiol.2018181224. doi:10.1148/radiol.2018180958.
Dorsey, E.R., Omberg, L., Waddell, E., Adams, J.L., Adams, R., Ali, M.R., Amodeo, K., Arky, A., Augustine, E.F., DInesh, K., Hoque, M.E., Glidden, A.M., Jensen-Roberts, S., Kabelac, Z., Katabi, D., Kieburtz, K., Kinel, D.R., Little, M.A., Lizarraga, K.J.,

Myers, T., Riggare, S., Rosero, S.Z., Saria, S., Schifitto, G., Schneider, R.B., Sharma, G., Shoulson, I., Stevenson, E.A., Tarolli, C.G., Luo, J., McDermott, M.P., 2020. Deep phenotyping of Parkinson's disease. J. Parkinsons Dis. 1877-718X. 10 (3), 855–873. Available from: http://www.iospress.nl/journal/journal-of-parkinsons-disease/. doi:10.3233/JPD-202006.

Eraslan, G., Avsec, Ž., Gagneur, J., Theis, F.J., 2019. Deep learning: new computational modelling techniques for genomics. Nat. Rev. Genet. 1471-0064. 20 (7), 389–403. Available from: http://www.nature.com/reviews/genetics. doi:10.1038/s41576-019-0122-6.

Esteva, A., Kuprel, B., Novoa, R.A., Ko, J., Swetter, S.M., Blau, H.M., Thrun, S., 2017. Dermatologist-level classification of skin cancer with deep neural networks. Nature. 1476-4687. 542 (7639), 115–118. Available from: http://www.nature.com/nature/index.html. doi:10.1038/nature21056.

Feng, Q., Dueva, E., Cherkasov, A., Ester, M., 2018. PADME: a deep learning-based framework for drug-target interaction prediction. arXiv. 2331-8422. Available from: https://arxiv.org. doi:10.48550/arxiv.1807.09741.

Frankart, A.J., Sadraei, N.H., Huth, B., Redmond, K.P., Barrett, W.L., Kurtzweil, N., Riaz, M.K., Wise-Draper, T., Rodriguez, C.P., Adelstein, D.J., Takiar, V., 2022. A phase I/II trial of concurrent immunotherapy with chemoradiation in locally advanced larynx cancer. Laryngoscope Investig. Otolaryngol. 2378-8038. 7 (2), 437–443. Available from: https://onlinelibrary.wiley.com/loi/23788038. doi:10.1002/lio2.780.

Fröhlich, H., Balling, R., Beerenwinkel, N., Kohlbacher, O., Kumar, S., Lengauer, T., Maathuis, M.H., Moreau, Y., Murphy, S.A., Przytycka, T.M., Rebhan, M., Röst, H., Schuppert, A., Schwab, M., Spang, R., Stekhoven, D., Sun, J., Weber, A., Ziemek, D., Zupan, B., 2018. From hype to reality: data science enabling personalized medicine. BMC Med. 1741-7015. 16 (1). Available from: http://www.biomedcentral.com/bmcmed/. doi:10.1186/s12916-018-1122-7.

Garnett, M.J., Edelman, E.J., Heidorn, S.J., Greenman, C.D., Dastur, A., Lau, K.W., Greninger, P., Thompson, I.R., Luo, X., Soares, J., Liu, Q., Iorio, F., Surdez, D., Chen, L., Milano, R.J., Bignell, G.R., Tam, A.T., Davies, H., Stevenson, J.A., Barthorpe, S., Lutz, S.R., Kogera, F., Lawrence, K., McLaren-Douglas, A., Mitropoulos, X., Mironenko, T., Thi, H., Richardson, L., Zhou, W., Jewitt, F., Zhang, T., O'Brien, P., Boisvert, J.L., Price, S., Hur, W., Yang, W., Deng, X., Butler, A., Choi, H.G., Chang, J.W., Baselga, J., Stamenkovic, I., Engelman, J.A., Sharma, S.V., Delattre, O., Saez-Rodriguez, J., Gray, N.S., Settleman, J., Futreal, P.A., Haber, D.A., Stratton, M.R., Ramaswamy, S., McDermott, U., Benes, C.H., 2012. Systematic identification of genomic markers of drug sensitivity in cancer cells. Nature. 1476-4687. 483 (7391), 570–575. doi:10.1038/nature11005.

Garraway, L.A., Verweij, J., Ballman, K.V., 2013. Precision oncology: an overview. J. Clin. Oncol. 1527-7755. 31 (15), 1803–1805. Available from: http://jco.ascopubs.org/content/31/15/1803.full.pdf+html. doi:10.1200/JCO.2013.49.4799.

Gayvert, K.M., Madhukar, N.S., Elemento, O., 2016. A data-driven approach to predicting successes and failures of clinical trials. Cell Chem. Biol. 2451-9448. 23 (10), 1294–1301. doi:10.1016/j.chembiol.2016.07.023.

Guinney, J., Dienstmann, R., Wang, X., De Reyniès, A., Schlicker, A., Soneson, C., Marisa, L., Roepman, P., Nyamundanda, G., Angelino, P., Bot, B.M., Morris, J.S., Simon, I.M., Gerster, S., Fessler, E., Sousa, F.D., Melo, E., Missiaglia, E., Ramay, H., Barras, D., Homicsko, K., Maru, D., Manyam, G.C., Broom, B., Boige, V., Perez-Villamil, B., Laderas, T., Salazar, R., Gray, J.W., Hanahan, D., Tabernero, J., Bernards, R., Friend, S.H., Laurent-Puig, P., Medema, J.P., Sadanandam, A., Wessels, L., Delorenzi, M., Kopetz, S., Vermeulen, L., Tejpar, S., 2015. The consensus molecular subtypes of colorectal cancer. Nat. Med. 1546-170X. 21 (11), 1350–1356. Available from: http://www.nature.com/nm/index.html. doi:10.1038/nm.3967.

Hampel, H., Williams, C., Etcheto, A., Goodsaid, F., Parmentier, F., Sallantin, J., Kaufmann, W.E., Missling, C.U., Afshar, M., 2020. A precision medicine framework using artificial intelligence for the identification and confirmation of genomic biomarkers of response to an Alzheimer's disease therapy: analysis of the blarcamesine (ANAVEX2-73) phase 2a clinical study. Alzheimers Dement. Transl. Res. Clin. Interv. 2352-8737. 6 (1). Available from: https://alz-journals.onlinelibrary.wiley.com/doi/full/10.1016/j.trci.2015.06.002. doi:10.1002/trc2.12013.

Hassan, M., Awan, F.M., Naz, A., Deandrés-Galiana, E.J., Alvarez, O., Cernea, A., Fernández-Brillet, L., Fernández-Martínez, J.L., Kloczkowski, A., 2022. Innovations in genomics and big data analytics for personalized medicine and health care: a review. Int. J. Mol. Sci. 1422-0067. 23 (9). Available from: https://www.mdpi.com/1422-0067/23/9/4645/pdf. doi:10.3390/ijms23094645.

Huang, B., Huang, H., Zhang, S., Zhang, D., Shi, Q., Liu, J., Guo, J., 2022. Artificial intelligence in pancreatic cancer. Theranostics. 1838-7640. 12 (16), 6931–6954. doi:10.7150/thno.77949.

Huang, C., Mezencev, R., McDonald, J.F., Vannberg, F., Liu, B., 2017. Open source machine-learning algorithms for the prediction of optimal cancer drug therapies. PLoS ONE. 1932-6203. 12 (10), e0186906. doi:10.1371/journal.pone.0186906.

Huang, J., Li, B., Wei, H., Li, C., Liu, C., Mi, H., Chen, S., 2024. Integrative analysis of gene expression profiles of substantia nigra identifies potential diagnosis biomarkers in Parkinson's disease. Sci. Rep. 2045-2322. 14 (1). doi:10.1038/s41598-024-52276-0.

Huang, S., Cai, N., Penzuti Pacheco, P., Narrandes, S., Wang, Y., Xu, W. , 2018. Applications of support vector machine (SVM) learning in cancer genomics. Cancer Genom. Proteom. 15 (1), 41–51. doi:10.21873/cgp.20063.

Hussein, M.A., Majumder, M.Z.H., 2023. Chronic kidney disease prediction based on machine learning algorithms. J. Pathol. Inform., 14, 100189.

Imrie, F., Cebere, B., McKinney, E.F., van der Schaar, M., Guillot, G., 2023. AutoPrognosis 2.0: democratizing diagnostic and prognostic modeling in healthcare with automated machine learning. PLOS Digit. Health. 2767-3170. 2 (6), e0000276. doi:10.1371/journal.pdig.0000276.

Ingelman-Sundberg, M., Pirmohamed, M., 2024. Precision medicine in cardiovascular therapeutics: evaluating the role of pharmacogenetic analysis prior to drug treatment. J. Intern. Med. 0954-6820. 295 (5), 583–598. doi:10.1111/joim.13772.

Ji, G.W., Jiao, C.Y., Xu, Z.G., Li, X.C., Wang, K., Wang, X.H., 2022. Development and validation of a gradient boosting machine to predict prognosis after liver resection for intrahepatic cholangiocarcinoma. BMC Cancer. 1471-2407. 22 (1). Available from: https://bmccancer.biomedcentral.com/. doi:10.1186/s12885-022-09352-3.

Jiang, L., Xu, C., Bai, Y., Liu, A., Gong, Y., Wang, Y.P., Deng, H.W., 2024. Autosurv: interpretable deep learning framework for cancer survival analysis incorporating clinical and multi-omics data. Npj Precis. Oncol. 2397-768X. 8 (1). Available from: https://www.nature.com/npjprecisiononcology/. doi:10.1038/s41698-023-00494-6.

Jones-Davis, D.M., Buckholtz, N., 2015. The impact of the Alzheimer's disease neuroimaging initiative 2: what role do public-private partnerships have in pushing the boundaries of clinical and basic science research on Alzheimer's disease?. Alzheimers Dement. 1552-5260. 11 (7), 860–864. doi:10.1016/j.jalz.2015.05.006.

Jung, H.C., Kim, C., Oh, J., Kim, T.H., Kim, B., Lee, J., Chung, J.H., Byun, H., Yoon, M.S., Lee, D.K., 2022. Position classification of the endotracheal tube with automatic segmentation of the trachea and the tube on plain chest radiography using deep convolutional neural network. J. Pers. Med. 2075-4426. 12 (9), 1363. doi:10.3390/jpm12091363.

Kamya, P., Ozerov, I.V., Pun, F.W., Tretina, K., Fokina, T., Chen, S., Naumov, V., Long, X., Lin, S., Korzinkin, M., Polykovskiy, D., Aliper, A., Ren, F., Zhavoronkov, A., 2024. PandaOmics: an AI-driven platform for therapeutic target and biomarker discovery. J. Chem. Inf. Model. 1549-960X. 64 (10), 3961–3969. Available from: http://pubs.acs.org/journal/jcisd8. doi:10.1021/acs.jcim.3c01619.

Katiyar, N., Thakur, H.K., Ghatak, A., 2024. Recent advancements using machine learning & deep learning approaches for diabetes detection: a systematic review. e-Prime—Adv. Electr. Eng., Electron. Energy. 2772-6711. 9, 100661. doi:10.1016/j.prime.2024.100661.

Kaushik, A.C., Mehmood, A., Wang, X., Wei, D.Q., Dai, X., 2021. Globally ncRNAs expression profiling of TNBC and screening of functional lncRNA. Front. Bioeng. Biotechnol. 2296-4185. 8. Available from: http://journal.frontiersin.org/journal/bioengineering-and-biotechnology#archive. doi:10.3389/fbioe.2020.523127.

Kaushik, A.C., Mehmood, A., Wei, D.Q., Dai, X., 2020. Robust biomarker screening using spares learning approach for liver cancer prognosis. Front. Bioeng. Biotechnol. 2296-4185. 8. Available from: http://journal.frontiersin.org/journal/bioengineering-and-biotechnology#archive. doi:10.3389/fbioe.2020.00241.

Kaushik, A.C., Zhao, Z., 2023. Machine learning-driven exploration of drug therapies for triple-negative breast cancer treatment. Front. Mol. Biosci. 2296-889X. 10. Available from: https://journal.frontiersin.org/journal/molecular-biosciences. doi:10.3389/fmolb.2023.1215204.

Khalifa, M., Albadawy, M., 2024. Artificial intelligence for diabetes: enhancing prevention, diagnosis, and effective management. Comput. Methods Programs Biomed. Update. 2666-9900. 5, 100141. doi:10.1016/j.cmpbup.2024.100141.

Komorowski, M., Celi, L.A., Badawi, O., Gordon, A.C., Faisal, A.A., 2018. The artificial intelligence clinician learns optimal treatment strategies for sepsis in intensive care. Nat. Med. 1546-170X. 24 (11), 1716–1720. Available from: http://www.nature.com/nm/index.html. doi:10.1038/s41591-018-0213-5.

Krishnan, G., Singh, S., Pathania, M., Gosavi, S., Abhishek, S., Parchani, A., Dhar, M., 2023. Artificial intelligence in clinical medicine: catalyzing a sustainable global healthcare paradigm. Front. Artif. Intell. 2624-8212. 6. doi:10.3389/frai.2023.1227091.

Kuenzi, B.M., Park, J., Fong, S.H., Sanchez K.S., Lee, J., Kreisberg, J.F., Ma, J., Ideker, T., 2020. Predicting drug response and synergy using a deep learning model of human cancer cells. Cancer Cell 38 (5), 672–684.e6. doi:10.1016/j.ccell.2020.09.014.

Kuenzi, B.M., Park, J., Fong, S.H., Sanchez, K.S., Lee, J., Kreisberg, J.F., Ma, J., Ideker, T., 2020. Predicting drug response and synergy using a deep learning model of human cancer cells. Cancer Cell. 1878-3686. 38 (5), 672. Available from: https://www.journals.elsevier.com/cancer-cell. doi:10.1016/j.ccell.2020.09.014.

Lee, C.H., Huh, J., Buckley, P.R., Jang, M., Pinho, M.P., Fernandes, R.A., Antanaviciute, A., Simmons, A., Koohy, H., 2022. A robust deep learning platform to predict CD8+ T-cell epitopes. bioRxiv. 2692-8205. Available from: https://www.biorxiv.org. doi:10.1101/2022.12.29.522182.

Leff, D.R., Yang, G.Z., 2015. Big data for precision medicine. Engineering. 2095-8099. 1 (3), 277–279. Available from: http://www.journals.elsevier.com/engineering/. doi:10.15302/J-ENG-2015075.

Lian, J., Luo, X., Shan, C., Han, D., Vardhanabhuti, V., Li, D., 2023. AdaMedGraph: adaboosting graph neural networks for personalized medicine. arXiv. 2331-8422. Available from: https://arxiv.org. doi:10.48550/arXiv.2311.14304.

Lind, A.P., Anderson, P.C., Olier, I., 2019. Predicting drug activity against cancer cells by random forest models based on minimal genomic information and chemical properties. PLoS ONE. 1932-6203. 14 (7), e0219774. doi:10.1371/journal.pone.0219774.

Litjens, G., Kooi, T., Bejnordi, B.E., Setio, A.A.A., Ciompi, F., Ghafoorian, M., van der Laak, J.A.W.M., van Ginneken, B., Sánchez, C.I., 2017. A survey on deep learning in medical image analysis. Med. Image Anal. 1361-8423. 42, 60–88. Available from: http://www.elsevier.com/inca/publications/store/6/2/0/9/8/3/index.htt. doi:10.1016/j.media.2017.07.005.

López-Martínez, F., Núñez-Valdez, E.R., García-Díaz, V., Bursac, Z., 2020. A case study for a big data and machine learning platform to improve medical decision support in population health management. Algorithms. 1999-4893. 13 (4), 102. doi:10.3390/a13040102.

Makarious, M.B., Leonard, H.L., Vitale, D., Iwaki, H., Saffo, D., Sargent, L., et al, , 2021. GenoML: Automated Machine Learning for Genomics. doi:10.48550/arXiv.2103.03221.

Malash, I., Mansour, O., Shaarawy, S., Abdellateif, M., Omar, A., Gaafer, R., Zekri, A.-R., Ahmed, O., Bahnassy, A., 2020. The role of CYP2D6 polymorphisms in determining response to tamoxifen in metastatic breast cancer patients: review and Egyptian experience. Asian Pac. J. Cancer Prev. 2476-762X. 21 (12), 3619–3625. doi:10.31557/apjcp.2020.21.12.3619.

Marek, K., Chowdhury, S., Siderowf, A., Lasch, S., Coffey, C.S., Caspell-Garcia, C., Simuni, T., Jennings, D., Tanner, C.M., Trojanowski, J.Q., Shaw, L.M., Seibyl, J., Schuff, N., Singleton, A., Kieburtz, K., Toga, A.W., Mollenhauer, B., Galasko, D., Chahine, L.M., Weintraub, D., Foroud, T., Tosun-Turgut, D., Poston, K., Arnedo, V., Frasier, M., Sherer, T., 2018. The Parkinson's progression markers initiative (PPMI) - establishing a PD biomarker cohort. Ann. Clin. Transl. Neurol. 2328-9503. 5 (12), 1460–1477. doi:10.1002/acn3.644.

Marques, L., Costa, B., Pereira, M., Silva, A., Santos, J., Saldanha, L., Silva, I., Magalhães, P., Schmidt, S., Vale, N., 2024. Advancing precision medicine: a review of innovative in silico approaches for drug development. Clin. Pharmacol. Pers. Healthc. Pharmaceutics. 1999-4923. 16 (3), 332. doi:10.3390/pharmaceutics16030332.

Menden, M.P., Iorio, F., Garnett, M., McDermott, U., Benes, C.H., Ballester, P.J., Saez-Rodriguez, J., 2013. Machine learning prediction of cancer cell sensitivity to drugs based on genomic and chemical properties. PLoS ONE. 1932-6203. 8 (4). Available from: http://www.plosone.org/article/fetchObjectAttachment.action?uri=info%3Adoi%2F10.1371%2Fjournal.pone.0061318&representation=PDF. doi:10.1371/journal.pone.0061318.

Mohsen, F., Al-Absi, H.R.H., Yousri, N.A., Hajj, N.E., Shah, Z., 2023. A scoping review of artificial intelligence-based methods for diabetes risk prediction. Npj Digit. Med. 2398-6352. 6 (1). Available from: https://www.nature.com/npjdigitalmed/. doi:10.1038/s41746-023-00933-5.

Mooi, J.K., Wirapati, P., Asher, R., Lee, C.K., Savas, P., Price, T.J., Townsend, A., Hardingham, J., Buchanan, D., Williams, D., Tejpar, S., Mariadason, J.M., Tebbutt, N.C., 2018. The prognostic impact of consensus molecular subtypes (CMS) and its predictive effects for bevacizumab benefit in metastatic colorectal cancer: molecular analysis of the AGITG MAX clinical trial. Ann. Oncol. 1569-8041. 29 (11), 2240–2246. Available from: https://www.journals.elsevier.com/annals-of-oncology. doi:10.1093/annonc/mdy410.

Naito, T., 2019. Predicting the impact of single nucleotide variants on splicing via sequence-based deep neural networks and genomic features. Hum. Mutat. 1059-7794. 40 (9), 1261–1269. doi:10.1002/humu.23794.

Nguyen-Ngoc, T., Bouchaab, H., Adjei, A.A., Peters, S., 2015. BRAF alterations as therapeutic targets in non-small-cell lung cancer. J. Thorac. Oncol. 1556-1380. 10 (10), 1396–1403. Available from: https://www.journals.elsevier.com/journal-of-thoracic-oncology/. doi:10.1097/JTO.0000000000000644.

Oikonomou, E.K., Spatz, E.S., Suchard, M.A., Khera, R., 2022. Individualising intensive systolic blood pressure reduction in hypertension using computational trial phenomaps and machine learning: a post-hoc analysis of randomised clinical trials. Lancet Digit. Health. 2589-7500. 4 (11), e796. Available from: https://www.sciencedirect.com/journal/the-lancet-digital-health. doi:10.1016/S2589-7500(22)00170-4.

Orth, M., Metzger, P., Gerum, S., Mayerle, J., Schneider, G., Belka, C., Schnurr, M., Lauber, K., 2019. Pancreatic ductal adenocarcinoma: biological hallmarks, current status, and future perspectives of combined modality treatment approaches.

Radiat. Oncol. 1748-717X. 14 (1). doi:10.1186/s13014-019-1345-6.
Ott, P.A., Hu, Z., Keskin, D.B., Shukla, S.A., Sun, J., Bozym, D.J., Zhang, W., Luoma, A., Giobbie-Hurder, A., Peter, L., Chen, C., Olive, O., Carter, T.A., Li, S., Lieb, D.J., Eisenhaure, T., Gjini, E., Stevens, J., Lane, W.J., Javeri, I., Nellaiappan, K., Salazar, A.M., Daley, H., Seaman, M., Buchbinder, E.I., Yoon, C.H., Harden, M., Lennon, N., Gabriel, S., Rodig, S.J., Barouch, D.H., Aster, J.C., Getz, G., Wucherpfennig, K., Neuberg, D., Ritz, J., Lander, E.S., Fritsch, E.F., Hacohen, N., Wu, C.J., 2017. An immunogenic personal neoantigen vaccine for patients with melanoma. Nature. 1476-4687. 547 (7662), 217–221. Available from: http://www.nature.com/nature/index.html. doi:10.1038/nature22991.
Öztürk, H., Özgür, A., Ozkirimli, E., 2018. DeepDTA: deep drug-target binding affinity prediction. Bioinformatics. 1460-2059. 34 (17), i821–i829. http://bioinformatics.oxfordjournals.org/. doi:10.1093/bioinformatics/bty593.
Papadakis, G., Karantanas, A., Tsikankis, M., Tsatsakis, A., Spandidos, D., Marias, K., 2019. Deep learning opens new horizons in personalized medicine (Review). Biomed. Rep. 2049-9434. 10 (4). doi:10.3892/br.2019.1199.
Parekh, A.-D.E., Shaikh, O.A., Simran, Manan, S., Hasibuzzaman, M.A., 2023. Artificial intelligence (AI) in personalized medicine: AI-generated personalized therapy regimens based on genetic and medical history: short communication. Ann. Med. Surg. 2049-0801. 85 (11), 5831–5833. doi:10.1097/ms9.0000000000001320.
Paul, D., Sanap, G., Shenoy, S., Kalyane, D., Kalia, K., Tekade, R.K., 2021. Artificial intelligence in drug discovery and development. Drug Discov. Today. 1878-5832. 26 (1), 80–93. Available from: www.elsevier.com/locate/drugdiscov. doi:10.1016/j.drudis.2020.10.010.
Preuer, K., Lewis, R.P.I., Hochreiter, S., Bender, A., Bulusu, K.C., Klambauer, G., 2018. DeepSynergy: predicting anti-cancer drug synergy with deep learning. Bioinformatics. 1460-2059. 34 (9), 1538–1546. Available from: http://bioinformatics.oxfordjournals.org/. doi:10.1093/bioinformatics/btx806.
Purcell, S., Neale, B., Todd-Brown, K., Thomas, L., Ferreira, M.A.R., Bender, D., Maller, J., Sklar, P., De Bakker, P.I.W., Daly, M.J., Sham, P.C., 2007. PLINK: a tool set for whole-genome association and population-based linkage analyses. Am. J. Hum. Genet. 0002-9297. 81 (3), 559–575. Available from: http://www.elsevier.com/wps/find/journaldescription.cws_home/713561/description#description. doi:10.1086/519795.
Qian, L., Lai, X., Gu, B., Sun, X., 2022. An immune-related gene signature for predicting neoadjuvant chemoradiotherapy efficacy in rectal carcinoma. Front. Immunol. 1664-3224. 13. Available from: https://www.frontiersin.org/journals/immunology#. doi:10.3389/fimmu.2022.784479.
Raies, A., Tulodziecka, E., Stainer, J., Middleton, L., Dhindsa, R.S., Hill, P., Engkvist, O., Harper, A.R., Petrovski, S., Vitsios, D., 2022. DrugnomeAI is an ensemble machine-learning framework for predicting druggability of candidate drug targets. Commun. Biol. 2399-3642. 5 (1). Available from: https://www.springer.com/journal/42003. doi:10.1038/s42003-022-04245-4.
Rajkomar, A., Dean, J., Kohane, I., 2019. Machine learning in medicine. N. Engl. J. Med. 0028-4793. 380 (14), 1347–1358. doi:10.1056/nejmra1814259.
Sahin, U., Derhovanessian, E., Miller, M., Kloke, B.P., Simon, P., Löwer, M., Bukur, V., Tadmor, A.D., Luxemburger, U., Schrörs, B., Omokoko, T., Vormehr, M., Albrecht, C., Paruzynski, A., Kuhn, A.N., Buck, J., Heesch, S., Schreeb, K.H., Müller, F., Ortseifer, I., Vogler, I., Godehardt, E., Attig, S., Rae, R., Breitkreuz, A., Tolliver, C., Suchan, M., Martic, G., Hohberger, A., Sorn, P., Diekmann, J., Ciesla, J., Waksmann, O., Brück, A.K., Witt, M., Zillgen, M., Rothermel, A., Kasemann, B., Langer, D., Bolte, S., Diken, M., Kreiter, S., Nemecek, R., Gebhardt, C., Grabbe, S., Höller, C., Utikal, J., Huber, C., Loquai, C., Türeci, Ö., 2017. Personalized RNA mutanome vaccines mobilize poly-specific therapeutic immunity against cancer. Nature. 1476-4687. 547 (7662), 222–226. Available from: http://www.nature.com/nature/

index.html. doi:10.1038/nature23003.
Sahu, M., Gupta, R., Ambasta, R.K., Kumar, P., 2022. Artificial intelligence and machine learning in precision medicine: a paradigm shift in big data analysis. Prog. Mol. Biol. Transl. Sci. 190, 57–100. Available from: http://www.elsevier.com/books/book-series/progress-in-molecular-biology-and-translational-science#. doi:10.1016/bs.pmbts.2022.03.002.
Selvaraj, C., Chandra, I., Singh, S.K., 2022. Artificial intelligence and machine learning approaches for drug design: challenges and opportunities for the pharmaceutical industries. Mol. Divers. 1573-501X. 26 (3), 1893–1913. Available from: https://www.springer.com/journal/11030. doi:10.1007/s11030-021-10326-z.
Sethi, Y., Patel, N., Kaka, N., Kaiwan, O., Kar, J., Moinuddin, A., Goel, A., Chopra, H., Cavalu, S., 2023. Precision medicine and the future of cardiovascular diseases: a clinically oriented comprehensive review. J. Clin. Med. 2077-0383. 12 (5), 1799. doi:10.3390/jcm12051799.
Shimizu, H., Nakayama, K.I., 2020. Artificial intelligence in oncology. Cancer Sci. 1349-7006. 111 (5), 1452–1460. Available from: http://onlinelibrary.wiley.com/journal/10.1111/(ISSN)1349-7006. doi:10.1111/cas.14377.
Singh, S., Gupta, H., Sharma, P., Sahi, S., 2024. Advances in artificial intelligence (AI)-assisted approaches in drug screening. Artif. Intell. Chem. 2949-7477. 2 (1), 100039. doi:10.1016/j.aichem.2023.100039.
Sun, B., Chen, L., 2023. Interpretable deep learning for improving cancer patient survival based on personal transcriptomes. Sci. Rep. 2045-2322. 13 (1). doi:10.1038/s41598-023-38429-7.
Tomczak, K., Czerwińska, P., Wiznerowicz, M., 2015. Review The Cancer Genome Atlas (TCGA): an immeasurable source of knowledge. Współczesna Onkologia. 1428-2526. 1A, 68–77. doi:10.5114/wo.2014.47136.
Tripathi, N., Goshisht, M.K., Sahu, S.K., Arora, C., 2021. Applications of artificial intelligence to drug design and discovery in the big data era: a comprehensive review. Mol. Divers. 1573-501X. 25 (3), 1643–1664. Available from: https://www.wkap.nl/journalhome.htm/1381-1991. doi:10.1007/s11030-021-10237-z.
Tripathi, S., Tabari, A., Mansur, A., Dabbara, H., Bridge, C.P., Daye, D., 2024. From machine learning to patient outcomes: a comprehensive review of AI in pancreatic cancer. Diagnostics. 2075-4418. 14 (2), 174. doi:10.3390/diagnostics14020174.
Uddin, S., Haque, I., Lu, H., Moni, M.A., Gide, E., 2022. Comparative performance analysis of K-nearest neighbour (KNN) algorithm and its different variants for disease prediction. Sci. Rep. 2045-2322. 12 (1). Available from: www.nature.com/srep/index.html. doi:10.1038/s41598-022-10358-x.
Viale, G., de Snoo, F.A., Slaets, L., Bogaerts, J., van 't Veer, L., Rutgers, E.J., Piccart-Gebhart, M.J., Stork-Sloots, L., Glas, A., Russo, L., Dell'Orto, P., Tryfonidis, K., Litière, S., Cardoso, F., 2018. Immunohistochemical versus molecular (BluePrint and MammaPrint) subtyping of breast carcinoma. Outcome results from the EORTC 10041/BIG 3-04 MINDACT trial. Breast Cancer Res. Treat. 0167-6806. 167 (1), 123–131. doi:10.1007/s10549-017-4509-9.
Vichianin, Y., Khummongkol, A., Chiewvit, P., Raksthaput, A., Chaichanettee, S., Aoonkaew, N., Senanarong, V., 2021. Accuracy of support-vector machines for diagnosis of Alzheimer's disease, using volume of brain obtained by structural MRI at Siriraj Hospital. Front. Neurol. 1664-2295. 12. Available from: http://www.frontiersin.org/Neurology. doi:10.3389/fneur.2021.640696.
Wong, C.H., Siah, K.W., Lo, A.W., 2019. Estimation of clinical trial success rates and related parameters. Biostatistics. 1468-4357. 20 (2), 273–286. Available from: http://biostatistics.oxfordjournals.org/. doi:10.1093/biostatistics/kxx069.

Xiao, X., Min, J.L., Lin, W.Z., Liu, Z., Cheng, X., Chou, K.C., 2015. IDrug-target: predicting the interactions between drug compounds and target proteins in cellular networking via benchmark dataset optimization approach. J. Biomol. Struct. Dyn. 1538-0254. 33 (10), 2221–2233. Available from: http://www.tandfonline.com/loi/tbsd20. doi:10.1080/07391102.2014.998710.

Xu, Z., Wang, X., Zeng, S., Ren, X., Yan, Y., Gong, Z., 2021. Applying artificial intelligence for cancer immunotherapy. Acta Pharm. Sin. B. 2211-3843. 11 (11), 3393–3405. Available from: http://www.elsevier.com/wps/find/journaldescription.cws_home/725753/description#description. doi:10.1016/j.apsb.2021.02.007.

Yang, C.Y., Shiranthika, C., Wang, C.Y., Chen, K.W., Sumathipala, S., 2023. Reinforcement learning strategies in cancer chemotherapy treatments: a review. Comput. Methods Programs Biomed. 1872-7565. 229. Available from: www.elsevier.com/locate/cmpb. doi:10.1016/j.cmpb.2022.107280.

Yang, K.D., Uhler, C., 2019. Multi-domain translation by learning uncoupled autoencoders. arXiv. 2331-8422. Available from: https://arxiv.org. doi:10.48550/arxiv.1902.03515.

Zehir, A., Benayed, R., Shah, R.H., Syed, A., Middha, S., Kim, H.R., Srinivasan, P., Gao, J., Chakravarty, D., Devlin, S.M., Hellmann, M.D., Barron, D.A., Schram, A.M., Hameed, M., Dogan, S., Ross, D.S., Hechtman, J.F., DeLair, D.F., Yao, J.J., Mandelker, D.L., Cheng, D.T., Chandramohan, R., Mohanty, A.S., Ptashkin, R.N., Jayakumaran, G., Prasad, M., Syed, M.H., Rema, A.B., Liu, Z.Y., Nafa, K., Borsu, L., Sadowska, J., Casanova, J., Bacares, R., Kiecka, I.J., Razumova, A., Son, J.B., Stewart, L., Baldi, T., Mullaney, K.A., Al-Ahmadie, H., Vakiani, E., Abeshouse, A.A., Penson, A.V., Jonsson, P., Camacho, N., Chang, M.T., Won, H.H., Gross, B.E., Kundra, R., Heins, Z.J., Chen, H.W., Phillips, S., Zhang, H., Wang, J., Ochoa, A., Wills, J., Eubank, M., Thomas, S.B., Gardos, S.M., Reales, D.N., Galle, J., Durany, R., Cambria, R., Abida, W., Cercek, A., Feldman, D.R., Gounder, M.M., Hakimi, A.A., Harding, J.J., Iyer, G., Janjigian, Y.Y., Jordan, E.J., Kelly, C.M., Lowery, M.A., Morris, L.G.T., Omuro, A.M., Raj, N., Razavi, P., Shoushtari, A.N., Shukla, N., Soumerai, T.E., Varghese, A.M., Yaeger, R., Coleman, J., Bochner, B., Riely, G.J., Saltz, L.B., Scher, H.I., Sabbatini, P.J., Robson, M.E., Klimstra, D.S., Taylor, B.S., Baselga, J., Schultz, N., Hyman, D.M., Arcila, M.E., Solit, D.B., Ladanyi, M., Berger, M.F., 2017. Mutational landscape of metastatic cancer revealed from prospective clinical sequencing of 10,000 patients. Nat. Med. 1546-170X. 23 (6), 703–713. Available from: http://www.nature.com/nm/index.html. doi:10.1038/nm.4333.

Zeng, X., Zhu, S., Liu, X., Zhou, Y., Nussinov, R., Cheng, F., 2019. DeepDR: a network-based deep learning approach to in silico drug repositioning. Bioinformatics. 1460-2059. 35 (24), 5191–5198. Available from: http://bioinformatics.oxfordjournals.org/. doi:10.1093/bioinformatics/btz418.

Zhao, L., Lee, V.H.F., Ng, M.K., Yan, H., Bijlsma, M.F., 2019. Molecular subtyping of cancer: current status and moving toward clinical applications. Brief. Bioinform. 1477-4054. 20 (2), 572–584. Available from: http://bib.oxfordjournals.org. doi:10.1093/bib/bby026.

Zhou, J., Theesfeld, C.L., Yao, K., Chen, K.M., Wong, A.K., Troyanskaya, O.G., 2018. Deep learning sequence-based ab initio prediction of variant effects on expression and disease risk. Nat. Genet. 1546-1718. 50 (8), 1171–1179. Available from: http://www.nature.com/ng/index.html. doi:10.1038/s41588-018-0160-6.

14

Artificial intelligence powered precision oncology

Bharti Pandey[a], Lakshmi Sonkusale[a], Naman Pratap Singh[b], and Tiratha Raj Singh[c]

[a]*Bioinformatics Lab, BTIS-Sub-Centre, Animal Biotechnology Division, ICAR—National Dairy Research Institute (Deemed University), Karnal, Haryana, India*
[b]*Department of Computer Science and Engineering, Jaypee University of Information Technology (JUIT), Solan, Himachal Pradesh, India*
[c]*Department of Biotechnology and Bioinformatics, Centre of Healthcare Technologies and Informatics (CEHTI), Jaypee University of Information Technology (JUIT), Solan, H.P., India*

1 Introduction

Cancer persists as a crucial health concern around the globe, being the leading cause of death at the global level. Worldwide, various kinds of cancers, such as those of the lungs and bronchi, prostate, skin, rectum, and female breast, represent the dominant cancer prevalence. For cancer-related deaths, bronchus and lung cancer are the primary causes, even in both sexes (Shams, 2024). Similar to other fields, the main objective of oncology therapy is to expand cancer control and reduce therapeutic toxicity. It also helps in improving the quality of life for patients (Kann et al., 2021). Despite significant advancements in cancer research and treatments, the disease remains challenging to cure completely, especially in high-risk patients. This emphasizes the urgent need for alternative therapeutic approaches. As a result, cancer research continues to be a critical focus for developing innovative and effective interventions (Tippur, 2023). Over the past decade, significant advancements in precision oncology have spurred the development of predictive tests for patient selection and stratification in cancer treatment. The intricate nature of cancer biology—encompassing complex signaling pathways and interactions between cancerous, stromal, and immune cells—poses challenges for creating biomarkers based on single genes or proteins. However, digital pathology has emerged as a powerful tool in this domain, where digitized tissue slides enable artificial intelligence (AI) and machine learning (ML) to examine

The AI Frontier in Molecular Modelling and Drug Designing. https://doi.org/10.1016/B978-0-443-40338-5.00008-1

subtle morphometric features, potentially improving patient care (Bera et al., 2019). Precision oncology is a personalized approach to cancer treatment that leverages genetic and molecular information to guide diagnosis, prognosis, and therapy decisions. The rise of high-throughput omics technologies has generated vast amounts of complex data, requiring advanced computational platforms for effective analysis (Bhalla and Laganà, 2022). AI, particularly ML, has proven highly effective in uncovering patterns in these large datasets, offering new insights and driving progress in precision oncology. Recently, the development of AI has accelerated the clinical adoption of AI-powered devices in healthcare. At present, the US Food and Drug Administration (FDA) has approved more than sixty AI-incorporated medical devices, and the growing integration of this technology is seen as an unavoidable trend in the future of medicine. The use of AI-driven medical devices, particularly in radiology, is already underway, with AI expected to become a central technology. Specifically, precision medicine, which focuses on tailoring treatments based on large volumes of medical data, including genomic information, has gained global prominence. AI is poised to play a key role in sifting through extensive datasets to extract clinically valuable insights that can enhance diagnosis and treatment (Hamamoto et al., 2020). The potential of AI in the healthcare system offers the ability to enhance clinical decision-making, streamline care processes, improve patient outcomes, and reduce healthcare costs. Over the past decade, AI's rapid growth in the healthcare sector has been remarkable. Its applications have demonstrated transformative potential by utilizing clinical data to extract valuable insights. AI assists healthcare providers in key tasks such as disease diagnosis, patient triage, risk assessment, and surgical support, becoming an indispensable tool in improving clinical care and patient outcomes. AI is now widely adopted across various fields, including remote patient monitoring, virtual assistants, drug discovery, medical diagnostics, medical imaging, risk management, wearable technology, and hospital administration (Mak et al., 2024). Its diverse applications highlight AI's transformative role in reshaping healthcare. As AI continues to evolve, its integration into healthcare practices promises to increase efficiency, improve accuracy, and elevate patient care (Fig. 14.1), ushering in a new era of medical development (Tippur, 2023).

2 Data sources

AI-powered precision oncology relies heavily on integrating diverse, high-quality datasets to understand cancer biology, predict treatment response, identify biomarkers, and personalize therapy. Here are various kinds of data sources commonly used in AI-driven precision oncology:

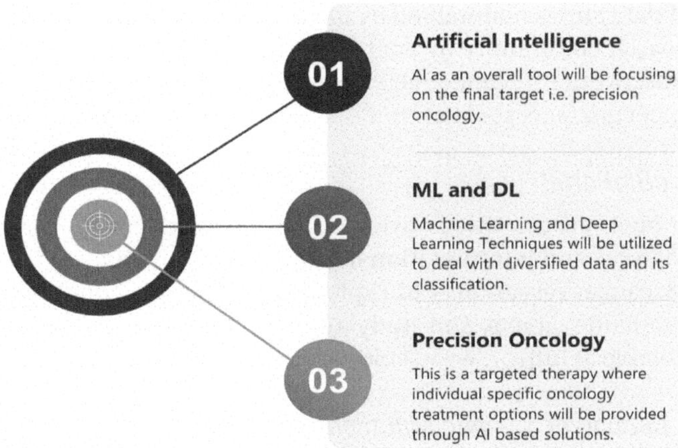

Fig. 14.1 An overview of three intrinsic technologies utilized for precision oncology to provide targeted personalized therapy and elevated patient care. Empowered by artificial intelligence, machine learning, and deep learning, precision oncology leverages cutting-edge tools like next-generation sequencing and liquid biopsy to deliver truly personalized, data-driven cancer care.

2.1 Genomic databases

Genomics databases in cancer provide valuable resources for researchers and clinicians by offering detailed information on genetic alterations, molecular profiles, and associated clinical data. These databases facilitate the study of cancer genomics by providing access to large-scale data sets and tools for analysis and interpretation. The genomics databases include.

2.1.1 OpenGDC

Next-generation sequencing (NGS) technologies have greatly expanded the availability of genomic data and associated clinical and biospecimen information. There is a growing need for new methodologies to facilitate easy access, integration, and effective searching of this vast amount of data (Cappelli et al., 2020). The accessible link is: https://geco.deib.polimi.it/opengdc/.

2.1.2 The Cancer Genome Atlas (TCGA)

It was developed in the US through the National Cancer Institute (NCI) and the National Human Genome Research Institute. The accessible link is: https://www.cancer.gov/ccg/access-data.

2.1.3 Genomics Data Commons (GDC)

It is a comprehensive data repository designed to support cancer research by providing access to a wide array of genomic as well as clinical data and is maintained by the NCI. It aims to support the cancer research community by enabling efficient data access and facilitating discoveries in cancer genomics. The accessible link is: https://gdc.cancer.gov/access-data.

2.1.4 cBioPortal

It is an open-access, interactive platform designed for the visualization, analysis, and interpretation of cancer genomics data. It is widely used by cancer researchers to explore large datasets, identify potential therapeutic targets, and study tumor biology at a molecular level. It is available at https://www.cbioportal.org/.

2.1.5 Catalog of Somatic Mutations in Cancer

World's largest and most comprehensive human cancer somatic mutations database. It is a valuable resource for understanding the molecular mechanisms driving cancer and supports research into cancer genetics and drug development. Available at: https://cancer.sanger.ac.uk/cosmic.

2.1.6 European Genome-Phenome Archive

It is a secure repository of genomic and phenotypic data designed to store and share information from biomedical research studies. It is intended to support research while maintaining the privacy of sensitive data. It serves as a vital resource for researchers seeking to understand the relationship between genetic and phenotypic variations, providing valuable data for studies in personalized medicine, disease mechanisms, and drug development. It is accessible through this link: https://ega-archive.org/datasets/.

2.1.7 Gene Expression Omnibus

A repository that openly distributes high-throughput gene expression data and other relevant datasets, which are publicly available. It is managed by the NCBINational Center for Biotechnology Information (NCBI). It is a crucial resource for genomics researchers, providing extensive gene expression data that can be used to explore biological processes, disease mechanisms, and potential therapeutic targets. It can be accessed through this link: https://www.ncbi.nlm.nih.gov/gds.

2.2 Proteomics databases

These databases, related to cancer research, provide a wealth of data for analyzing protein expressions, modifications, and interactions, often used for identifying biomarkers and therapeutic targets.

2.2.1 Clinical proteomic tumor analysis consortium

Sponsored by NCI, it aims to characterize the proteomes of cancer specimens, integrating proteomic and genomic data to understand cancer biology. It can be accessed through this link: https://gdc.cancer.gov/about-gdc/contributed-genomic-data-cancer-research/clinical-proteomic-tumor-analysis-consortium-cptac.

2.2.2 Human protein atlas

It is an open-access database that provides protein expression data and localization in normal and cancer tissues. It is available at this link: https://www.proteinatlas.org/about/download.

2.2.3 ProteomicsDB

A platform that integrates proteomics data, providing information on proteins across different human tissues, including cancer samples. It is available at this link: https://www.proteomicsdb.org/proteomicsdb/.

2.2.4 Proteomics identifications database

It is hosted and managed by the European Bioinformatics Institute. It is one of the largest public repositories for mass spectrometry-based proteomics data. It can be accessed via this link: https://www.ebi.ac.uk/pride/.

2.2.5 Cancer proteome variation database

This database focuses on cancer-related proteome variation, mapping protein variations to mutations observed in cancer patients. These databases provide valuable resources for exploring protein expression, modifications, and interactions in cancer, which can help identify potential biomarkers, drug targets, and mechanisms driving cancer progression. It can be accessed via this link: http://canprovar2.zhang-lab.org/.

2.3 Steps to access data

To access this database, here is the step-by-step guide in addition to the flowchart portrayed in Fig. 14.2, which can help to understand how to access the database and interpret the results. Fig. 14.2 displays the flowchart for accessing the data, as well as for analysis and result interpretation.

3 AI in precision oncology and cancer genomics

The emergence of NGS technologies and a surge in biomedical research outputs have ushered in a fresh era of big data in cancer genomics (Xu et al., 2019). Managing as well as interpreting this

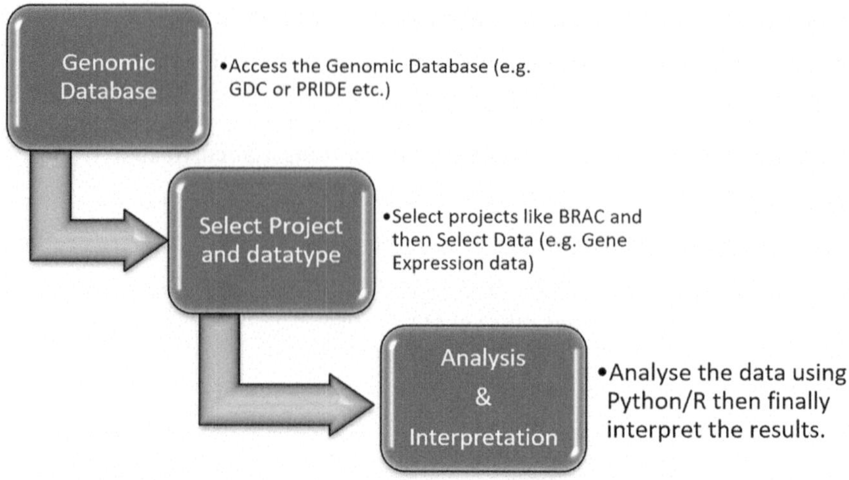

Fig. 14.2 Flowchart for accessing the data, analysis and result interpretation. A streamlined workflow for accessing oncology datasets, performing AI-driven analysis, and interpreting clinically actionable results for precision cancer care.

massive and complex data landscape requires robust computational approaches, with AI playing a pivotal role (Dlamini et al., 2020). Techniques such as deep learning (DL), ML, and natural language processing are increasingly employed to make sense of the vast genomic datasets (Dlamini et al., 2022). In the context of precision oncology, AI is particularly valuable for analyzing genomic information to uncover cancer-specific mutations. Through approaches such as supervised and unsupervised learning, and DL, researchers can identify links between genetic alterations and therapeutic responses (Kalia and Singh, 2025). Furthermore, AI models can forecast the progression of genetic mutations, aiding oncologists in modifying treatment strategies as cancers evolve and develop resistance to existing therapies.

4 AI in drug discovery and development

AI is transforming the landscape of drug discovery along with developments in biomedicine by employing sophisticated algorithms to enhance treatment strategies, reduce development time, and improve patient care (Afrose et al., 2024). By analyzing multiomics data, AI can uncover molecular mechanisms, identify potential drug targets, and detect relevant biomarkers. Tools such as virtual screening, predictive modeling, and high-throughput analysis powered by AI are streamlining and advancing the process of drug development. DL and ML techniques improve predictions related to drug-target interactions, pharmacodynamics, and experimental outcomes

(Farghali et al., 2021). In addition, structure-based drug design is becoming more efficient with the help of AI, enabling faster discovery of promising therapeutic candidates. Personalized medicine also benefits from AI, as it allows for customized treatment strategies based on individual genetic and clinical profiles. When integrated with pharmacogenomics and predictive analytics, AI supports greater accuracy in the selection of drugs, dosage adjustment, and prediction of treatment outcomes, ultimately enhancing efficacy and minimizing adverse effects (Mak et al., 2024).

5 Predicting patient response to treatment

A critical component of precision oncology involves forecasting a patient's response to a particular treatment. AI, especially DL models, is increasingly being used to process various types of data, including genomic profiles, healthcare imaging, and electronic health records (EHR), to predict clinical outcomes. These insights assist healthcare professionals in selecting the most effective treatment options while reducing the risk of prescribing therapies that may be ineffective or harmful (Abajian et al., 2018). Similarly, in psychotherapy, patient outcome predictions are made using baseline clinical data. Participants completed surveys prior to their initial session and at regular intervals throughout treatment. By applying hierarchical linear modeling, researchers estimated each patient's expected progress. Patients were then categorized based on whether their treatment outcomes aligned with or surpassed these projections. Discriminant function analysis revealed that initial clinical characteristics could reliably distinguish between these groups, with higher discriminant scores indicating a greater probability of achieving predicted outcomes. The robustness of these findings was supported through cross-validation techniques (Leon et al., 1999). There are several such case studies where the prediction of patient response toward treatment is a priority, and the outcomes of these studies have helped biomedical scientists make crucial decisions at different disease stages.

6 Medical imaging and AI

Besides genomics, AI has had a significant impact on medical imaging, a critical component of oncology. AI algorithms are able to analyze computed tomography (CT) scans, MRIs, and additional imaging data to detect tumors earlier and more accurately than traditional methods (Fig. 14.3 and Table 14.1). DL, a recent advancement in AI and ML, has garnered significant interest for its medical applications in recent years (Ting et al., 2018). DL models can identify subtle

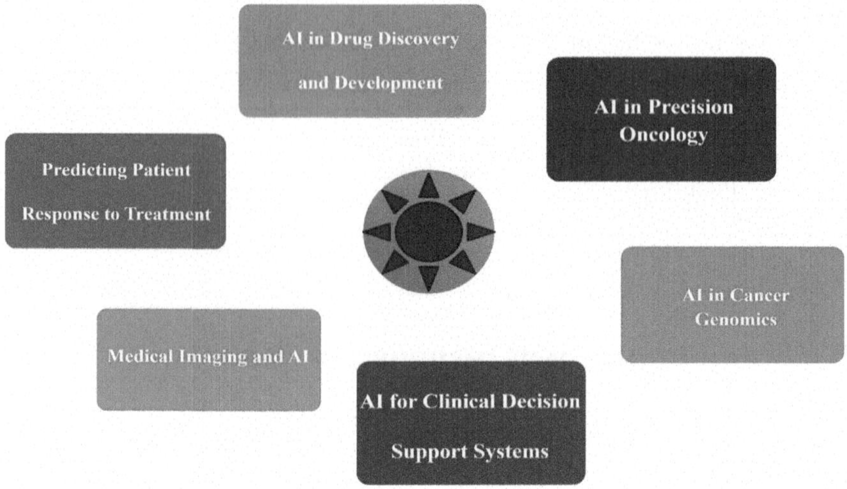

Fig. 14.3 AI-based sub domains specifically involved in personalized therapy and enhanced patient care. These range from genomics to drug discovery, utilizing clinical data, images, and decision support systems.

Table 14.1 AI/ML-based analysis in precision oncology.

Task	Methods Used	In *situ* examples
Subtype identification	Clustering, t-SNE, autoencoders	Identification of molecular subtypes in breast/ glioblastoma
Biomarker discovery	Random forest, SHAP, feature ranking	Immune, metabolic, or DNA repair biomarkers for prognosis
Drug response prediction	Gradient boosting, deep learning, matrix factorization	Predicted response of tumors to immunotherapy or kinase inhibitors
Radiogenomics	CNNs, multimodal fusion	Linking imaging features with mutational status
Survival prediction	Cox models, deep survival networks	Personalized risk models for overall survival or progression
Resistance mechanisms	Temporal modeling, omics comparison	Detection of acquired mutations or transcriptomic shifts

changes in tumor size, shape, and texture, which helps in tracking treatment response over time. Radiomics, a field that extracts quantitative features from medical images, has further expanded with AI tools, allowing oncologists to better understand tumor behavior. Biomedical imaging has transformed medical practice by enabling the diagnosis of diseases through detailed imaging and high-resolution visualization of pathological specimens (Panayides et al., 2020).

7 AI for clinical decision support systems: Transforming evidence-based medicine

AI-driven clinical decision support systems (CDSS) play a major role in precision oncology. These systems assist oncologists by delivering data-informed recommendations, drawing from integrated genomic, clinical, and lifestyle information to support choices regarding treatment plans, dosages, and timing. Extracting useful insights from complicated clinical information has become much easier thanks to recent developments in AI, especially in DL. Diagnostic tools based on the analysis of histopathological and radiological images can now identify critical diagnostic, prognostic, and predictive features that inform patient care (like in Fig. 14.4, chest X-ray data is used for pneumonia detection using the ChexNet tool (Rajpurkar et al., 2017), developed by Stanford University). While AI-based CDSS show great promise in fields such as hepatology, their widespread adoption still requires rigorous clinical validation and regulatory clearance (Nam et al., 2022). In parallel, the analysis of individual patient data from clinical trials, such as those for rheumatoid arthritis, is being used to uncover variables that influence treatment outcomes. For instance, patient responses are often measured using the American College of Rheumatology (ACR) improvement criteria, also known as the "ACR response." AI tools are now being applied to identify the predictors

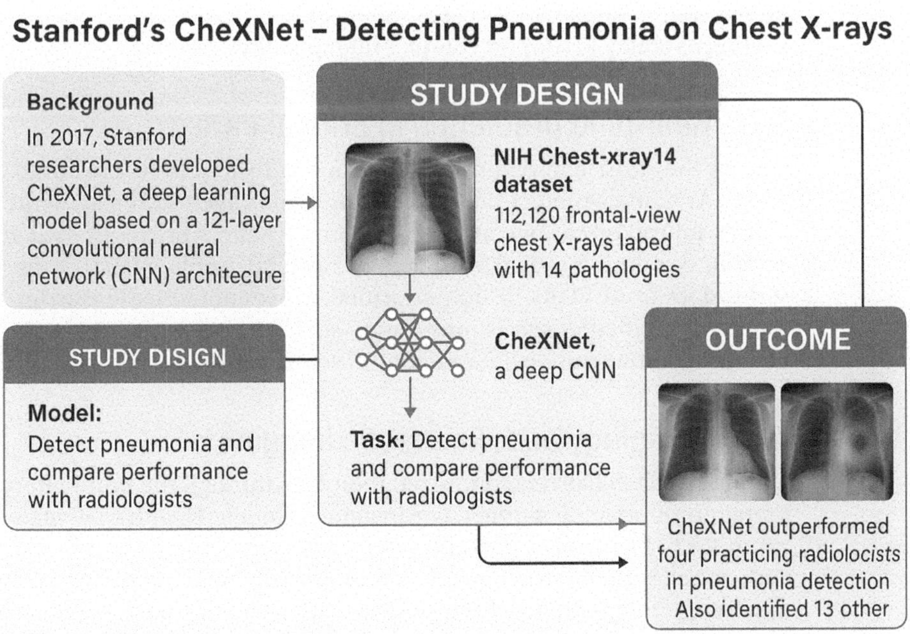

Fig. 14.4 Detecting pneumonia on chest X-rays using CheXNet. A prime example of AI for clinical decision support systems.

of these responses, potentially enhancing personalized treatment approaches across a range of diseases (Anderson et al., 2000). AI-based prediction methods for cancer and other diseases are powerful tools for decision-making and overall management of these diseases (Kapoor et al., 2021; Shukla and Singh, 2021, 2024).

AI is rapidly redefining the landscape of clinical decision-making by augmenting CDSS with data-driven precision, real-time analytics, and context-aware recommendations. Traditional CDSS relied on static, rule-based logic and expert-defined heuristics. In contrast, AI-enabled CDSS leverages ML, DL, and Natural Language Processing (NLP) to derive actionable insights from vast, heterogeneous clinical data sources, including genomics, electronic health records (EHRs), medical imaging, and real-time patient monitoring (Rajkomar et al., 2019).

7.1 From rule-based to intelligence-augmented systems

AI-enhanced CDSS transcends the limitations of static rule engines by learning continuously from patient populations and evolving medical knowledge. For example, IBM Watson for Oncology uses NLP to process clinical notes and peer-reviewed literature to generate individualized treatment options. In multicenter validations in India and Thailand, Watson's treatment concordance with oncologist panels exceeded 90% in breast and colon cancer cases (Somashekhar et al., 2018), demonstrating its ability to support complex therapeutic decisions.

7.2 Real-time prediction in critical care

One of the most compelling applications is in intensive care units, where AI models predict life-threatening events such as sepsis, acute kidney injury, or cardiac arrest hours in advance. The *Sepsis Watch* system, developed at Duke University Hospital, applies DL to time-series data from EHRs. It outperformed conventional early warning scores by predicting sepsis onset up to six hours earlier, allowing clinicians to initiate timely interventions (Sendak et al., 2020).

7.3 Radiology and diagnostic imaging

DL-based CDSS has revolutionized radiology through the rapid interpretation of imaging studies. For instance, Google Health's DL algorithm for breast cancer detection demonstrated performance on par with or better than radiologists in a report involving more than 25,000 mammograms, reducing false positives by 5.7% and false negatives by 9.4% (McKinney et al., 2020). Such systems can be deployed as second readers or triage assistants, improving both diagnostic accuracy and workflow efficiency.

7.4 Personalized decision support in genomics and precision medicine

As mentioned earlier, the integration of AI-CDSS with genomics is central to precision medicine. FoundationOne CDx and Tempus xT are AI-driven platforms that interpret tumor genomics and suggest targeted therapies. These platforms use supervised learning algorithms trained on clinical trial data and outcomes from thousands of patients to provide evidence-graded therapeutic options based on individual molecular profiles (Topol, 2019). The ability to dynamically match patients to therapies or clinical trials exemplifies the paradigm shift toward personalized care.

7.5 Natural language processing and unstructured clinical data

Over 80% of clinical information in EHRs exists in unstructured formats such as progress notes, discharge summaries, and pathology reports. AI-based CDSS with NLP capabilities can extract relevant clinical variables, detect drug interactions, or identify missed diagnoses. For instance, the AI system developed by Johns Hopkins University applied NLP to flag patients with undiagnosed hypertension from physician notes, outperforming traditional methods by 26% (Shickel et al., 2018).

7.6 Ethical, regulatory, and operational challenges

As we had numerous Ethical, Legal and Social Issues (ELSI) challenges during the Human Genome Project, similarly, despite their promise, AI-CDSS must navigate significant challenges. These include algorithmic transparency ("black-box" models), data bias, explainability, interoperability with hospital IT systems, and regulatory oversight (Artificial Intelligence/Machine Learning (AI/ML)-Based Software as a Medical Device (SaMD) Action Plan, 2021). To regulate adaptive AI-based medical devices, the FDA has proposed a total product lifecycle approach, which emphasizes transparency and postdeployment monitoring (Total Product Life Cycle for medical devices, 2023).

7.6.1 Practical challenges of AI in healthcare

Making AI work across hospitals

Primary difficulties in implementing AI in medicine are related to something that typically goes unnoticed when a person is in a hospital: how information is stored and distributed. Different health organizations record patient information differently. For example, a simple blood test is called "Hemoglobin" in one hospital and "Hb" in another. Although doctors can understand such variations, AI systems cannot—unless trained extensively to recognize them. To enable AI to provide consistent and secure recommendations, it is imperative to establish consistent communication regarding data among healthcare facilities. This calls for executing systematic approaches and leveraging the capacity of AI to address discrepancies that emerge between hospitals, regions, and even nations.

It's as though it's trying to solve a puzzle in which every hospital adds a piece—and only when the pieces are assembled can AI view the complete picture.

Does AI work for everyone?

Most AI algorithms are trained on data from specific groups of patients. If the training data predominantly consist of middle-aged patients in big city hospitals, then what happens when you use the same AI in a rural hospital or with older patients who have comorbidities? There is indeed a danger that AI will produce worse choices for others who are different from those it has been trained on. That does create quite serious moral issues: medicine must be available to everyone on an equal basis, not solely to those best represented in the data.

To correct this problem, researchers and health organizations are working together to ensure AI is trained on diverse patient populations, tested in different settings, and regularly updated to respond to the changing environment.

Testing AI before using it on real patients

Even before drugs are administered to patients, they are tested for years. So then, what happens to AI systems? Shouldn't they be tested similarly? Yes is the answer. Too many AI devices are tested in laboratories or at a single institution only, before they are used in a bigger setting. This can be risky. AI may function flawlessly in one setting but not in another. Thus, AI systems must be tested in numerous hospitals, under numerous conditions, and with actual data before they are relied upon in daily care. Health ministries and governments are now establishing standards so that AI is safe, dependable, and helpful—just like any medical device.

Integrating AI with hectic hospital life

Even the best AI systems are useless if they are not easy to use. Doctors and nurses are already working extended shifts while dealing with complicated computing systems. If AI makes their tasks even more complicated or takes too much time to execute, it will never help anyone. The source of the problem is how AI can be implemented into the healthcare institution's business processes so that it complements doctors rather than hinders them. It demands developing tools that are accessible to everyone, effective in performance, and able to provide timely advice—similar to an experienced assistant providing subtle but worthwhile tips.

7.6.2 Human—AI collaboration

Human-AI collaboration is revolutionizing the diagnosis, treatment, and care of patients by doctors. The collaboration is not a plan to replace doctors with AI but to support their abilities and enhance decision-making. The following is a comprehensive breakdown of how doctors and AI collaborate, with an emphasis on trust, role changes, and integration on a daily basis.

Trust between doctor and AI recommendations

Doctors don't inherently trust AI results—instead, they assess them in a clinical context. Trust develops over time through the following aspects shown in Fig. 14.5.

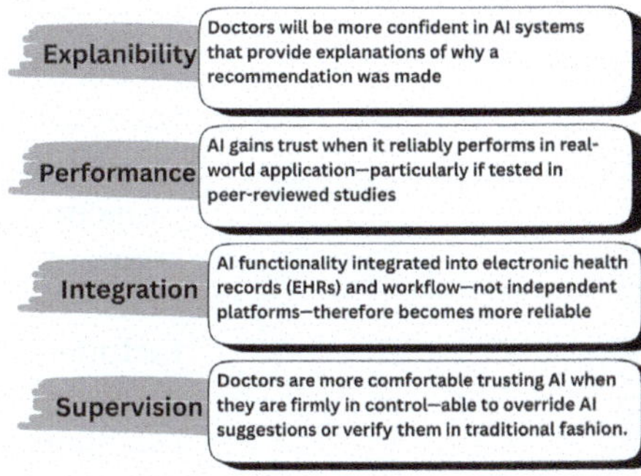

Fig. 14.5 Aspects that develop trust between doctors and AI. Involving healthcare experts in AI development, protecting data privacy, and coordinating AI with medical ethics are all significant. When these elements work together, they create a cooperative setting where medical professionals see AI as a reliable collaborator in providing better, more knowledgeable patient care rather than as a substitute.

Changing roles of doctors in the AI era

As AI becomes more prevalent, the role of doctors is shifting from being sole decision-makers to augmented decision-makers. Key changes are illustrated in Fig. 14.6.

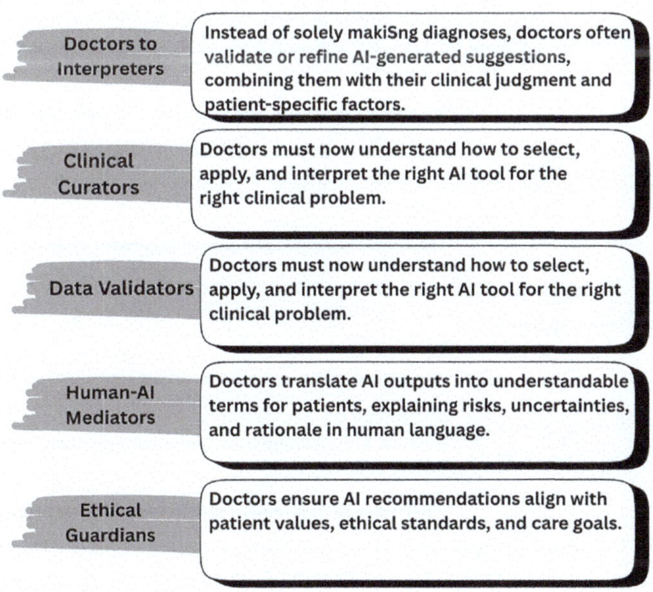

Fig. 14.6 Key changes in the roles of doctors. AI is an efficient tool that improves their capacity to decipher intricate data, spot trends, and reach better clinical conclusions.

Leveraging AI tools in daily clinical practice

AI becomes more and more embedded in the day-to-day work of many doctors in subtle but important ways, as referred to in Fig. 14.7.

AI-powered CDSS marks a fundamental shift from reactive to proactive healthcare by enabling early diagnosis, personalized interventions, and evidence-aligned treatment planning. As these systems (Table 14.2) continue to mature, the focus must also expand to include ethical AI, human-AI collaboration, and clinical validation across diverse populations. When thoughtfully integrated, AI-CDSS can elevate the standard of care and fulfill the long-envisioned goal of intelligent, precision-driven medicine.

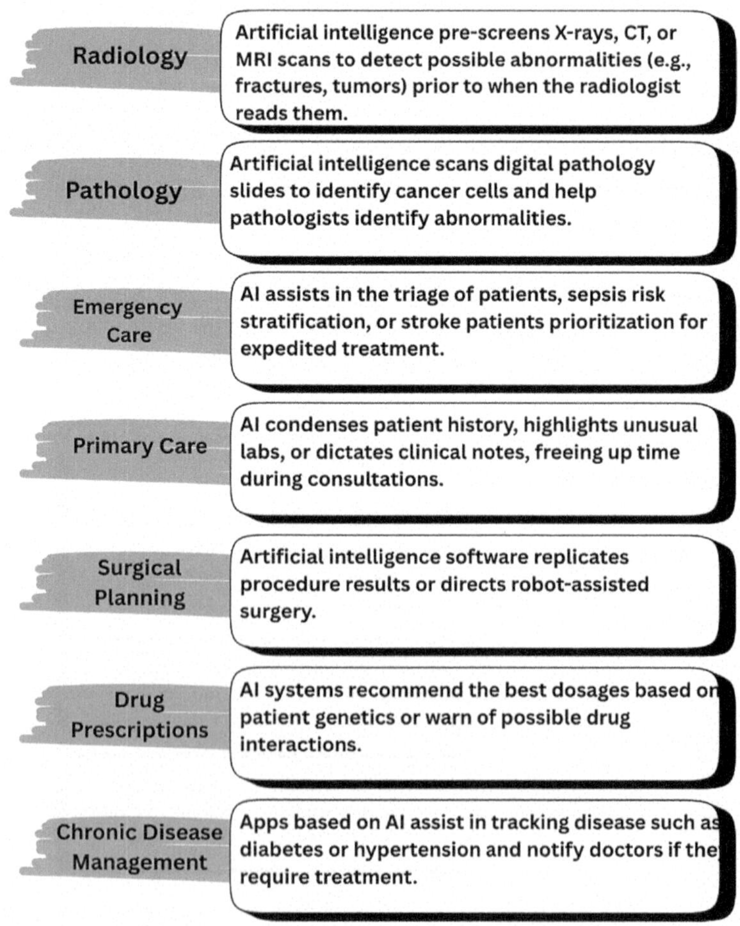

Fig. 14.7 Use of AI in daily clinical practices AI improves the quality of treatment while freeing up physicians to concentrate more on patient engagement and intricate medical decisions by blending seamlessly with daily routines.

Table 14.2 AI-based clinical decision support systems across healthcare, biomedical, and bioinformatics domains.

Domain	Application	AI/ML methods	CDSS/Platform name	Key features/output	References/Notes
Critical care	Early sepsis prediction	Deep learning on EHR time-series	*Sepsis Watch* (Duke University)	Real-time alerts up to 6 hours in advance	Sendak et al. (2020)
Oncology	Personalized cancer treatment	NLP, supervised learning	*Watson for Oncology* (IBM)	Treatment recommendations based on clinical notes and literature	Somashekhar et al. (2018)
Radiology	Breast cancer detection from mammograms	CNNs (Deep Learning)	*Google AI Breast Cancer System*	Outperformed radiologists in detection accuracy	McKinney et al. (2020)
Ophthalmology	Retinal disease diagnosis	Deep learning (CNN)	*DeepMind Health AI*	Identifies 50+ retinal diseases with expert-level accuracy	De Fauw et al. (2018)
Genomics/ Precision medicine	Molecular diagnostics and therapy matching	ML on genomic data	*FoundationOne CDx, Tempus xT*	Gene variant analysis and therapy recommendations	Topol (2019)
Primary Care/ Dermatology	Skin cancer screening	Mobile CNNs	*SkinVision, DermAssist*	Risk assessment via mobile apps from lesion images	Esteva et al. (2017)
Nephrology	AKI (Acute kidney injury) prediction	Recurrent neural networks (RNN)	*DeepAKI*	Predictive alerts for kidney injury using ICU data	Tomašev et al. (2019)
Cardiology	Arrhythmia detection	CNN on ECG signals	*AliveCor KardiaAI*	Detects atrial fibrillation using a smartphone ECG	FDA-cleared tool
Pathology	Automated histopathology review	Vision transformers, CNNs	*Paige.AI, PathAI*	AI-guided biopsy interpretation	Improving speed and consistency of diagnosis
EHR Analysis	Extracting clinical insights from unstructured notes	NLP+ deep learning	Johns Hopkins NLP Engine	Flags missed diagnoses (e.g., hypertension)	Shickel et al. (2018)
Bioinformatics (Genomic)	Variant annotation, biomarker prediction	ML, SVM, Random Forest	*PolyPhen, SIFT, MutPred*	Pathogenicity prediction of genomic variants	Used widely in GWAS and personalized genomics
Biomedical Imaging	Multimodal image fusion for diagnosis	Multimodal deep learning	Research-based platforms	Combines MRI, CT, and histology for precision diagnostics	Ongoing in translational research
Drug Discovery	Drug-target interaction prediction	Graph neural networks, DTI models	*DeepDTI, DeepPurpose*	Predicts molecule-protein binding affinity	Used in repurposing and lead optimization
Public health surveillance	Disease outbreak prediction and resource allocation	Time-series + spatial ML	*BlueDot, HealthMap*	Monitors outbreaks and alerts based on data mining	Used in early COVID-19 alerts
Mental health	Depression risk screening	NLP + sentiment analysis	*Woebot, Wysa*	Conversational agents for mental health monitoring	Real-time behavioral support
Rare disease diagnosis	Suggesting potential rare genetic conditions	Bayesian + DL	*Face2Gene, AMELIE*	Analyzes phenotypic features for diagnostic support	Phenotype-genotype matching

8 AI algorithms used in cancer research

AI and ML are increasingly impacting biomedical research and healthcare, particularly in cancer research and oncology. Their applications span detection, subtype classification, diagnosis, along with treatment optimization and the discovery of novel therapeutic targets for cancer. While vast datasets exist for training ML models, fully harnessing AI's potential in research and clinical practice requires overcoming major challenges (Elemento et al., 2021). Some AI algorithms used in cancer research are described below:

8.1 Convolutional neural network

DL architecture is particularly effective for analyzing visual data, such as medical images. In oncology, convolutional neural networks (CNNs) have been widely used for detecting and classifying cancer in histopathological slides, CT scans, and mammograms (Dabeer et al., 2019). Their ability to accurately extract and determine spatial characteristics from large datasets makes them ideal for identifying patterns indicative of cancer (Al-Yasriy et al., 2020). CNNs have demonstrated dermatologist-level accuracy in skin cancer classification and have been applied effectively to breast, lung, esophageal, and brain cancer diagnostics (Begum et al., 2022).

8.2 Support vector machine (SVM)

A ML technique that classifies data by finding the optimal boundary separating different categories. It performs well in high-dimensional data spaces like gene expression or multiomics data. In cancer research, support vector machines (SVMs) are widely used for classifying tumor types and predicting patient outcomes. Their ability to choose the best hyperplane for classifying data into distinct groups makes them appropriate for accurate diagnostic categorization. SVMs have shown excellent performance in breast and liver cancer classification and have been used for survival prediction using integrated clinical and genomic data (Kumar and Kamalraj, 2022a).

8.3 K-nearest neighbors (KNN)

A simple and intuitive ML algorithm that classifies data based on the properties of its closest neighbors (Zadeh Shirazi et al., 2024). It works well for early cancer detection tasks when the dataset has clear cluster patterns. It has demonstrated competitive accuracy in the classification of lung and breast cancer. Although it lacks model interpretability compared to other techniques, its simplicity and effectiveness in handling labeled datasets make it useful for basic diagnostic tasks in oncology (Bhuvaneswari and Therese, 2015).

8.4 Decision tree

Decision trees (DT) are tree-like structures that model decisions based on feature values. A feature is represented by each node, and a decision rule is represented by each branch. In cancer classification, DTs help identify critical features contributing to malignancy. They are easy to understand and visualize, making them a popular choice in clinical settings where interpretability is essential. DTs have been applied in breast cancer classification, often in combination with ensemble techniques for improved accuracy (Kumar and Kamalraj, 2022).

8.5 Back propagation Network

Artificial neural networks are trained using backpropagation. They are effective in modeling complex, nonlinear relationships between features and outcomes. In cancer diagnosis, BPNNs have been used to process features from mammography and histopathological data. Although more computationally intensive than traditional models, BPNNs can improve classification accuracy when trained on large, labeled datasets (Al-Hadidi et al., 2017).

8.6 Logistic regression (Lr)

This classic statistical approach is applied to issues involving binary categorization, such as distinguishing between cancerous and non-cancerous cases. It is particularly favored for its interpretability and simplicity. It has been applied to breast cancer detection, often as a baseline model. While it may not perform as well as DL algorithms on complex datasets, it remains valuable for smaller datasets and provides insights into feature importance (Sukari et al., 2016).

8.7 Survival CNN

A specialized form of CNN is designed to predict survival outcomes by integrating histopathological images and genomic data. Survival CNN (SCNNs) have been applied to brain cancer prognosis, providing predictions that align with molecular subtypes and clinical histologic grades. This model enhances prognostic accuracy by incorporating both visual and molecular biomarkers, making it highly valuable for precision oncology (Mobadersany et al., 2018).

8.8 Shallow deep CNN

A hybrid DL model that combines the strengths of shallow and deep convolutional layers. In cancer diagnostics, particularly breast cancer, SD-CNNs have demonstrated high diagnostic accuracy by effectively capturing both low-level and high-level features. This balance enables SD-CNNs to generalize well on smaller datasets while maintaining high precision, making them an advanced tool in medical imaging analysis (Gao et al., 2018).

8.9 Long short-term memory

It is a kind of recurrent neural network that is used to describe long-range dependencies in sequential data. In cancer applications, long short-term memories (LSTMs) are often used alongside CNNs and other models for the analysis of time-series data, such as patient history or gene expression changes over time. When integrated into hybrid systems, LSTMs contribute to high accuracy and improved classification performance in breast cancer studies (Begum et al., 2022).

8.10 Random Forest

In order to increase classification accuracy and robustness, this ensemble learning technique builds several DTs during training and combines their outputs. In cancer research, random forest is particularly useful for feature selection and handling complex, nonlinear relationships. Its ability to manage large datasets with many features makes it a popular choice in clinical data analysis (Begum et al., 2022).

Advancements in AI are revolutionizing cancer research by enhancing detection, prognosis, and treatment outcomes. This includes a tabular summary of major studies, offering a quick reference for researchers and clinicians (Table 14.3).

9 AI-based biomarkers for cancer screening

Biomarkers are crucial tools used to assess biological and pathological states, particularly in cancer detection, progression monitoring, and treatment efficacy. With recent advances in high-throughput proteomic technology, researchers can now process vast amounts of protein data from biological samples, providing opportunities to identify new biomarkers that reflect the molecular changes in diseases. When combined with AI, these technologies are driving the development of next-generation biomarkers, revolutionizing clinical practice (Xiao et al., 2021; Mikdadi et al., 2022).

Nam et al. (2021) developed an AI-powered IBM to predict tumor invasiveness from mammograms (shown in Fig. 14.8) and validated its performance in an external cohort. The AI model was trained using 151,764 mammograms from five institutions, including 31,776 cancer exams. Initially designed for breast cancer detection, the model was fine-tuned to predict invasiveness (ductal carcinoma in situ [DCIS], DCIS microinvasive [DCIS-MI], invasive ductal

Table 14.3 Overview of AI algorithms applied in cancer detection, diagnosis, and prognosis.

AI application	Data	Algorithm/Method	Cancer type	Results	References
Classification	129,450 clinical images from Stanford Hospital	Convolutional neural networks (CNN)	Skin cancer	CNNs are the foundation of an AI system that can classify skin cancer with an accuracy level on par with dermatologists	Esteva et al. (2017)
Detection	TCGA and NC	CNN	breast cancer	The average area under the curve (AUC) increased for the classifier to 0.9018 ± 0.0093, demonstrating high accuracy in distinguishing cancerous from noncancerous tissue	Cruz-Roa et al. (2017)
	Breast malignant growth dataset	K-nearest neighbor (KNN), Support Vector Machine (SVM), Decision Tree Classifier (DT)	breast cancer	SVM performs best execution in the context of exactness, accuracy, and review	Kumar and Kamalraj (2022)
	Mammography images	K-NN, Back Propagation Neural Network (BPNN), Logistic Regression (LR)	breast cancer	LR model utilized more features than the BPNN	Sukari et al. (2016)
	CT lung images	K-nearest neighbour (K-NN), Genetic algorithm	Lung	Classification accuracy of 90% is achieved as fitness	Bhuvaneswari and Therese (2015)
Survival prediction	TCGA	Support vector machine (SVM)	liver cancer	The approach provides a new avenue for personalized treatment strategies in liver cancer, supporting precision oncology through multidimensional data integration	Chaudhary et al. (2018)
Prognosis	Whole-slide images, clinical, and genomic data were obtained from TCGA via the Genomic Data Commons (https://gdc.cancer.gov/)	Survival convolutional neural network (SCNN)	Brain	SCNN predictions correlate with molecular subtypes and manual histologic grade, improving prognostic accuracy by integrating genomic biomarkers	Mobadersany et al. (2018)
Diagnosis	384 patients' 8428 esophageal cancer pictures from the Cancer Institute Hospital in Japan	Esophageal cancer	CNN	The CNN has a 98% accuracy rate in differentiating between superficial and advanced esophageal cancer	Horie et al. (2019)
	Histopathological stained images	Breast cancer	CNN	Accuracy of CNN: 99.86%	Dabeer et al. (2019)
	Institutional dataset from Mayo Clinic Arizona, INbreast public dataset	Breast cancer	Shallow-Deep CNN (SD-CNN)	SD-CNN improves the diagnostic accuracy to 0.90 (AUC = 0.92)	Gao et al. (2018)
	CT scans	Lung cancer	CNN	Accuracy (93.548%), Precision (97.1015%), Recall (97.1015%), Specificity (~95%)	Al-Yasriy et al. (2020)
	UCI Repository's Wisconsin Breast Cancer Database (WBCD)	Breast cancer	CNN, Long Short-Term Memory (LSTM), Random Forest (RF)	The proposed system accomplishes accuracy: 100%, sensitivity: 99%, recall: 99%, and F1-score: 98%	Begum et al. (2022)

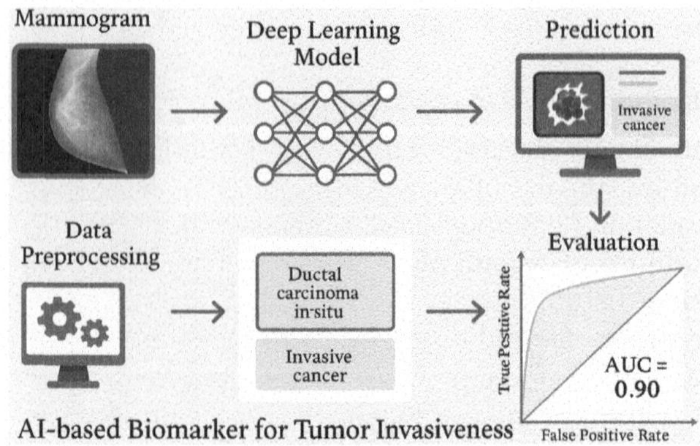

Fig. 14.8 Imaging biomarker in mammography (IBM) driven by AI to forecast tumor invasiveness. It enables early and accurate forecasting of tumor invasiveness, transforming breast cancer diagnosis and personalized treatment planning.

carcinoma [IDC]) using 8251 cancer exams for development and 886 for internal validation. A total of 699 cancer tests that had been confirmed by surgical biopsy were subjected to external testing. The AI-powered IBM achieved an AUC of 0.968 for the detection of breast cancer and 0.898 for distinguishing IDC from DCIS. It had a similar performance in predicting invasiveness and diagnosed cancer in the external cohort with an AUC of 0.952.

10 Precision oncology data, analysis, and market-based predictions

Precision oncology leverages individual patient data, such as molecular, clinical, and environmental information, to tailor cancer diagnostics and treatment. This field is driven by the integration of multiomics datasets and AI/ML tools that uncover hidden patterns, optimize therapy, and predict outcomes. This data is multimodal in nature and serves as an accompaniment to the currently available resources. Digital pathology has enabled high-throughput analysis of histopathological slides. AI models, particularly CNNs, display great promise in recognizing cancerous regions, grading tumors, and predicting outcomes based on tissue morphology. NGS provides vast genomic data used to identify cancer-associated mutations. AI helps interpret this data to detect oncogenes, tumor suppressor genes, and actionable variants relevant for targeted therapy. Genetic profiling data can help researchers and biomedical scientists look for standard genetic parameters associated with various stages of cancer. A thorough understanding of tumor biology is provided by multiomics techniques, which include transcriptomics, proteomics,

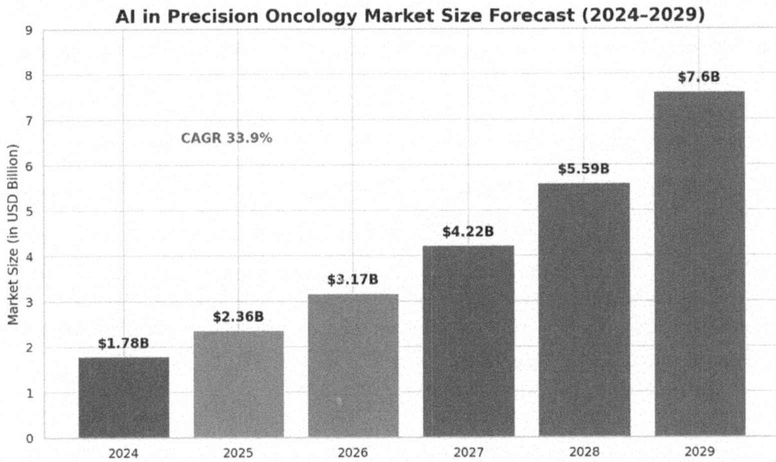

Fig. 14.9 Predictions for AI-based precision oncology for the future market size and projections through standard metrics such as Compound Annual Growth Rate (CAGR). A growing market and improved predictive tools help oncologists streamline data collection, analysis, and interpretation for personalized treatment.

metabolomics, and genomics. AI methods, including DL and ensemble models, facilitate the fusion of these data types for tasks like drug ranking, cancer subtype classification, and prediction of therapy response. Spatial transcriptomics will also be part of this and utilized in association with AI to provide crucial insights into region-specific predictions. A huge market size and better predictions can help precision oncologists plan and execute resources for data collection, analysis, and interpretation (Fig. 14.9).

Precision oncology, driven by multidimensional data and advanced analytics, represents a transformative shift in cancer diagnosis, treatment, and management. Integrating high-throughput omics technologies (metabolomics, proteomics, transcriptomics, and genomics) and clinical data has enabled the development of personalized therapies tailored to individual tumor profiles. The application of AI and ML in analyzing these complex datasets has significantly improved biomarker discovery, drug response prediction, and treatment optimization. These technologies facilitate early detection, precise classification of cancer subtypes, and adaptive treatment strategies, reducing trial-and-error approaches in oncology.

10.1 Real-world example: Foundation medicine

A high-visibility real-world use case is FoundationOne CDx, developed by Foundation Medicine, which employs comprehensive genomic profiling to detect actionable mutations in solid tumors.

The platform combines NGS data with a vast cancer therapy and biomarker knowledge base. AI models help interpret the data, guiding oncologists to targeted therapies and clinical trials. This is a good example of how combining omics data with AI streamlines precision decision-making.

10.2 Multiomics integration

Multiomics approaches—combining transcriptomics, genomics, metabolomics, and proteomics—offer a holistic understanding of tumor biology. AI/ML techniques, including DL, graph neural networks, and ensemble models, facilitate the merging and analysis of these heterogeneous data sets for:

1. Cancer subtype classification
2. Drug ranking and repositioning
3. Prediction of therapy response
4. Long-term monitoring of tumor progression

Spatial transcriptomics, when integrated with AI, provides region-specific gene expression information, allowing for more accurate resolution in tumor behavior prediction and therapy response.

10.3 Most frequently used open-source tools and databases

TCGA: A comprehensive database with genomic, epigenomic, transcriptomic, and proteomic data for various cancers.

1. **cBioPortal:** An open-source, interactive platform to study cancer genomics data.
2. **Xena browser:** Offers graphical exploration and analysis of public and private cancer genomics datasets.
3. **GDC data portal:** Provides access to TARGET and TCGA program data.
4. **DeepBio & DeepPath:** Open-source digital pathology AI-enabled platforms.
5. **PyRadiomics:** For radiomic feature extraction from medical image data.

Caption: A growing market and improved predictive tools help oncologists streamline data collection, analysis, and interpretation for personalized treatment.

From a market perspective, the global landscape for AI-enabled precision oncology is experiencing exponential growth. Multiple independent market analyses project the AI-in-oncology sector to expand from approximately USD 1.3–1.8 billion in 2024 to USD 10–19 billion by 2030–2034, with the Compound Annual Growth Rate (CAGR) ranging between 17% and 34%, depending on scope and segmentation. In parallel, the broader precision oncology market, encompassing diagnostics, targeted therapies, and companion technologies, is predicted to increase at a more moderate CAGR of about 10%, from USD 120.97 billion in 2024 to over USD 312 billion by 2034 (several open sources). These projections reflect an increasing demand for personalized cancer care, a rising incidence of cancer, supportive regulatory frameworks, and the proliferation of AI along with big data solutions. As precision oncology continues to evolve, its convergence with the future of cancer care will be significantly shaped by AI-driven analytics, which offer both clinical promise and robust commercial potential.

11 Conclusion

AI-powered precision oncology represents the convergence of two transformative technologies: AI and genomics. By leveraging AI's ability to analyze massive datasets and uncover hidden patterns, we are getting closer to an era when cancer can be treated in a way that is personalized to each patient's unique genetic and molecular profile. The amazing promise of AI to transform cancer treatment has been demonstrated by this chapter's exploration of its applications in genomics, medical imaging, clinical decision support, biomarker identification, and drug development. Plausible market-based predictions were also included to provide a financial perspective on the problem. As we continue to overcome current challenges and refine these tools, AI in precision oncology has enormous potential to reduce medical expenses and save lives by improving patient outcomes.

12 Future directions in precision oncology with AI

As AI and biomedical sciences continue to converge, the future of precision oncology is rapidly unfolding. Several new technologies and strategies are set to revolutionize the field over the coming years:

12.1 Integration of new omics technologies

Advances in single-cell and spatial transcriptomics are revolutionizing our understanding of tumor heterogeneity and communication within the microenvironment. These new technologies produce high-resolution molecular portraits of individual tumor cells, providing detailed insights that earlier bulk sequencing technologies cannot.

AI strategies, particularly DL and graph neural networks, are most likely to be at the center of interpreting these complex datasets, discovering novel biomarkers, and revealing hitherto hidden therapeutic targets.

12.2 Improving liquid biopsy analysis

Liquid biopsies, such as circulating tumor DNA (ctDNA) and exosomal RNA profiling, provide noninvasive means of cancer diagnosis and monitoring. The tests' specificity and sensitivity remain heterogeneous, however. AI can enhance performance through the integration of heterogeneous data types (genomic, proteomic, and clinical) and the detection of subtle longitudinal sample patterns. Training of ML models that can aid in earlier diagnosis will be achieved by these big multimodal datasets, real-time monitoring of treatment, and therapeutic resistance prediction.

12.3 Privacy-preserving AI through federated learning

The training of collaborative AI across various healthcare facilities is frequently constrained by privacy regulations and data silos. Federated learning presents a groundbreaking solution: it facilitates the creation of resilient models by utilizing decentralized datasets without the need to transfer sensitive patient data. In the field of oncology, this methodology permits multiinstitutional AI models to assimilate knowledge from diverse populations and uncommon cancer subtypes while ensuring adherence to stringent data privacy legislation. This framework is particularly advantageous for international cancer research and clinical trials.

With the development of these technologies, a new generation of smart, patient-centric oncology solutions that are equitable and accurate will emerge.

Step-wise-step example of TCGA

Step 1: Access the Database: Navigate to the GDC Portal.

Step 2: Select and download the required data: Search for ***"TCGA-BRAC"*** in Projects, under Data Category, select Gene Expression Quantification, and choose ***"HTSeq—Counts"*** as the type of file.

Step 3: Download the Data: Click *"Add to Cart"*, go to the cart, and download.

Step 3: Analyze the data: Load the file in Python using Pandas (see the code snippet below).

```
import pandas as pd
df = pd.read_csv("HTSeq_counts.csv", sep = "\t")
print(df.head())
#Apply any model or algorithm that you want to apply.
```

Case Study: IBM Watson for Oncology (WTO) Optimal Cancer Treatment Prediction

Background: IBM Watson for Oncology (WTO) was developed together with Memorial Sloan Kettering Cancer Center (MSKCC) to help provide individualized recommendations for cancer treatment to patients based on their clinical and genomic data.

Study Design: WFO was trained on a large corpus of clinical guidelines, research literature, and anonymized patient data from MSKCC. The system utilized natural language processing, as well as ML, to analyze treatment options.

It contrasts a patient's genomic markers, tumor characteristics, and clinical history with established treatments and ongoing clinical trials.

Real-World Application: Used in Indian hospitals (Apollo Hospitals and Manipal Hospitals). In a retrospective survey conducted at Gachon University Gil Medical Center, Korea, Watson's recommendations for breast, colon, and gastric cancers concurred with oncologists' in 93% of instances.

Conclusion: WFO helped reduce time in treatment decision-making. It provided oncologists with access to up-to-date research and trials, enabling evidence-based practice, which was especially useful in situations where expert knowledge might be in short supply.

A Real-World Case Study: Prediction of Breast Cancer Invasiveness by AI-Augmented Imaging Biomarkers (Nam et al., 2021)

Background:- Traditional biomarkers like HER2 and Ki-67 require invasive biopsy methods and laboratory tests. Nam et al. (2021) proposed a new noninvasive imaging biomarker (IBM) based on AI, using mammographic information to predict the invasiveness of the tumor, e.g., distinguishing between DCIS and IDC.

Tools and Algorithms Used:-

Input Data:

151,764 mammograms from 5 institutions, of which 31,776 were cancer cases, were used. Digital mammograms marked by radiologists and validated by pathology were included.

Preprocessing:

Standardization and alignment of the images. Identification of the region of interest (ROI) with lesions.

Model structure:- Based on a state-of-the-art deep CNN. Fine-tuned ResNet or EfficientNet backbone, learned with supervised learning, to predict images to:

a. DCIS (nonsurgical)

b. DCIS-MI (microinvasive)

c. IDC (invasive)

Continued

Training:- For internal validation, 8251 images from 886 cases are used, and for external testing, 699 cancer samples are used; all were confirmed through surgical biopsy.

Results:-

1. Breast Cancer Detection AUC was 0.968 (Excellent).
2. Invasiveness Prediction AUC was 0.898 (separating IDC from DCIS).
3. External Cohort Generalizability.

AUC = 0.952 for detecting cancer using unseen data.

Interpretability:- Applied Grad-CAM heatmaps to highlight lesion areas impacting predictions, thereby enhancing radiologists' confidence.

References

Artificial Intelligence/Machine Learning (AI/ML)-Based Software as a Medical Device (SaMD) Action Plan, 2021. Available from: https://www.fda.gov/media/145022/download.

Total product life cycle for medical devices, 2023. Available from: https://www.fda.gov/about-fda/cdrh-transparency/total-product-life-cycle-medical-devices.

Abajian, A., Murali, N., Savic, L.J., Laage-Gaupp, F.M., Nezami, N., Duncan, J.S., Schlachter, T., Lin, M.D., Geschwind, J.F., Chapiro, J., 2018. Predicting treatment response to intra-arterial therapies for hepatocellular carcinoma with the use of supervised machine learning—an artificial intelligence concept. J. Vasc. Interv. Radiol. 1535-7732. 29 (6), 850. Available from: http://www.elsevier.com. doi:10.1016/j.jvir.2018.01.769.

Afrose, N., Chakraborty, R., Hazra, A., Bhowmick, P., Bhowmick, M., 2024. AI-driven drug discovery and development. In: Future of AI in Biomedicine and Biotechnology. IGI Global, India, pp. 259–277. Available from: https://www.igi-global.com/book/future-biomedicine-biotechnology/336539. doi:10.4018/979-8-3693-3629-8.ch013.

Al-Hadidi, M.R., Alarabeyyat, A., Alhanahnah, M. 2017 Breast cancer detection using K-nearest neighbor machine learning algorithm. In: Proceedings—2016 9th International Conference on Developments in eSystems Engineering, DeSE 2016. 9781509054879. Institute of Electrical and Electronics Engineers Inc., Jordan, pp. 35–39doi:10.1109/DeSE.2016.8.

Al-Yasriy, H.F., Al-Husieny, M.S., Mohsen, F.Y., Khalil, E.A., Hassan, Z.S., 2020. Diagnosis of lung cancer based on CT scans using CNN. IOP Conf. Ser. Mater. Sci. Eng. 1757-899X. 928 (2). https://iopscience.iop.org/journal/1757-899X. doi:10.1088/1757-899X/928/2/022035.

Anderson, J.J., Wells, G., Verhoeven, A.C., Felson, D.T., 2000. Factors predicting response to treatment in rheumatoid arthritis: the importance of disease duration. Arthritis Rheum. 0004-3591. 43 (1), 22–29. doi:10.1002/1529-0131(200001)43:1<22::aid-anr4>3.0.co;2-9.

Begum, A., Kumar, V.D., Asghar, J., Hemalatha, D., Arulkumaran, G., Ahmad, M., 2022. A combined deep CNN: LSTM with a random forest approach for breast cancer diagnosis. Complexity. 1076-2787. 2022 (1). doi:10.1155/2022/9299621.

Bera, K., Schalper, K.A., Rimm, D.L., Velcheti, V., Madabhushi, A., 2019. Artificial intelligence in digital pathology—new tools for diagnosis and precision oncology. Nat. Rev. Clin. Oncol. 1759-4782. 16 (11), 703–715. Available from: http://www.nature.com/nrclinonc/archive/index.html. doi:10.1038/s41571-019-0252-y.

Bhalla, S., Laganà, A., 2022. Artificial intelligence for precision oncology. In: Advances in Experimental Medicine and Biology, Vol. 1361. Springer Science and Business Media LLC, pp. 249–268. doi:10.1007/978-3-030-91836-1_14.

Bhuvaneswari, P., Therese, A.B., 2015. Detection of cancer in lung with K-NN classification using genetic algorithm. Procedia Mater. Sci. 2211-8128. 10, 433–440. doi:10.1016/j.mspro.2015.06.077.

Cappelli, E., Cumbo, F., Bernasconi, A., Canakoglu, A., Ceri, S., Masseroli, M., Weitschek, E., 2020. OpenGDC: unifying, modeling, integrating cancer genomic data and clinical metadata. Appl. Sci. 2076-3417. 10 (18), 6367. doi:10.3390/app10186367.

Chaudhary, K., Poirion, O.B., Lu, L., Garmire, L.X., 2018. Deep learning–based multi-omics integration robustly predicts survival in liver cancer. Clin. Cancer Res. 1557-3265. 24 (6), 1248–1259. Available from: http://clincancerres.aacrjournals.org/content/24/6/1248.full-text.pdf. doi:10.1158/1078-0432.CCR-17-0853.

Cruz-Roa, A., Gilmore, H., Basavanhally, A., Feldman, M., Ganesan, S., Shih, N.N.C., Tomaszewski, J., González, F.A., Madabhushi, A., 2017. Accurate and reproducible invasive breast cancer detection in whole-slide images: a deep learning approach for quantifying tumor extent. Sci. Rep. 2045-2322. 7 (1). doi:10.1038/srep46450.

Dabeer, S., Khan, M.M., Islam, S., 2019. Cancer diagnosis in histopathological image: CNN based approach. Inform. Med. Unlocked. 2352-9148. 16. Available from: https://www.sciencedirect.com/science/journal/23529148. doi:10.1016/j.imu.2019.100231.

De Fauw, J., Ledsam, J.R., Romera-Paredes, B., Nikolov, S., Tomasev, N., Blackwell, S., Askham, H., Glorot, X., O'Donoghue, B., Visentin, D., van den Driessche, G., Lakshminarayanan, B., Meyer, C., Mackinder, F., Bouton, S., Ayoub, K., Chopra, R., King, D., Karthikesalingam, A., Hughes, C.O., Raine, R., Hughes, J., Sim, D.A., Egan, C., Tufail, A., Montgomery, H., Hassabis, D., Rees, G., Back, T., Khaw, P.T., Suleyman, M., Cornebise, J., Keane, P.A., Ronneberger, O., 2018. Clinically applicable deep learning for diagnosis and referral in retinal disease. Nat. Med. 1546-170X. 24 (9), 1342–1350. Available from: http://www.nature.com/nm/index.html. doi:10.1038/s41591-018-0107-6.

Dlamini, Z., Francies, F.Z., Hull, R., Marima, R., 2020. Artificial intelligence (AI) and big data in cancer and precision oncology. Comput. Struct. Biotechnol. J. 2001-0370. 18, 2300–2311. Available from: https://www.csbj.org. doi:10.1016/j.csbj.2020.08.019.

Dlamini, Z., Skepu, A., Kim, N., Mkhabele, M., Khanyile, R., Molefi, T., Mbatha, S., Setlai, B., Mulaudzi, T., Mabongo, M., Bida, M., Kgoebane-Maseko, M., Mathabe, K., Lockhat, Z., Kgokolo, M., Chauke-Malinga, N., Ramagaga, S., Hull, R., 2022. AI and precision oncology in clinical cancer genomics: from prevention to targeted cancer therapies-an outcomes based patient care. Inform. Med. Unlocked. 2352-9148. 31, 100965. doi:10.1016/j.imu.2022.100965.

Elemento, O., Leslie, C., Lundin, J., Tourassi, G., 2021. Artificial intelligence in cancer research, diagnosis and therapy. Nat. Rev. Cancer. 1474-175X. 21 (12), 747–752. doi:10.1038/s41568-021-00399-1.

Esteva, A., Kuprel, B., Novoa, R.A., Ko, J., Swetter, S.M., Blau, H.M., Thrun, S., 2017. Dermatologist-level classification of skin cancer with deep neural networks. Nature. 14764687. 542 (7639), 115–118. Available from: http://www.nature.com/nature/index.html. doi:10.1038/nature21056.

Farghali, H., Canová, N.K., Arora, M., 2021. The potential applications of artificial intelligence in drug discovery and development. Physiol. Res. 1802-9973. 70, 715–722. Available from: http://www.biomed.cas.cz/physiolres/. doi:10.33549physiolres.934765.

Gao, F., Wu, T., Li, J., Zheng, B., Ruan, L., Shang, D., Patel, B., 2018. SD-CNN: a shallow-deep CNN for improved breast cancer diagnosis. Comput. Med. Imaging Graph. 0895-6111. 70, 53–62. doi:10.1016/j.compmedimag.2018.09.004.

Hamamoto, R., Suvarna, K., Yamada, M., Kobayashi, K., Shinkai, N., Miyake, M., Takahashi, M., Jinnai, S., Shimoyama, R., Sakai, A., Takasawa, K., Bolatkan, A., Shozu, K., Dozen, A., Machino, H., Takahashi, S., Asada, K., Komatsu, M., Sese, J., Kaneko, S., 2020. Application of artificial intelligence technology in oncology: towards the establishment of precision medicine. Cancers. 2072-6694. 12 (12), 3532. doi:10.3390/cancers12123532.

Horie, Y., Yoshio, T., Aoyama, K., Yoshimizu, S., Horiuchi, Y., Ishiyama, A., Hirasawa, T., Tsuchida, T., Ozawa, T., Ishihara, S., Kumagai, Y., Fujishiro, M., Maetani, I., Fujisaki, J., Tada, T., 2019. Diagnostic outcomes of esophageal cancer by artificial intelligence using convolutional neural networks. Gastrointest. Endosc. 0016-5107. 89 (1), 25–32. doi:10.1016/j.gie.2018.07.037.

Kalia, D., Singh, T.R., 2025. Asthma and chronic obstructive pulmonary disease (COPD) prediction using PEEP expiratory occlusion data: a hybrid approach with random forest and feedforward neural network. In: Proceedings of IEEE International Conference on Signal Processing,Computing and Control. 9798331538934. Institute of Electrical and Electronics Engineers Inc., India, pp. 539–544. doi:10.1109/ISPCC66872.2025.11039525.

Kann, B.H., Hosny, A., Aerts, H.J.W.L., 2021. Artificial intelligence for clinical oncology. Cancer Cell. 1878-3686. 39 (7), 916–927. Available from: https://www.journals.elsevier.com/cancer-cell. doi:10.1016/j.ccell.2021.04.002.

Kapoor, M., Kapoor, M., Shukla, R., Raj, S.T. 2021. Early diagnosis of Alzheimer's disease using machine learning based methods. In: ACM International Conference Proceeding Series. Association for Computing Machinery, India, pp. 70–76. http://portal.acm.org/. doi:10.1145/3474124.3474134. 9781450389204.

Kumar, S., Kamalraj, R., 2022. Breast cancer detection using machine learning algorithms. Int. J. Adv. Eng. Manag. 4 (3) , 987–994.

Leon, S.C., Kopta, S.M., Howard, K.I., Lutz, W., 1999. Predicting patients' responses to psychotherapy: are some more predictable than others?. J. Consult. Clin. Psychol. 0022-006X. 67 (5), 698–704. doi:10.1037/0022-006X.67.5.698.

Mak, K.K., Wong, Y.H., Pichika, M.R., 2024. Artificial Intelligence in drug discovery and development. In: Drug Discovery and Evaluation: Safety and Pharmacokinetic Assays, vols. 1-3. Vol. 2, third Ed. Springer International Publishing, Malaysia, pp. 1461–1498. Available from: https://link.springer.com/book/9783031355295. doi:10.1007/978-3-031-35529-5_92.

McKinney, S.M., Sieniek, M., Godbole, V., Godwin, J., Antropova, N., Ashrafian, H., Back, T., Chesus, M., Corrado, G.C., Darzi, A., Etemadi, M., Garcia-Vicente, F., Gilbert, F.J., Halling-Brown, M., Hassabis, D., Jansen, S., Karthikesalingam, A., Kelly, C.J., King, D., Ledsam, J.R., Melnick, D., Mostofi, H., Peng, L., Reicher, J.J., Romera-Paredes, B., Sidebottom, R., Suleyman, M., Tse, D., Young, K.C., De Fauw, J., Shetty, S., 2020. International evaluation of an AI system for breast cancer screening. Nature. 1476-4687. 577 (7788), 89–94. Available from: http://www.nature.com/nature/index.html. doi:10.1038/s41586-019-1799-6.

Mikdadi, D., O'connell, K.A., Meacham, P.J., Dugan, M.A., Ojiere, M.O., Carlson, T.B., Klenk, J.A., 2022. Applications of artificial intelligence (AI) in ovarian cancer, pancreatic cancer, and image biomarker discovery. Cancer Biomark. 1875-8592. 33 (2), 173–184. Available from: www.iospress.nl/journal/cancer-biomarkers/. doi:10.3233/CBM-210301.

Mobadersany, P., Yousefi, S., Amgad, M., Gutman, D.A., Barnholtz-Sloan, J.S., Velázquez Vega, J.E., Brat, D.J., Cooper, L.A.D., 2018. Predicting cancer outcomes from histology and genomics using convolutional networks. Proc. Natl. Acad. Sci. U. S. A. 1091-6490. 115 (13), E2970. Available from: http://www.pnas.org/content/pnas/115/13/E2970full.pdf. doi:10.1073/pnas.1717139115.

Nam, D., Chapiro, J., Paradis, V., Seraphin, T.P., Kather, J.N., 2022. Artificial intelligence in liver diseases: improving diagnostics, prognostics and response prediction.

JHEP Rep. 2589-5559. 4 (4). Available from: https://www.journals.elsevier.com/jhep-reports. doi:10.1016/j.jhepr.2022.100443.

Nam, H., Kim, K.H., Ock, C.-Y., 2021. AI-based imaging biomarker in mammography for prediction of tumor invasiveness. J. Clin. Oncol. 0732-183X. 39 (15_suppl), 1568. doi:10.1200/jco.2021.39.15_suppl.1568.

Panayides, A.S., Amini, A., Filipovic, N.D., Sharma, A., Tsaftaris, S.A., Young, A., Foran, D., Do, N., Golemati, S., Kurc, T., Huang, K., Nikita, K.S., Veasey, B.P., Zervakis, M., Saltz, J.H., Pattichis, C.S., 2020. AI in medical imaging informatics: current challenges and future directions. IEEE J. Biomed. Health Inform. 2168-2208. 24 (7), 1837–1857. Available from: http://ieeexplore.ieee.org/xpl/RecentIssue.jsp?punumber=6221020. doi:10.1109/JBHI.2020.2991043.

Rajkomar, A., Dean, J., Kohane, I., 2019. Machine learning in medicine. New England Journal of Medicine 380 (14), 1347–1358.

Rajpurkar, P., Irvin, J., Zhu, K., Yang, B., Mehta, H., Duan, T., Ding, D., Bagul, A., Ball, R.L., Langlotz, C., Shpanskaya, K., Lungren, M.P., Ng, A.Y., 2017. CheXNet: radiologist-level pneumonia detection on chest X-rays with deep learning. arXiv. 2331-8422. Available from: https://arxiv.org. doi:10.48550/arxiv.1711.05225.

Sendak, M.P., D'Arcy, J., Kashyap, S., 2020. A path for translation of machine learning products into healthcare delivery. NPJ Digit. Med. 3, 1. doi:10.1038/s41746-020-0231-0.

Shams, A., 2024. Leveraging state-of-the-art AI algorithms in personalized oncology: from transcriptomics to treatment. Diagnostics. 2075-4418. 14 (19), 2174. doi:10.3390/diagnostics14192174.

Shickel, B., Tighe, P.J., Bihorac, A., Rashidi, P., 2018. Deep EHR: a survey of recent advances in deep learning techniques for electronic health record (EHR) analysis. J. Biomed. Health Inform. 2168-2208. 22 (5), 1589–1604. Available from: http://ieeexplore.ieee.org/xpl/RecentIssue.jsp?punumber=6221020. doi:10.1109/JBHI.2017.2767063.

Shukla, A., Singh, T.R., 2021. Structure based inference of functional single nucleotide polymorphism and its role in TGFβ1 allied colorectal cancer (CRC). Int. J. Bioinform. Res. Appl. 1744-5493. 17 (1), 80–99. http://www.inderscience.com/ijbra. doi:10.1504/IJBRA.2021.113965.

Shukla, R., Singh, T.R., 2024. AlzGenPred—CatBoost-based gene classifier for predicting Alzheimer's disease using high-throughput sequencing data. Sci. Rep. 2045-2322. 14 (1). Available from: https://www.nature.com/srep/. doi:10.1038/s41598-024-82208-x.

Somashekhar, S.P., Sepúlveda, M.-J., Puglielli, S., Norden, A.D., Shortliffe, E.H., Kumar, C.R., Rauthan, A., Kumar, N.A., Patil, P., Rhee, K., Ramya, Y., 2018. Watson for oncology and breast cancer treatment recommendations: agreement with an expert multidisciplinary tumor board. Ann. Oncol. 0923-7534. 29 (2), 418–423. doi:10.1093/annonc/mdx781.

Sukari, A., Nagasaka, M., Al-Hadidi, A., Lum, L.G., 2016. Cancer immunology and immunotherapy. Anticancer Res. 1791-7530. 36 (11), 5593–5606. Available from: http://ar.iiarjournals.org/content/36/11/5593.full.pdf+html. doi:10.21873/anticanres.11144.

Ting, D.S.W., Liu, Y., Burlina, P., Xu, X., Bressler, N.M., Wong, T.Y., 2018. AI for medical imaging goes deep. Nat. Med. 1546-170X. 24 (5), 539–540. Available from: http://www.nature.com/nm/index.html. doi:10.1038/s41591-018-0029-3.

Tippur, A., 2023. AI-powered precision oncology: computational insights redefining therapeutic landscapes. DHR Proc. 2689-839X. doi:10.47488/dhrp.v3is1.95.

Tomašev, N., Glorot, X., Rae, J.W., Zielinski, M., Askham, H., Saraiva, A., Mottram, A., Meyer, C., Ravuri, S., Protsyuk, I., Connell, A., Hughes, C.O., Karthikesalingam, A., Cornebise, J., Montgomery, H., Rees, G., Laing, C., Baker, C.R., Peterson, K., Reeves, R., Hassabis, D., King, D., Suleyman, M., Back, T., Nielson, C., Ledsam, J.R., Mohamed, S., 2019. A clinically applicable approach to continuous prediction of

future acute kidney injury. Nature. 1476-4687. 572 (7767), 116–119. Available from: http://www.nature.com/nature/index.html. doi:10.1038/s41586-019-1390-1.
Topol, E., 2019. Deep medicine: how artificial intelligence can make healthcare human again.
Xiao, Q., Zhang, F., Xu, L., Yue, L., Kon, O.L., Zhu, Y., Guo, T., 2021. High-throughput proteomics and AI for cancer biomarker discovery. Adv. Drug Deliv. Rev. 0169-409X. 176, 113844. doi:10.1016/j.addr.2021.113844.
Xu, J., Yang, P., Xue, S., Sharma, B., Sanchez-Martin, M., Wang, F., Beaty, K.A., Dehan, E., Parikh, B., 2019. Translating cancer genomics into precision medicine with artificial intelligence: applications, challenges and future perspectives. Hum. Genet. 1432-1203. 138 (2), 109–124. Available from: http://www.springerlink.com/content/100421/. doi:10.1007/s00439-019-01970-5.
Zadeh Shirazi, A., Tofighi, M., Gharavi, A., Gomez, G.A., 2024. The application of artificial intelligence to cancer research: a comprehensive guide. Technol. Cancer Res. Treat. 1533-0338. 23. Available from: https://journals.sagepub.com/home/TCT. doi:10.1177/15330338241250324.

15

Artificial intelligence emergence in nanomedicine, pharmacogenomics and biotechnology

Kirtan Dave[a], Shriya Joshi[b], and Ruchita Shelat[c]
[a]*Bioinformatics Laboratory, Research and Development Cell, Parul University, Vadodara, Gujarat, India*
[b]*Parul Institute of Applied Sciences, Parul University, Vadodara, Gujarat, India*
[c]*Department of Physiology, The University of Tennessee Health Science Center, Memphis, TN, United States*

1 Introduction

Artificial intelligence, or AI, can be described as a simulation of human intelligence by a machine or computer (Xu et al., 2021). A machine that is capable of thinking and portraying itself as human by being able to perceive, reason, learn, plan, anticipate, and respond to its surroundings is an ideal example of AI. AI should be capable of demonstrating cognizance, logical reasoning, and should have the competence to adapt based on experience over time (Bhardwaj et al., 2022). The main goal of using AI is to reduce the manpower required to perform labor-intensive tasks. It is able to automate repetitive tasks, saving time, improving resource allocation, and enabling people to concentrate on innovative and creative work. AI research encompasses search algorithms, evolution algorithms, data graphs, natural language processing (NLP), machine learning (ML), sophisticated systems, and deep learning (DL) techniques, enabling the development of intelligent networks capable of performing tasks requiring human intellect (Xu et al., 2021). ML is a type of AI that learns and refines its assessments through the use of computational algorithms. It trains independent recommendations by identifying patterns in huge data sets. Following iteration and adjustment, the algorithm generates predictions, which are then checked for accuracy against known results (Helm et al., 2020).

The AI Frontier in Molecular Modelling and Drug Designing. https://doi.org/10.1016/B978-0-443-40338-5.00009-3

1.1 Need for artificial intelligence

High-throughput sequencing technology revolutionizes genomic data generation, enabling researchers to analyze individual genetic makeup on a large scale, providing extensive information about population genetic variants. Technologies such as next generation sequencing (NGS) and genome wide association studies generate a huge volume of genomics, proteomics, and transcriptomics data that are too large for humans to process and understand. These datasets often consist of millions of data points, capturing complex relationships between genes, proteins, and other molecular elements. Large datasets generated by clinical and experimental setups sometimes provide a major difficulty for academics since managing ever-increasing volumes of data becomes an exhausting effort. Furthermore, in order to properly analyze, comprehend, and derive significant insights from the data, sophisticated and advanced analytical methods and computational tools are needed (Lin and Ngiam, 2023).

1.2 Machine learning

The use of ML to manage large volumes of data has become essential across various fields, as it not only handles vast datasets efficiently but also uncovers insights that extend beyond our current understanding of the entities being studied. Furthermore, by learning from the experience gathered from training data, ML models naturally improve (Caudai et al., 2021). AI has the power to identify complex and interesting patterns or trends in huge datasets, which might be overlooked by humans. This helps researchers gain in-depth insights and allows them to improve the accuracy with which they make predictions, such as predicting phenotypic expression from genetic sequences and predicting protein structure from its amino acid sequence, etc. (Halagali et al., 2025).

1.3 Deep learning

A subset of ML is DL, which can be described as a complex architecture of artificial neural networks (ANNs). DL has the ability to encode and simulate many types of complex datasets (Grapov et al., 2018). Neurons, which are mathematical operations grouped in numerous layers connected to one another, are inspired by human brain layers and excel in learning complex tasks. DL methods are incredibly useful in analyzing various types of information, particularly while working with textual data, images, numeric data, or audio data types. They are also capable of processing nonlinear relationships, which are highly complex (Caudai et al., 2021). DL has the power to learn and process data to extract meaningful features and patterns by passing the data through multiple hidden layers in a neural network, as compared to traditional ML models. Currently, DL has many applications in the field of genomics, such as the identification of novel biomarkers and new and alternate drug targets, homology modeling, prediction of protein structure from its amino acid sequence, pathway analysis, gene expression analysis, single-nucleotide polymorphism (SNP) tagging, cancer genome analysis, etc. The consistent interface of this class of models to data encoding and integration is one of the most promising aspects of DL techniques (Caudai et al., 2021).

2 AI for targeted therapies and disease treatment

2.1 Introduction

There has been a significant change in traditional healthcare organizations in recent years due to the realization that every individual needs unique treatment. Traditional approaches often utilize a one-size-fits-all model, but the integration of AI into healthcare has completely transformed treatment modalities for patients. This new field of personalized medicine, powered by AI, offers more effective and tailored treatments for patients. This approach utilizes an individual's genetic profile to guide decisions with respect to disease prevention, diagnosis, and treatment (Mathur and Sutton, 2017; O'Shea et al., 2022). The overall aim of personalized medicine is to provide the right care to the right patients (based on their genetic information) at the right time. Personalized medicine is often referred to as precision medicine by many. There is an overlap between the two; however, as per the US National Security Council, personalized medicine is often considered an innovative approach that is individually developed for each patient, whereas precision medicine focuses on treatment approaches that are effective for patients based on their genetic, environmental, and lifestyle factors (Committee on A Framework for Developing a New Taxonomy of Disease Board on Life Sciences Division on Earth and Life Studies, 2011). Precision medicine will help transform the overall healthcare industry (Parekh et al., 2023). Hence, it is imperative to understand various parameters that may affect the future of precision medicine, directly or indirectly (Fig. 15.1).

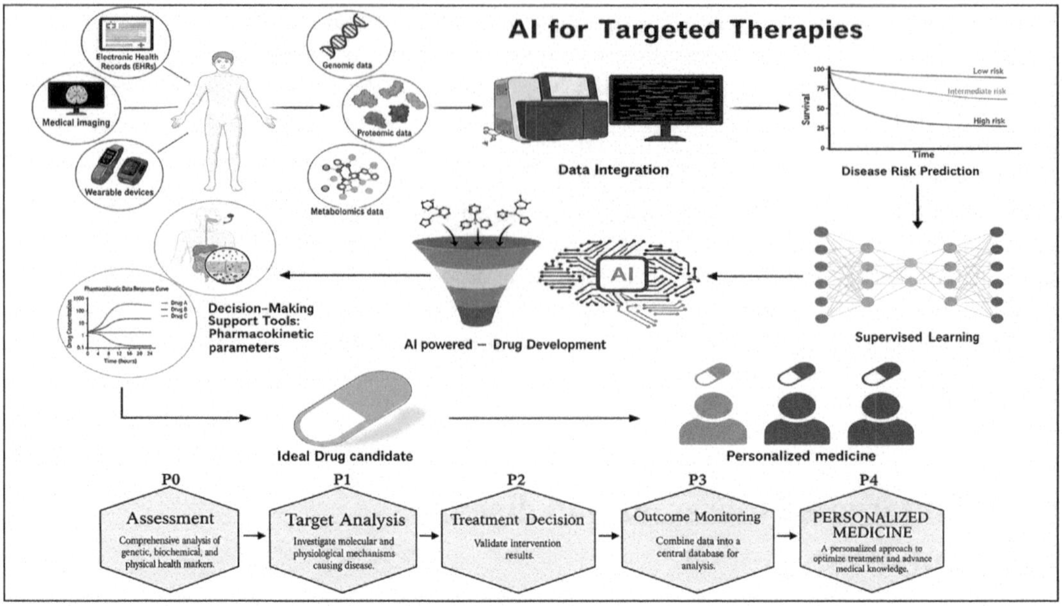

Fig. 15.1 Personalized medicine (upper) and personalized drug discovery (lower), which will benefit the individual patient.

2.1.1 Understanding individual variability in health

In healthcare, every individual is different and responds in a unique manner when treated together. This phenomenon is referred to as 'individual variability,' which plays an important role in patient response to treatments (Abdelhalim et al., 2022). The term 'individual variability' refers to the inherent differences among individuals with respect to their genetic makeup, physiological traits, lifestyle conditions, environmental exposures, and other personal characteristics.

Genetic factors

Genetic variations can substantially impact an individual's response to medications and treatments. Genetic differences can affect the process of drug metabolism, their interaction with target molecules, and the process of elimination from the body. These variations can make certain individuals susceptible to adverse drug reactions, while others may experience an enhanced treatment effect.

Physiological factors

Various physiological factors like age, sex, hormonal levels, body type, and composition can contribute to individual variability in response to a treatment. Differences in all of these may influence drug metabolism and thereby therapeutic outcomes (Pinto and Eileen Dolan, 2011).

Lifestyle and environmental factors

Various lifestyle factors like diet, exercise, smoking, alcohol, and environmental factors like toxin or pollutant exposure may change the way an individual responds to a particular treatment. People with a sedentary lifestyle and poor habits may observe reduced effectiveness of certain medications or therapies, which might work very well for individuals with a healthy lifestyle. Similarly, environmental toxins can lead to a reduced therapeutic outcome.

2.2 Role of AI in healthcare

AI is a generic term for computer tools and technologies that can simulate human intelligence without human intervention. AI systems can simulate human learning, creative thinking, and problem-solving abilities, making them suitable in any field. The last decade has seen a remarkable rise in the field of AI in many work sectors, but mainly in the healthcare industry (Johnson et al., 2021). This is due to the various AI technologies (e.g., DL-based information systems and robotic assemblies) that may assist healthcare providers in active decision-making and also assist surgeons during surgery. In addition, many AI tools are powerful enough to recognize hidden structures and difficult patterns better than clinicians and hence can be used for image detection and diagnostics.

2.2.1 AI in biotechnology

The area of biotechnology is advancing rapidly due to the integration of technologies like AI and big data analysis, which can analyze vast amounts of data to identify variations, predict treatment responses, and offer treatment plans (Johnson et al., 2021). The ongoing research in fields like pharmacogenomics and systems biology will help healthcare providers understand the underlying mechanisms in a better way to offer personalized treatment approaches. Given below are a few examples of how AI is transforming the biotechnology domain.

Data analysis and Integration

Reports from "The European Bioinformatics Institute (EMBL-EBI)" show a trend where in nucleotide and proteomics data generation is emerging exponentially, considering that the quantity of databases doubles every year (Howe, 2021) The increasing amount of data poses a significant challenge for organizations that deal with storing and organizing data. Despite this, the ever-increasing data also presents opportunities for biotechnology researchers to explore and exploit the growing information. The process of combining data generated and merging it with individually generated data is known as data integration. This procedure may be classified as either eager or sluggish, based on whether machine-readable interfaces are available. Web services that use protocols like Asynchronous JavaScript and XML, Simple Object Access Protocol, or Representational State Transfer (Khan and Abbasi, 2015) automate data integration techniques. However, the coexistence of several standards makes data integration difficult. Large-scale genomic initiatives, drug development, chemical characteristics, pathway effect evaluation, electronic health record (EHR) mining, genome analysis, personal genomics, automated experiments, and experiment design are important fields where innovation can lead to the transformation of the world of biotechnology. Drug development, recycling, and safety studies are all aided by AI, which also saves manual work and optimizes data collection, storage, and processing (Oliveira, 2019).

Genomic medicine

By revolutionizing disease diagnosis and prognosis, AI has driven genomic medicine in a new direction. The use of AI algorithms has enabled the precise and accurate identification of genetic mutations and health risks associated with various mutations. ML models can analyze genetic data to predict an individual's susceptibility to various diseases, such as cancer, cardiovascular conditions, and neurodegenerative disorders. AI models can also identify specific genetic mutations linked to breast cancer, facilitating early detection and improving patient outcomes. Support vector machines (SVMs), neural networks, and decision trees are examples of supervised learning techniques that are frequently used to predict treatment outcomes and disease susceptibility based on genetic data. They can also predict disease progression by analyzing longitudinal genetic data, helping clinicians develop personalized monitoring and treatment plans. AI is also enhancing drug development and personalized treatment by uncovering new drug targets and predicting individual responses to therapies (Felici et al., 2025).

Treatment personalization

Emerging strategies and AI techniques could lead to more holistic and efficient treatments for individual patients. A unified procedure that integrates diagnosis, treatment, and follow-up monitoring provides the best environment for individualized medicine and healthcare. The development of cell replacement treatments for a range of ailments serves as an excellent example of this. Harvesting and sensitizing cells to identify neoantigens enable the manufacture of treatments in real time in immune-modulating cell-based therapies for cancer (Schork, 2019).

Predictive analysis

Predictive biotechnology uses data, such as more than two billion sequences of proteins and two million experimentally determined crystal structures, to create new proteins. Comprehensive predictions are now possible thanks to developments in structure prediction that have resolved issues with small molecule cofactors. The selection of a specific protein for the targeted catalytic process may be advised by combining virtual prediction algorithms with protein sequences, which allow us to anticipate gene expression. Beyond cost savings, cloud computing is providing biotechnology with new commercial opportunities. With over 214 million entries, the AlphaFold DB presents opportunities for creative predictive biotechnological initiatives. Numerous biotechnology subfields, including functional annotation, enzyme structure prediction, cellular processes, modeling, and downstream processing, currently make good use of predictive techniques (Nestl et al., 2024).

Image analysis and prediction

By integrating clinical data with noninvasive measures from blood, urine, or radiological imaging, AI can enhance clinical outcomes and treatment monitoring. While imaging and genetic data can offer complementary information for the creation of biomarkers, deep neural networks (DNNs) can extract additional information from radiological images. Projects like tumor and lymph node delineation may be automated with AI techniques, especially DNNs, which improve consistency and save time in clinical settings. Clinical notes can contain discrete data pieces that can be extracted using NLP techniques, providing context to other data types (Holzinger et al., 2019).

AI algorithms in personalized healthcare are key contributors in the field, as they have the ability to analyze, process, and incorporate large volumes of patient data, including patients' genetic information, health records, imaging data, and wearable device data. This integration assists healthcare providers in gaining a deeper insight into patients' health, allowing them to make accurate diagnoses and treatment decisions. Given below is a detailed explanation of how AI has transformed the domain of biotechnology.

2.2.2 AI in precise diagnostics

AI can transform various aspects of healthcare, including accurate diagnosis, which is still considered a significant challenge globally. This accuracy is possible with the help of various ML tools (Alowais et al., 2023). Specifically, ML utilizes information as a resource that is highly contingent upon the quality and quantity of input data, capable of addressing the complexities and obstacles of diagnosis. In summary, ML may facilitate prompt decision-making, optimize workflow management, and automate numerous operations efficiently and economically. Numerous DL technologies, including convolutional neural networks (CNNs) and data mining approaches, facilitate the identification of disease patterns within large datasets. These instruments are utilized for the prediction and diagnosis of many diseases. Notwithstanding this, AI remains underutilized, with the exception of certain tumors.

A study indicated the incorporation of mammography into AI for breast cancer diagnosis. The outcome demonstrated a total decrease in false positives and false negatives of 5.7% and 9.4%, respectively. A comparable study correlated AI diagnosis of breast cancer with those of radiologists. The study revealed that AI-assisted diagnosis was more effective at detecting early breast cancer (91%) compared to radiologists (74%). The former approach demonstrated greater sensitivity in diagnosing breast cancer compared to the latter (90% vs. 78%). A separate study employed a DL model, namely a CNN, to identify skin cancer, demonstrating accuracy in diagnosis relative to dermatologists and even suggesting treatment options. Research has indicated the application of AI in identifying several disease modalities, such as diabetic retinopathy and electrocardiogram (EKG) abnormalities. DL algorithms have identified pneumonia in chest radiographs with superior sensitivity (96% vs. 50%) and specificity (64% vs. 73%) relative to radiologists (Alowais et al., 2023).

AI tools have an edge over traditional diagnostic methods with respect to improved accuracy and reasonable cost, which saves time and also reduces the risk of human errors. Researchers are trying to analyze various medical images like X-rays, computed tomography (CT) scans, and magnetic resonance imaging (MRIs). By exploiting various ML tools, AI can help identify abnormalities, detect fractures or other conditions, and provide quantitative measurements for faster and more accurate medical diagnosis.

The role of AI in the clinical laboratory is progressing and expanding. Various ML tools have been developed to detect, identify, and quantify microorganisms, diagnose diseases, and predict outcomes. These tools extract information from gene sequencing, metagenomic sequencing, and microscopic imaging of the organisms. Moreover, gram staining results of these organisms also increase the sensitivity and specificity (Dhaarani and Reddy, 2025).

2.2.3 AI in targeted therapies

Targeted therapy has become a popular treatment option in precision medicine. It is a challenging process, starting from target identification to targeted drug therapy based on single-omics data. Thus, AI holds great potential here by integrating vast datasets along with the information collected through genes and gene products. With AI, it is easier to develop and validate newer drugs with minimal side effects. Targeted cancer therapies in oncology aim to prevent particular genetic or molecular changes that contribute to tumor development, resulting in fewer adverse effects and more effective treatments. Immunotherapy is another area of personalized healthcare where biotechnology is essential in utilizing the body's immune response to fight against illnesses (Calvino et al., 2025). Precision medicine reduces the trial-and-error method of choosing a therapy by emphasizing prevention and early detection determined by individual risk factors. Clinicians can select therapies with fewer chances of adverse responses by understanding the genetic and molecular components influencing medication response. This improves patient health and ease of use by predicting and mitigating side effects (Anyanwu et al., 2024).

Drug development

Recently, unusual N6-methyladenosine (m6A) regulators have emerged as novel anticancer drug targets (You et al., 2022). Modification of these regulators can lead to the occurrence, development, progression, and prognosis of cancer. It has been reported that AI-assisted synthesis of Fat mass and obesity-associated protein (FTO) and ethyltransferase-like 3 (METL3) inhibitors has an edge over natural compounds. Hence, AI assistance can help open up newer drug targets. The information about the drug mode of action (MoA) is crucial for formulating anticancer drugs. A similar study was published wherein the authors predicted the MoA of novel drugs in prostate cancer cells through metabolomics data, along with ML tools, and validated the results in various cancer types (Wang et al., 2023). In addition, researchers have also identified compound UM-164 as a potent TIPE2 inhibitor (Zhang et al., 2021). Table 15.1 provides a glimpse of a few anticancer drugs that have entered clinical trial phases.

Drug selection

Selecting the suitable medication for targeted therapy postdrug development is a critical stage. A DL framework known as the Siamese Response Deep Factorization Machines Network was introduced for tailored recommendations of anticancer treatments, leveraging the gene expression profiles of cancer cell lines and the chemical structures of anticancer agents. This network may assess the drug based on its specificity and determine the most effective drug. In a similar study, authors developed a DL network, scDEAL, to predict and select drugs (Su et al., 2022). A DL neural network utilizing contrastive learning, named GraphCDR, was developed for predicting cancer medication

Table 15.1 Few anticancer drugs designed by AI that have successfully entered phase II/III clinical trials in the last 5 years.

Name	Chemical Structure	Company	Therapeutic Area	Target/ Function	Phase
REC-2282	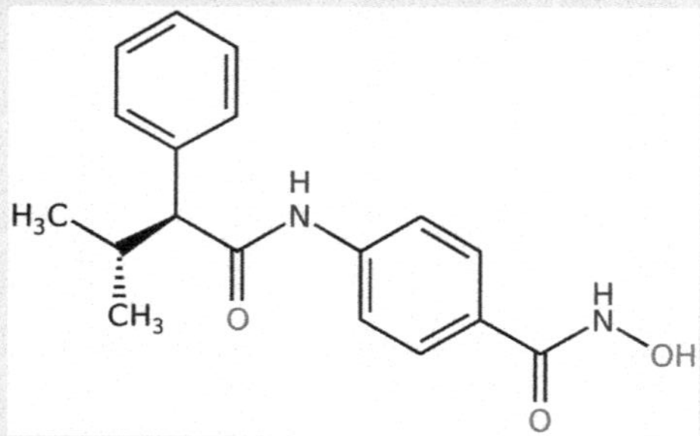	Recursion	Neurofibromatosis Type 2	HDAC	Phase 2/3
RLY-4008	Not disclosed	Relay Therapeutics	Solid tumour	FGFR	Phase 2
BPM31510	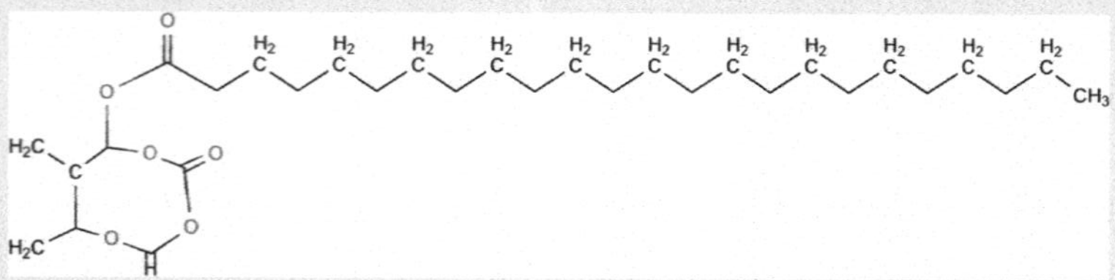	Berg	Solid tumour	Protein cbcl2 modulators	Phase 2
EXS-21,546	Not disclosed	Exscientia	Solid tumour	A2aR	Phase 1
PHI-101	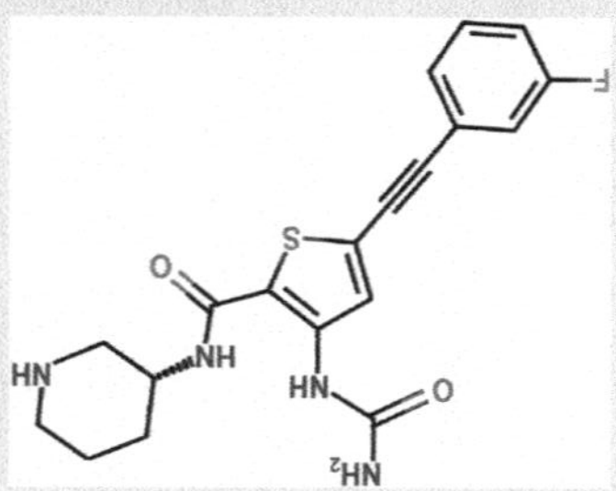	Pharos iBio	Ovarian cancer Breast cancer	Flt3 tyrosine kinase inhibitor	Phase 1

response (CDR). This approach employs multiomics data from cancer cell lines, the chemical structures of medicines, and established drug responses of cancer cell lines for cancer drug response prediction (Wang et al., 2023).

Drug application

In order to enhance efficacy and minimize toxicity, researchers have proposed single-cell therapy along with single-cell transcriptomics to prioritize multitargeted therapeutic options for cancer patients. In a recent Pan cancer analysis of five cancer types, 19% of the treatments offered were patient-specific. A system called REcurrent Features LEveraged for Combination Therapy (REFLECT) was developed by integrating cancer informatics and ML methods for choosing proper drug combinations (Ianevski et al., 2024) In another study, authors proposed a graph neural network, GraphRepur, for repurposing drugs against breast cancer (Cui et al., 2021). This method was based on gene expression and drug exposure gene expression (Wang et al., 2023). Thus, AI definitely contributes to drug combination, repurposing, and drug delivery.

2.2.4 AI-powered wearables

AI-powered wearables facilitate convenient patient monitoring of vital signs, including heart rate, blood pressure, blood glucose, and oxygen saturation. Furthermore, these gadgets furnish data on electrocardiography of the heart, electroencephalography of the brain, and photoplethysmography of blood variations, thus presenting a comprehensive overview of the patient's health. These gadgets are highly beneficial in managing chronic illnesses like diabetes. Patients can consistently assess their blood glucose levels to prevent any critical situations. Likewise, these gadgets can analyze the gathered data and forecast any problems before they escalate. These wearables can analyze heart rate variations, cardiac biomarkers, and sleep patterns to forecast the likelihood of cardiovascular diseases and sleep problems, thereby facilitating early preventive intervention. When coupled with other applications, these devices can provide individualized care recommendations, medication alerts, and appropriate exercise suggestions based on patient data and current health status. AI/ML systems analyze complex relationships among pharmaceutical properties, formulation components, and physiological factors. This promotes the advancement of efficient medication delivery systems and enhances comprehension of drug delivery mechanisms. It assists in forecasting the medication's stability, in vitro drug release profile, and physicochemical properties (Shajari et al., 2023).

Virtual nursing assistance

Virtual nursing aid provides ongoing monitoring and patient support, ultimately improving the efficiency of patient care. These programs provide continuous assistance, including health-related alerts, medication reminders, and appointment scheduling, thereby aiding both patients and healthcare professionals. Virtual assistants can monitor patients' health status and symptoms, alerting doctors when necessary to avert problems and minimize hospital admissions. They can also gather and analyze patient data, providing insights into healthcare trends. Challenges associated with this approach include data privacy and information accuracy. Nonetheless, advancements in this domain are anticipated to significantly enhance virtual nursing assistants, heralding a future of accessible, personalized, and efficient healthcare. A DL neural network utilizing contrastive learning, named GraphCDR, was developed for predicting CDR. This approach employs multiomics data from cancer cell lines, the chemical structures of medicines, and established drug responses of cancer cell lines for the prediction of CDR (Liu et al., 2022).

AI in telemedicine

The integration of AI with telemedicine is revolutionizing healthcare accessibility and efficiency for patients. AI enhances telehealth platforms by providing sophisticated diagnostic and consulting services, enabling physicians to remotely assess patients. AI-enabled chatbots and virtual assistants facilitate the appointment scheduling process for patients. The role of AI in remote patient monitoring is to forecast and analyze chronic conditions and to streamline this process for patients. A study developed a medical chatbot called PROSCA for educating individuals about prostate cancer. This involved ten men with suspected prostate cancer. The chatbot improved participants' awareness of prostate cancer, and they expressed a willingness to use and recommend the chatbot again. Some challenges in this field include data privacy and accuracy. Nonetheless, the incorporation of AI into telemedicine is essential and offers more accessible and personalized health plans (Görtz et al., 2023).

2.3 Improving treatment personalization

It is important to comprehend variability in an individual patient's response to treatments for better outcomes. Here, in this section, we have provided a few implications that can help a healthcare provider optimize the treatment plan for the individual with maximum efficacy and minimum adverse effects. Major differences exist between the conventional drug discovery process and personalized, patient-based drug discovery, which will benefit the individual patient rather than the entire population (Schork, 2019).

2.3.1 Pharmacogenomics

Pharmacogenomics, or pharmacogenetics, is a rapidly growing branch of precision medicine that studies how a person's genetic profile may affect the way their body processes certain medications. Many times, drugs lead to adverse events rather than improving the disease condition due to genetic variability in certain individuals. With the advent of science, it is now possible to study how an individual's genes may respond to administered drugs. The term pharmacogenomics is used interchangeably with 'pharmacogenetics' and is derived from pharmacology (the study of drugs) and genomics (the study of genes) to develop safe medications and dosages tailored to variations in an individual's genetic profile. Currently, pharmacogenomics is used only for conditions like HIV, certain cancers (breast, colon, and acute lymphoblastic leukemia), depression, and heart issues (Nathanson, 2010).

2.4 Tools in AI-enhanced pharmacogenomics

AI and ML offer favorable solutions to the challenges posed by the fast-growing, high volume of data. These tools have the ability to independently detect and analyze any abnormal patterns within the data, study the pharmaceutical properties of drugs Absorption, Distribution, Metabolism, Excretion, and Toxicity (ADMET), which is helpful to healthcare providers in clinical settings (Pun et al., 2023). Both these tools can analyze and merge data from genomics and pharmacokinetics and hence are well-suited for drug discovery applications. For example, AI and ML assist in the virtual screening of compounds from the vast compound library, in in silico drug targeting, and in identifying risk factors leading to diseases. Thus, all of these features speed up the entire drug discovery process (Taherdoost and Ghofrani, 2024). Due to all these reasons, AI is widely utilized in pharmacology research and in clinical settings, starting from drug discovery to bedside applications (You et al., 2022).

2.4.1 ML and DL

ML and DL have shown promising results in analyzing vast amounts of data in pharmacology, making them well-suited for drug discovery applications. DL, which is a part of the ML toolkit, has improved the overall analysis even in genomics and the drug discovery area (Kalinin et al., 2018).

2.4.2 Big data analytics

Big data analytics in pharmacogenomics has completely transformed the healthcare industry by efficiently managing and analyzing large volumes of data. This integration can test multiple drugs at a time and provide vital information ahead of time, which can impact a large population.

2.5 Applications of AI in pharmacogenomics

ML models are widely utilized in cancer therapy for predicting drug responses. These models use different parameters to record drug responses in order to classify them. For example, a DL model, DrugCell, was developed to assess drug response in human cancer cells and obtained great predictability by analyzing the drug response determinants (Kuenzi et al., 2020). ML models are a great choice for investigating the efficacy of multiple drug molecules in various cancer therapies. This involves drug response evaluation and quantification, molecule selection from a large pool, cellular measurements, and overall efficacy. These datasets are based on the results obtained from high-throughput screening (HTS) performed on various cancer cell lines (Kallal et al., 2021; Adam et al., 2020). A recent study evaluated the outcomes obtained from both ML and DL models to be used in cancer studies. Two different datasets were designed (a gene expression and mutation dataset) to understand individual drug responses, which helped in identifying the major genomic factors affecting drug sensitivity. The study highlighted the potential of these models for personalized medicine in cancer therapies (Kuenzi et al., 2020; Park et al., 2023a). They narrate how integrating data with different types uses ML algorithms to assist in decision-making in cancer treatments and pharmacogenomics, as shown in Fig. 15.2.

2.5.1 Challenges of using ML in pharmacogenomics

The incorporation of AI into healthcare has numerous potential benefits; however, there are certain limitations and challenges which need to be addressed, too.

Data privacy

It is very important to maintain patients' data private and secure. The program must adhere to the guidelines laid down by the health authorities. Also, the quality of data is very crucial. Any glitch in the healthcare data may affect the overall prediction and may lead to errors (Tembhare et al., 2019).

Ethical issues

Ethical considerations may come into the picture when AI tools handle patient data. It is critical to ensure that AI algorithms align with ethical guidelines to avoid any harm to the patient.

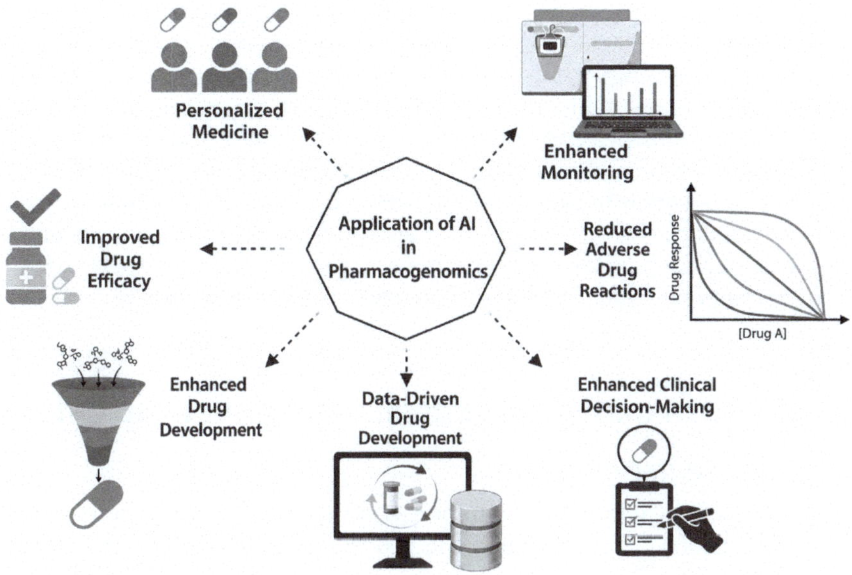

Fig. 15.2 Integration of AI into pharmacogenomics.

Regulatory bodies

With the prompt integration of AI into healthcare, it is now significant to have clear guidelines and regulations for its appropriate use. This will ensure patient safety, data security, data privacy, and will guarantee innovation.

Human-AI collaboration

It follows that AI tools are available to assist healthcare providers and not to replace them. These tools will only help in better decision-making and save a lot of lives. Human intervention should be prioritized, as human judgment and expertise help significantly in critical cases (Bajwa et al., 2021).

Mitigation of challenges

The digital infrastructure and networked protocols for communication play an integral part in the processing, analysis, and sharing of biological data via laboratory automation systems, next-generation sequencing platforms, and bioinformatics tools. Combining these technologies, however, also creates additional cybersecurity risks, such as the potential for unauthorized access to genetic data, manipulation of experimental results, or disruption of important research procedures.

The cooperation between cybersecurity and biosafety protocols, together with the development of a security awareness and preparedness culture, can help businesses become more resilient to emerging threats and vulnerabilities. This includes public education and outreach, cross-training and cooperation, risk assessment and mitigation, secure-by-design principles, and regulatory harmonization and alignment. Organizations may strengthen themselves against complex and ever-changing security issues by recognizing the mutual impact of biological and cyber threats and leveraging the synergies between biosafety and cybersecurity policies. To share threat intelligence, best practices, and lessons learned from cyber events, research institutions, governmental agencies, and business sector partners can collaborate more closely (AL-Eitan et al., 2025).

3 AI in analyzing genomic and proteomic data

3.1 AI in genomics

The human genome is 3 billion base pairs long and encodes for over 20,000 genes. Through the process of transcription, the information encoded by DNA is passed onto mRNA. mRNA (messenger RNA) is a small, single-stranded chain of nucleotides that carries the genetic instructions from the DNA in the nucleus to the ribosomes in the cytoplasm, where proteins are synthesized via translation. Proteins are the functional molecules that drive the complexity of life. Their diverse roles in structure, function, and regulation are fundamental to the maintenance and growth of living organisms. Proteins are essential for carrying out the vast majority of biological functions in cells, including catalyzing biochemical reactions, providing structural support, and regulating processes like cell division and gene expression. Even small changes in DNA can result in serious consequences, such as disease or the death of organisms. Sequencing DNA is a significant step in understanding the development of organisms and potential diseases that might harm them (Murray, 2018).

3.1.1 History

Genomics can be described as the study of a complete set of genes present in an organism and any possible relationship between the environment and genes. Thomas Roderick first used the phrase in 1986 to refer to the emerging field of genome sequencing, mapping, annotation, and analysis. The field can be divided into four main categories—functional genomics, metagenomics, epigenomics, and structural genomics. Three phases are usually involved in genomic analysis. The first step is genome sequencing, which can be done through low-throughput techniques (Sanger sequencing, etc.) or high-throughput techniques (NGS, whole genome sequencing [WGS], etc.); the second is sequence assembly, which involves aligning and combining all of the sequenced DNA to recreate the primary sequence. This typically requires computational software (Sanger reads, Euler, etc.); and the third is gene annotation, which consists of giving the sequence biological meaning. Many different tools are available online (GenMark, MAKER, etc.) (Giani et al., 2020; Dias and Torkamani, 2019).

HTS is a scientific method for the rapid evaluation of chemical substances against biological targets in drug development, especially in the pharmaceutical sector. It makes it possible to conduct experiments with greater efficiency and identify potential therapeutic candidates. HTS is essential to modern biomedical research because of its contributions to data quality, functionality, technical improvements, and broad applications (Macarron et al., 2011). ChIP-seq refers to a DNA-based test that is utilized in gene expression, disease diagnosis, and the development of customized therapies. The largest library of sequencing-based methods, such as ChIP-seq, is the Encyclopedia of DNA Elements (ENCODE). In addition to using tools like the Scythe utility, BWA, IGB, MAC/Peakseq, SAMTools, MEME suites, MAST suite, and Fastx tools, it encompasses stages I and II, sequencing, gene mining, and normalization. ENCODE provides documented standards for every stage of the research and encodes ChIP-seq summary data (Muhammad et al., 2019).

3.1.2 Challenges

The Human Genome Project was a groundbreaking international initiative aimed at sequencing the entire human genome with high-quality results. The advancements in techniques to sequence DNA were brought about, and new methods like WGS and next-generation sequencing were developed. As a result, the speed of sequencing increased exponentially, leading to the generation of a vast amount of data consisting of DNA sequences, coding and noncoding regions, promoters, operators, etc. With ever-developing technologies, new challenges emerge. It becomes challenging to manage the vast amount of data generated. Among others, these challenges include data storage, processing and analysis, data integration, data interpretation, privacy and security, infrastructure scalability, standardization, and cost (Dziuda, 2010).

Storing this vast amount of data requires immense capacity, as the human genome can produce hundreds of gigabytes of raw data. As more and more data are generated with each organism, it makes the task of interpreting this data even harder for researchers. Analyzing every nucleotide change is a time-consuming process that is prone to human error. It also requires expertise to differentiate between harmless mutations and deadly ones. That is why it demands a significant workforce to meticulously examine each nucleotide. This is a computationally intensive task, which requires highly sophisticated and advanced computers with high processing power. In addition, the program must be able to correctly differentiate between various sequences on its own, without assistance from a person. These challenges have prompted the creation and development of novel and advanced bioinformatics techniques and computational tools, which should be able to handle, analyze, and derive meaningful insights from the rapidly growing volume of genomic data. In addition to paving the way for several developments in biotechnology, medicine, and personalized health, the Human Genome Project has revolutionized our understanding of genetics and disease, especially with the integration of AI to analyze complex genomic data and uncover novel insights (Dziuda, 2010).

3.1.3 Application of AI

The introduction of AI in the field of genomics has allowed researchers to understand complex biological networks and infer information from vast amounts of data. ML and DL both have applications in genomics for addressing different problems encountered while analyzing the genome. First, we will take a look at how ML is utilized in the field of genomics. One of the main features of ML is its ability to learn from previous information or data and apply it to make predictions or choices when faced with new, unknown data. Through a process called training, the ML model is exposed to historical data, which allows the model to recognize patterns and relationships between data set points. Using large samples as reference data points, any ML model can be trained to recognize specific elements in any unknown data (Libbrecht and Noble, 2015).

Application of ML

For example, an ML model could be trained to identify the position of key transcription start locations in the genome sequence. Ohler, Uwe, and his team trained the ML model "McPromoter" on data obtained from Drosophila genome sequences about transcription start sites by analyzing their core promoter motifs and discovered new motifs like DNA-replication-related element (DRE). The accuracy of the model's promoter predictions increased as a result of this training, and these predictions were subsequently contrasted with those of vertebrates (Ohler et al., 2002). Similarly, the study team headed by Degroeve, Sven, developed splice site prediction models for *Arabidopsis thaliana* using supervised learning algorithms. They chose features based on the occurrence of particular nucleotides close to splice sites. The results demonstrated that a wrapper-based feature subset selection technique employing naive Bayes or SVMs performed better than conventional techniques by selecting more pertinent features and increasing prediction speed and accuracy (Degroeve et al., 2002).

ML is generally divided into two types—supervised and unsupervised. In supervised ML, the data given as input features and corresponding target outputs are known. Whereas in unsupervised ML, the model is trained on an unlabeled dataset. In supervised ML, the main objective is to make predictions or classifications based on labeled data. On the other hand, unsupervised ML is used when the objective is to explore and identify patterns or structures within an unlabeled dataset. It can help identify hidden patterns in gene expression data, which can lead to insights about disease mechanisms or biological processes (for example, the discovery of biomarkers) (Williams et al., 2018). Another application of ML is the annotation of genes. The conventional methods of assigning functions to genes (gene ontology) have been manual, labor-intensive, and overpriced. By utilizing ML to elucidate gene function, a comprehensive matrix representing probability interactions between genes is created by evaluating, weighting, and integrating data from several trials. The model uses large-scale datasets to construct probabilistic networks of gene interactions, inferring gene functions iteratively, and accounting for complexities like pleiotropy and experimental noise (Fraser and Marcotte, 2004). Finally, yet importantly, ML techniques are being used to understand gene expression mechanisms, predicting gene expression levels using DNA sequences, or incorporating data like ChIP-seq profiles (Libbrecht and Noble, 2015).

Application of DL

DL methods are able to offer higher accuracy in predicting complex promoter sequences compared to traditional approaches (e.g., chromatin immunoprecipitation (ChIP)) by learning patterns from datasets. These methods can process and analyze much larger and more complex datasets. For instance, Basset uses a CNN to learn the function of genes from genomics data, detecting cell-type-specific accessible chromatin regions (Libbrecht and Noble, 2015). Predicting Enhancers with a Deep Learning-based Algorithmic framework (PEDLA), created by Liu et al., predicts enhancers from a variety of datasets. It consistently generalizes predictions across various cell types and tissues and captures universal patterns. DeepSEA predicts the effects of noncoding variants directly from DNA sequences. In addition, Sequence-based Promoter-Enhancer Interaction with Deep learning (SPEID) achieves higher accuracy in predicting enhancer-promoter interactions by using sequence features, outperforming the best methods (Liu et al., 2020) that use features from genomic data not directly based on DNA sequences (Liu et al., 2020).

3.2 AI in proteomics

3.2.1 Introduction to the role of proteomics

Proteins are one of the most important molecules in all biological processes. They are directly responsible for the main processes that occur in cells. They help by catalyzing chemical reactions by acting as enzymes, transporting oxygen (hemoglobin), providing structural support in the form of actin/myosin fibers, and also play an important role in cell-to-cell communication with the help of receptors or cell surface markers. In addition, they defend cells from foreign invaders by stimulating the immune response, aiding in the detection and labeling of pathogens with antibodies, and facilitating the elimination of pathogens such as viruses and bacteria. Furthermore, proteins regulate gene expression by functioning as transcription factors and orchestrating various cellular processes, making them vital for growth, repair, and adaptation to environmental changes. Proteins are essentially responsible for all aspects of life, including cell development and division, tissue repair, and environmental response. Proteins are essential to life because, without them, cells could not operate correctly (Petsko and Ringe, 2009).

Consequently, it has become more important to study and characterize essential proteins. The field which deals with the study of the structure, function, and interactions of proteins within a cell, tissue, or organism is called 'Proteomics.' After the Human Genome Project was completed, scientists had the complete blueprint of the genome of human cells. They then shifted their focus to the entire set of proteins produced by an organism, called the proteome. They believed that the proteome would more accurately depict the workings of a cell and its functioning in a tissue or an organism. Protein levels are not always reflected by RNA quantification, and DNA sequence analysis cannot predict a protein's active form. After the translation of mRNA into peptides, these peptides undergo posttranslational modifications, which pose a problem when analyzing DNA/RNA. Another challenge arises due to the process of alternative splicing, wherein a single gene can code for many different proteins. Understanding the proteome requires the identification and quantification of proteins, which provide information on biological processes, disease mechanisms, and possible treatment strategies. Together, these complexities make the study of the proteome essential for a more accurate understanding of biological processes (Gobena et al., 2024).

3.2.2 Techniques for protein analysis in proteomics

To study the structure and function of proteins, many advanced and sophisticated techniques are utilized. Two-dimensional polyacrylamide gel electrophoresis (2D PAGE) is the most common technique to separate proteins from cell/tissue samples. However, the process of

2D PAGE requires a lot of work and time. Liquid chromatography is another method for separating compounds in a sample. One of the most popular techniques in proteomic research is mass spectrometry, which utilizes electron beams to ionize biomolecules in samples and is useful for protein identification and determining protein mass. It is quite effective and is becoming more and more well-liked in proteomics studies because of its capacity to examine large, delicate biomolecules (Cho, 2007).

3.2.3 Challenges in proteomics data analysis

This field of study also experiences the challenges faced by traditional approaches to genomics. The data generated by techniques like mass spectrometry (MS) is huge and complex. The process of analyzing proteomics data involves multiple steps in a well-defined pipeline. The data is received in the form of spectral signals, which have to be converted to peptide sequences. The peptides then have to be reassembled into proteins. The results can be stored in the database after they are validated. The data obtained has high dimensionality, noise, and dynamic range. The samples contain a vast number of proteins and their complex interactions. Since proteins are involved in numerous cellular processes, the data often includes thousands of variables (proteins, peptides, modifications, etc.), making it challenging to interpret and analyze (Kidwai-Khan et al., 2022)

Most proteins exert their effect by interacting with other proteins, forming a protein-protein complex. The protein-protein interaction allows cells to communicate with other cells and control metabolic processes, cell growth, and development. protein-protein interactions (PPIs) control an extensive scope of organic processes, such as cell-to-cell interactions and metabolic and developmental control. Despite this, it is very hard to study PPI networks under in vitro conditions, considering that the interaction between these proteins depends upon their 3D structure, which is susceptible to breakage during isolation.

3.2.4 Application of AI in proteomics

AI, in particular ML, has found many applications and uses in studying proteomics. The use of ML allows researchers to predict the structure and function of peptides and proteins with higher accuracy and less expenditure of resources. A peculiar characteristic of proteins is that their structure dictates their function, and their function dictates their structure. Traditionally, techniques such as X-ray crystallography and nuclear magnetic resonance have been used to resolve protein structures from their crystals. Understanding how a protein chain folds into its unique 3D structure, how chains interact in quaternary complexes, and predicting spatial arrangements from primary sequences is made possible by the essential information provided by all resolved protein structures. ML models are developed and improved by utilizing the enormous amount of data produced by these resolved structures. This enables researchers to discover intricate correlations and forecast protein properties with previously unheard-of efficiency and accuracy (AlQuraishi, 2021).

Advancements in protein structure prediction using ML

The goal of protein structure prediction is to infer many different features of proteins, such as secondary structures, domains of proteins, binding sites, functional sites, and how they interact with other biomolecules (proteins, peptides, small compounds, etc.). Researchers map the primary structure of amino acids according to their classification and deduce unique features of secondary structures. A significant advancement was made in the 1980s with the development of feedforward neural networks, which increased prediction accuracy to 60–70%. Over time, improved algorithms and the expansion of protein sequence databases like Research Collaboratory for Structural Bioinformatics Protein Data Bank (RCSB PDB) and SwissProt led to an increase in accuracy to 78%–80% (Cheng et al., 2008).

With modern algorithms, there are four main components of any ML model. First, an input module that uses a single protein sequence to generate additional features; second, a neural network comprising 'trunks' to transform these features into spatial information; third, an output module that transforms this spatial information into an initial 3D structure; and fourth, a refinement module that refines the structure and generates atomic coordinates. By (AlQuraishi, 2021) taking advantage of (ML models, 2021), many distinct characteristics of proteins, such as stability, solubility, sites where posttranslational modifications occur (e.g., sites for phosphorylation, acetylation, etc.), and the specific location or compartment within a cell where a protein performs its biological function, can be predicted. This will reduce the load on experimental results and improve the pipeline for computer-aided drug design (Cheng et al., 2008).

3.2.5 Application of ML in proteomics

One of the innovative ways that ML is used is to predict 1D features of membrane proteins, such as identifying and characterizing the proteins involved in the cell membrane, determining the presence of α-helices or β-strands, and analyzing the placement of loops as intracellular or extracellular. ML models can be trained and utilized in protein 3D structure prediction, including processes such as identifying folding patterns, creating structural models, and assessing their accuracy. By correlating the structure of an unknown protein with the structure of a protein that has been experimentally validated, the ML models can recognize different folding patterns. ML techniques, including fold identification, model creation, and model assessment, are crucial for predicting protein 3D structures, a challenging task. Beyond conventional experimental approaches, this all-encompassing methodology enables researchers to reliably predict protein structures, supporting applications such as medicine formulation and disease mechanism comprehension (Cheng et al., 2008).

ML models are emerging as a powerful tool in proteomics, particularly for the discovery of biomarkers. Biomarkers are characteristics that can be quantified, representing the progress of any biological process (Strimbu and Tavel, 2010). These biomarkers, which are experimentally proven to be linked to a disease, can be used for early diagnosis or for monitoring the effectiveness of therapies. Biomarkers should be specific to a disease, and even low concentrations of biomarkers in blood should be measurable.

3.2.6 Alphafold: Revolutionizing protein structure prediction

The fact that proteins are involved in every biological function and that their expression levels can indicate an organism's state of health or illness makes them perfect biomarkers. Analyzing experimental demographics with similar physiological settings and comparing the outcomes to control groups is the initial step in finding new and novel biomarkers. ML models are then trained using this data. The ML models analyze the data and assist in locating pertinent and helpful patterns in the datasets. This thorough examination contributes to the robustness, dependability, and disease-specificity of biomarkers. Potential biomarkers are chosen, and decision boundaries are established using ML approaches. To make sure the biomarkers found are precise and applicable to various patient populations, the effectiveness of these models is assessed using data that hasn't been seen before. The most revolutionary tool in the field of proteomics is a software called AlphaFold. It has been able to surpass all tools to date and achieve unprecedented accuracy while predicting protein structures. This was followed by the creation of The AlphaFold Protein Structure Database in 2021 by DeepMind and EMBL-EBI to provide the scientific community with an unparalleled quantity of trustworthy protein structure predictions (Varadi and Velankar, 2023).

4 Nanorobots and AI in drug delivery

4.1 Introduction

The incorporation of AI into nanotechnology has revolutionized various biomedical and energy sectors. Advancements in these domains have led to the development of intelligent nanorobots, which can transform fields like drug delivery and personalized medicine. One major challenge with the current drug delivery methods is their inability to reach the targeted sites while avoiding healthy tissues, and to address this problem, high amounts of medications are administered, which may lead to toxicity and various side effects (Adepu and Ramakrishna, 2021). Nanorobots have the ability to overcome these issues by transporting drugs or any other biological material directly to the targeted tissues in vivo. In order to completely understand the capability of nanorobots, it is important to consider various in vivo parameters that may affect the overall outcome. This is where AI comes into play by assisting nanorobots with advanced settings like sensing, navigation, and decision-making.

4.2 Nanorobots

Nanorobots are tiny microscopic tools (1–100 nm) that are engineered for targeted drug delivery and various therapeutic and diagnostic purposes (Subramani and Mehta, 2018). They are composed of organic materials like proteins/polynucleotides or inorganic materials like carbon nanotubes or metals (Calderón-Jiménez et al., 2017). The surface properties of these tiny robots play a significant role in determining their interaction with other cellular surfaces and macromolecules. In addition, size and shape also affect their reactivity and permeabilization. Thus, it is important to optimize the size, shape, and surface properties of the nanorobots for maximum efficacy.

In contrast to the conventional drug delivery mechanism, which relies on the internal blood circulation for drug transport, these nanorobots have independent mobility, enabling drug transport to various inaccessible parts of the body (Das and Sultana, 2024; Nance et al., 2021). In addition, these robots are driven externally by magnetic fields, electric fields, or acoustics, and internally by various chemical reactions. We will discuss both the exogenous and endogenous power systems, which allow nanorobots to autonomously move within the body.

4.2.1 *Exogenous power assisted nanorobots*

Since the nanorobots have a size that is in the nanoscale, it is important for them to overcome Brownian motion to possess independent movement within the body fluids. For this reason, external power is attached, which can control the movement of these tiny robots (Hu et al., 2020).

Magnetic field assisted nanorobots

The application of a magnetic field is the most popular as it mimics the same model as bacterial flagella or helically shaped appendages. These helically shaped nanorobots can be propelled via a corkscrew mechanism due to the interaction between the external magnetic field and their helical shape. Magnetic field-powered nanorobots have several advantages, including position accuracy, directional control, and an extensive motion range. These nanorobots can move even under a small magnetic field, making them safe and compatible. However, the metals used for the development of nanorobots may limit their use for some in vivo applications (Zhou et al., 2021).

Electric field assisted nanorobots

Electric field is often used for nanorobots as it is easily available. However, the penetration rate of the electric field is not as strong as that of the magnetic field, and hence higher intensities are required for better penetration inside the body. This raises questions as to how feasible it is to provide electric current to the body. In addition, the usage of metallic material for the design is similar, and hence it poses additional harm to the body.

Light energy assisted nanorobots

This is an alternative mode for power generation in tiny robots. Light energy is nontoxic, biocompatible, environmentally friendly, and hence is a good source for nanorobots. Apart from ultraviolet rays, which may harm the cells, other forms of light energy are considered safe. Light energy not only helps in nanorobot movement but can also regulate endogenous chemical reactions, which additionally help in propulsion.

4.2.2 Endogenous power system in nanorobots

Endogenous power is generated using various chemical or biological reactions taking place inside the body which helps in nanorobot propulsion. This type of nanorobots is often coated with catalyzers which can continuously obtain energy from the chemical reactions happening in the surrounding environment. This nanorobots are often asymmetric with shapes like rods, vesicular polymer, etc. Even though, chemical reactions may propel nanorobots, they still need external power like magnetic/electric field for precise positioning and control of the robots. Also, chemical reactions may produce certain gases which might pose some problem in vivo. All of these should be considered before the use of this methodology (Hu et al., 2020).

4.3 AI and ML in nanorobots

Incorporation of AI and ML in nanotechnology has improved a lot of parameters, enabling its use in drug delivery aspects. Both AI and ML can design nanorobots with enhanced capability and intelligence. AI can develop nanorobots that are capable of identifying targeted sites with enhanced specificity, and ML can train these robots to perform complicated tasks. These improved nanorobots are a great alternative to the traditional drug delivery mechanisms and their associated limitations, such as inefficient targeting, poor drug release kinetics, and potential side effects (Xu et al., 2024).

4.3.1 AI-enabled nanorobots for drug delivery

AI has completely transformed the pharmacology and drug delivery area. Given below are some of the ways in which AI and ML have changed the drug delivery mechanisms.

Targeting efficiency

AI algorithms and tools have the ability to analyze patient data, such as medical history, genomics, and other related factors, in order to determine the most effective delivery route, drug dosage, and time. This ensures precise targeting of the drugs to diseased sites (Zhong et al., 2018; Ori et al., 2024). Another advancement in precision targeting is the development of a sophisticated navigation framework that utilizes magnetic/acoustic fields or chemical reactions. For example, these navigation systems enable nanorobots to reach the specific location, and the magnetic field can be manipulated to direct nanorobots to the tumor area. This will ensure the release of the drugs directly to the cancerous cells, thereby minimizing their effects on the normal cells (Biswas, 2024). Surface modification is another way to achieve target efficiency. Surface coating with antibodies or ligands specific to the surface markers may help in effective targeting. All these approaches can help achieve efficient and precise targeting.

Precise and optimized formulations

Various ML tools possess the capability to envisage the best possible nanoparticle design and formulation for various drugs by taking into consideration factors like drug solubility, kinetics, drug release, etc. (Zhong et al., 2018). In addition, nanorobots integrated with AI can analyze the surrounding environment through chemical reactions and can avoid areas with high toxicity in order to reach their specific target site. Reinforcement learning is another tool in AI that learns strategies over time. This is especially useful for navigating in complex body fluids where there is constant change with respect to flow rate, cell type, density, etc. This tool enables nanorobots to optimize their performance in such complex fluids. This is called real-time adaptation and helps nanorobots achieve enhanced performance (Biswas, 2024).

Enhanced drug release

AI-powered systems have the capability to regulate the drug release rates as per the patient's response and drug release kinetics data. This option helps in controlled drug release, thereby achieving maximum therapeutic output and minimal side effects. Fig. 15.3 illustrates how the integration of AI with nanotechnology will provide useful chemical compounds that facilitate advanced medication production.

4.4 Nanorobots in drug delivery

Nanorobots promise precise targeting and controlled release of drugs within the body compared to conventional nanomaterials. These tiny robots offer various key advantages in drug delivery, including: (1) these robots can easily navigate complex biological environments and deliver drugs directly to the target site, thereby minimizing off-target effects and reducing drug dosage (Das and Sultana, 2024); (2) these robots propose exceptional precision in controlled and on-demand drug release, which is valuable in disorders with fluctuating symptoms; (3) these robots can carry poorly water-soluble drugs, thereby increasing their solubility and bioavailability and improving therapeutic outcomes; (4) these nanorobots can minimize toxicity by reducing systemic exposure, thereby improving patient tolerance to treatment; (5) these robots can facilitate the release of multiple drugs at a time or in sequence, enabling successful combination drug delivery; and (6) these robots can easily pass through inaccessible organs like the blood-brain barrier.

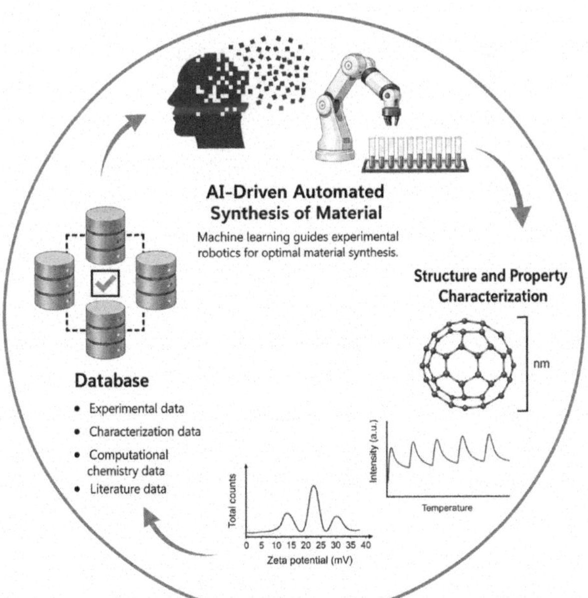

Fig. 15.3 AI in advancing nanotechnology.

4.4.1 Current applications of nanorobots in drug delivery

Various in vivo studies of tiny robots have been performed to validate the use of nanorobots in drug delivery (Table 15.2).

Several researchers have started using micro/nanorobots for their experiments. We will be discussing all such current applications and findings of nanorobots in the field of drug delivery. The gastrointestinal tract is easier to enter for nanorobots due to the acidic pH in the stomach, which propels them further. A study published in Nature Communications developed a magnesium (Mg)-based microrobot filled with clarithromycin for treating mice with gastric infections. Mice infected with *Helicobacter pylori* were administered microrobots orally and showed a reduced bacterial load compared to the negative control group, without any toxicity in the mice. Another study utilized zinc-based microrobots with gold nanoparticles as a core drug against mice stomach infections. The study confirmed the retention of the robots and their compatibility, validating their use for future experiments (Gao et al., 2015). Recent advancements in micro/nanorobot design have led to newer versions. A similar microrobot was developed based on sperm motor movement, and another one featured multifunctional micro rollers for targeted drug delivery (Hu et al., 2020). Photoacoustic computed tomography (PACT) was utilized to assist microrobot investigation in the intestines of mice. This

Table 15.2 In vivo studies of nanorobots in drug delivery.

Animal model used	Type of nanorobot used	Drug loaded	Target region	Key findings	References
Mice	Gold	Doxorubicin	Tumor	Improved drug delivery, along with tumor shrinkage.	Elbialy et al. (2015))
Rats	Magnetic	Paclitaxel	Bloodstream	Enhanced drug circulation and efficacy	Dilnawaz et al. (2012)
Rabbits	Polymer	Methotrexate	Joints	Targeted therapy and reduced inflammation	Ha et al. (2020)
Guinea pigs	Lipid	Insulin	Gastrointestinal	Controlled release of insulin	Mohammadpour et al. (2022)
Monkeys	DNA nanorobots	Antiviral drug	Brain	Improved drug delivery	Self-Assembly of DNA Molecules: Toward DNA Nanorobots for Biomedical Applications

approach allows visualization of the microrobots in real time through PACT. Near-infrared light further breaks down the microrobots to release the drug, paving the way for biomedical applications using such technology (de Ávila et al., 2017). Along with the experimental data, various companies are also investing in nanorobots to be used in clinical trials. One such company, called Bionaut in Los Angeles, invested 43 million dollars in January 2023 to progress its nanorobots to phase I clinical trials. Another US based company is focused on developing a nanorobot specific to a rare genetic disease, "Dandy-Walker syndrome," which affects neural development in children.

4.5 Challenges

Along with the rapid advancement in this field, there are still a few challenges that may limit its use for human trials. A few of them include the viscosity of human blood, which may interfere with the flow rate of the tiny robots. Another issue could be the safety of the material used for the development of nanorobots. Any metallic material may pose toxicity, and hence biodegradable-based nanorobots should be designed. The size of the nanorobots is crucial, as it may directly hamper their entry into the cell. All of these factors must be considered for their optimum use.

4.6 Designing nanoparticle using AI

4.6. 1 Introduction

The advancement in nanotechnology has completely transformed the drug delivery field. Nanoparticle-based drug delivery mechanisms provide precise targeting, optimized formulations, improved bioavailability, and reduced side effects (Kapoor et al., 2024). However, designing nanoparticles specific to drugs and disease targets is still not completely optimized and remains a major challenge. The integration of AI into nanoparticle drug delivery has innovated various approaches, resulting in higher efficacy. In this section, we will first explore the nanoparticle-based drug delivery mechanisms and later examine how AI helps in nanoparticle design for better outcomes (Herdiana, 2025).

Nanoparticle drug delivery system

The conventional drug delivery systems (DDS) were associated with poor targeting and absorption, increased cure time, and many systemic side effects. To address this problem, nanoparticles were introduced. Nanomaterial-based DDS have a better edge over conventional DDS as they improve targeting efficiency, bioavailability, drug solubility, and hence possess fewer side effects (Cheng et al.,

2023). Targeted drug delivery is another approach for delivering therapeutic agents to selected sites within the body. Incorporating life-saving drugs with nanoparticles and designing a suitable pathway for their delivery has helped in delivering various drugs/molecules/genes to different sites of the body (Cheng et al., 2023; Jahan et al., 2017). This approach requires higher retention times for precise targeting, maximum drug release, and evasion of immune system recognition, which is achieved with nanoparticles. In addition, nanoparticles can also pass through the bloodstream and access internal blood vessels to treat intravascular diseases. Along with this, nanoparticles can reach the endothelium of blood vessels and treat various endothelium-related ailments. Thus, nanoparticle-based DDS can deliver drugs to both intravascular as well as extravascular sites (Cheng et al., 2023). Despite this, there are many off-target effects associated with nanoparticle-based DDS. This area needs further research for an enhanced DDS.

Integration of AI in nanoparticle drug delivery

Various off-target effects associated with nanoparticle DDS have led to a deeper investigation in this area. AI and ML are advanced tools that have transformed the healthcare organization, including the drug delivery field. Both AI and ML have the capability to identify various patterns, envisage outcomes, and enhance processes of large datasets, which are far beyond human reach (Jena et al., 2024). Drug designing, which is the first and critical step in drug development, depends on the data obtained from several hit-and-trial results, which is an extensive process. This issue can be addressed by AI tools like DL, which can predict the drug target, their molecular interaction, and the possible toxicity triggered by various compounds. This has enabled testing multiple compounds in a very short time, thereby reducing the time of the entire drug discovery phase (Jena et al., 2024).

Currently, the research is focused more on personalized medicine. This is possible with the integration of AI with drug delivery. AI has the ability to tailor medications specific to an individual based on their genomic and proteomic data (Awwalu et al., 2015). Moreover, ML can predict how these drug molecules will be processed by different individuals based on their genomic variations, lifestyle, and environmental factors. This approach helps in diminishing side effects, thereby achieving maximum efficacy. AI-based drug delivery methods are constantly evolving in the fields of drug design, drug release, clinical trials, and much more. Here, we will focus on the role of AI in nanoparticle designing and its associated challenges.

4.6.2 AI tools in nanoparticle design

4.6.3.1 AI algorithms in nanoparticle synthesis

Various AI tools like ML, DL, neural networks, and optimization algorithms assist in developing nanoparticles with desired size, shape, surface properties, and drug release patterns. This results in the precise selection of initial drug molecules that can be tested experimentally. A recent study reported the identification of drugs that can cross the blood-brain barrier using a ML approach. This prediction was based on the chemical properties and indications of drugs (Adir et al., 2020). In another study, an ANN was used to envisage the size and burst rates of polylactic-co-glycolic acid (PLGA) nanoparticles. The process involved inputting the molecular weight, concentration, and sonication rates of PLGA along with poly vinyl alcohol. The algorithm processed all the information provided and resulted in the size and initial burst size of PLGA nanoparticles (Adir et al., 2020). A study by (Stillman et al., 2021) presented a unique platform named evolvable platform for programmable nanoparticle-based cancer therapies (EVONANO) for developing nanomedicines against cancer. This platform allows researchers to grow tumors and observe nanoparticle transport to tumor sites using simulation models. In addition, nanoparticle designs are augmented using ML to develop the best anticancer medicine (Stillman et al., 2021). A similar study by Lin et al. (2022) utilized a DNN to predict the targeting efficiency of various nanoparticles to tumor sites. This study offers a quantitative tool based on physiology-based pharmacokinetic modeling to improve the design of nanoparticles with greater tumor delivery efficacy.

Various ML algorithms are employed for nanoparticle synthesis owing to their precise prediction. Some of the pivotal tools include SVM and ANN. Table 15.3 describes the utilization of various AI algorithms for nanoparticle design.

AI algorithms for nanoparticle size, shape, and surface properties

Various studies have shown the utilization of AI and ML for predicting the effective size, shape, and surface properties of NPs that can provide better outcomes. A recent study focused on otitis media, which is more commonly seen in children, but its identification is sometimes critical. This issue was addressed by a group of researchers who employed an ANN to improve the efficacy of NPs in the automated detection of otitis media (Kapoor et al., 2024). Silver nanoparticles (AgNPs) were synthesized using an ANN approach. This model predicted the size of AgNPs using an ANN while saving both time and money in extensive research. A similar approach was

Table 15.3 AI algorithms for determining nanoparticle size, shape, design, and properties.

Sr. No	Type of NPs	AI model used	Key findings	References
1	Can be used for all NPs	Deep Neural Network (DNN)	Developed a physiology-based pharmacokinetic model (PBPK) to predict the NPs' efficiency at various tumor sites	Lin et al. (2022)
2	Pullulan conjugated $AgTiO_2$	Artificial neural network (ANN)	This method efficiently produced a high yield of pullulan and successfully conjugated AgTiO2 NPs for enhanced stability and masking against human pathogens	Eldadamony et al. (2024)
3	Lecithin/chitosan NPs, Silymarin	Quality by design, ANN	This approach helped the NPs load a poorly water-soluble drug, Silymarin, for carcinoma treatment	Dawoud et al. (2023)
4	Fucoidan and polyethyleneimine-based sorafenib NPs	ANN	The model confirmed high accuracy and predictability	Chaurawal et al. (2024)
5	In-situ nanoparticles (ISNs) for Piroxicam delivery	Design Expert	AI tools helped in developing ISNs for piroxicam delivery via intra-articular injection in arthritis	Yacoub et al. (2022), Xu et al. (2021)
6	Polystyrene NPs	ML	AI tools, like genetic algorithms, can help researchers envisage the progression of cancer stem cells	Ramović Hamzagić et al. (2024)
7	Silver NPs	ML	AI approach can achieve accurate size differentiation of NPs at the individual level	Xu et al. (2024)

used in another study, where the authors utilized a hybrid method, including ANN and particle swarm optimization, to envisage the size of AgNPs synthesized using a green method (Kapoor et al., 2024).

4.6.3 Clinical applications of AI-based NP design

Various studies have utilized AI, which has helped them overcome many challenges faced otherwise. One recent study used AI to design and optimize lipid nanoparticles (LNPs), as the earlier method of synthesis faced issues like poor delivery efficacy, immune activation, and toxicity. AI also helped to envisage LNP properties and performance (Yuan et al., 2024). Another recent study employed AI tools like design of experiments and ANN for predicting the physicochemical properties of progesterone-loaded solid LNPs. The formulation demonstrated high accuracy and was used for transdermal delivery, which showed no toxicity (Suriyaamporn et al., 2024).

5 Combination drug delivery and AI predictions

5.1 Challenges in drug development and delivery

Drug development is a challenging, cost-intensive, and demanding process by nature because of a number of interrelated issues. Drugs are integral to modern healthcare, serving as critical tools for the prevention, management, and treatment of a wide range of diseases. Drugs target specific molecules that are involved in specific disease progression, which might be upregulated, downregulated, or mutated. Protein-protein or protein-nucleic acid interactions allow these biomolecules to interact with one another, spreading signaling events and altering metabolic processes. Drugs prevent and treat diseases by blocking their function with small compounds that have a higher binding affinity, blocking interactions between biomolecules, or stimulating biomolecules that are functionally dysregulated in specific diseases (Mandal et al., 2009) The procedure for producing an ideal and efficient medication is time-consuming, costly, and extensive. Finding potent drugs that are safe for human use and may halt the progression of a disease requires an exhaustive amount of investigation. The potential drug candidates have to be rigorously evaluated and tested for their safety and effects in animal models and clinical trials (Mandal et al., 2009).

5.1.1 Role of DSS in enhancing therapeutic efficacy

AI has significantly transformed drug design and delivery, playing a vital role in the entire drug development process. The process of absorption, distribution, metabolism, and elimination is a main feature that has to be evaluated for the efficacy of drugs in the system, drug safety, and possible side effects. Binding scores, the balance between hydrophilicity and lipophilicity, electrophilicity, nucleophilicity, and the toxicity of parent molecules and products as a result of biotransformation in various metabolism phases also have to be evaluated (Oualikene-Gonin et al., 2024).

Another major factor in determining the effectiveness of a drug is the method of delivery. DSS have demonstrated their ability to elevate success in treating diseases with the help of drugs in various ways, such as enhancing therapeutic effectiveness, minimizing toxicity, improving patient adherence, and paving the way for groundbreaking medical therapies. Each drug requires a unique delivery system, as the delivery system has a significant influence on the bioavailability and pharmacokinetic properties of drugs. Previously, the main candidates (Gao et al., 2023) for drugs were small molecules, where research focused on increasing the time it took for drugs to release from gels. Many compounds were used, such as cellulose derivatives, poly(acrylic acid) hydrogels, or biodegradable polymers, which were employed to entrap the drugs (Mandal et al., 2009). The development of novel therapeutics, like proteins, peptides, and nucleic acids, has expanded treatment options. Yet, these breakthroughs also bring unique challenges, including stability concerns, intracellular delivery hurdles, and cell viability issues, driving innovation in DSS. There are five main classes of drugs available—small molecules, proteins/peptides, DNA, antibodies, and live cells. The main challenge in delivering any class of drugs is maintaining the pharmacokinetic parameters, solubility, bioavailability, and permeability while reducing off-target toxicity as well as any negative side effects of the drugs (Vargason et al., 2021)

5.2 Computational pharmacokinetics: Integrating AI with DSS

Computational pharmacokinetics is a novel and innovative scientific discipline that has arisen from the integration of AI with drug delivery methods. Researchers utilize AI to formulate pharmaceuticals for consistent and timely medication release. They use extensive databases of substances with experimentally determined characteristics to train ML and AI models. AI aggregates data from diverse sources (patient information, pharmacokinetic characteristics of medications, target cell/tissue evaluations, etc.) and assists researchers in evaluating alternative scenarios and enhancing DSS by simulating drug formulation and distribution methodologies (Jiang et al., 2022).

If done experimentally, this process is a trial-and-error method with potentially many test runs until an effective, stable, and safe drug is formulated. But the use of AI/ML shortens the time required to research and develop new pharmaceuticals, reduces expenses, and increases the number of therapies for common and rare diseases. DSS for all classes of drugs can be modeled in computational pharmaceutics. To predict medication behavior at every scale (from molecular interaction to physiological effects), AI/ML systems examine complex relationships between pharmaceutical traits, formulation components, and physiological measures. This promotes the advancement of efficient medication delivery systems and enhances comprehension of drug delivery mechanisms. It assists in forecasting the medication's stability, in vitro drug release profile, and physicochemical properties (Jiang et al., 2022; Vora et al., 2023). By identifying possible risks in DSS early on, AI algorithms allow for rapid modifications and adjustments for maximum performance. Fig. 15.4 illustrates the workflow of AI-driven drug design, highlighting how AI accelerates and refines the drug discovery process.

5.2.1 Advantages of ANN in drug delivery optimization

Another facet of ML is DL, specifically ANNs or ANNs. They are made up of artificial neurons, which are interconnected and act as basic units for processing information. ANNs are essential for pharmaceutical research in order to predict the behavior of active pharmaceutical ingredients (APIs) and optimize the release of drugs into the system. They possess fault tolerance, immense information storage capacity, and simultaneous multitasking capabilities (Vora et al., 2023). In the study by Obeid et al. (2021), ANNs were employed to

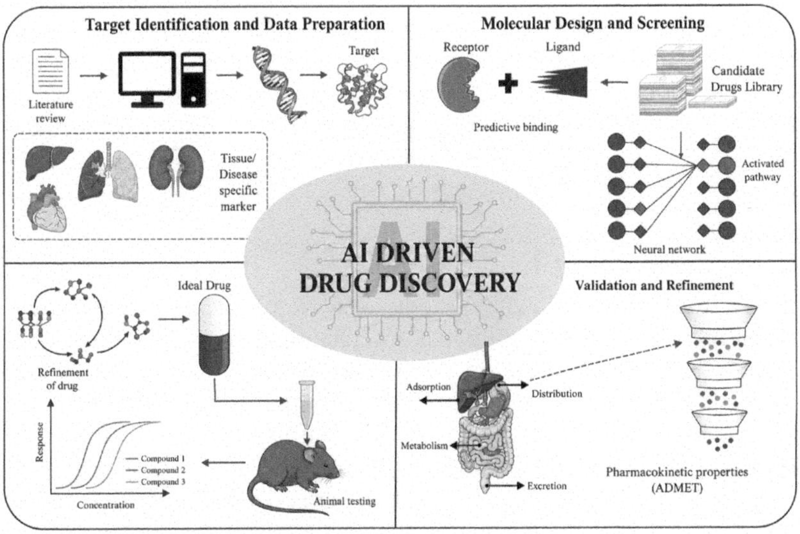

Fig. 15.4 AI-driven drug design.

predict and optimize the drug release properties of 3D-printed diazepam tablets. The model was used to examine connections between processing factors (such as surface-to-volume ratio and parameters for printing tablets) and drug release behavior with respect to time using multilayer perceptron networks and self-organizing maps. The study found that a zigzag infill pattern and lower infill densities resulted in higher disintegration rates, demonstrating the precision of ANNs in pharmaceutical manufacturing (Obeid et al., 2021).

5.2.2 Challenges of ANN in drug delivery optimization

However, it is extremely difficult to design complex architectures that ANNs might require for different tasks. They may need advanced computational resources and significant hardware. This makes them expensive and requires regular maintenance. The method is time-consuming. Regardless of these difficulties, ANNs continue to be an effective tool in drug research, especially for applications such as API optimization and drug release prediction (Vora et al., 2023). By identifying possible risks in DSS early on, AI algorithms allow for rapid modifications and adjustments for maximum performance. Fig. 15.4 illustrates the workflow of AI-driven drug design, highlighting how AI accelerates and refines the drug discovery process.

6 Case studies and real-world applications

AI has revolutionized the field of personalized medicine, nanomedicine, and targeted therapies by allowing researchers to fast-track the complete pipeline, from discovering a drug and designing tailored formulations to predicting the most effective route of administration. AI has profound and versatile applications, some of which are yet to be discovered. There are many real-world applications of the use of AI/ML to create a novel therapeutic drug for treating rare diseases. The tool has been utilized to transform theoretical possibilities into effective and functional models.

6.1 Case study 1

(Feng, 2025; Ren et al., 2025) reported in *Nature Biotechnology* that a small-molecule TRAF2- and NCK-interacting kinase (TNIK) inhibitor effectively targets fibrosis in both preclinical and clinical models. The article focused on developing a novel small-molecule drug acting as an inhibitor with antifibrotic and antiinflammatory effects. Idiopathic pulmonary fibrosis (IPF), a severe interstitial lung disease with a high death rate, could potentially be treated with the drug created using AI. This led to the discovery of a new and novel molecule called INS018_055, which is a small-molecule with the potential to halt disease progression (Ren et al., 2023, 2025). Fig. 15.5 depicts the sequential steps involved in the AI-driven discovery of therapeutic targets for IPF. The process begins with the integration of multiomics datasets.

A novel AI platform was used for the discovery of potential drugs to target antifibrotic molecules. PandaOmics is a platform integrating data from various omics studies, literature reviews, and network biology. The most promising option for treating fibrosis was found to be TNIK. Following that, small-molecule candidates targeting TNIK were generated using the Chemistry42 platform. One such candidate, called INS018_055, which targets the ATP-binding site and a nearby allosteric pocket for enhanced selectivity and efficacy, was created and refined by AI-driven Chemistry42. Predictive modeling further supported the potential of TNIK inhibition to disrupt key fibrosis-related pathways, including TGF-β, WNT, and YAP-TAZ, offering a strong foundation for therapeutic development (Ren et al., 2023). Fig. 15.6 illustrates the stages of the AI-driven drug development process, highlighting the application of ML in designing novel inhibitors targeting TNIK.

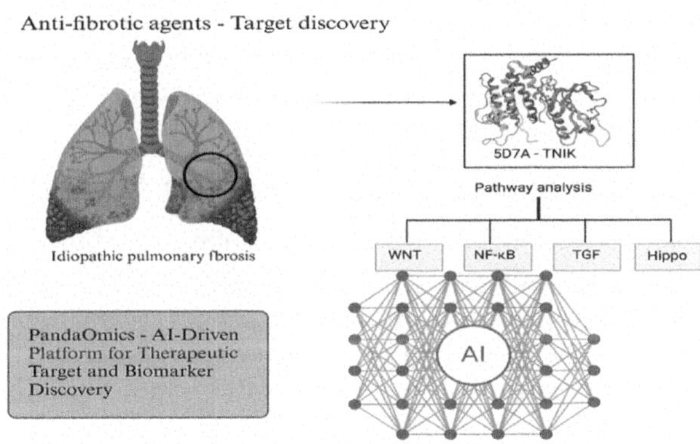

Fig. 15.5 AI-driven discovery of IPF.

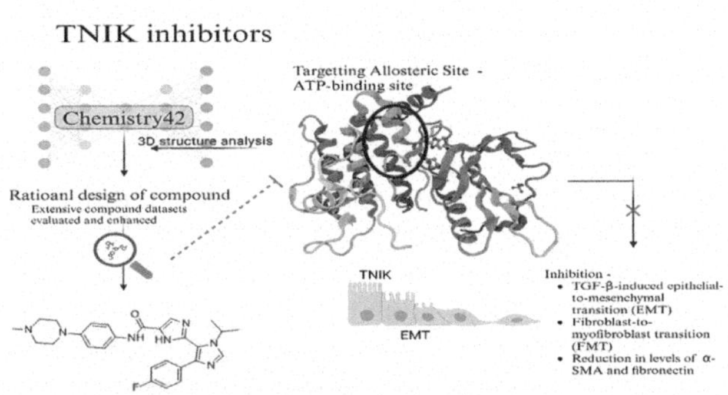

Fig. 15.6 Use of machine learning to generate TNIK inhibitors.

7 Challenges and ethical consideration

AI has led the future of the scientific field, and it has been able to open new and interesting avenues for the development of novel, innovative, and cutting-edge tools, which allow researchers to personalize and treat rare diseases. However, along with great benefits, new challenges and ethical concerns also arise. As the field of AI progresses, it is important to carefully address these concerns and ensure that AI is used for the betterment of society with responsibility and ethics.

7.1 Risks of misclassification in AI-driven analysis

Many issues arise when AI is used to decipher patterns from data, which can significantly affect the outcomes. When data is classified, the model can miscalculate and make an assignment error. It can either assign a nonmember element to a class or miss an element that belongs to the class. The former can lead to false positive results, and the latter can result in false negative results. False positive results can lead to unnecessary difficulties and financial strain through unwarranted screenings and tests, while false negatives can delay accurate diagnoses, with serious implications for diseases (Chen et al., 2025).

7.2 Impact of biased training data on AI models

The data used to train the AI model can be biased and unstable. This can often lead to misdiagnoses based on the data. It has been historically noted that privileged groups are more represented in datasets, while underprivileged groups are discriminated against, leading to discriminatory behavior from the model when presented with biased data, thereby worsening inequalities in healthcare (González Sendino et al., 2024).

7.3 Privacy concerns and data security in AI applications

Another concern is the privacy of data belonging to patients and participants. Data shared by participants is personal and sensitive. AI models often require huge datasets to train and achieve accuracy in pattern recognition. AI algorithms, like DL neural networks, are complex and difficult to interpret, making their decision-making processes challenging for experts to understand. Participants may be unaware of how their data is used, the insights generated, or the decisions made based on the information they provide (Cheng et al., 2023). To give informed consent, participants must understand the potential risks and benefits of sharing their data, and if they don't, they may not be fully aware of the implications of their participation, raising ethical concerns about whether they are truly providing consent under these conditions. It can be difficult to monitor how data is used across many platforms or research studies after it has been utilized to train AI models, which could result in unethical or unlawful use (Char et al., 2018).

References

Abdelhalim, H., Berber, A., Lodi, M., Jain, R., Nair, A., Pappu, A., Patel, K., Venkat, V., Venkatesan, C., Wable, R., Dinatale, M., Fu, A., Iyer, V., Kalove, I., Kleyman, M., Koutsoutis, J., Menna, D., Paliwal, M., Patel, N., et al., 2022. Artificial intelligence, healthcare, clinical genomics, and pharmacogenomics approaches in precision medicine. Front. Genet. 13. doi:10.3389/fgene.2022.929736.

Adam, G., Rampášek, L., Safikhani, Z., Smirnov, P., Haibe-Kains, B., Goldenberg, A., 2020. Machine learning approaches to drug response prediction: challenges and recent progress. NPJ Precis. Oncol. 4 (1), 19. doi:10.1038/s41698-020-0122-1.

Adepu, S., Ramakrishna, S., 2021. Controlled drug delivery systems: current status and future directions. Molecules 26 (19), 5905. doi:10.3390/molecules26195905.

Adir, O., Poley, M., Chen, G., Froim, S., Krinsky, N., Shklover, J., Shainsky-Roitman, J., Lammers, T., Schroeder, A., 2020. Integrating artificial intelligence and nanotechnology for precision cancer medicine. Adv. Mater. 32 (13). doi:10.1002/adma.201901989.

AL-Eitan, L., Jaouni, H., Mihyar, A., 2025. Addressing Cyberbiosecurity Challenges in the Modern Era of Biotechnology and Artificial Intelligence. Global Biosecurity. doi:10.31646/gbio.282.

Alowais, S.A., Alghamdi, S.S., Alsuhebany, N., Alqahtani, T., Alshaya, A.I., Almohareb, S.N., Aldairem, A., Alrashed, M., Bin Saleh, K., Badreldin, H.A., Al Yami, M.S., Al Harbi, S., Albekairy, A.M., 2023. Revolutionizing healthcare: The role of artificial intelligence in clinical practice. BMC Medical Education 23 (1), 689. doi:10.1186/s12909-023-04698-z.

AlQuraishi, M., 2021. Machine learning in protein structure prediction. Curr. Opin. Chem. Biol. 65, 1–8. doi:10.1016/j.cbpa.2021.04.005.

Anyanwu, E.C., Arowoogun, J.O., Odilibe, I.P., Akomolafe, O., Onwumere, C., Ogugua, J.O., 2024. The role of biotechnology in healthcare: a review of global trends. World J. Adv. Res. Rev. 21 (1), 2740–2752. doi:10.30574/wjarr.2024.21.1.0382.

Awwalu, J., Garba, A.G., Ghazvini, A., Atuah, R., 2015. Artificial intelligence in personalized medicine application of AI algorithms in solving personalized medicine problems. Int. J. Comput. Theory Eng. 7 (6), 439–443. doi:10.7763/IJCTE.2015.V7.999.

Bajwa, J., Munir, U., Nori, A., Williams, B., 2021. Artificial intelligence in healthcare: transforming the practice of medicine. Future Healthcare Journal 8 (2), e188–e194. doi:10.7861/fhj.2021-0095.

Bhardwaj, A., Kishore, S., Pandey, D.K., 2022. Artificial intelligence in biological sciences. Life 12 (9). doi:10.3390/life12091430.

Biswas, M., 2024. AI-powered nanorobots: a mini review on innovations in healthcare. J. Artif. Intell. Robot. doi:10.61577/jaiar.2024.100007.

Calderón-Jiménez, B., Johnson, M.E., Montoro Bustos, A.R., Murphy, K.E., Winchester, M.R., Vega Baudrit, J.R., 2017. Silver Nanoparticles: Technological Advances, Societal Impacts, and Metrological Challenges. Front. Chem. 5. doi:10.3389/fchem.2017.00006.

Calvino, G., Farro, J., Zampatti, S., Peconi, C., Megalizzi, D., Trastulli, G., Andreucci, S., Cascella, R., Strafella, C., Caltagirone, C., Grifalchi, F., Giardina, E., 2025. From Genomics to AI: Revolutionizing Precision Medicine in Oncology. Applied Sciences 15 (12), 6578. doi:10.3390/app15126578.

Caudai, C., Galizia, A., Geraci, F., le Pera, L., Morea, V., Salerno, E., Via, A., Colombo, T., 2021. AI applications in functional genomics. Comput. Struct. Biotechnol. J. 19, 5762–5790. doi:10.1016/j.csbj.2021.10.009.

Char, D.S., Shah, N.H., Magnus, D., 2018. Implementing machine learning in health care—addressing ethical challenges. N. Engl. J. Med. 378 (11), 981–983. doi:10.1056/nejmp1714229.

Chaurawal, N., Quadir, S.S., Joshi, G., Barkat, M.A., Alanezi, A.A., Raza, K., 2024. Development of fucoidan/polyethyleneimine based sorafenib-loaded self-assembled nanoparticles with machine learning and DoE-ANN implementation: optimization, characterization, and in-vitro assessment for the anticancer drug delivery. Int. J. Biol. Macromol. 279, 135123. doi:10.1016/j.ijbiomac.2024.135123.

Chen, L., Song, Y., Guo, J., Sun, L., Childs, P., Yin, Y., 2025. How generative AI supports human in conceptual design. Des. Sci. 11. doi:10.1017/dsj.2025.2.

Cheng, J., Tegge, A.N., Baldi, P., 2008. Machine learning methods for protein structure prediction. IEEE Rev. Biomed. Eng. 1, 41–49. doi:10.1109/RBME.2008.2008239.

Cheng, X., Xie, Q., Sun, Y., 2023. Advances in nanomaterial-based targeted drug delivery systems. Front. Bioeng. Biotechnol. 11. doi:10.3389/fbioe.2023.1177151

Cho, W.C.S., 2007. Proteomics technologies and challenges. Genom., Proteom. Bioinform. 5 (2), 77–85. doi:10.1016/S1672-0229(07)60018-7.

Committee on A Framework for Developing a New Taxonomy of Disease Board on Life Sciences Division on Earth and Life Studies [Internet], 2011. Available from: http://www.nap.edu.

Cui, C., Han, X., Jin, Y., Wang, X., Zhang, J., Lei, X., 2021. Drug repurposing against breast cancer by integrating drug-exposure expression profiles and drug–drug links based on graph neural network. Bioinformatics 37 (18), 2930–2937. doi:10.1093/bioinformatics/btab191.

Das, T., Sultana, S., 2024. Multifaceted applications of micro/nanorobots in pharmaceutical drug delivery systems: a comprehensive review. Future J. Pharm. Sci. 10 (1), 2. doi:10.1186/s43094-023-00577-y.

Dawoud, M.H.S., Mannaa, I.S., Abdel-Daim, A., Sweed, N.M., 2023. Integrating artificial intelligence with quality by design in the formulation of Lecithin/Chitosan nanoparticles of a poorly water-soluble drug. AAPS PharmSciTech 24 (6), 169. doi:10.1208/s12249-023-02609-5.

de Ávila, B.E.-F., Angsantikul, P., Li, J., Angel Lopez-Ramirez, M., Ramírez-Herrera, D.E., Thamphiwatana, S., Chen, C., Delezuk, J., Samakapiruk, R., Ramez, V., Obonyo, M., Zhang, L., Wang, J., 2017. Micromotor-enabled active drug delivery for in vivo treatment of stomach infection. Nat. Commun. 8 (1), 272. doi:10.1038/s41467-017-00309-w.

Degroeve, S., de Baets, B., van de Peer, Y., Rouzé, P., Rouzé, R., 2002. Feature subset selection for splice site prediction. Bioinformatics 18, 75–83. http://bioinformatics.oxfordjournals.org/.

Dhaarani, R., Reddy, M.K., 2025. Progressing microbial genomics: Artificial intelligence and deep learning driven advances in genome analysis and therapeutics. Intelligence-Based Medicine 11, 100251. doi:10.1016/j.ibmed.2025.100251.

Dias, R., Torkamani, A., 2019. Artificial intelligence in clinical and genomic diagnostics. Genome Med. 11 (1), 70. doi:10.1186/s13073-019-0689-8.

Dilnawaz, F., Singh, A., Mewar, S., Sharma, U., Jagannathan, N., Sahoo, S.K., 2012. The transport of non-surfactant based paclitaxel loaded magnetic nanoparticles across the blood brain barrier in a rat model. Biomaterials 33 (10), 2936–2951. doi:10.1016/j.biomaterials.2011.12.046.

Dziuda, D.M. (2010). Data Mining for Genomics and Proteomics: analysis of Gene and Protein Expression Data (Wiley Series on Methods and Applications in Data Mining).

Elbialy, N.S., Fathy, M.M., Khalil, W.M., 2015. Doxorubicin loaded magnetic gold nanoparticles for in vivo targeted drug delivery. International Journal of Pharmaceutics 490 (1-2), 190–199. doi:10.1016/j.ijpharm.2015.05.032.

Eldadamony, N.M., Ghoniem, A.A., Al-Askar, A.A., Attia, A.A., El-Hersh, M.S., Elattar, K.M., Alrdahi, H., Saber, W.I.A., 2024. Optimization of pullulan production by *Aureobasidium pullulans* using semi-solid-state fermentation and artificial neural networks: characterization and antibacterial activity of pullulan impregnated with Ag-TiO_2 nanocomposite. Int. J. Biol. Macromol. 269, 132109. doi:10.1016/j.ijbiomac.2024.132109.

Felici, A., Peduzzi, G., Pellungrini, R., Campa, D., 2025. Artificial intelligence to predict cancer risk, are we there yet? A comprehensive review across cancer types. European Journal of Cancer 222, 115440. doi:10.1016/j.ejca.2025.115440.

Fraser, A.G., Marcotte, E.M., 2004. A probabilistic view of gene function. Nat. Genet. 36 (6), 559–564. doi:10.1038/ng1370.

Gao, J., Karp, J.M., Langer, R., Joshi, N., 2023. The future of drug delivery. Chem. Mater. 35 (2), 359–363. doi:10.1021/acs.chemmater.2c03003.

Gao, W., Dong, R., Thamphiwatana, S., Li, J., Gao, W., Zhang, L., Wang, J., 2015. Artificial micromotors in the mouse's stomach: a step toward in vivo use of synthetic motors. ACS Nano 9 (1), 117–123. doi:10.1021/nn507097k.

Giani, A.M., Gallo, G.R., Gianfranceschi, L., Formenti, G., 2020. Long walk to genomics: history and current approaches to genome sequencing and assembly. Comput. Struct. Biotechnol. J. 18, 9–19. doi:10.1016/j.csbj.2019.11.002.

Gobena, S., Admassu, B., Kinde, M.Z., Gessese, A.T., Del Hierro, I., 2024. Proteomics and Its Current Application in Biomedical Area: Concise Review. The Scientific World Journal 2024, 1–13. doi:10.1155/2024/4454744.

González Sendino, R., Serrano, E., Bajo, J., Novais, P., 2024. A Review of Bias and Fairness in Artificial Intelligence. IJIMAI 9 (1), 5–17. doi:10.9781/ijimai.2023.11.001.

Görtz, M., Baumgärtner, K., Schmid, T., Muschko, M., Woessner, P., Gerlach, A., Byczkowski, M., Sültmann, H., Duensing, S., Hohenfellner, M., 2023. An artificial intelligence-based chatbot for prostate cancer education: Design and patient evaluation study. DIGITAL HEALTH 9. doi:10.1177/20552076231173304.

Grapov, D., Fahrmann, J., Wanichthanarak, K., Khoomrung, S., 2018. Rise of deep learning for genomic, proteomic, and metabolomic data integration in precision medicine. OMICS J. Integr. Biol. 22 (10), 630–636. doi:10.1089/omi.2018.0097.

Ha, Y., Lee, S., Mun, C.H., Kim, H.J., Bae, Y., Lim J., Park, K., Lee, S., Yoo, K., Park, Y., 2020. Methotrexate-loaded multifunctional nanoparticles with near-infrared irradiation for the treatment of rheumatoid arthritis. Arthritis Res Ther 22(1). doi:10.1186/s13075-020-02230-y.

Halagali, P., Nayak, D., Seenivasan, R., Manikkath, J., Rathnanand, M., Tippavajhala, V.K., 2025. Artificial intelligence revolution in pharmaceutical sciences: advancements, clinical impacts, and applications. Curr. Pharm. Biotechnol. 26. doi:10.2174/0113892010356115241224104018

Helm, J.M., Swiergosz, A.M., Haeberle, H.S., Karnuta, J.M., Schaffer, J.L., Krebs, V.E., Spitzer, A.I., Ramkumar, P.N., 2020. Machine learning and artificial intelligence: definitions, applications, and future directions. Curr. Rev. Musculoskelet. Med. 13 (1), 69–76. doi:10.1007/s12178-020-09600-8.

Herdiana, Y., 2025. Nanoparticles of natural product-derived medicines: beyond the pandemic. Heliyon 11 (4), e42739. doi:10.1016/j.heliyon.2025.e42739.

Holzinger, A., Haibe-Kains, B., Jurisica, I., 2019. Why imaging data alone is not enough: AI-based integration of imaging, omics, and clinical data. Eur. J. Nucl. Med. Mol. Imaging 46 (13), 2722–2730. doi:10.1007/s00259-019-04382-9.

Howe, K.L., et al., 2021. Ensembl 2021. Nucleic Acids Research 49(D1), D884–D891. doi:10.1093/nar/gkaa942.
Hu, M., Ge, X., Chen, X., Mao, W., Qian, X., Yuan, W.-E., 2020. Micro/Nanorobot: a promising targeted drug delivery system. Pharmaceutics 12 (7), 665. doi:10.3390/pharmaceutics12070665.
Ianevski, A., Kushnir, A., Nader, K., Miihkinen, M., Xhaard, H., Aittokallio, T., Tanoli, Z., 2024. RepurposeDrugs: an interactive web-portal and predictive platform for repurposing mono- and combination therapies. Briefings in Bioinformatics 25 (4). doi:10.1093/bib/bbae328.
Jahan, S.T., Sadat, S.M.A., Walliser, M., Haddadi, A., 2017. Targeted therapeutic nanoparticles: an immense promise to fight against cancer. J. Drug Deliv. 1–24. doi:10.1155/2017/9090325.
Jena, G.K., Patra, C.N., Jammula, S., Rana, R., Chand, S., 2024. Artificial intelligence and machine learning implemented drug delivery systems: a paradigm shift in the pharmaceutical industry. J. Bio-X Res. 7. doi:10.34133/jbioxresearch.0016
Jiang, J., Ma, X., Ouyang, D., Williams, R.O., 2022. Emerging artificial intelligence (AI) technologies used in the development of solid dosage forms. Pharmaceutics 14 (11). doi:10.3390/pharmaceutics14112257.
Johnson, K.B., Wei, W., Weeraratne, D., Frisse, M.E., Misulis, K., Rhee, K., Zhao, J., Snowdon, J.L., 2021. Precision medicine, AI, and the future of personalized health care. Clin. Transl. Sci. 14 (1), 86–93. doi:10.1111/cts.12884.
Kalinin, A.A., Higgins, G.A., Reamaroon, N., Soroushmehr, S., Allyn-Feuer, A., Dinov, I.D., Najarian, K., Athey, B.D., 2018. Deep learning in pharmacogenomics: from gene regulation to patient stratification. Pharmacogenomics 19 (7), 629–650. doi:10.2217/pgs-2018-0008.
Kallal, L.A., Waszkiewicz, A., Jaworski, J.P., Della Pietra, A., Berrodin, T., Brady, P., Jurewicz, A.J., Zeng, X., Payne, L., Medina, J.R., Doepner-Buser, C., Mangatt, B., 2021. High-throughput screening and triage assays identify small molecules targeting c-MYC in cancer cells. SLAS Discovery 26 (2), 216–229. doi:10.1177/2472555220985457.
Kapoor, D.U., Sharma, J.B., Gandhi, S.M., Prajapati, B.G., Thanawuth, K., Limmatvapirat, S., Sriamornsak, P., 2024. AI-driven design and optimization of nanoparticle-based drug delivery systems. Sci., Eng. Health Stud. 24010003. doi:10.69598/sehs.18.24010003.
Khan, M.W., Abbasi, E., 2015. Differentiating parameters for selecting simple object access protocol (SOAP) vs. representational state transfer (REST) based architecture. J. Adv. Comput. Netw. 3 (1), 63–66. doi:10.7763/JACN.2015.V3.143.
Kidwai-Khan, F., Rentsch, C.T., Pulk, R., Alcorn, C., Brandt, C.A., Justice, A.C., 2022. Pharmacogenomics driven decision support prototype with machine learning: a framework for improving patient care. Front. Big Data 5. doi:10.3389/fdata.2022.1059088
Kuenzi, B.M., Park, J., Fong, S.H., Sanchez, K.S., Lee, J., Kreisberg, J.F., Ma, J., Ideker, T., 2020. Predicting drug response and synergy using a deep learning model of human cancer cells. Cancer Cell 38 (5), 672–684.e6. doi:10.1016/j.ccell.2020.09.014.
Libbrecht, M.W., Noble, W.S., 2015. Machine learning applications in genetics and genomics. Nat Rev Genet 16 (6), 321–332. doi:10.1038/nrg3920.
Lin, J., Ngiam, K.Y., 2023. How data science and AI-based technologies impact genomics. Singapore Med. J. 64 (1), 59–66. doi:10.4103/singaporemedj.SMJ-2021-438.
Lin, Z., Chou, W.-C., Cheng, Y.-H., He, C., Monteiro-Riviere, N.A., Riviere, J.E., 2022. Predicting nanoparticle delivery to tumors using machine learning and artificial intelligence approaches. Int. J. Nanomed. 17, 1365–1379. doi:10.2147/IJN.S344208.
Liu, J., Li, J., Wang, H., Yan, J., 2020. Application of deep learning in genomics. Sci. China Life Sci. 63 (12), 1860–1878. doi:10.1007/s11427-020-1804-5.

Liu, X., Song, C., Huang, F., Fu, H., Xiao, W., Zhang, W., 2022. GraphCDR: a graph neural network method with contrastive learning for cancer drug response prediction. Briefings in Bioinformatics 23(1). doi:10.1093/bib/bbab457.

Macarron, R., Banks, M.N., Bojanic, D., Burns, D.J., Cirovic, D.A., Garyantes, T., Green, D.V.S., Hertzberg, R.P., Janzen, W.P., Paslay, J.W., Schopfer, U., Sittampalam, G.S., 2011. Impact of high-throughput screening in biomedical research. Nat. Rev. Drug Discov. 10 (3), 188–195. doi:10.1038/nrd3368v.

Mandal, S., Moudgil, M., Mandal, S.K., 2009. Rational drug design. Eur. J. Pharmacol. 625 (1–3), 90–100. doi:10.1016/j.ejphar.2009.06.065.

Mathur, S., Sutton, J., 2017. Personalized medicine could transform healthcare. Biomed. Rep. 7 (1), 3–5. doi:10.3892/br.2017.922.

Mohammadpour, F., Kamali, H., Gholami, L., McCloskey, A.P., Kesharwani, P., Sahebkar, A., 2022. Solid lipid nanoparticles: a promising tool for insulin delivery. Expert Opinion on Drug Delivery 19 (12), 1577–1595. doi:10.1080/17425247.2022.2138328.

Muhammad, I.I., Kong, S.L., Akmar Abdullah, S.N., Munusamy, U., 2019. RNA-seq and ChIP-seq as complementary approaches for comprehension of plant transcriptional regulatory mechanism. Int. J. Mol. Sci. 21 (1), 167. doi:10.3390/ijms21010167.

Murray, M.F., 2018. The Path to Routine Genomic Screening in Health Care. Ann Intern Med 169 (6), 407–408. doi:10.7326/M18-1722.

Nance, E., Pun, S.H., Saigal, R., Sellers, D.L., 2021. Drug delivery to the central nervous system. Nat. Rev. Mater. 7 (4), 314–331. doi:10.1038/s41578-021-00394-w.

Nathanson, K.L., 2010. Using genetics and genomics strategies to personalize therapy for cancer: Focus on melanoma. Biochemical Pharmacology 80 (5), 755–761. doi:10.1016/j.bcp.2010.04.017.

Nestl, B.M., Nebel, B.A., Resch, V., Schürmann, M., Tischler, D., 2024. The development and opportunities of predictive biotechnology. ChemBioChem 25 (13). doi:10.1002/cbic.202300863.

O'Shea, J., Ledwidge, M., Gallagher, J., Keenan, C., Ryan, C., 2022. Pharmacogenetic interventions to improve outcomes in patients with multimorbidity or prescribed polypharmacy: a systematic review. Pharmacogenomics J. 22 (2), 89–99. doi:10.1038/s41397-021-00260-6.

Obeid, S., Madžarević, M., Krkobabić, M., Ibrić, S., 2021. Predicting drug release from diazepam FDM printed tablets using deep learning approach: influence of process parameters and tablet surface/volume ratio. Int. J. Pharm. 601. doi:10.1016/j.ijpharm.2021.120507

Ohler, U., Liao, G.-C., Niemann, H., Rubin, G.M., 2002. Computational analysis of core promoters in the Drosophila genome. http://genomebiology.com/2002/3/12/research/0087.1.

Oliveira, A.L., 2019. Biotechnology, big data and artificial intelligence. Biotechnol. J. 14 (8). doi:10.1002/biot.201800613.

Ori, M.O., Ekpan, F.M., Samuel, H.S., Egwuatu, O.P., 2024. Integration of artificial intelligence in nanomedicine. Eurasian J. Sci. Technol 4 (2), 88–104. doi:10.48309/EJST.2024.422419.1105.

Oualikene-Gonin, W., Jaulent, M.-C., Thierry, J.-P., Oliveira-Martins, S., Belgodère, L., Maison, P., Ankri, J., Scientific Advisory Board of ANSM, 2024. Artificial intelligence integration in the drug lifecycle and in regulatory science: policy implications, challenges and opportunities. Front. Pharmacol. 15, 1437167. doi:10.3389/fphar.2024.1437167.

Parekh, A.-D.E., Shaikh, O.A., Simran, Manan, S., Hasibuzzaman, M.A., 2023. Artificial intelligence (AI) in personalized medicine: AI-generated personalized therapy regimens based on genetic and medical history: short communication. Ann. Med. Surg. 85 (11), 5831–5833. doi:10.1097/MS9.0000000000001320.

Park, A., Lee, Y., Nam, S., 2023a. A performance evaluation of drug response prediction models for individual drugs. Sci. Rep. 13 (1), 11911. doi:10.1038/s41598-023-39179-2.

Petsko, G.A., Ringe, D., 2009. Protein Structure and Function, Oxford University Press; Distributed inside North America by Sinauer Associates.

Pinto, N., Eileen Dolan, M., 2011. Clinically Relevant Genetic Variations in Drug Metabolizing Enzymes. CDM 12 (5), 487–497. doi:10.2174/138920011795495321.

Pun, F.W., Ozerov, I.V., Zhavoronkov, A., 2023. AI-powered therapeutic target discovery. Trends Pharmacol. Sci. 44 (9), 561–572. doi:10.1016/j.tips.2023.06.010.

Ramović Hamzagić, A., Gazdić Janković, M., Cvetković, D., Nikolić, D., Nikolić, S., Milivojević Dimitrijević, N., Kastratović, N., Živanović, M., Miletić Kovačević, M., Ljujić, B., 2024. Machine learning model for prediction of development of cancer stem cell subpopulation in tumurs subjected to polystyrene nanoparticles. Toxics 12 (5), 354. doi:10.3390/toxics12050354.

Ren, F., Aliper, A., Chen, J., Zhao, H., Rao, S., Kuppe, C., Ozerov, I.V., Zhang, M., Witte, K., Kruse, C., Aladinskiy, V., Ivanenkov, Y., Polykovskiy, D., Fu, Y., Babin, E., Qiao, J., Liang, X., Mou, Z., Wang, H., et al., 2025. A small-molecule TNIK inhibitor targets fibrosis in preclinical and clinical models. Nat. Biotechnol. doi:10.1038/s41587-024-02143-0.

Ren, F., Ding, X., Zheng, M., Korzinkin, M., Cai, X., Zhu, W., Mantsyzov, A., Aliper, A., Aladinskiy, V., Cao, Z., Kong, S., Long, X., Man Liu, B.H., Liu, Y., Naumov, V., Shneyderman, A., Ozerov, I.V., Wang, J., Pun, F.W., et al., 2023. AlphaFold accelerates artificial intelligence powered drug discovery: efficient discovery of a novel CDK20 small molecule inhibitor. Chem. Sci. 14 (6), 1443–1452. doi:10.1039/d2sc05709c.

Schork, N.J., 2019. Artificial intelligence and personalized medicine. In: Cancer Treatment and Research, pp. 265–283. doi:10.1007/978-3-030-16391-4_11.

Shajari, S., Kuruvinashetti, K., Komeili, A., Sundararaj, U., 2023. The Emergence of AI-Based Wearable Sensors for Digital Health Technology: A Review. Sensors 23 (23), 9498. doi:10.3390/s23239498.

Stillman, N.R., Balaz, I., Tsompanas, M., Kovacevic, M., Azimi, S., Lafond, S., Adamatzky, A., Hauert, S., 2021. Evolutionary computational platform for the automatic discovery of nanocarriers for cancer treatment. npj Comput Mater 7 (1). doi:10.1038/s41524-021-00614-5.

Strimbu, K., Tavel, J.A., 2010. What are biomarkers?. Curr. Opin. HIV AIDS 5 (6), 463–466. doi:10.1097/COH.0b013e32833ed177.

Su, R., Huang, Y., Zhang, D., Xiao, G., Wei, L., 2022. SRDFM: Siamese Response Deep Factorization Machine to improve anti-cancer drug recommendation. Briefings in Bioinformatics 23 (2). doi:10.1093/bib/bbab534.

Subramani, K., Mehta, M., 2018. Nanodiagnostics in microbiology and dentistry. In: Emerging Nanotechnologies in Dentistry. Elsevier, pp. 391–419. doi:10.1016/B978-0-12-812291-4.00019-4.

Suriyaamporn, P., Pamornpathomkul, B., Wongprayoon, P., Rojanarata, T., Ngawhirunpat, T., Opanasopit, P., 2024. The artificial intelligence and design of experiment assisted in the development of progesterone-loaded solid-lipid nanoparticles for transdermal drug delivery. Pharmacia 71, 1–12. doi:10.3897/pharmacia.71.e123549.

Taherdoost, H., Ghofrani, A., 2024. AI's role in revolutionizing personalized medicine by reshaping pharmacogenomics and drug therapy. Intell. Pharm. 2 (5), 643–650. doi:10.1016/j.ipha.2024.08.005.

Tembhare, A., Sibi Chakkaravarthy, S., Sangeetha, D., Vaidehi, V., Venkata Rathnam, M., 2019. Role-based policy to maintain privacy of patient health records in cloud. J Supercomput 75 (9), 5866–5881. doi:10.1007/s11227-019-02887-6.

Varadi, M., Velankar, S., 2023. The impact of AlphaFold protein structure database on the fields of life sciences. Proteomics 23 (17). doi:10.1002/pmic.202200128.

Vargason, A.M., Anselmo, A.C., Mitragotri, S., 2021. The evolution of commercial drug delivery technologies. Nat. Biomed. Eng. 5 (9), 951–967. doi:10.1038/s41551-021-00698-w.

Vora, L.K., Gholap, A.D., Jetha, K., Thakur, R.R.S., Solanki, H.K., Chavda, V.P., 2023. Artificial intelligence in pharmaceutical technology and drug delivery design. Pharmaceutics 15 (7). doi:10.3390/pharmaceutics15071916.

Wang, L., Song, Y., Wang, H., Zhang, X., Wang, M., He, J., Li, S., Zhang, L., Li, K., Cao, L., 2023. Advances of artificial intelligence in anti-cancer drug design: a review of the past decade. Pharmaceuticals 16 (2), 253. doi:10.3390/ph16020253.

Williams, A.M., Liu, Y., Regner, K.R., Jotterand, F., Liu, P., Liang, M., 2018. Artificial intelligence, physiological genomics, and precision medicine. Physiol. Genomics 50 (4), 237–243. doi:10.1152/physiolgenomics.00119.2017.

Xu, Y., Jiang, W.-J., Bai, -Y.-Y., Yang, Y.-J., Zhang, Z.-L., 2024. Artificial intelligence-assisted multiparameter size discrimination of silver nanoparticles through electrochemical collision. Anal. Chem. 96 (16), 6195–6201. doi:10.1021/acs.analchem.3c05115.

Xu, Y., Liu, X., Cao, X., Huang, C., Liu, E., Qian, S., Liu, X., Wu, Y., Dong, F., Qiu, C.W., Qiu, J., Hua, K., Su, W., Wu, J., Xu, H., Han, Y., Fu, C., Yin, Z., Liu, M., et al., 2021. Artificial intelligence: a powerful paradigm for scientific research. Innov. 2 (4), 100179. doi:10.1016/J.XINN.2021.100179.

Yacoub, A.S., Ammar, H.O., Ibrahim, M., Mansour, S.M., El Hoffy, N.M., 2022. Artificial intelligence-assisted development of in situ forming nanoparticles for arthritis therapy via intra-articular delivery. Drug Deliv. 29 (1), 1423–1436. doi:10.1080/10717544.2022.2069882.

You, Y., Lai, X., Pan, Y., Zheng, H., Vera, J., Liu, S., Deng, S., Zhang, L., 2022. Artificial intelligence in cancer target identification and drug discovery. Signal Transduct. Target. Ther. 7 (1), 156. doi:10.1038/s41392-022-00994-0.

Yuan, Y., Wu, Y., Cheng, J., Yang, K., Xia, Y., Wu, H., Pan, X., 2024. Applications of artificial intelligence to lipid nanoparticle delivery. Particuology 90, 88–97. doi:10.1016/j.partic.2023.11.014.

Zhang, H., Li, J., Saravanan, K.M., Wu, H., Wang, Z., Wu, D., Wei, Y., Lu, Z., Chen, Y.H., Wan, X., Pan, Y., 2021. An Integrated Deep Learning and Molecular Dynamics Simulation-Based Screening Pipeline Identifies Inhibitors of a New Cancer Drug Target TIPE2DataSheet1.docx. Front. Pharmacol. 12. doi:10.3389/fphar.2021.772296.

Zhong, F., Xing, J., Li, X., Liu, X., Fu, Z., Xiong, Z., Lu, D., Wu, X., Zhao, J., Tan, X., Li, F., Luo, X., Li, Z., Chen, K., Zheng, M., Jiang, H., 2018. Artificial intelligence in drug design. Sci. China Life Sci. 61 (10), 1191–1204. doi:10.1007/s11427-018-9342-2.

Zhou, H., Mayorga-Martinez, C.C., Pané, S., Zhang, L., Pumera, M., 2021. Magnetically Driven Micro and Nanorobots. Chem. Rev. 121(8), 4999–5041. doi:10.1021/acs.chemrev.0c01234.

16

Artificial intelligence in medical image processing and translational science

Kushagra Kashyap and Darshana Zujam
Department of Life Sciences, School of Science and Mathematics, DES Pune University, Pune, Maharashtra, India

1 Introduction

The development of artificial intelligence (AI) has undergone many ups and downs since the term was initially coined by John McCarthy in 1955. The big data revolution, advancements in wearable medical devices, and mobile health applications have empowered the biomedical community to leverage AI and machine learning (ML) for large scale data analysis. Significant advancements have recently been observed in predictive analytics. Notable progress has recently been made in the field of predictive analytics (Dixon et al., 2024), precision medicine (Carini and Seyhan, 2024), virtual diagnosis (Zeltzer et al., 2023), patient monitoring (Jeddi and Bohr, 2020), and drug discovery (Kashyap et al., 2023b, 2023a; Kashyap and Siddiqi, 2021), drawing the interest of governmental organizations alongside academia and industry, offering practitioners novel technologies.

Development of AI models requires training, validating, and testing their network weights and parameters. Data sets are important for this and must be collected in a manner that ensures interdependence between them. This approach reduces overfitting and underfitting issues by increasing the model's ability to generalize effectively. Before 2000, insufficient computational power, limited datasets, and a smaller number of research groups hindered progress a great deal. The domain of AI/ML observed exceptional progress after 2012 owing to the significant achievements in computer vision and the emergence of innovative deep learning (DL) models (Fig. 16.1). These developments were made possible not only by algorithmic advancements but also by the growing availability of huge, well organized digital datasets and the rapid evolution of computational hardware,

The AI Frontier in Molecular Modelling and Drug Designing. https://doi.org/10.1016/B978-0-443-40338-5.00004-4

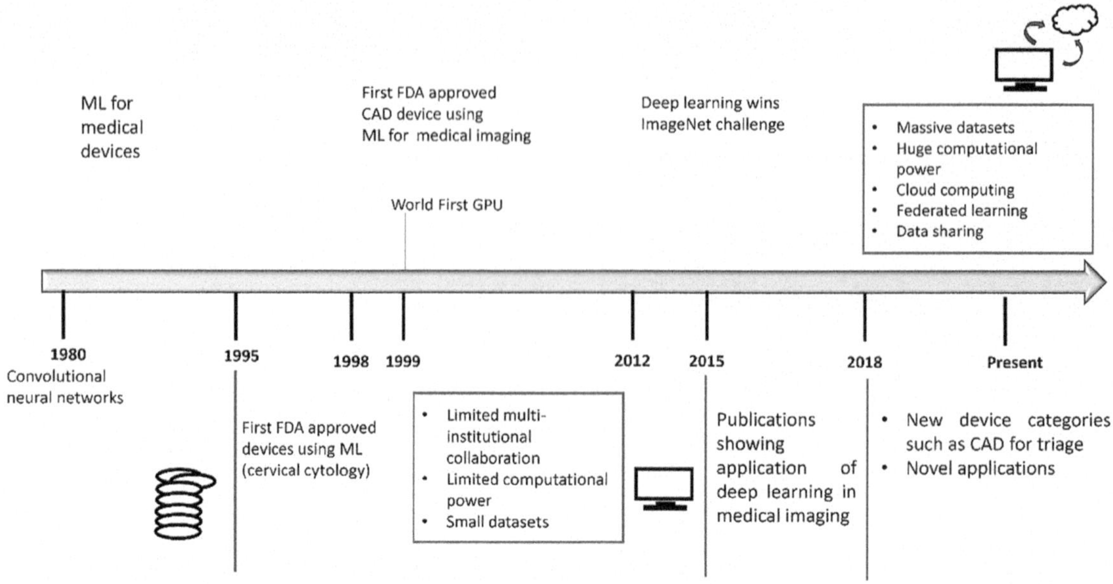

Fig. 16.1 Evolution of artificial intelligence and machine learning technologies in the field of medical imaging. The timeline highlights key milestones in the integration of AI and ML technologies into medical imaging workflows.

particularly the graphics processing units (GPUs), which were later proved to be inadequate due to the ever increasing complexity of AI models. To solve these problems, Google created the Tensor Processing Unit (TPU), a specialized hardware accelerator intended for incorporation into its TensorFlow AI framework (Xu et al., 2021). TPUs are engineered for handling neural network computations and provide an ultra fast and efficient solution for ML. Their potential extends beyond general AI applications, with promising implications for medical imaging, diagnostics, and research.

These technological advancements paved the way for AI to enter the medical field. The expert systems, which support health care professionals in making clinical decisions, are the best known early applications. Due to its capability of detecting, classifying, and segmenting malignant lesions in medical images, the neural network emerged as a powerful tool (Rayed et al., 2024). Interestingly, the idea of integrating AI with medical imaging is not new; the earliest references date back to 1993, when researchers described the development of an “intelligent workstation for computer aided diagnosis” (CAD) (Giger et al., 1993).

While traditional computer vision techniques for CAD in radiology have been studied for many years, it is the advent of DL that has truly transformed the field in recent years. Among the leading AI based technologies in image analysis, convolutional neural networks (CNNs) stand out for their noteworthy contribution to achieving unparalleled accuracy. Today, the increasing reliability and accessibility of ML tools are speeding up their integration into clinical workflows.

The advancement of present ML tools has paved the way for their incorporation in clinical settings. Joint efforts between research teams, clinicians, and industries are now driving the growth of clinical AI solutions. With AI's clinical implementation becoming increasingly imminent, a foundational understanding of AI and its underlying learning techniques, including their development and present state of the art, is crucial for all medical professionals. Equipping the medical physics community with this expertise will not only raise research quality but also empower new researchers and create innovative research directions within the field.

2 Artificial intelligence technologies in medical imaging

2.1 AI in radiology

ML based models have been in use since the 1980s. In medical imaging, the characteristics of the image are of utmost concern. Images collected from different sources are segregated into training and testing. During the training stage, a wide range of ML models, like the traditional—**random forests (RFs)** and **support vector machine (SVM),** along with more sophisticated DL frameworks like **CNN, U-Net,** and **ResNet,** are employed to learn significant image features. The trained models are subsequently utilized to find features present in the test sets and to also perform classification. The strength of an ML model lies in its ability to generalize beyond the training data while still proficiently identifying intricate features across different image categories. A strong model not only captures fundamental geometric characteristics, such as shapes and areas, but also discerns nuanced patterns within the pixel level data, which is essential for identifying abnormal or pathological areas.

While creating high quality medical imaging datasets like the **Curated Breast Imaging Subset of Digital Database for Screening Mammography (DDSM)** (Lee et al., 2017), **INbreast** (Moreira et al., 2012), the **Mammographic Image Analysis Society Digital Mammogram Database** (Suckling, 1994) and the **OPTIMAM Medical Image Database** (Halling-Brown et al., 2021), it is always recommended to segment the area of the image that includes only the tumor. However, it has always been a challenge to manually select the features when building ML models, as these features can vary significantly due to differences among patients and users. Previously, ML models were utilized on imaging modalities such as computed tomography, magnetic resonance imaging, and mammography scans. Despite making several efforts, it was concluded after many trials that computer based detection delivered no benefit and also reduced radiology accuracy, leading to higher recall and biopsy rates.

Initially, when AI was being integrated into the health care field, ML based models were mainly applied to imaging techniques like computed tomography scans, magnetic resonance imaging, and mammography. These efforts demonstrated the capabilities of AI integration in the medical imaging field; however, they still face several challenges and limitations, as identified by large scale studies and trials. Specifically, early computer based detection systems were hardly able to enhance diagnostic accuracy. On the contrary, they sometimes contributed to increased recall rates and unnecessary biopsies, which reduced overall radiology efficiency.

Recent technological advancements have propelled the progress of deep neural networks in the past few years. These models are made up of many interconnected neurons and multiple hidden layers, allowing them to automatically identify and extract intricate, high level features from unprocessed clinical images. The widespread application of **DL** in medical imaging has been enabled by advancements in computational resources, particularly high performance GPUs and enhanced memory capacities.

A remarkable illustration of this advancement is the emergence of DL algorithms that can evaluate both current and previous CT scans to predict lung cancer occurrence with a 94.4% area under the curve. AI driven models, in comparison to traditional low dose CT screening methods—which, according to cancer.gov—are not risk free as they cause false positives, overdiagnosis, increased lung cancer related deaths, and radiation exposure—have demonstrated potential in alleviating several of these issues. Furthermore, research has shown that DL-based approaches outperform conventional ML based methods (Paul et al., 2016). Much of this success is attributed to the enormous amount of image data required to achieve more accurate predictions (Hosny et al., 2018). The ongoing success of models based on DL is anticipated to continue leading image research in radiology. Given their ongoing success, these models are likely to continue shaping the trajectory of radiological imaging research.

The relatively recent **foundation models** are increasingly being adopted in medical imaging. These are large scale AI models trained on extensive datasets, which can be customized or fine tuned for numerous downstream applications, including image classification, segmentation, lesion detection, and report generation. **Segment Anything** (Kirillov et al., 2023) by Meta is one such foundation model for universal image segmentation. It does not require fine tuning; however, its performance on complex medical segmentation tasks, like those involving the pancreas and spine, was unsatisfactory. To address these limitations,

SAM (Segment Anything Model) was tailored to be more medical domain-specific, leading to the creation of **Medical SAM 2** (Zhu et al., 2024). **CXR Foundation Models** are self supervised models (https://huggingface.co/google/cxr-foundation) developed for chest X-ray image analysis. Another significant innovation is **UniverSeg**, a universal segmentation model trained on a wide range of medical image types. Unlike traditional models, UniverSeg can generalize to previously unseen anatomical structures and segmentation tasks.

2.2 AI in radiation oncology

Beyond its application in radiology, AI has been widely applied in radiation oncology, particularly for tasks such as image registration, radiomics analysis, segmentation of organs and lesions, and detection of markers. Scholars have widely employed DL based models for segmenting different organs, including the brain, prostate, lung, pelvis, kidney, and regions of the head and neck. The **U-Net** architecture is a frequently utilized approach for these tasks. U-Net features a contracting pathway (a mix of convolution and pooling layers) and an expanding pathway (employing transposed convolutions), resulting in its U shaped structure.

Recent developments have investigated the application of **U-Net-generative adversarial** (U-Net-GAN) networks for segmenting various organs in CT images. In this method, the generator (U-Nets) and discriminator (convolutional networks) collaborate to create the best segmentation maps for various organs. Likewise, another study utilized **CNNs** for segmenting thoracic organs from 3D medical images for risk evaluation (Feng et al., 2019).

In radiation therapy, image registration is frequently required either between different imaging modalities (multimodal) or within the same modality captured at different time points (monomodal). This process entails locating matching points across two or more imaging datasets (CT, PET, MR, SPECT) to establish a precise geometric relationship between them. In one study, a convolutional stacked auto encoder network was employed to capture the inherent features within image patches (Wu et al., 2016). The algorithm demonstrated better results and can be utilized for multimodal as well as monomodal image registrations. A few years ago, a new CNN based method was proposed that regresses the transformation parameters, and this also can be applied to mono and multimodal applications.

For tracking the real time treatment area during delivery, the automatic fiducial or marker detection is crucial. In traditional methods, the design of a detection template is usually dependent on prior information about the marker's characteristics. In contrast to those conventional methods, the recently proposed CNN based models do not depend on predefined marker properties. Instead, they are capable of learning to automatically detect and segment fiducial markers of varying shapes, including cylindrical and irregularly shaped markers, directly from imaging data (Mylonas et al., 2019).

Similarly, AI has also been used in the field of radiomics assisted radiation oncology. It consists of two steps: extraction of features following image segmentation and incorporation of those features into the AI models. For the first part, the extracted features include tumor volume, shape, density, pixel intensity, geometric information, and texture. In the second step, the feature-fitted models were used to predict the tumor outcome. This capability of radiomics can help in predicting the survival time prior to treatment, which, in turn, can help in selecting suitable treatment regimens. In a research study, scientists developed a radiomics signature and demonstrated strong associations between radiomic features and gene expression profiles across different types of cancer (Aerts et al., 2014). In addition to lung cancer, there have been reported applications concerning head and neck (Marcu et al., 2019) and prostate cancers (Perez-Lopez et al., 2019).

iSeg is Northwestern Medicine's tool that precisely segments lung tumors in 3D and also captures respiratory motion (Sarkar et al., 2025). AI supports adaptive radiotherapy by constantly evaluating a patient's imaging and clinical information during the course of treatment, enabling real time modifications to the treatment plan (Dona Lemus et al., 2024). Several Food and Drug Administratio approved AI tools are transforming clinical workflows in medical imaging and radiation oncology. MVision AI Oy, Medical Image Merge (MIM) ProtégéAI+, VBrain by Vysioneer, and Radiation Planning Assistant are a few examples of such tools.

MVision AI Oy is a cloud based DL software solution specifically designed for the automatic segmentation of organs at risk (OAR) in CT images (Li et al., 2023). The software provides high quality contours quickly with minimal manual input and thus enables greater consistency and efficiency in treatment planning through reduced time and effort.

MIM ProtégéAI+, developed by MIM Software Inc., is an advanced auto contouring tool that particularly focuses on the delineation of lymph nodes and various OARs. The zero click automation is the main feature of MIM ProtégéAI+, by which the contouring starts as soon as the imaging is available, thus greatly decreasing the time required for manual segmentation and making the workflow more efficient (Urago et al., 2021).

Vysioneer's **VBrain** employs DL techniques to automatically identify and outline metastatic brain tumors (Wang et al., 2023). In addition to improving the accuracy of lesion detection, it also makes the contouring process faster, thus allowing clinicians more time to deal with complex brain metastasis cases.

The Radiation Planning Assistant is an AI based platform dedicated to facilitating the radiotherapy treatment planning process. It combines both treatment planning AI tools and contouring aids. It excels in low resource environments. This tool not only helps to speed up the process of treatment plan generation with higher precision, but it also supports worldwide initiatives to increase fair access to quality cancer care (Court et al., 2023).

2.3 Generative models for medical image synthesis

Generative models, especially **Generative Adversarial Networks** (GANs), have shown significant promise in advancing medical imaging applications, encompassing augmentation or data synthesis (Toda et al., 2021). These models are composed of two main parts: a generator and a discriminator (Fig. 16.2). The goal during training is to optimize the generator so effectively that it creates highly realistic images capable of deceiving the discriminator into classifying them as authentic.

Its one application involves generating pseudo healthy images from pathological scans. These are synthetic images depicting what a patient's anatomy would look like in the absence of disease. By visualizing this negative image alongside the actual patient's scan, radiologists can more easily detect and characterize lesions (Wolterink et al., 2021). In addition, synthetic virtual patient groups can be created to conduct virtual clinical trials for evaluating new medications, treatments, or diagnostic methods, thus lowering the costs associated with human clinical trials (Acosta et al., 2022).

GANs showcase amazing capabilities in MRI image reconstruction, especially because they can effectively capture subtle textures and

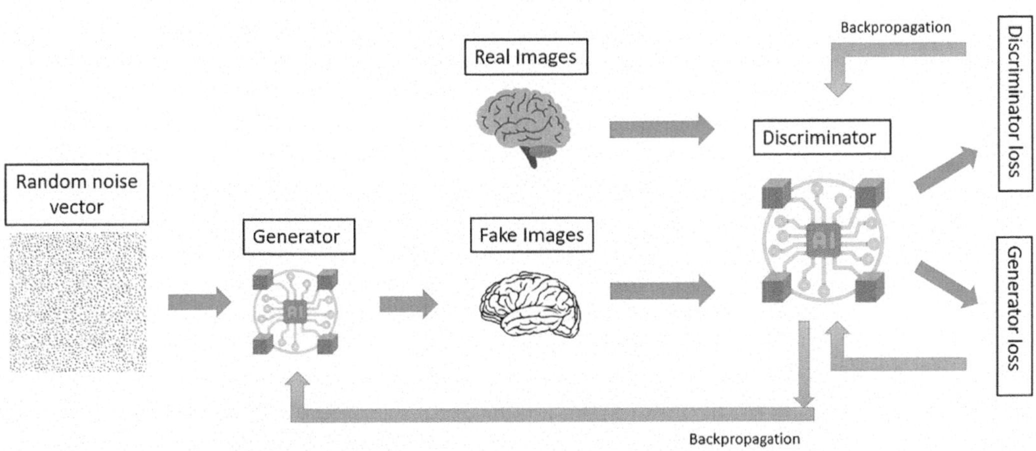

Fig. 16.2 General architecture of a GAN model. A schematic representation of a typical generative adversarial network (GAN) comprising the generator and discriminator networks.

intricate structural details (Lee, 2021). **CycleGAN** (https://github.com/junyanz/CycleGAN) is a GAN algorithm that translates between image modalities without paired data (e.g., MRI ↔ CT). It serves as a tool for cross modality synthesis and harmonization of MRI. **Superresolution GAN** (https://github.com/leftthomas/SRGAN) is employed to enhance image resolution, particularly for improving the quality of low resolution MRI, CT, or ultrasound images. Deep Convolutional GANs are used as foundational models for generating medical images of synthetic nature. **Conditional GANs** extend the deep convolutional GAN approach by incorporating label or image conditions. They allow for targeted synthesis, such as generating tumor containing regions (Sindhura et al., 2024). **Laplacian Pyramid GAN** can produce high quality images in a progressive manner from low to high resolution. It is suitable for applications in histopathology and dermoscopy, where fine details are very important. **NVIDIA Clara** (https://www.nvidia.com/en-in/clara/) is a suite of computing tools and services that provides GPU accelerated tools. It supports GAN based image enhancement, which includes tasks such as superresolution, denoising, and modality translation that are vital in improving image quality and harmonizing data across different scanners or protocols.

Similarly, the **CNNs** have found successful applications in both rigid (Sloan et al., 2018) and deformable image registration (Fourcade et al., 2022), a crucial step for precise voxel level dose tracking in radiotherapy (Avanzo et al., 2017). A promising emerging architecture, neural fields, offers a unified approach by efficiently parameterizing the physical properties of images, enabling it to effectively handle tasks like image reconstruction and registration (Sun et al., 2024).

Variational autoencoders (VAE) are generative models that learn to encode input medical images into a latent space and then reconstruct them using a decoder, making them useful for modeling healthy anatomy. Lesions or abnormalities can be identified as deviations in reconstruction, thus enabling lesion detection. VAE variants, like the **Conditional VAE**, allow image generation that is conditioned on labels and can reconstruct missing image regions, making them suitable for large scale medical images. **Vector quantized VAE** further enhances image quality by making use of discrete latent embeddings. A more advanced approach is the combination of VAEs with GANs (**VAE-GAN**) (Celard et al., 2023). It combines the structured latent representation of VAE with the image sharpness capabilities of GAN by integrating a discriminator. This hybrid framework supports high quality, diverse image generation and has been effectively used in brain tumor synthesis, as demonstrated by (Ahmad et al., 2022).

In addition to GAN and VAE, **diffusion models** and **autoregressive models** are emerging as powerful generative techniques in medical imaging. Denoising Diffusion Probabilistic Models are diffusion models that work by learning to reverse a noise process, thus generating high quality images with fewer artifacts and better mode coverage than GANs (Khader et al., 2023). Autoregressive models generate images by modeling the joint distribution of pixels or patches as a sequence of conditional probabilities (Wang et al., 2025). Their use is limited due to slower generation, but they can be used in segmentation map generation and patch based image generation. For example, **VoxelCNN** is an autoregressive model.

2.4 Integrating natural language processing and large language models in biomedical data analysis

Natural language processing (NLP) (Steinkamp and Cook, 2021), a branch of AI that allows computers to comprehend, interpret, and produce human language, has gained significant popularity in recent years, particularly within the healthcare sector. The quantity of research concentrating on employing NLP to create diagnostic models utilizing both structured and unstructured data from electronic health records is swiftly rising (Kreimeyer et al., 2017; Ravuri et al., 2018).

One of the noteworthy advancements in NLP was the introduction of the Transformer architecture. By leveraging the self attention mechanism, this architecture can effectively model long distance relationships in input sequences and perform computations in parallel. The Transformers serve as the foundation for powerful **large language models** (LLMs) like GPT (OpenAI) (Currie et al., 2023) and Bidirectional Encoder Representations from Transformers (BERT) (Google) (Talebi et al., 2024). Trained on vast datasets sourced from the internet, these models demonstrate impressive capabilities in text generation, including translation, summarization, sentence completion, and even producing creative content that is tailored to user defined domains. LLMs are seen to possess the ability to act as effective decision support systems, suggesting suitable imaging techniques according to a patient's symptoms and medical background. The GPT-4, a powerful generative LLM that OpenAI recently released, demonstrates significant advancements. GPT-4's ability to analyze images indicates its potential application in radiology, where it could assist radiologists by generating preliminary diagnostic interpretations and acting as a virtual aide (Langlotz, 2023). **Vision Transformers** (ViTs), a specialized subset of Transformer architectures, have gained recognition as powerful tools in computer vision (Wu et al., 2023). Unlike their NLP counterparts that process sequences of words, ViTs effectively process image patches, enabling them to perform well in numerous medical imaging applications, such as lesion detection, image segmentation, registration, and classification (Attention is All You Need). Using

Vision Transformers (ViTs) to analyze diagnostic images alongside LLMs to interpret clinical reports has the potential to create a powerful, comprehensive image based decision support system. See Table 16.1 for a comparative overview.

Table 16.1 Comparative overview of AI models used in medical imaging.

Approach	AI Model	Strengths	Weaknesses	Applications	References
Traditional ML	RF, SVM (SVM), Logistic regression	Interpretable, lower potential for overfitting	Need manual feature extraction	Basic classification and risk prediction	Ravuri et al. (2018)
DL	CNN, ResNet, U-Net, SegNet	Automated feature extraction, high accuracy	Black- box nature	Lesion detection, image classification, segmentation	Rayed et al. (2024)
Generative AI	Generative Adversarial Networks (GANs), Variational Autoencoders (VAEs), Diffusion models, Autoregressive models	Data augmentation, realistic image reconstruction	Training instability and complexity issues	Image synthesis, virtual clinical trials	Wolterink et al. (2021), Wang et al. (2025), et al. (2025), Celard et al. (2023), Khader et al. (2023)
Foundation models	RadImageNet, pretrained DL models	Reduced data requirements with easy transferability	Limited to predefined tasks	Medical image classification, fine tuning	Mei et al. (2022)
Explainable AI (XAI)	Saliency maps, Heatmaps	Model transparency and enhanced interpretability of the models.	Their interpretability is still evolving; the explanations may be incomplete or misleading.	Visual explanation of the AI predictions, building clinical trust.	Neri et al. (2023)
Self-supervised learning	Contrastive learning frameworks	Learning from unlabeled data	Limited clinical validation	Multimodal image incorporation	
NLP	LLM	Summarization of texts, patient friendly explanations	May generate factually incorrect or misleading text; struggles with domain specific terminology.	Automatic medical report drafting	Kreimeyer et al. (2017), Steinkamp and Cook (2021).
Neural fields	Neural representations	Efficient parameterization of image properties	High computational demands	Image reconstruction, registration tasks	Sun et al. (2024)

3 Transformative applications of AI in diagnostic imaging

3.1 Leveraging AI for disease detection and diagnosis

AI's implementation in medical imaging has revolutionized healthcare, playing a crucial role in the early identification and accurate diagnosis of various diseases. Imaging methods like X-ray, MRI, CT, ultrasound, and PET generate large quantities of complex data. Radiologists and clinicians have heavily depended on their knowledge and personal judgment to analyze these images. AI, on the other hand, offers a data driven, unbiased, and extremely scalable solution for mining significant information from medical images. By integrating imaging, clinical, and genomic data, AI can help in making personalized treatment decisions. Radiomics and predictive models can sort out patients based on likely treatment responses, enabling tailored therapy.

3.1.1 AI in oncology imaging

AI is revolutionizing the field of oncologic imaging by enabling more precise detection, characterization, and prognostic assessment of various cancer types, thereby supporting personalized treatment planning. AI utilizes advanced algorithms, especially DL and radiomics, to find complex patterns and quantitative features in medical images obtained from mammography, CT, MRI, and PET. Such AI powered methods allow for more precise identification and characterization of tumors, often surpassing human performance in terms of speed and consistency.

DL algorithms, especially CNNs like **VGGNet** and **RESNet,** have demonstrated great success in identifying breast cancer in mammography, ultrasound, and MRI images. Tools relying on AI, such as **Google's LYNA** (Lymph Node Assistant), have reached accuracy at the level of pathologists in finding metastatic breast cancer in lymph node biopsies (Liu et al., 2019). Likewise, **CAD** systems support radiologists by marking questionable regions in mammograms, thereby decreasing false negatives. **INBreast** is a popular dataset for training and testing ML and DL models (Moreira et al., 2012). The standardized labels and varied image collection render it an essential asset for creating and assessing computer aided detection systems, particularly for enhancing the precision and dependability of automated breast cancer screening tools.

Due to its aggressive behavior and the occurrence of diagnosis at a late stage, lung cancer imaging and detection have been a focus for a long time. Various DL models can scan chest X-rays, CT scans, and PET scans, and they are able to find lung nodules automatically as well as determine if the lesions are of a benign or malignant nature.

3.1.2 AI in ophthalmology imaging

Retinal diseases have become a significant problem worldwide. They rank among the primary factors contributing to substantial vision loss and blindness globally. Timely identification and proper intervention are necessary to prevent vision loss. Ocular imaging is crucial for diagnosis, monitoring, treatment planning, and managing retinal diseases, particularly diabetic eye diseases. Advancements in imaging technologies have significantly improved our understanding of disease progression and strengthened our capacity to make well informed clinical decisions. Current imaging methods for the diagnosis of retinopathies include the use of fundus photography, optical coherence tomography (OCT), and fluorescein angiography, which offer comprehensive information on retinal anatomy and physiology. A wide array of retinal diseases can be diagnosed using these imaging modalities. The list of diseases includes diabetic retinopathy (DR), diabetic macular edema (DME), age related macular degeneration (AMD), retinal artery occlusion (RAO), retinal tears, epiretinal membranes, macular holes, and retinitis pigmentosa (Saleh et al., 2022).

In the recent past, the use of AI has considerably increased for the diagnosis, grading, and severity assessment of retinal diseases. AI powered algorithms, specifically DL based models, are capable of accomplishing retinal image analysis with remarkable accuracy, sometimes even on par with or better than experts. Traditional ML techniques formed the basis of automated screening of retinal images; however, DL models have shown better results by capturing complex image patterns across diverse imaging modalities. Traditional ML methods like **SVM, RFs, decision trees, logistic regression, gradient boost, AdaBoost, Gaussian naïve Bayes**, etc., have been widely used either individually or in combination. Recently, DL technologies, including **multilayer CNN, deep CNN networks, VGGNet, ResNet,** and also specialized architectures such as **OCDT_Net,** have proven their ability to automatically learn complicated image features and boost diagnostic accuracy.

Among the most notable tools in ophthalmology image analysis is **IDx-DR** by Digital Diagnostics. It is recognized as the first FDA approved AI based system for the autonomous detection of diabetic retinopathy using retinal fundus images (Khan et al., 2025). IDx-DR has the ability to make clinical decisions without requiring any input from an ophthalmologist. This makes it useful in primary care settings and weaker regions where access to specialists may be limited. Another tool, **EyeArt** by Eyenuk, is a fully automated AI system that is designed for rapid and accurate diabetic retinopathy screening, thus helping in early intervention and reducing the risk of irreversible vision damage (Li et al., 2023). In addition, AI is also making strides in age related macular degeneration (AMD) detection. For example,

DeepSeeNet is a DL model made to assess the severity by analyzing retinal images (Peng et al., 2019).

3.1.3 AI in neural imaging

AI speeds up neuroimaging by improving compressed sensing MRI scans (CS-MRI). For example, the synthetic multiorientation resolution enhancement method, along with deep residual learning AI, not only eliminates aliasing but also increases the resolution of CS-MRI, which is crucial for conditions like multiple sclerosis (Zhao et al., 2019). Further developments, such as GANs with improved loss functions, retain high image quality while drastically reducing reconstruction times. Sparse coding methods offer additional time savings with lightweight, online processing.

Specific AI systems, like the **Grad-CAM** (gradient weighted class activation mapping), are able to detect conditions such as intracranial hemorrhage. The **Viz.ai Viz LVO** system quickly detects large vessel occlusions on CT angiograms, notifies stroke teams, and enables rapid interventions (Hassan, 2021). AI tools, like **Medtronic RAPID,** provide automated, quantitative assessments of ischemic brain regions, which are essential for stroke treatment decisions based on parameters like cerebral blood flow and ASPECT scores. Moreover, various FDA approved AI technologies for brain structure quantification assist in analyzing anatomical and functional changes in conditions like dementia, MS, seizures, and brain trauma, using both MRI and PET scans (Monsour, 2022).

3.2 AI in image segmentation

Image segmentation involves dividing an image into several segments or regions to create a simplified representation that aids in easier analysis and interpretation. Medical image segmentation aids in more precise and efficient tracing of anatomical structures and pathological regions. DL models, especially **CNNs** and their variants like **U-Net** and **SegNet,** automatically segment complicated structures from imaging techniques like MRI, CT, PET, and ultrasound. This automated segmentation minimizes the requirement for radiologists' manual annotation, a process that is quite time intensive, thereby decreasing manual errors and guaranteeing consistency along with high quality outcomes.

Explainable AI (XAI)-powered segmentation is conducted to help improve diagnosis, monitoring, and treatment planning across various specialties like oncology, neurology, gastroenterology, dermatology, and more (Gipiškis et al., 2024). In dermatology, methods like **Grad-CAM**, CAM-based explainability, and attention based CNN are used to segment and explain skin lesions, especially melanoma. They utilize datasets like ISIC 2018 and ISIC 2019. Oncology continues to be a key area where methods like DeepDream inspired approaches, radiomic feature analysis, SUNet, region guided attention, ProtoSeg, and SHAP are applied to liver, brain, and breast tumor segmentation using datasets like LiTS, BraTS, and INbreast. Ophthalmology employs XAI methods like Importance Activation Mapping (IAM) and Seg-Grad-CAM for retinal layer and optic disc segmentation. In pancreas segmentation, perturbation based methods like U-Noise, Grad-CAM, and dynamic noise maps help identify key regions.

3.3 AI in surgical planning

Imaging that is AI assisted, along with 3D modeling and 3D printing, is revolutionizing surgical planning. These technologies increase precision, personalization and efficiency. Using medical imaging data from CT scans, MRI, and echocardiography, AI can generate very detailed 3D models of a patient's anatomy (Takeuchi and Kitagawa, 2024). This allows the surgeon to understand the anatomy more clearly before a complex operation. For instance, a DL based tool, which is a combination of **YOLOv7** (a real time object detection algorithm) and **U-Net,** has been created to extract the left heart structures from echocardiographic inputs, thus aiding in cardiac surgery planning (Mortada et al., 2023).

Besides the virtual models, **3D printing** also makes it possible for these AI generated anatomical models to be physically produced. This helps surgeons visualize complex structures, anticipate challenges, and plan more effectively. Surgical guides and implants that are 3D printed and customized to the patient's specific anatomical features serve as an additional resource to increase surgical accuracy and reduce operating time.

4 The evolving role of AI in medical imaging research

Growth of DL techniques in medical imaging research has been fueled by several important elements, including advancements in GPUs and the widespread availability of openly shared DL libraries and pretrained models. These advancements greatly reduce technical barriers, making DL tools more accessible. This has led to worldwide global users contributing to enhancing AI for radiology. The users need not be domain experts in developing models; however, to make an impact, domain knowledge is necessary.

As the volume of digital health data continues to expand, a plethora of multimodal datasets is emerging, integrating medical imaging with diverse sources of information such as genomic data, laboratory results, clinical notes, and even real time health data collected from wearable devices. To address this, AI based models, particularly those leveraging self supervised learning, are emerging as powerful tools. These models can learn from vast amounts of uncategorized data, greatly minimizing reliance on manual, effort driven annotation methods. These models enable associations that surpass human cognitive limits, revealing how imaging features correlate with specific genomic patterns, biomarkers, and laboratory values. The incorporation of these multimodal AI systems is anticipated to greatly enhance healthcare by enabling more precise quantification of disease burden and delivering highly accurate predictions of disease progression, ultimately supporting personalized medicine and improving patient outcomes.

In past years, LLMs have made a considerable impact on the medical landscape. They are drafting medical reports and even clarifying medical guidelines. However, despite their impressive language capabilities, LLMs still face limitations, particularly in areas requiring logical reasoning or basic mathematical calculations. This shortcoming has, at times, led to inaccuracies in tasks like differential diagnosis, highlighting the need for cautious and supervised deployment. Nevertheless, LLMs are soon expected to be applied to various medical imaging tasks.

To make the reports comprehensive and understandable, they can help by summarizing the information in a very basic, patient readable language. For example, when asked to explain the blood brain barrier at a fifth grade reading level, ChatGPT (an LLM developed by OpenAI) provided the following response: "The blood brain barrier is like a security system for your brain that keeps it safe. It's made up of special cells that form a tight barrier around the blood vessels in your brain. This barrier decides what can pass through and what needs to stay out. For example, it lets in good things like oxygen and nutrients, which your brain needs to work properly, but blocks harmful things like germs, toxins, and certain chemicals. Think of it as a smart filter that protects your brain from getting hurt. Even though it is very selective, it still makes sure your brain gets everything it needs to stay healthy. Without the blood brain barrier, your brain could easily get damaged by things in your blood that don't belong there. It's one of the reasons your brain can keep working so hard every day to help you think, move, and feel!". This simple, readable response will make patients feel more comfortable with medical reports and, in turn, bring radiologists and patients closer.

The recent surge in AI innovation has largely been propelled by the use of the ImageNet database, which has created a benchmark for computer vision algorithms. There is also the availability of other imaging datasets, and one can assemble these large medical image datasets; however, the full potential of such datasets remains underutilized due to privacy concerns, regulatory restrictions, and challenges related to data sharing. These limitations often hinder the development of diverse, reliable, and generalizable medical AI algorithms, raising concerns about fairness and applicability across different populations.

To counter this, the newer approaches are in line:

- The National COVID Cohort Collaboration (N3C) is the largest open access U.S. database for ongoing COVID 19 research (**https://covid.cd2h.org/**). This national resource has been utilized by researchers and clinicians to detect risk factors for Long COVID, assist healthcare providers in selecting effective treatments, and support a wide range of other critical studies.
- Similarly, the **Medical Imaging and Data Resource Center (MIDRC)** (https://www.midrc.org/) serves as a leading open access platform for medical imaging and associated data. Sponsored by the **National Institute of Biomedical Imaging and Bioengineering (NIBIB)** and conducted at the **University of Chicago**, MIDRC is a collaborative effort led in partnership with the **American College of Radiology® (ACR®)**, the **Radiological Society of North America (RSNA)**, and the **American Association of Physicists in Medicine (AAPM)**. It has released over **100,000 imaging studies**, encompassing diverse techniques like **computed tomography scans, X-rays, magnetic resonance imaging**, and **ultrasound images**, collected from healthcare institutions across the United States. MIDRC serves as a model for building large, diverse, and publicly accessible medical imaging datasets.
- In addition, the **RadImageNet** database (https://www.radimagenet.com/) is an open access repository specifically designed to advance **transfer learning** for downstream medical imaging applications. Aggregating **CT, MRI**, and **ultrasound examinations** from approximately **130,000 patients**, RadImageNet enables researchers to leverage pretrained models to enhance efficiency in numerous clinical imaging tasks (Mei et al., 2022)
- In India, a joint initiative by ICMR, IISc, and ARTPARK led to the creation of Medical Imaging Datasets for India (MIDAS) (**https://artpark.in/health/midas**). The database uses a standardized process for curating, annotating, and storing data, ensuring quality control and consistency throughout.

5 AI in translational science

Translational science is the discipline that seeks to connect laboratory research with its practical applications. The most prominent feature of AI is its ability to quickly handle and accurately analyze extensive data sets, identifying patterns that are unnoticed by

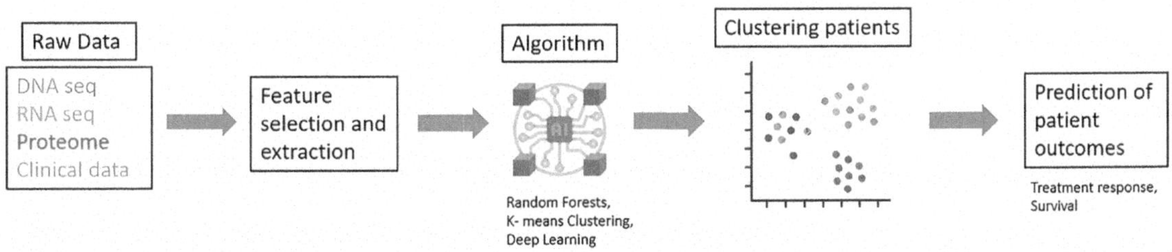

Fig. 16.3 Depiction of the application of AI/ML in Translational Science. Depiction of AI/ML applications bridging gaps between omics data, preclinical studies, and patient centered outcomes.

humans (Fig. 16.3). AI has become a significant factor in this sector. AI enables researchers and doctors to make sense of the huge amounts of data and locate hidden connections within, thus helping in disease prediction and diagnosis. It has made computational drug discovery and personalized medicine a reality. Instead of testing thousands of compounds manually, AI can rapidly scan huge chemical libraries and flag promising candidates for new drugs.

5.1 Medical imaging

This chapter talks a lot about the applications of AI in medical imaging. The creation of ML models, whether for medical imaging or other uses, relies heavily on large datasets for training. These datasets are frequently gathered in academic or research environments. After successful training, these models detect subtle patterns in the new data provided or predict disease progression. However, real impact is realized when these models are integrated into clinical workflows, assisting radiologists, surgeons, and physicians in making more accurate and faster decisions. This transition from research and development to their utilization in clinical practice is quite a challenging task. AI tools must initially be tested and validated on diverse, real world patient data for safety, fairness, and reliability. They need to work seamlessly with the hospital systems, adhering to the rules and regulatory standards. Moreover, the clinicians and patients must trust these tools and not see them as black boxes.

5.2 Drug discovery

Drug discovery traditionally has been a lengthy, costly, and complicated process. Bringing a simple drug to the market often takes decades and requires huge amounts of money and resources. AI is reshaping this process by accelerating each stage of drug development, from target identification to clinical trials.

5.2.1 Identification of target

Target identification serves as a vital and initial phase in the drug discovery process. Traditionally, target identification relies on a range of experimental techniques like affinity pull down, photoaffinity labeling, cell based assays, thermal shift assays, whole-genome knockdown screening, high-throughput screening, mass spectrometry, X-ray crystallography, electron microscopy, and more. These techniques, however, are time consuming, expensive, and labor intensive. The advent of AI and its subset, ML, is transforming the process of identifying targets by forecasting likely druggable candidates through various innovative computational methods.

Proteins are the most common drug targets. Knowledge of protein structure is important for target identification and the overall drug discovery process. Experimental methods like X-ray crystallography, nuclear magnetic resonance (NMR) spectroscopy, and cryo-electron microscopy (cryo-EM) for protein structure determination are powerful but, at the same time, costly, time consuming, and have limitations. When experimental data is unavailable, computational methods such as homology modeling, threading, and AI-driven tools are employed to predict protein structures. **AlphaFold 3** (Abramson et al., 2024) and **AlphaFold-Multimer** (Evans et al., 2021) by DeepMind, **ESMFold** (Li et al., 2023) by Meta AI, **RoseTTAFold** (Lisanza et al., 2024) and **RoseTTAFold All-Atom** (Marchal, 2024) by the Baker lab, **HelixFold-Multimer** (Fang et al., 2024), **ColabFold** (Mirdita et al., 2022), **OmegaFold** (Wu et al., 2022), **OpenFold** (Ahdritz et al., 2022) and **DMPFold** (Greener et al., 2019) are the various AI based protein structure prediction tools available. Moreover, protein language models like **ProtGPT2** and **ESM-2**, graph neural networks, and protein diffusion models show the capability to predict novel proteins and folds.

In addition to protein structure determination, AI plays a vital role in many other tasks within target identification, including binding site prediction, allosteric site detection, cryptic pocket prediction, de novo ligand generation, and network based target prediction. These processes are important for understanding the molecular interactions and druggability of targets. Novel therapeutic opportunities can be uncovered by utilization utilization of advanced AI algorithms that leverage structural, biochemical, and omics level data. Table 16.2 summarizes various AI based tools and algorithms for target identification.

5.2.2 Virtual screening

Virtual screening is a powerful computational approach in drug discovery that helps identify promising bioactive compounds from vast chemical libraries. This method is cost effective and time efficient compared to traditional high throughput screening. It computationally

Table 16.2 Summary of AI based tools and algorithms for target identification.

Method	AI tools/algorithms
Binding site prediction	• EquiBind (Li et al., 2023) • ProBiS tools (Konc and Janežič, 2017) • Uni-Mol (Alcaide et al., 2024) • GNN (Graph Neural Networks)
Allosteric site prediction	• AlloReverse (Zha et al., 2023) • AlloSigMA 2 (Tan et al., 2020) • AlloPred (Greener and Sternberg, 2015) • Allosite (Huang et al., 2013)
Cryptic pocket prediction	• PocketMiner (Meller et al., 2023) • CryptoSite by Andrej Sali Lab (Cimermancic et al., 2016)
De novo ligand generation	• GAN (Generative adversarial networks) • VAE (Variational autoencoders)RNN (Recurrent neural networks)
Network- based target prediction	• DeepDTnet (Zeng et al., 2020) • BANDIT (Madhukar et al., 2019)

simulates the interaction between a target protein or any other disease related biomolecule with a large and diverse chemical library. Predictive algorithms, often AI based, are used to evaluate which compounds are more likely to bind effectively to the target's active site or regulatory sites and regulate its function. This enables the quick identification of potential drug candidates from millions and billions of chemical structures. Virtual screening primarily consists of two approaches: structure based virtual screening (SBVS) and ligand based virtual screening (LBVS). SBVS involves docking candidate compounds into the three dimensional structure of a target protein to predict their binding affinity and interaction patterns. In contrast, LBVS depends on the known activity profiles or structural characteristics of previously identified ligands. **Deep Docking** (Gentile et al., 2020), **DeepChem** (https://github.com/deepchem/deepchem), **GINNA** (McNutt et al., 2025), **MolPal** (Graff et al., 2021), and **AtomNet** by Atomwise are various AI based tools for virtual screening. ML models like **SVMs, RFs, k-nearest neighbors, artificial neural networks, and naïve Bayesian classifiers** are also used.

5.2.3 ADMET

ADMET is short for absorption, distribution, metabolism, excretion, and toxicity. It is a fundamental set of pharmacokinetic and pharmacodynamic properties that determine a drug candidate's safety and efficacy profile. Late stage drug failures can be prevented by accurate prediction of ADMET characteristics. Due to the expensive and time inefficient nature of in vitro and in vivo experiments, the development of AI based tools for ADMET property prediction is in progress. Wet lab evaluations are required for clinical approval, but early stage in silico ADMET predictions can significantly reduce failures due to poor pharmacokinetic properties. Various ML algorithms, like RFs, SVM, and gradient boosting, are commonly used to build models to predict ADMET properties. **Bayer's in silico ADMET platform** is one such tool that uses these ML models (Göller et al., 2020). Modern approaches now use neural networks (like CNN, GNN, and transformers) and their subset, DL based techniques, to automatically extract meaningful patterns from raw inputs such as SMILES and molecular graphs. **GeoGNN** (Fang et al., 2022), **ADMET-AI** (Swanson et al., 2024) and **ADMETlab 3.0** (Fu et al., 2024) are some ADMET predicting tools that make use of such technologies.

The utilization of all these AI powered tools and algorithms in real world settings requires navigating the various regulatory frameworks, ensuring biological relevance, and demonstrating efficacy in clinical settings. They must be validated not just in silico but through wet lab experiments, preclinical studies, and ultimately human trials.

5.3 Digital twin technology

Digital twin technology is the creation of a virtual representation of a physical system, process, or object that continuously synchronizes with real time data from its real world equivalent. In the healthcare and biomedical area, digital twins represent organs, patients, or even whole physiological systems, thus enabling predictive simulations and personalized treatment strategies. The fusion of AI and digital twin technology has profoundly impacted the healthcare and biomedical fields by providing innovative solutions for personalized medicine, predictive analytics, and real time clinical decision making. In unison, they form a powerful framework that replicates, comprehends, and improves biological and clinical systems. AI driven digital twins are being designed for use in cancer treatment planning, cardiac modeling, surgical simulations, and more, allowing clinicians to test interventions in silico before applying them to real patients. The development of AI has been transforming digital twin technology from simple static representations to more interactive, dynamic, self-updating systems that can assist in decision-making, increase productivity, and facilitate personalized treatment.

Application of AI enabled digital twins in personalized medicine helps simulate patient responses to drugs or treatments and tailor therapies based on predictions from the virtual twin. Several healthcare institutions and companies are advancing the use of digital twin technology to enhance clinical treatment and device development. GE Health Systems developed a hospital level digital twin platform known as Care Command (Katsoulakis et al., 2024). In the medical domain, digital twin technology is used for advanced organ modeling and virtual simulations. A prominent example is the **SIMULIA Living Heart Project**. It is a collaboration between Dassault Systèmes and the FDA that is aimed at developing a validated digital twin of the human heart to study organ drug interactions and enhance cardiac device design (Baillargeon et al., 2014). During the COVID 19 pandemic, **Project BreathEasy** by OnScale created a digital twin model of COVID affected lungs to optimize ventilator use and improve outcomes in severely impacted areas. Digital health twin technology uses advanced tools like CT/MRI imaging, 3D modeling, virtual and augmented reality, and ML to produce extremely accurate, patient specific virtual copies of organs and systems. These replicas enable users to visualize anatomy in detail, help surgeons plan surgeries beforehand, and virtually experiment with procedures in order to better localize lesions, prevent complications, and achieve an optimal surgical outcome (Lareyre et al., 2020). In neurosurgery, digital health twin technology integrated with neuronavigation and intraoperative electrostimulation supports precision brain mapping, while in organ transplantation, it aids in preoperative evaluation, donor recipient matching, and posttransplant monitoring using implantable sensors and predictive AI algorithms. In addition, digital health twin technology is instrumental in designing custom implants and prosthetics that are tailored to patient anatomy, thus making patient care more personalized, predictive, and precise (Cellina et al., 2023).

5.4 Challenges in the of AI in translational science

It is worth pointing out here that, in order to advance the progression of AI/ML technologies from research and development to clinical application, there should be a collaboration between expert teams of AI/ML, clinicians, physicists, patient advocacy groups, payors, and hospital administrators. However, this process is not without challenges. Practical issues, like clearly defining the key information to be communicated and specifying the target audience, are critical to ensuring patient safety and preventing bias in automation, which can arise from overreliance on AI systems during clinical decision making. Therefore, transparency is a crucial aspect here across every phase of the AI/ML development cycle that cannot be emphasized enough. A lack of transparency undermines trust in AI/ML systems, limits their clinical adoption, and hinders their ability to function as reliable decision support tools. Moreover, ongoing monitoring of AI/ML performance in clinical settings demands a high level of transparency. This includes systematically identifying potential biases that may affect specific patient subgroups and detecting deviations in system behavior that could compromise safety or effectiveness.

Despite AI making significant advancements during the past decades, its varied applicability also presents considerable difficulties in developing a robust quality management and acceptance testing system for ensuring assured safety and efficacy. Furthermore, unaddressed issues surrounding judicial responsibility in cases of AI system errors remain a concern. Establishing a comprehensive structure to oversee all phases—from development to clinical application—is crucial, particularly as the field of medical imaging moves toward a groundbreaking AI driven transformation. Collaborative quality assurance approaches may offer an effective solution, where healthcare organizations work together to develop practical quality assurance methods and share data, allowing for efficient risk assessment and tailored control measures specific to individual AI tools.

6 Ethical issues

The integration of AI in healthcare brings significant concerns and moral challenges, with fairness and bias mitigation being key issues. AI systems may display biases when trained on unbalanced datasets. A few years ago, a study revealed that an AI tool created to diagnose diabetic retinopathy was found to have a lower accuracy rate for individuals with darker skin due to the training dataset, which was mostly composed of individuals with lighter skin (Burlina et al., 2021). This example highlights the essential necessity of tackling bias in AI development and deployment to ensure equitable and reliable healthcare outcomes for all.

A major risk stems from the potential for a discrepancy between the training data utilized to create the AI model and the real world patient data encountered in actual clinical settings, a phenomenon known as 'data shift.' This difference can result from variations in patient demographics, evolving disease patterns, or technical differences in imaging acquisition protocols, treatment approaches, and equipment over time or between healthcare institutions (Mahmood et al., 2024).

To address these risks and ensure responsible implementation, the regulatory environment in the European Union (EU) imposes strict oversight. **The European Medical Devices Regulation (EU MDR) 2017/745** and the **General Data Protection Regulation 2016/679** lay down the foundational legal frameworks that highlight patient safety, data confidentiality, and ethical governance in the application of AI in healthcare (Zanca et al., 2022). The EU has also explicitly addressed the challenges AI technology presents and its rapid growth by proposing the Artificial Intelligence Act (AI Act) as a further step. This new legislation aims to create a clear, comprehensive, unified regulatory structure specifically for AI. It is designed to direct the development, deployment, and continuous evaluation of AI applications across all sectors—including healthcare—by classifying AI systems based on risk and enforcing requirements for transparency, accountability, and performance validation.

7 Challenges

Robustness and generalizability of algorithms are crucial elements for effectively implementing AI in clinical imaging and translational sciences. The robustness of an AI model refers to its ability to deliver stable, dependable results despite fluctuations in the input data. For example, models that are trained on high resolution CT scans may struggle with noisy or lower resolution images, leading to unreliable outcomes. The differences caused by various equipment manufacturers or different settings make it even more challenging for the AI to be robust, as it has to handle these discrepancies without significant degradation in performance.

Despite significant achievements in AI/ML medical imaging, a few challenges always remain, and if they are not adequately tackled, they will negatively impact patient care and raise ethical and privacy considerations. An analysis of 320 recently published studies highlighted these concerns, revealing that a significant proportion of ML based models developed for evaluating COVID 19 using chest radiographs and CT scans suffered from design flaws and potential biases (Roberts et al., 2021).

Generalizability refers to a model's capability to maintain strong performance on new, unseen datasets, including those from different populations or institutions not part of the original training data (Eche et al., 2021). Many AI algorithms, however, are trained on data from limited sources, leading to overfitting and reduced effectiveness when applied to varied real world situations. For example, a model that has been created using data from a single geographic region may not be able to generalize if it is applied to other populations due to underlying differences in disease prevalence or imaging practices. Addressing these challenges requires diverse, representative datasets, domain specific augmentation techniques, and rigorous cross institutional validation to ensure models are both robust and generalizable.

Image analysis algorithms face several problems in efficiently, accurately, and consistently extracting significant information from tissue images. Tissue images are very different from many other imaging modalities since they carry an enormous amount of information encoded across multiple spatial scales. The scales range from individual pixels to distinct cellular structures like cells and nuclei, to larger sections including tumor areas, stromal tissues, and other microenvironmental components. This complexity is further intensified by variations in tissue morphology and textural features, which can vary widely across different disease regions, tumor subtypes, and patient populations. Classifications can depend on the fraction of the specimen exhibiting specific patterns of tissue abnormality. In such instances, the evaluation of classifications relies on accurately quantifying these patterns within the specimen. Traditionally, when interpretations were confined to glass slides, efforts to reduce differences between observers relied on several pathologists independently reviewing the same slides and reaching a consensus. Nonetheless, these approaches are quite time consuming and are still limited by personal bias in interpretation (Table 16.3).

These limitations have led to the growth of automated image analysis techniques, particularly those applied to whole slide pathology images. By leveraging computational tools, these methods aim to improve diagnostic consistency, accuracy, and efficiency, offering the potential to enhance pathology workflows and support more objective, reproducible assessments of complex tissue specimens.

While advancements have been made in developing automated methods for analyzing tissue microarray (TMA) images, many existing systems still remain constrained. TMA technology allows researchers to take small, cylindrical tissue cores from histological specimens and

Table 16.3 Key challenges and solutions in AI for medical imaging.

Challenge	Description	Solution
Data shift	Difference in the patient data as compared to the training data	Continuous monitoring, Diverse datasets
Bias and fairness	AI model performs inconsistently across the demographics	Bias detection and use of inclusive datasets
Lack of interpretability	Black- box decision making	XAI tools like saliency maps, heatmaps
Regulatory and legal barriers	Absence of clear legal frameworks is a major problem	Setting of AI specific rules and regulations (e.g., EU AI Act)
Computational load	Managing large imaging datasets	Scalable infrastructure and cloud solutions

arrange them in a matrix format on a recipient paraffin block in a systematic manner (Bubendorf et al., 2001). This setup enables the simultaneous analysis of hundreds of tissue samples, significantly increasing efficiency and throughput in studies. However, they are often closed and proprietary, fail to leverage advanced computer vision techniques, and lack alignment with emerging data standards. Beyond these analytical limitations, the immense quantity of data, text, and image based content generated by even small scale TMA studies presents significant computational and data management challenges, underscoring the necessity for stronger, scalable, and compatible solutions.

8 Conclusion

AI leads the way in medical innovation, driven by its versatility, effectiveness, and the growth of open source platforms alongside advanced high performance computing resources. Traditional ML approaches, such as RF, are able to successfully solve specific challenges in medical imaging, are less prone to overfitting, and provide improved model interpretability compared to DL based models, which are often described as black boxes and can, therefore, be challenging to comprehend in terms of their predictions (Neri et al., 2023). Notably, DL has reached expert level accuracy in lesion detection, classification, and image segmentation. In addition, foundation models, initially trained on extensive datasets, can be effectively adapted for various fields through fine tuning, minimizing the need for large domain specific datasets.

Several critical factors need to be addressed for AI powered tools to be optimally used in medical practice. First, rigorous, large scale clinical studies are indispensable to validate the effectiveness, efficacy, and generalizability of these advanced technologies across diverse clinical settings and patient populations. Without such robust validation, the reliability of AI systems in real world healthcare remains uncertain.

Secondly, a significant obstacle in incorporating AI into clinical practice is the "black box" nature of many AI models in general, and particularly of DL systems. DL networks' intricate and complex decision making processes generally lack transparency, making it difficult for clinicians to understand how the system reaches specific conclusions. Hence, to address this, there is a growing emphasis on developing interpretable and XAI approaches. For instance, techniques such as saliency maps and heatmaps are increasingly used in image based models to visually emphasize the parts of an image that have more impact on the performance of the models. These techniques offer critical insights into AI decision making, fostering greater trust and accountability (Neri et al., 2023).

Finally, the ethical deployment of AI in healthcare still requires careful attention to issues of fairness, bias mitigation, and reliability. AI models must be extensively evaluated to ensure they deliver equitable outcomes across different demographic groups, so that no unintended disparities are created in healthcare delivery.

Collectively, the implementation of these steps, clinical validation, enhancing explainability, and addressing ethical concerns ensures that AI can be appropriately incorporated into routine medical practice, ultimately improving patient care and outcomes.

References

Abramson, J., Adler, J., Dunger, J., Evans, R., Green, T., Pritzel, A., Ronneberger, O., Willmore, L., Ballard, A.J., Bambrick, J., Bodenstein, S.W., Evans, D.A., Hung, C.C., O'Neill, M., Reiman, D., Tunyasuvunakool, K., Wu, Z., Žemgulytė, A., Arvaniti, E., Beattie, C., Bertolli, O., Bridgland, A., Cherepanov, A., Congreve, M., Cowen-Rivers, A.I., Cowie, A., Figurnov, M., Fuchs, F.B., Gladman, H., Jain, R., Khan, Y.A., Low, C.M.R., Perlin, K., Potapenko, A., Savy, P., Singh, S., Stecula, A., Thillaisundaram, A., Tong, C., Yakneen, S., Zhong, E.D., Zielinski, M., Žídek, A., Bapst, V., Kohli, P., Jaderberg, M., Hassabis, D., Jumper, J.M., 2024. Accurate structure prediction of biomolecular interactions with AlphaFold 3. Nature. 1476-4687. 630 (8016), 493–500. Available from: https://www.nature.com/nature/. doi:10.1038/s41586-024-07487-w.

Acosta, J.N., Falcone, G.J., Rajpurkar, P., Topol, E.J., 2022. Multimodal biomedical AI. Nat. Med. 1546-170X. 28 (9), 1773–1784. Available from: http://www.nature.com/nm/index.html. doi:10.1038/s41591-022-01981-2.

Aerts, H.J.W.L., Velazquez, E.R., Leijenaar, R.T.H., Parmar, C., Grossmann, P., Cavalho, S., Bussink, J., Monshouwer, R., Haibe-Kains, B., Rietveld, D., Hoebers, F., Rietbergen, M.M., Leemans, C.R., Dekker, A., Quackenbush, J., Gillies, R.J., Lambin, P., 2014. Decoding tumour phenotype by noninvasive imaging using a quantitative radiomics approach. Nat. Commun. 2041-1723. 5. Available from: http://www.nature.com/ncomms/index.html. doi:10.1038/ncomms5006.

Ahdritz, G., Bouatta, N., Floristean, C., Kadyan, S., Xia, Q., Gerecke, W., O'Donnell, T.J., Berenberg, D., Fisk, I., Zanichelli, N., Zhang, B., Nowaczynski, A., Wang, B., Stepniewska-Dziubinska, M.M., Zhang, S., Ojewole, A., Guney, M.E., Biderman, S., Watkins, A.M., Ra, S., Lorenzo, P.R., Nivon, L., Weitzner, B., Ban, Y.E.A., Sorger, P.K., Mostaque, E., Zhang, Z., Bonneau, R., AlQuraishi, M., 2022. OpenFold: retraining AlphaFold2 yields new insights into its learning mechanisms and capacity for generalization. bioRxiv. 2692-8205. Available from: https://www.biorxiv.org. doi:10.1101/2022.11.20.517210.

Ahmad, B., Sun, J., You, Q., Palade, V., Mao, Z., 2022. Brain tumor classification using a combination of variational autoencoders and generative adversarial networks. Biomedicines. 2227-9059. 10 (2), 223. doi:10.3390/biomedicines10020223.

Alcaide, E., Gao, Z., Ke, G., Li, Y., Zhang, L., Zheng, H., Zhou, G., 2024, Uni-Mol Docking V2: Towards Realistic and Accurate Binding Pose Prediction. Avalibale from:https://arxiv.org/abs/2405.11769. doi:arXiv:2405.11769.

Avanzo, M., Barbiero, S., Trovo, M., Bissonnette, J.P., Jena, R., Stancanello, J., Pirrone, G., Matrone, F., Minatel, E., Cappelletto, C., Furlan, C., Jaffray, D.A., Sartor, G., 2017. Voxel-by-voxel correlation between radiologically radiation induced lung injury and dose after image-guided, intensity modulated radiotherapy for lung tumors. Phys. Med. 1724-191X. 42, 150–156. Available from: https://www.fisicamedica.org. doi:10.1016/j.ejmp.2017.09.127.

Baillargeon, B., Rebelo, N., Fox, D.D., Taylor, R.L., Kuhl, E., 2014. The living heart project: a robust and integrative simulator for human heart function. Eur. J. Mech., A/Solids. 0997-7538. 48 (1), 38–47. Available from: https://www.journals.elsevier.com/european-journal-of-mechanics-a-solids. doi:10.1016/j.euromechsol.2014.04.001.

Bubendorf, L., Nocito, A., Moch, H., Sauter, G., 2001. Tissue microarray (TMA) technology: miniaturized pathology archives for high-throughputin situ studies. J. Pathol. 0022-3417. 195 (1), 72–79. doi:10.1002/path.893.

Burlina, P., Joshi, N., Paul, W., Pacheco, K.D., Bressler, N.M., 2021. Addressing artificial intelligence bias in retinal diagnostics. Transl. Vis. Sci. Technol. 2164-2591. 10 (2), 1–13. Available from: https://tvst.arvojournals.org/article.aspx?articleid=2772266. doi:10.1167/tvst.10.2.13.

Carini, C., Seyhan, A.A., 2024. Tribulations and future opportunities for artificial intelligence in precision medicine. J. Transl. Med. 1479-5876. 22 (1), 411. doi:10.1186/s12967-024-05067-0.

Celard, P., Iglesias, E.L., Sorribes-Fdez, J.M., Romero, R., Vieira, A.S., Borrajo, L., 2023. A survey on deep learning applied to medical images: from simple artificial neural networks to generative models. Neural Comput. Appl. 1433-3058. 35 (3), 2291–2323. Available from: https://www.springer.com/journal/521. doi:10.1007/s00521-022-07953-4.

Cellina, M., Cè, M., Alì, M., Irmici, G., Ibba, S., Caloro, E., Fazzini, D., Oliva, G., Papa, S., 2023. Digital twins: the new frontier for personalized medicine?. Appl. Sci. 2076-3417. 13 (13), 7940. doi:10.3390/app13137940.

Cimermancic, P., Weinkam, P., Rettenmaier, T.J., Bichmann, L., Keedy, D.A., Woldeyes, R.A., Schneidman-Duhovny, D., Demerdash, O.N., Mitchell, J.C., Wells, J.A., Fraser, J.S., Sali, A., 2016. CryptoSite: expanding the druggable proteome by characterization and prediction of cryptic binding sites. J. Mol. Biol. 1089-8638. 428 (4), 709–719. Available from: https://www.journals.elsevier.com/journal-of-molecular-biology. doi:10.1016/j.jmb.2016.01.029.

Court, L.E., Aggarwal, A., Burger, H., Cardenas, C., Chung, C., Douglas, R., du Toit, M., Jhingran, A., Mumme, R., Muya, S., Naidoo, K., Ndumbalo, J., Netherton, T., Nguyen, C., Olanrewaju, A., Parkes, J., Shaw, W., Trauernicht, C., Xu, M., Yang, J., Zhang, L., Simonds, H., Beadle, B.M., 2023. Radiation planning assistant—a web-based tool to support high-quality radiotherapy in clinics with limited resources. J. Vis. Exp. 1940-087X. 2023 (200). Available from: https://www.jove.com/pdf/65504/radiation-planning-assistant-web-based-tool-to-support-high-quality. doi:10.3791/65504.

Currie, G., Singh, C., Nelson, T., Nabasenja, C., Al-Hayek, Y., Spuur, K., 2023. ChatGPT in medical imaging higher education. Radiography. 1078-8174. 29 (4), 792–799. doi:10.1016/j.radi.2023.05.011.

Dixon, D., Sattar, H., Moros, N., Kesireddy, S.R., Ahsan, H., Lakkimsetti, M., Fatima, M., Doshi, D., Sadhu, K., Hassan, M.J., 2024. Unveiling the influence of AI predictive analytics on patient outcomes: a comprehensive narrative review. Cureus. 2168-8184. 16 (5). doi:10.7759/cureus.59954.

Dona Lemus, O.M., Cao, M., Cai, B., Cummings, M., Zheng, D., 2024. Adaptive radiotherapy: next-generation radiotherapy. Cancers. 2072-6694. 16 (6). Available from: http://www.mdpi.com/journal/cancers/. doi:10.3390/cancers16061206.

Eche, T., Schwartz, L.H., Mokrane, F.Z., Dercle, L., 2021. Toward generalizability in the deployment of artificial intelligence in radiology: role of computation stress testing to overcome underspecification. Radiol. Artif. Intell. 2638-6100. 3 (6). Available from: https://pubs.rsna.org/doi/pdf/10.1148/ryai.2021210097. doi:10.1148/ryai.2021210097.

Evans, R., O'Neill, M., Pritzel, A., Antropova, N., Senior, A., Green, T., Žídek, A., Bates, R., Blackwell, S., Yim, J., Ronneberger, O., Bodenstein, S., Zielinski, M., Bridgland,

A., Potapenko, A., Cowie, A., Tunyasuvunakool, K., Jain, R., Clancy, E., Kohli, P., Jumper, J., Hassabis, D., 2021. Protein complex prediction with AlphaFold-multimer. bioRxiv. 2692-8205. Available from: https://www.biorxiv.org. doi:10.1101/2021.10.04.463034.

Fang, X., Gao, J., Hu, J., Liu, L., Xue, Y., Zhang, X., Zhu, K., 2024. Helixfold-multimer: elevating protein complex structure prediction to new heights. arXiv. 2331-8422. Available from: https://arxiv.org. doi:10.48550/arXiv.2404.10260.

Fang, X., Liu, L., Lei, J., He, D., Zhang, S., Zhou, J., Wang, F., Wu, H., Wang, H., 2022. Geometry-enhanced molecular representation learning for property prediction. Nat. Mach. Intell. 2522-5839. 4 (2), 127–134. doi:10.1038/s42256-021-00438-4.

Feng, X., Qing, K., Tustison, N.J., Meyer, C.H., Chen, Q., 2019. Deep convolutional neural network for segmentation of thoracic organs-at-risk using cropped 3D images. Med. Phys. 0094-2405. 46 (5), 2169–2180. doi:10.1002/mp.13466.

Fourcade, C., Ferrer, L., Moreau, N., Santini, G., Brennan, A., Rousseau, C., Lacombe, M., Fleury, V., Colombié, M., Jézéquel, P., Rubeaux, M., Mateus, D., 2022. Deformable image registration with deep network priors: a study on longitudinal PET images. Phys. Med. Biol. 0031-9155. 67 (15), 155011. doi:10.1088/1361-6560/ac7e17.

Fu, L., Shi, S., Yi, J., Wang, N., He, Y., Wu, Z., Peng, J., Deng, Y., Wang, W., Wu, C., Lyu, A., Zeng, X., Zhao, W., Hou, T., Cao, D., 2024. ADMETlab 3.0: an updated comprehensive online ADMET prediction platform enhanced with broader coverage, improved performance, API functionality and decision support. Nucleic Acids Res. 0305-1048. 52 (W1), W422. doi:10.1093/nar/gkae236.

Gentile, F., Agrawal, V., Hsing, M., Ton, A., Ban, F., Norinder, U., Gleave, M.E., Cherkasov, A., 2020. Deep Docking: A Deep Learning Platform for Augmentation of Structure Based Drug Discovery. ACS Cent. Sci. 6 (6), 939–949. doi:10.1021/acscentsci.0c00229.

Giger, M.L., Doi, K., MacMahon, H., Nishikawa, R.M., Hoffmann, K.R., Vyborny, C.J., Schmidt, R.A., Jia, H., Abe, K., Chen, X., 1993. An "intelligent" workstation for computer-aided diagnosis. Radiographics. 0271-5333. 13 (3), 647–656. doi:10.1148/radiographics.13.3.8316671.

Gipiškis, R., Tsai, C.W., Kurasova, O., 2024. Explainable AI (XAI) in image segmentation in medicine, industry, and beyond: a survey. ICT Express. 2405-9595. 10 (6), 1331–1354. Available from: https://www.sciencedirect.com/science/journal/24059595. doi:10.1016/j.icte.2024.09.008.

Göller, A.H., Kuhnke, L., Montanari, F., Bonin, A., Schneckener, S., ter Laak, A., Wichard, J., Lobell, M., Hillisch, A., 2020. Bayer's in silico ADMET platform: a journey of machine learning over the past two decades. Drug Discov. Today. 1878-5832. 25 (9), 1702–1709. Available from: https://www.elsevier.com/locate/drugdiscov. doi:10.1016/j.drudis.2020.07.001.

Graff, D.E., Shakhnovich, E.I., Coley, C.W., 2021. Accelerating high-throughput virtual screening through molecular pool-based active learning. Chem. Sci. 12 (22), 7866–7881. doi:10.1039/D0SC06805E.

Greener, J.G., Kandathil, S.M., Jones, D.T., 2019. Deep learning extends de novo protein modelling coverage of genomes using iteratively predicted structural constraints. Nat. Commun. 2041-1723. 10 (1). Available from: http://www.nature.com/ncomms/index.html. doi:10.1038/s41467-019-11994-0.

Greener, J.G., Sternberg, M.J.E., 2015. AlloPred: prediction of allosteric pockets on proteins using normal mode perturbation analysis. BMC Bioinformatics. 1471-2105. 16 (1). Available from: http://www.biomedcentral.com/bmcbioinformatics/. doi:10.1186/s12859-015-0771-1.

Halling-Brown, M.D., Warren, L.M., Ward, D., Lewis, E., Mackenzie, A., Wallis, M.G., Wilkinson, L.S., Given-Wilson, R.M., McAvinchey, R., Young, K.C., 2021. OPTIMAM mammography image database: a large-scale resource of mammography images and clinical data. Radiol. Artif. Intell. 2638-6100. 3 (1). Available from: https://pubs.rsna.org/doi/pdf/10.1148/ryai.2020200103. doi:10.1148/ryai.2020200103.

Hassan, A.E., 2021. New technology add-on payment (NTAP) for Viz LVO: a win for stroke care. J. Neurointerv. Surg. 1759-8486. 13 (5), 406–408. Available from: http://jnis.bmj.com/. doi:10.1136/neurintsurg-2020-016897.

Hosny, A., Parmar, C., Quackenbush, J., Schwartz, L.H., Aerts, H.J.W.L., 2018. Artificial intelligence in radiology. Nat. Rev. Cancer. 1474-1768. 18 (8), 500–510. Available from: http://www.nature.com/cancer/. doi:10.1038/s41568-018-0016-5.

Huang, W., Lu, S., Huang, Z., Liu, X., Mou, L., Luo, Y., Zhao, Y., Liu, Y., Chen, Z., Hou, T., Zhang, J., 2013. Allosite: a method for predicting allosteric sites. Bioinformatics. 1367-4811. 29 (18), 2357–2359. doi:10.1093/bioinformatics/btt399.

Jeddi, Z., Bohr, A., 2020. Remote patient monitoring using artificial intelligence. In: Artificial Intelligence in Healthcare. Elsevier, Morocco, pp. 203–234. Available from: https://www.elsevier.com/books/artificial-intelligence-in-healthcare/bohr/978-0-12-818438-7. doi:10.1016/B978-0-12-818438-7.00009-5.

Kashyap, K., Mahapatra, P.P., Ahmed, S., Buyukbingol, E., Siddiqi, M.I., 2023b. Identification of potential aldose reductase inhibitors using convolutional neural network-based in silico screening. J. Chem. Inf. Model. 1549-960X. 63 (20), 6261–6282. Available from: http://pubs.acs.org/journal/jcisd8. doi:10.1021/acs.jcim.3c00547.

Kashyap, K., Panigrahi, L., Ahmed, S., Siddiqi, M.I., 2023a. Artificial neural network models driven novel virtual screening workflow for the identification and biological evaluation of BACE1 inhibitors. Mol. Inform. 1868-1751. 42 (3). Available from: http://onlinelibrary.wiley.com/journal/10.1002/(ISSN)1868-1751. doi:10.1002/minf.202200113.

Kashyap, K., Siddiqi, M.I., 2021. Recent trends in artificial intelligence-driven identification and development of anti-neurodegenerative therapeutic agents. Mol. Divers. 1573-501X. 25 (3), 1517–1539. Available from: www.wkap.nl/journalhome.htm/1381-1991. doi:10.1007/s11030-021-10274-8.

Katsoulakis, E., Wang, Q., Wu, H., Shahriyari, L., Fletcher, R., Liu, J., Achenie, L., Liu, H., Jackson, P., Xiao, Y., Syeda-Mahmood, T., Tuli, R., Deng, J., 2024. Digital twins for health: a scoping review. Npj Digit. Med. 2398-6352. 7 (1). doi:10.1038/s41746-024-01073-0.

Khader, F., Müller-Franzes, G., Arasteh, S.T., Han, T., Haarburger, C., Schulze-Hagen, M., Schad, P., Engelhardt, S., Baeßler, B., Foersch, S., Stegmaier, J., Kuhl, C., Nebelung, S., Kather, J.N., Truhn, D., 2023. Denoising diffusion probabilistic models for 3D medical image generation. Sci. Rep. 2045-2322. 13 (1). Available from: https://www.nature.com/srep/. doi:10.1038/s41598-023-34341-2.

Khan, Z., Gaidhane, A.M., Singh, M., Ganesan, S., Kaur, M., Sharma, G.C., Rani, P., Sharma, R.S.K., Thapliyal, S., Kushwaha, M., Kumar, H., Agarwal, R.K., Shabil, M., Verma, L., Sidhu, A., Manan, N.B.A., Bushi, G., Mehta, R., Sah, S., Satapathy, P., Samal, S.K., 2025. Diagnostic accuracy of IDX-DR for detecting diabetic retinopathy: a systematic review and meta-analysis. Am. J. Ophthalmol. 1879-1891. 273, 192–204. Available from: https://www.sciencedirect.com/science/journal/00029394. doi:10.1016/j.ajo.2025.02.022.

Kirillov, A., Mintun, E., Ravi, N., Mao, H., Rolland, C., Gustafson, L., Xiao, T., Whitehead, S., Berg, A., Lo, W.Y., Dollár, P., Girshick, R., 2023. Segment Anything. Available from: https://arxiv.org/abs/2304.02643. doi:arXiv:2304.02643 arXiv:2304.02643.

Konc, J., Janežič, D., 2017. ProBiS tools (algorithm, database, and web servers) for predicting and modeling of biologically interesting proteins. Prog. Biophys. Mol. Biol. 0079-6107. 128, 24–32. doi:10.1016/j.pbiomolbio.2017.02.005.

Kreimeyer, K., Foster, M., Pandey, A., Arya, N., Halford, G., Jones, S.F., Forshee, R., Walderhaug, M., Botsis, T., 2017. Natural language processing systems for capturing and standardizing unstructured clinical information: a systematic review. J. Biomed. Inform. 1532-0464. 73, 14–29. Available from: http://www.elsevier.com/inca/publications/store/6/2/2/8/5/7/index.htt. doi:10.1016/j.jbi.2017.07.012.

Langlotz, C.P., 2023. The future of AI and informatics in radiology: 10 predictions. Radiology. 1527-1315. 309 (1). Available from: https://pubs.rsna.org/doi/epdf/10.1148/radiol.231114. doi:10.1148/radiol.231114.

Lareyre, F., Adam, C., Carrier, M., Raffort, J., 2020. Using digital twins for precision medicine in vascular surgery. Ann. Vasc. Surg. 0890-5096. 67, e577. doi:10.1016/j.avsg.2020.04.042.

Lee, J.S., 2021. A review of deep-learning-based approaches for attenuation correction in positron emission tomography. IEEE Trans. Radiat. Plasma Med. Sci. 2469-7311. 5 (2), 160–184. Available from: http://ieeexplore.ieee.org/xpl/RecentIssue.jsp?punumber=7433213. doi:10.1109/TRPMS.2020.3009269.

Lee, R.S., Gimenez, F., Hoogi, A., Miyake, K.K., Gorovoy, M., Rubin, D.L., 2017. A curated mammography data set for use in computer-aided detection and diagnosis research. Sci. Data. 2052-4463. 4 (1). doi:10.1038/sdata.2017.177.

Li, Y., Li, L., Wang, S., Tang, X., 2023. EQUIBIND: a geometric deep learning-based protein-ligand binding prediction method. Drug Discov. Ther. 1881-7831. 17 (5), 363–364. doi:10.5582/ddt.2023.01063.

Lisanza, S.L., Gershon, J.M., Tipps, S.W.K., Sims, J.N., Arnoldt, L., Hendel, S.J., Simma, M.K., Liu, G., Yase, M., Wu, H., Tharp, C.D., Li, X., Kang, A., Brackenbrough, E., Bera, A.K., Gerben, S., Wittmann, B.J., McShan, A.C., Baker, D., 2024. Multistate and functional protein design using RoseTTAFold sequence space diffusion. Nat. Biotechnol. 1546-1696. Available from: https://www.nature.com/nbt/. doi:10.1038/s41587-024-02395-w.

Liu, Y., Kohlberger, T., Norouzi, M., Dahl, G.E., Smith, J.L., Mohtashamian, A., Olson, N., Peng, L.H., Hipp, J.D., Stumpe, M.C., 2019. Artificial intelligence–based breast cancer nodal metastasis detection insights into the black box for pathologists. Arch. Pathol. Lab. Med. 1543-2165. 143 (7), 859–868. Available from: https://www.archivesofpathology.org/doi/pdf/10.5858/arpa.2018-0147-OA. doi:10.5858/arpa.2018-0147-OA.

Madhukar, N.S., Khade, P.K., Huang, L., Gayvert, K., Galletti, G., Stogniew, M., Allen, J.E., Giannakakou, P., Elemento, O., 2019. A Bayesian machine learning approach for drug target identification using diverse data types. Nat. Commun. 2041-1723. 10 (1). Available from: http://www.nature.com/ncomms/index.html. doi:10.1038/s41467-019-12928-6.

Mahmood, U., Shukla-Dave, A., Chan, H.-P., Drukker, K., Samala, R.K., Chen, Q., Vergara, D., Greenspan, H., Petrick, N., Sahiner, B., Huo, Z., Summers, R.M., Cha, K.H., Tourassi, G., Deserno, T.M., Grizzard, K.T., Näppi, J.J., Yoshida, H., Regge, D., Mazurchuk, R., Suzuki, K., Morra, L., Huisman, H., Armato, S.G., Hadjiiski, L., 2024. Artificial intelligence in medicine: mitigating risks and maximizing benefits via quality assurance, quality control, and acceptance testing. BJR Artif. Intell. 2976-8705. 1 (1). doi:10.1093/bjrai/ubae003.

Marchal, I., 2024. RoseTTAFold expands to all-atom for biomolecular prediction and design. Nat. Biotechnol. 1087-0156. 42 (4), 571. doi:10.1038/s41587-024-02211-5.

Marcu, L.G., Boyd, C., Bezak, E., 2019. Feeding the data monster: data science in head and neck cancer for personalized therapy. J. Am. Coll. Radiol. 1558-349X. 16 (12), 1695–1701. Available from: http://www.elsevier.com/wps/find/journaldescription.cws_home/699814/description#description. doi:10.1016/j.jacr.2019.05.045.

McNutt, A.T., Li, Y., Meli, R., Aggarwal, R., Koes, D.R., 2025. GNINA 1.3: the next increment in molecular docking with deep learning. J. Cheminform. 17 (1). doi:10.1186/s13321-025-00973-x.

Mei, X., Liu, Z., Robson, P.M., Marinelli, B., Huang, M., Doshi, A., Jacobi, A., Cao, C., Link, K.E., Yang, T., Wang, Y., Greenspan, H., Deyer, T., Fayad, Z.A., Yang, Y., 2022.

RadImageNet: an open radiologic deep learning research dataset for effective transfer learning. Radiol. Artif. Intell. 2638-6100. 4 (5). Available from: https://pubs.rsna.org/journal/ai. doi:10.1148/ryai.210315.

Meller, A., Ward, M., Borowsky, J., Kshirsagar, M., Lotthammer, J.M., Oviedo, F., Ferres, J.L., Bowman, G.R., 2023. Predicting locations of cryptic pockets from single protein structures using the PocketMiner graph neural network. Nat. Commun. 2041-1723. 14 (1). Available from: https://www.nature.com/ncomms/. doi:10.1038/s41467-023-36699-3.

Mirdita, M., Schütze, K., Moriwaki, Y., Heo, L., Ovchinnikov, S., Steinegger, M., 2022. ColabFold: making protein folding accessible to all. Nat. Methods. 1548-7091. 19 (6), 679–682. doi:10.1038/s41592-022-01488-1.

Monsour, R., 2022. Neuroimaging in the era of artificial intelligence: current applications. Fed. Pract. 39 (39 (Suppl 1)). doi:10.12788/fp.0231.

Moreira, I.C., Amaral, I., Domingues, I., Cardoso, A., Cardoso, M.J., Cardoso, J.S., 2012. INbreast: toward a full-field digital mammographic database. Acad. Radiol. 1878-4046. 19 (2), 236–248. doi:10.1016/j.acra.2011.09.014.

Mortada, M.J., Tomassini, S., Anbar, H., Morettini, M., Burattini, L., Sbrollini, A., 2023. Segmentation of anatomical structures of the left heart from echocardiographic images using deep learning. Diagnostics. 2075-4418. 13 (10). Available from: http://www.mdpi.com/journal/diagnostics/. doi:10.3390/diagnostics13101683.

Mylonas, A., Keall, P.J., Booth, J.T., Shieh, C.C., Eade, T., Poulsen, P.R., Nguyen, D.T., 2019. A deep learning framework for automatic detection of arbitrarily shaped fiducial markers in intrafraction fluoroscopic images. Med. Phys. 2473-4209. 46 (5), 2286–2297. Available from: http://aapm.onlinelibrary.wiley.com/hub/journal/10.1002/(ISSN)2473-4209/issues/. doi:10.1002/mp.13519.

Neri, E., Aghakhanyan, G., Zerunian, M., Gandolfo, N., Grassi, R., Miele, V., Giovagnoni, A., Laghi, A., 2023. Explainable AI in radiology: a white paper of the Italian Society of Medical and Interventional Radiology. La Radiologia Medica. 1826-6983. 128 (6), 755–764. doi:10.1007/s11547-023-01634-5.

Paul, R., Hawkins, S., Balagurunathan, Y., Schabath, M., Gillies, R., Hall, L., Goldgof, D., 2016. Deep feature transfer learning in combination with traditional features predicts survival among patients with lung adenocarcinoma. Tomography. 2379-139X. 2 (4), 388–395. doi:10.18383/j.tom.2016.00211.

Peng, Y., Dharssi, S., Chen, Q., Keenan, T.D., Agrón, E., Wong, W.T., Chew, E.Y., Lu, Z., 2019. DeepSeeNet: a deep learning model for automated classification of patient-based age-related macular degeneration severity from color fundus photographs. Ophthalmology. 1549-4713. 126 (4), 565–575. Available from: www.elsevier.com/locate/ophtha. doi:10.1016/j.ophtha.2018.11.015.

Perez-Lopez, R., Tunariu, N., Padhani, A.R., Oyen, W.J.G., Fanti, S., Vargas, H.A., Omlin, A., Morris, M.J., De Bono, J., Koh, D.M., 2019. Imaging diagnosis and follow-up of advanced prostate cancer: clinical perspectives and state of the art. Radiology. 1527-1315. 292 (2), 273–286. Available from: https://pubs.rsna.org/doi/pdf/10.1148/radiol.2019181931. doi:10.1148/radiol.2019181931.

Ravuri, M., Kannan, A., Tso, G.J., Amatriain, X. 2018 Learning from the experts: from expert systems to machine-learned diagnosis models. In: Proceedings of Machine Learning Research, Vol. 85. 2640-3498. ML Research Press, pp. 227–243 https://proceedings.mlr.press/.

Rayed, M.E., Islam, S.M.S., Niha, S.I., Jim, J.R., Kabir, M.M., Mridha, M.F., 2024. Deep learning for medical image segmentation: state-of-the-art advancements and challenges. Inform. Med. Unlocked. 2352-9148. 47. Available from: https://www.sciencedirect.com/science/journal/23529148. doi:10.1016/j.imu.2024.101504.

Roberts, M., Driggs, D., Thorpe, M., Gilbey, J., Yeung, M., Ursprung, S., Aviles-Rivero, A.I., Etmann, C., McCague, C., Beer, L., Weir-McCall, J.R., Teng, Z., Gkrania-Klotsas, E., Ruggiero, A., Korhonen, A., Jefferson, E., Ako, E., Langs, G., Gozaliasl, G.,

Yang, G., Prosch, H., Preller, J., Stanczuk, J., Tang, J., Hofmanninger, J., Babar, J., Sánchez, L.E., Thillai, M., Gonzalez, P.M., Teare, P., Zhu, X., Patel, M., Cafolla, C., Azadbakht, H., Jacob, J., Lowe, J., Zhang, K., Bradley, K., Wassin, M., Holzer, M., Ji, K., Ortet, M.D., Ai, T., Walton, N., Lio, P., Stranks, S., Shadbahr, T., Lin, W., Zha, Y., Niu, Z., Rudd, J.H.F., Sala, E., Schönlieb, C.B., 2021. Common pitfalls and recommendations for using machine learning to detect and prognosticate for COVID-19 using chest radiographs and CT scans. Nat. Mach. Intell. 2522-5839. 3 (3), 199–217. Available from: https://www.nature.com/natmachintell/. doi:10.1038/s42256-021-00307-0.

Saleh, G.A., Batouty, N.M., Haggag, S., Elnakib, A., Khalifa, F., Taher, F., Mohamed, M.A., Farag, R., Sandhu, H., Sewelam, A., El-Baz, A., 2022. The role of medical image modalities and AI in the early detection, diagnosis and grading of retinal diseases: a survey. Bioengineering. 2306-5354. 9 (8). Available from: www.mdpi.com/journal/bioengineering. doi:10.3390/bioengineering9080366.

Sarkar, S., Teo, P.T., Abazeed, M.E., 2025. Deep learning for automated, motion-resolved tumor segmentation in radiotherapy. Npj Precis. Oncol. 2397-768X. 9 (1). Available from: https://www.nature.com/npjprecisiononcology/. doi:10.1038/s41698-025-00970-1.

Sindhura, D.N., Pai, R.M., Bhat, S.N., Pai, M.M.M., 2024. A review of deep learning and generative adversarial networks applications in medical image analysis. Multimed. Syst. 1432-1882. 30 (3). Available from: https://www.springer.com/journal/530. doi:10.1007/s00530-024-01349-1.

Sloan, J.M., Goatman, K.A., Siebert, J.P. 2018 Learning rigid image registration utilizing convolutional neural networks for medical image registration. In: BIOIMAGING 2018 - 5th International Conference on Bioimaging, Proceedings; Part of 11th International Joint Conference on Biomedical Engineering Systems and Technologies, BIOSTEC 2018. Vol. 2 9789897582783. SciTePress, United Kingdom. pp. 89–99. http://www.scitepress.org/DigitalLibrary/HomePage.aspx. doi:10.5220/0006543700890099.

Steinkamp, J., Cook, T.S., 2021. Basic artificial intelligence techniques. Radiol. Clin. North Am. 0033-8389. 59 (6), 919–931. doi:10.1016/j.rcl.2021.06.003.

Suckling, J., 1994. The mammographic images analysis society digital mammogram database. In: Exerpta Medica International Congress Series. Vol. 1069, pp. 375–378.

Sun, S., Han, K., You, C., et al., 2024. Medical image registration via neural fields. Med. Image. Anal. 97, 103249. doi:10.1016/j.media.2024.103249.

Swanson, K., Walther, P., Leitz, J., Mukherjee, S., Wu, J.C., Shivnaraine, R.V., Zou, J., 2024. ADMET-AI: a machine learning ADMET platform for evaluation of large-scale chemical libraries. Bioinformatics. 1367-4811. 40 (7). Available from: http://bioinformatics.oxfordjournals.org/. doi:10.1093/bioinformatics/btae416.

Takeuchi, M., Kitagawa, Y., 2024. Artificial intelligence and surgery. Ann. Gastroenterol. Surg. 2475-0328. 8 (1), 4–5. doi:10.1002/ags3.12766.

Talebi, S., Tong, E., Li, A., Yamin, G., Zaharchuk, G., Mofrad, M.R.K., 2024. Exploring the performance and explainability of fine-tuned BERT models for neuroradiology protocol assignment. BMC Med. Inform. Decis. Mak. 1472-6947. 24 (1). Available from: https://bmcmedinformdecismak.biomedcentral.com/. doi:10.1186/s12911-024-02444-z.

Tan, Z.W., Guarnera, E., Tee, W.V., Berezovsky, I.N., 2020. AlloSigMA 2: paving the way to designing allosteric effectors and to exploring allosteric effects of mutations. Nucleic Acids Res. 1362-4962. 48 (1), W116. Available from: https://academic.oup.com/nar/issue. doi:10.1093/NAR/GKAA338.

Toda, R., Teramoto, A., Tsujimoto, M., Toyama, H., Imaizumi, K., Saito, K., Fujita, H., 2021. Synthetic CT image generation of shape-controlled lung cancer using semi-conditional InfoGAN and its applicability for type classification. Int. J. Comput. Assist. Radiol. Surg. 1861-6410. 16 (2), 241–251. doi:10.1007/s11548-021-02308-1.

Urago, Y., Okamoto, H., Kaneda, T., Murakami, N., Kashihara, T., Takemori, M., Nakayama, H., Iijima, K., Chiba, T., Kuwahara, J., Katsuta, S., Nakamura, S., Chang, W., Saitoh, H., Igaki, H., 2021. Evaluation of auto-segmentation accuracy of cloud-based artificial intelligence and atlas-based models. Radiat. Oncol. 1748-717X. 16 (1). doi:10.1186/s13014-021-01896-1.

Wang, J.Y., Qu, V., Hui, C., Sandhu, N., Mendoza, M.G., Panjwani, N., Chang, Y.C., Liang, C.H., Lu, J.T., Wang, L., Kovalchuk, N., Gensheimer, M.F., Soltys, S.G., Pollom, E.L., 2023. Stratified assessment of an FDA-cleared deep learning algorithm for automated detection and contouring of metastatic brain tumors in stereotactic radiosurgery. Radiat. Oncol. 1748-717X. 18 (1). Available from: https://ro-journal.biomedcentral.com/. doi:10.1186/s13014-023-02246-z.

Wang, S., Wang, C., Gao, F., Su, L., Zhang, F., Wang, Y., Yu, Y., 2025. Autoregressive sequence modeling for 3D medical image representation. Proc. AAAI Conf. Artif. Intell. 2374-3468. 39 (8), 7871–7879. doi:10.1609/aaai.v39i8.32848.

Wolterink, J.M., Mukhopadhyay, A., Leiner, T., Vogl, T.J., Bucher, A.M., Išgum, I., 2021. Generative adversarial networks: a primer for radiologists. Radiographics. 1527-1323. 41 (3), 840–857. Available from: https://pubs.rsna.org/doi/pdf/10.1148/rg.2021200151. doi:10.1148/rg.2021200151.

Wu, G., Kim, M., Wang, Q., Munsell, B.C., Shen, D., 2016. Scalable high-performance image registration framework by unsupervised deep feature representations learning. IEEE Trans. Biomed. Eng. 1558-2531. 63 (7), 1505–1516. Available from: http://ieeexplore.ieee.org/xpl/RecentIssue.jsp?reload=true&punumber=10. doi:10.1109/TBME.2015.2496253.

Wu, J.H., Koseoglu, N.D., Jones, C., Liu, T.Y.A., 2023. Vision transformers: the next frontier for deep learning-based ophthalmic image analysis. Saudi J. Ophthalmol. 2542-6680. 37 (3), 173–178. Available from: http://www.saudijophthalmol.org/. doi:10.4103/sjopt.sjopt_91_23.

Wu, R., Ding, F., Wang, R., Shen, R., Zhang, X., Luo, S., Su, C., Wu, Z., Xie, Q., Berger, B., Ma, J., Peng, J., 2022. High-resolution de novo structure prediction from primary sequence. bioRxiv. 2692-8205. Available from: https://www.biorxiv.org. doi:10.1101/2022.07.21.500999.

Xu, Y., Liu, X., Cao, X., Huang, C., Liu, E., Qian, S., Liu, X., Wu, Y., Dong, F., Qiu, C.-W., Qiu, J., Hua, K., Su, W., Wu, J., Xu, H., Han, Y., Fu, C., Yin, Z., Liu, M., Roepman, R., Dietmann, S., Virta, M., Kengara, F., Zhang, Z., Zhang, L., Zhao, T., Dai, J., Yang, J., Lan, L., Luo, M., Liu, Z., An, T., Zhang, B., He, X., Cong, S., Liu, X., Zhang, W., Lewis, J.P., Tiedje, J.M., Wang, Q., An, Z., Wang, F., Zhang, L., Huang, T., Lu, C., Cai, Z., Wang, F., Zhang, J., 2021. Artificial intelligence: a powerful paradigm for scientific research. Innov. 2666-6758. 2 (4), 100179. doi:10.1016/j.xinn.2021.100179.

Zanca, F., Brusasco, C., Pesapane, F., Kwade, Z., Beckers, R., Avanzo, M., 2022. Regulatory aspects of the use of artificial intelligence medical software. Semin. Radiat. Oncol. 1053-4296. 32 (4), 432–441. doi:10.1016/j.semradonc.2022.06.012.

Zeltzer, D., Herzog, L., Pickman, Y., Steuerman, Y., Ber, R.I., Kugler, Z., Shaul, R., Ebbert, J.O., 2023. Diagnostic accuracy of artificial intelligence in virtual primary care. Mayo Clin. Proc. Digit. Health. 2949-7612. 1 (4), 480–489. Available from: https://www.sciencedirect.com/journal/mayo-clinic-proceedings-digital-health. doi:10.1016/j.mcpdig.2023.08.002.

Zeng, X., Zhu, S., Lu, W., Liu, Z., Huang, J., Zhou, Y., Fang, J., Huang, Y., Guo, H., Li, L., Trapp, B.D., Nussinov, R., Eng, C., Loscalzo, J., Cheng, F., 2020. Target identification among known drugs by deep learning from heterogeneous networks. Chem. Sci. 2041-6539. 11 (7), 1775–1797. Available from: http://pubs.rsc.org/en/journals/journal/sc. doi:10.1039/c9sc04336e.

Zha, J., Li, Q., Liu, X., Lin, W., Wang, T., Wei, J., Zhang, Z., Lu, X., Wu, J., Ni, D., Song, K., Zhang, L., Lu, X., Lu, S., Zhang, J., 2023. AlloReverse: multiscale understanding among hierarchical allosteric regulations. Nucleic Acids Res. 0305-1048. 51 (W1), W33. doi:10.1093/nar/gkad279.

Zhao, C., Shao, M., Carass, A., Li, H., Dewey, B.E., Ellingsen, L.M., Woo, J., Guttman, M.A., Blitz, A.M., Stone, M., Calabresi, P.A., Halperin, H., Prince, J.L., 2019. Applications of a deep learning method for anti-aliasing and super-resolution in MRI. Magn. Reson. Imaging. 1873-5894. 64, 132–141. Available from: https://www.elsevier.com/locate/mri. doi:10.1016/j.mri.2019.05.038.

Zhu, J., Hamdi, A., Qi, Y., Jin, Y., Wu, J., 2024. Medical SAM 2: segment medical images as video via segment anything model 2. arXiv. 2331-8422. Available from: https://arxiv.org. doi:10.48550/arXiv.2408.00874.

Index

Note: Page numbers followed by "*f*" indicate figures, "*b*" indicate boxes, "*t*" indicate tables.

W

X

Printed and bound by CPI Group (UK) Ltd, Croydon, CR0 4YY
17/09/2026
02218538-0011